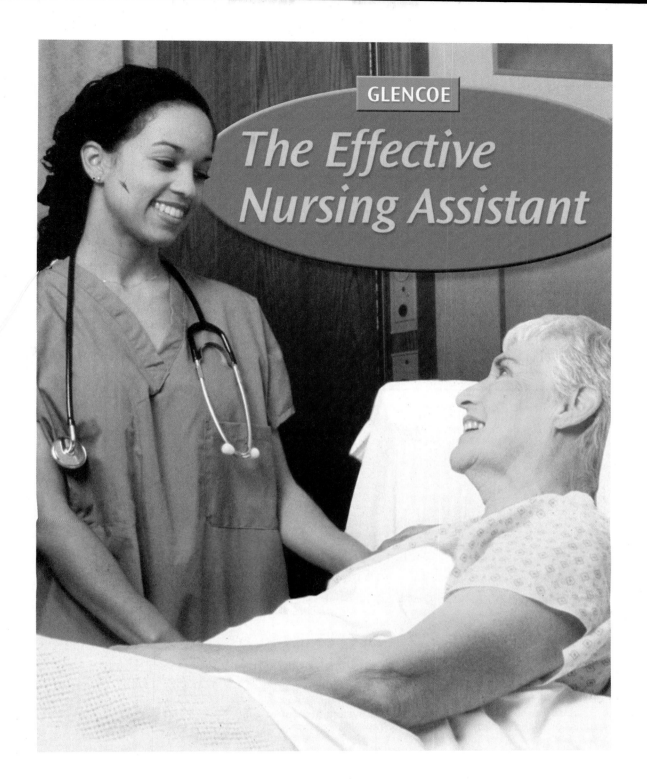

GLENCOE

The Effective Nursing Assistant

Ruth Ann Stratton, RN
Roanne Mancari, MSN, RN

Y0-ARL-710

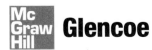 **Glencoe**

New York, New York   Columbus, Ohio   Chicago, Illinois   Peoria, Illinois   Woodland Hills, California

Safety Notice

The reader is expressly advised to consider and use all safety precautions described in *The Effective Nursing Assistant* or that might also be indicated by undertaking the activities described herein. In addition, common sense should be exercised to help avoid all potential hazards. Publisher assumes no responsibility for the activities of the reader or for the subject matter experts who prepared this text. Publisher makes no representation or warranties of any kind, including but not limited to, the warranties of fitness for particular purpose or merchantability, nor for any implied warranties related thereto, or otherwise. Publisher will not be liable for damages of any type, including any consequential, special or exemplary damages resulting, in whole or in part, from reader's use or reliance upon the information, instructions, warnings or other matter contained in *The Effective Nursing Assistant*.

Brand Disclaimer

Publisher does not necessarily recommend or endorse any particular company or brand name product that may be discussed or pictured in *The Effective Nursing Assistant*. Brand name products are used because they are readily available, likely to be known to the reader, and their use may aid in the understanding of the text. Publisher recognizes that other brand name or generic products may be substituted and work as well or better than those featured in *The Effective Nursing Assistant*.

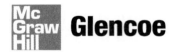

Send all inquiries to:
Glencoe/McGraw-Hill
3008 W. Willow Knolls Drive
Peoria, IL 61614

13-digit ISBN 978-0-07-874477-8
10-digit ISBN 0-07-874477-6

Printed in the United States of America
2 3 4 5 6 7 8 9 10   079   10 09 08 07 06

Contents in Brief

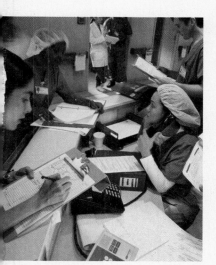

Unit 1 Health Care Workplace Basics

Chapter 1 The Nursing Assistant
Chapter 2 Workplaces in the Health Care Industry
Chapter 3 Getting a Job as a Nursing Assistant
Chapter 4 Legal Rights and Ethics
Chapter 5 Patient Needs
Chapter 6 Safety
Chapter 7 Vital Signs

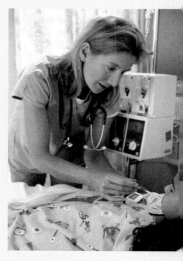

Unit 2 The Human Body

Chapter 8 Human Growth and Development
Chapter 9 Health and the Human Body
Chapter 10 Anatomy and Physiology
Chapter 11 Infection Control and Standard Precautions

Unit 3 Medical Communication

Chapter 12 Medical Terminology
Chapter 13 Observing, Reporting, and Recording

Unit 4 Patient Care

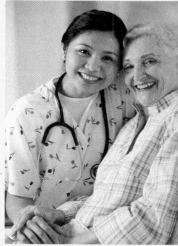

Chapter 14 Care of the Patient's Room
Chapter 15 Admission, Transfer, and Discharge
Chapter 16 Body Mechanics
Chapter 17 Emergency Care
Chapter 18 Examinations and Therapies
Chapter 19 Elimination and Sample Collection
Chapter 20 Caring for the Surgical Patient
Chapter 21 Patient Rehabilitation

Unit 5 Long-Term Care

Chapter 22 Personal Care in a Long-Term Care Facility
Chapter 23 Caring for Patients with Chronic Illnesses
Chapter 24 Assisting the Elderly in Long-Term Care

Unit 6 Home and Special Care

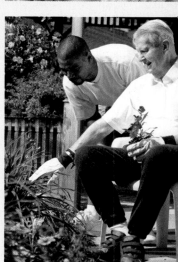

Chapter 25 Home Health Care
Chapter 26 Nutrition
Chapter 27 Understanding Mental Health
Chapter 28 Nursing Assistant Specialties
Chapter 29 Caring for the Terminally Ill
Chapter 30 Death and Postmortem Care

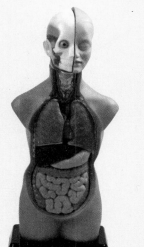

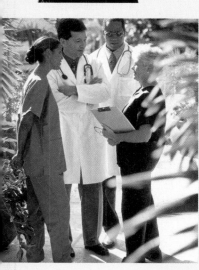

ABOUT THE AUTHORS

Ruth Ann Stratton, RN, is a consultant for Emergency Resource Staffing and Health Services, Inc., where she is developing the Home Health Care Division. She has 15 years of experience in community health and in hospital nursing as the nurse manager of a busy medical/respiratory floor. In addition to her consulting work, Ms. Stratton maintains a position as an adjunct faculty member at Illinois Central College, East Peoria, teaching in the Nurse Assistant program. Over the course of her nursing career, she has developed a niche working with the geriatric population.

Roanne Mancari, MSN, RN, is an instructor of clinical nursing at the College of Southern Idaho, Twin Falls. She received a BSN degree from the University of Nevada, Las Vegas, and a MS degree in Nursing Education from the University of California, Dominguez Hills. She is a member of the Idaho Alliance of Leaders in Nursing. She has been a practicing nurse for 27 years, has been involved in clinical education for 15 years, and has taught at the academic level for 4 years. Her background includes clinical expertise in emergency nursing, infection control, and home health care. At the academic level, she is involved in curriculum design, simulation usage as an instructional strategy, and fundamental nursing theory.

CONTRIBUTORS AND REVIEWERS

Deborah Bille, RN, JD
Utilization Review Nurse
Zurich North American
Colorado Springs, Colorado

Susan Chaffee-Hall, RN, BA
Director of Health Services
Montebello On Academy HC
Albuquerque, New Mexico

M. Grace Decken
Health Science Technology Instructor
Daniel Morgan Technology Center
Spartanburg, South Carolina

Genevieve Gipson, RN, MEd, RNC Director
National Network of Career Nursing Assistants
Norton, Ohio

Annette Heist, MA
Freelance Writer
Kunkletown, Pennsylvania

Penny Howard
Health Care Instructor
Mary Persons High School
Forsyth, Georgia

Sally Carroll Keating, RN, MS, ARNP
Ponte Vedra Beach, Florida

Deborah Larson
Health Science Technology Instructor
Pendleton High School
Pendleton, South Carolina

Joanne Mullen, RN
San Diego, California

Maureen Onischuck
Health Science and Practical Nursing
Broward County Schools
Cooper City, Florida

Linda Pelli, RN
Health Careers/CNA Instructor
Houghton County Medical Care Facility
Hancock, Michigan

Jon Zonderman
Naugatuck Valley Community College
Waterbury, Connecticut

Contents

Unit 1 Health Care Workplace Basics

Chapter 1 The Nursing Assistant **18**

The Nursing Assistant and Caregiving, 20 •
OBRA and State Testing, 30 • Understanding the
Health Care Team, 33 • Chain of Command, 36 •
Choosing a Career as a Nursing Assistant, 37

Chapter 1 Review **38**

CNA Certification Exam Prep **41**

Chapter 2 Workplaces in the Health Care Industry **42**

The Health Care Delivery System, 44 • Health
Care Facilities, 45 • Workplace Management, 52 •
Paying for Health Care, 54 • Regulating Health
Care, 55

Chapter 2 Review **58**

CNA Certification Exam Prep **61**

Chapter 3 Getting a Job as a Nursing Assistant **62**

Organizing Your Job Search, 64 • Applying for
Jobs, 69 • Interviewing, 71 • Starting Your New
Job, 75 • Personal and Professional Growth, 77

Chapter 3 Review **80**

CNA Certification Exam Prep **83**

Chapter 4 Legal Rights and Ethics **84**

Protecting Patients' Legal Rights, 86 • Violations
of the Law, 93 • Protecting Yourself, 99

Chapter 4 Review **100**

CNA Certification Exam Prep **103**

Chapter 5 Patient Needs **104**

Basic Human Needs, 106 • Meeting Patient Needs, 107 • Valuing Diversity, 114 • Interacting with Visitors, 115

Chapter 5 Review **118**

CNA Certification Exam Prep................................. **121**

Chapter 6 Safety **122**

Creating a Safe Environment, 124 • Fire Safety, 128 • Disaster Preparedness, 132 • Routine Patient Safety, 134 • Incident Reports, 148

Chapter 6 Review... **150**

CNA Certification Exam Prep................................. **153**

Chapter 7 Vital Signs **154**

Working with Vital Signs, 156 • Measuring Body Temperature, 156 • Measuring a Patient's Pulse Rate, 166 • Measuring Respirations, 169 • Measuring Blood Pressure, 171 • Pulse Oximetry, 173 • Determining Pain Level, 174 • Measuring Height and Weight, 175

Chapter 7 Review **182**

CNA Certification Exam Prep................................. **185**

Unit 2 The Human Body

Chapter 8 Human Growth and Development **188**

Stages of Growth and Development, 190 • Personality Development, 200

Chapter 8 Review **202**

CNA Certification Exam Prep................................. **205**

Chapter 9 Health and the Human Body **206**

Body Structure, 208 • Major Organs of the
Body, 213

Chapter 9 Review **222**

CNA Certification Exam Prep.................................. **225**

Chapter 10 Anatomy and Physiology............................**226**

Systems of the Body, 228 • The Cardiovascular
System, 228 • The Respiratory System, 231 • The
Digestive System, 232 • The Urinary System, 234 •
The Endocrine System, 235 • The Reproductive
Systems, 236 • The Nervous System, 239 • The
Sensory System, 240 • The Musculoskeletal
System, 241 • The Integumentary System, 243 •
The Lymphatic System, 244

Chapter 10 Review **246**

CNA Certification Exam Prep **249**

**Chapter 11 Infection Control and
Standard Precautions**...................................**250**

Microorganisms and Disease, 252 • The Infection
Process, 253 • Infection Control, 256 • Caring for
the Patient in Isolation, 265 • Infection Control
in Home Care, 268 • Infectious Diseases, 269 •
Staying Healthy on the Job, 271

Chapter 11 Review.. **274**

CNA Certification Exam Prep **277**

Unit 3 Medical Communication

Chapter 12 Medical Terminology **280**

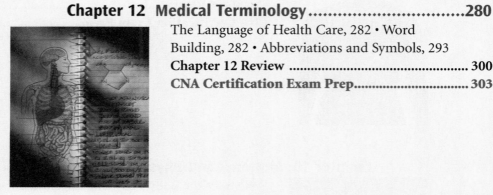

The Language of Health Care, 282 • Word
Building, 282 • Abbreviations and Symbols, 293
Chapter 12 Review 300
CNA Certification Exam Prep.................................. 303

Chapter 13 Observing, Reporting, and Recording **304**

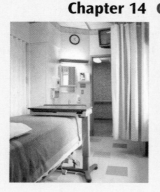

Communication, 306 • Observing, 313 •
Reporting, 317 • Recording, 318
Chapter 13 Review.. 324
CNA Certification Exam Prep 327

Unit 4 Patient Care

Chapter 14 Care of the Patient's Room **330**

A Safe, Pleasant Environment, 332 • Bed Linens
and Bedmaking, 335
Chapter 14 Review.. 346
CNA Certification Exam Prep.................................. 349

Chapter 15 Admission, Transfer, and Discharge **350**

Admission, 352 • Transfer, 358 • Discharge, 361

Chapter 15 Review **366**

CNA Certification Exam Prep **369**

Chapter 16 Body Mechanics **370**

Using Proper Body Mechanics, 372 • Positioning and Draping Patients, 373 • Safely Moving Patients in Bed, 376 • Transferring Patients, 385 • Transporting Patients, 393

Chapter 16 Review **394**

CNA Certification Exam Prep **397**

Chapter 17 Emergency Care **398**

Responding to an Emergency, 400 • Basic Life Support, 402 • Airway Obstructions, 410 • Shock, 412 • Stroke, 413 • Hemorrhage, 414 • Seizures, 416 • Burns, 418 • Poisoning, 420 • Weather Emergencies, 421

Chapter 17 Review **424**

CNA Certification Exam Prep **427**

Chapter 18 Examinations and Therapies **428**

Assisting with Examinations, 430 • Warm Therapy, 432 • Cold Therapy, 440 • Dressings and Support Devices, 444

Chapter 18 Review **450**

CNA Certification Exam Prep **453**

Chapter 19 Elimination and Sample Collection **454**

Elimination, 456 • Assisting with Elimination, 459 •
Collecting and Testing Urine Samples, 477 •
Collecting and Testing Stool Samples, 485 •
Collecting Other Specimens, 488

Chapter 19 Review **490**

CNA Certification Exam Prep 493

Chapter 20 Caring for the Surgical Patient **494**

Caring for the Preoperative Patient, 496 • Caring
for the Postoperative Patient, 502 • Ambulatory
Surgery, 511

Chapter 20 Review **512**

CNA Certification Exam Prep 515

Chapter 21 Patient Rehabilitation **516**

The Rehabilitation Program, 518 • Restoring
Range of Motion, 520 • Helping a Patient Walk,
524 • Orthopedic Care, 531

Chapter 21 Review **534**

CNA Certification Exam Prep 537

Unit 5 Long-Term Care

**Chapter 22 Personal Care in a
Long-Term Care Facility** **540**

Helping Residents with Hygiene, 542 • Oral
Hygiene, 542 • Hair Care, 549 • Bathing and
Showering, 551 • Perineal Care, 558 • Nail Care, 560 •
The Role of Massage, 562 • Shaving, 563 • Dressing,
566 • Providing Skin Care, 567 • Caring for Eye
Appliances, 569 • Caring for a Hearing Aid, 571

Chapter 22 Review **572**

CNA Certification Exam Prep 575

Chapter 23 Caring for Patients with Chronic Illnesses ..576

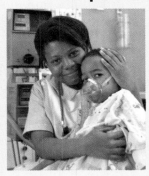

Chronic Illness, 578 • Patients with Diabetes Mellitus, 579 • Patients with Cardiovascular Disease, 584 • Patients with Respiratory Disorders, 587 • Patients with Neurological Disorders, 590 • Patients with Cancer, 594 • Patients with AIDS, 596 • Patients with Kidney Failure, 598

Chapter 23 Review..**600**

CNA Certification Exam Prep...............................**603**

Chapter 24 Assisting the Elderly in Long-Term Care......604

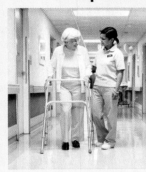

Care of the Elderly, 606 • Resident Exercises and Activities, 606 • Geriatric Care, 611

Chapter 24 Review..**618**

CNA Certification Exam Prep...............................**621**

Unit 6 Home and Special Care

Chapter 25 Home Health Care **624**

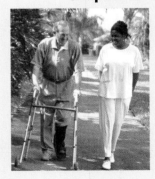

The Home Health Aide, 626 • The Client's Progress, 630 • Interacting with the Family, 632 • Recording and Reporting, 633 • Infection Control and Housekeeping, 636 • Food Preparation, 638 • A Safe Environment, 640

Chapter 25 Review..**644**

CNA Certification Exam Prep...............................**647**

Chapter 26 Nutrition **648**

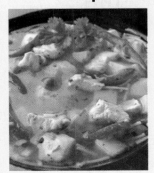

Food, 650 • Serving Food, 653 • Fluid Balance in the Body, 660 • Alternative Methods to Meet Food and Fluid Needs, 664 • Dietary Preferences and Restrictions, 667

Chapter 26 Review..**670**

CNA Certification Exam Prep...............................**673**

Chapter 27 Understanding Mental Health **674**

Mental Health, 676 • Mental Disorders, 676 •
Depression, 680 • Schizophrenia and Psychosis,
681 • Dementias, 683 • Substance-Related
Disorders, 689 • Treatment Planning, 690 • Mental
Retardation, 690

Chapter 27 Review **692**
CNA Certification Exam Prep 695

Chapter 28 Nursing Assistant Specialties **696**

Expanded Roles of Nursing Assistants, 698 •
Assistance with Medications, 698 • Pregnancy,
Labor, and Postpartum Care, 701 • Newborn
Care, 706

Chapter 28 Review **710**
CNA Certification Exam Prep 713

Chapter 29 Caring for the Terminally Ill **714**

The Terminally Ill Patient, 716 • Care Options for
Terminally Ill Patients, 717 • Physical Care, 718 •
Psychological Needs, 720 • Helping the Patient's
Family, 722

Chapter 29 Review **724**
CNA Certification Exam Prep 727

Chapter 30 Death and Postmortem Care **728**

Grieving with the Person Who Is Dying, 730 •
Signs of Approaching Death, 730 • Signs of Death,
732 • Postmortem Care, 733

Chapter 30 Review **736**
CNA Certification Exam Prep 739

Glossary **740**

Credits **756**

Index **758**

Vital Skills READING

Vital Skills: Reading features teach you the reading skills that are so critical in the health care workplace. You'll learn comprehension skills, such as previewing, activating prior knowledge, summarizing, clarifying, questioning, predicting, and evaluating. You'll learn to interpret a variety of texts, including patient medical records, graphic charts, flow sheets, and nurses' notes.

Summarizing Information 35
Determining What Is Important.....................57
Collaborative Questions...............................77
Fact vs. Opinion 97
Make Personal Connections........................108
MSDS: Using the Dictionary. 126
Reading Strategy 165
Making Connections 201
Visualizing Directional Terms 213
Keeping a Vocabulary Log 237
Comparing and Contrasting........................254
Using Context Clues. 283
Objective vs. Subjective Information 314
Skimming and Scanning 333
Concept Map or Web 365

Asking Questions 373
Analyzing Advance Directives 403
Making Predictions.....................................444
Two-Column Notes 458
Identifying Confusing Parts 496
Identifying Key Concepts 532
Reading Aloud to Residents.........................565
Identifying New Words 589
Setting a Purpose for Reading 613
Monitoring Comprehension. 636
Paraphrasing 651
Set Aside Time to Read 677
Be a Critical Reader....................................701
Vary Your Reading Rate 723
Reading Circle 733

Vital Skills WRITING

Vital Skills: Writing features teach the writing skills you'll need on the job. From creating a simple paragraph to composing a five-paragraph essay, you'll develop the skills needed to present your ideas clearly and concisely. You'll learn how to produce end-of-shift reports, incident reports, and other documents used in health care.

Main Idea and Supporting Details 25
Idea Maps...46
Proofreading 66
Clear, Concise Writing.................................98
Creative Writing...109
Writing an Incident Report 149
Learning Log..157
The Five-Paragraph Essay 194
Writing Sentences Using New Words 216
Peer Editing...245
Creating Summary Notes 270
Using a Dictionary......................................290
Sequencing Ideas.......................................322
Process Analysis List 340
Creative Writing—Keeping a Journal 353

Read Your Writing Out Loud 377
Writing Concisely 401
Using Words and Word Parts Correctly..........441
Using Spell-Checkers...................................485
Brainstorming Essay Topics..........................511
Deleting Unnecessary Words........................527
The Six-Step Writing Process 570
Using Active Verbs 579
Creating an Outline 615
Avoiding Plagiarism.....................................632
Compare and Contrast.................................665
Varying Sentence Length and Structure 682
Taking Notes 709
Avoiding Common Writing Mistakes 722
Creative Writing: Poetry...............................730

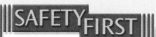

SAFETY FIRST

Safety First features emphasize information you need to follow proper safety procedures on the job, keep yourself and patients safe, and prevent the spread of infection.

FOCUS ON

Focus On features provide additional information about issues discussed in the chapters. They highlight skills and attitudes you need on the job.

Vital Skills MATH

Vital Skills: Math features offer the chance to put practical math skills right to work. Features present an on-the-job math problem with the solution and then provide a Practice activity to give you more experience in solving the same type of problem.

Calculating Calorie Requirements...................28

Calculating Insurance Payments.....................56

Calculating Time...72

Using 24-Hour Time 91

Calculating Distance 111

Reading an Oxygen Pressure Gauge 138

Reading an Upright Scale 176

Converting Inches to Feet and Inches...........198

Cell Division: Exponential Functions.............209

Calculating Urinary Output............................235

Calculating Vaccination Schedules................273

Determining Medication Times 293

Working Out a Schedule 323

Converting Fractions to Percentages.............345

Counting Money 359

Estimating Angles 374

Converting Temperatures 422

Calculating Therapy Times.............................440

Averaging Hourly Urine Output 466

Calculating Exercise Repetitions 510

Calculating Walking Distance.........................525

Bath Temperatures 560

Percentage of Meals Eaten............................581

Calculating Exercise Times.............................611

Calculating Weekly Earnings 629

Converting Liquid Measures 662

Calculating Fluid Intake.................................684

Mixing Formula for Bottle Feeding...............708

Subtraction with Months 719

Calculating Frequency of Respirations..........732

Vital Skills (COMMUNICATION)

Vital Skills: Communication features encompass a variety of scenarios that teach specific communication strategies, including listening and speaking effectively. You'll have the opportunity to practice communication skills in role-playing situations with patients, coworkers, supervisors, and your family members.

Characteristics of a Good Communicator 24

Courtesy 54

Sender-Receiver Model 74

Active Listening 89

Language Barriers 117

Communicating in Emergencies 134

Using Plain Language 174

Communicating with a Pediatric Patient 196

Feeding a Patient with Sensory Deficits........221

Communicating with Patients with Speech
Impairments...240

Communication and Standard Precautions...266

Pronunciation of Medical Terms....................288

End-of-Shift Report...318

Giving and Following Directions....................337

Teaching a Patient About the Call Signal 356

Pressure Sores: Explaining Planned
Movement 384

Nonverbal Messages 416

Asking Questions 436

Communicating with Sensitivity 464

Taking Telephone Messages...........................502

Being Observant. 519

Communicating with Visitors.........................552

Giving an Oral Presentation...........................599

Discussing Levels of Long-Term Care 616

Conducting a Formal Meeting 643

Communicating with Visually Impaired
Patients 658

Validation Therapy 687

Working in a Team 704

Reminiscing Therapy 721

Teaching Others 734

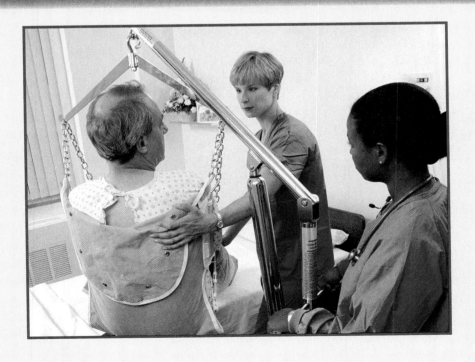

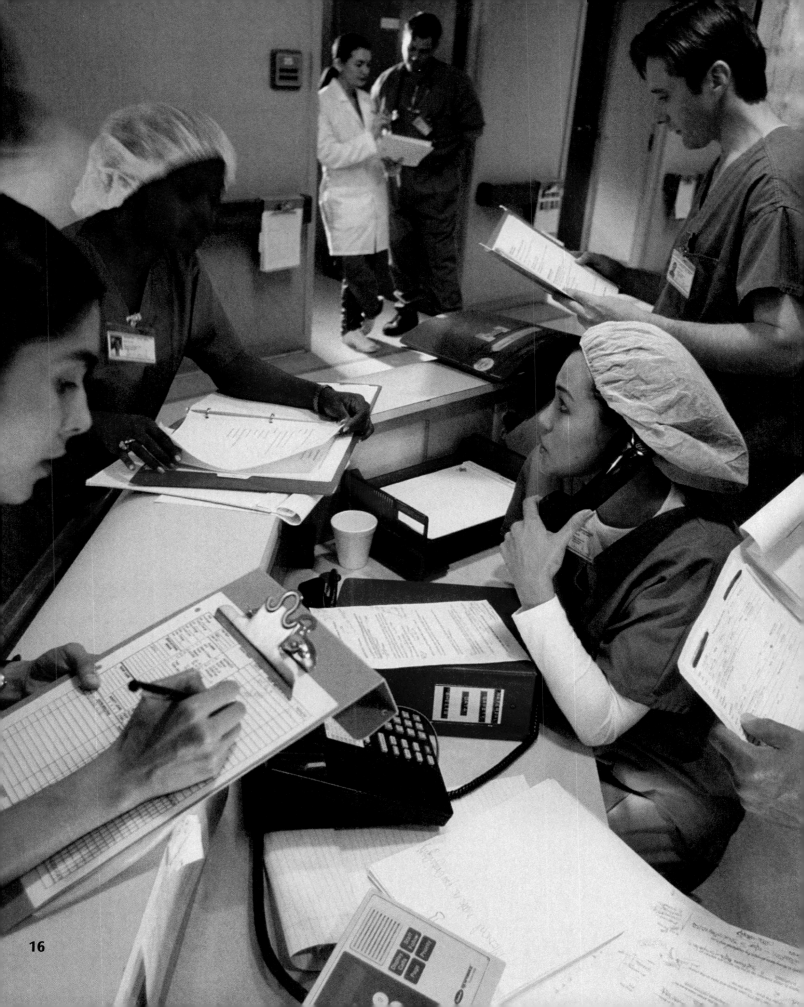

Health Care Workplace Basics

Chapter 1 **The Nursing Assistant**

Chapter 2 **Workplaces in the Health Care Industry**

Chapter 3 **Getting a Job as a Nursing Assistant**

Chapter 4 **Legal Rights and Ethics**

Chapter 5 **Patient Needs**

Chapter 6 **Safety**

Chapter 7 **Vital Signs**

Unit 1 introduces you to the role and working environment of a nursing assistant. These seven chapters provide you with the foundation you need to become an effective nursing assistant. In addition to an overview of workplaces and duties, this unit provides a look at safety techniques, legal and ethical considerations, and a few basic skills, such as checking vital signs.

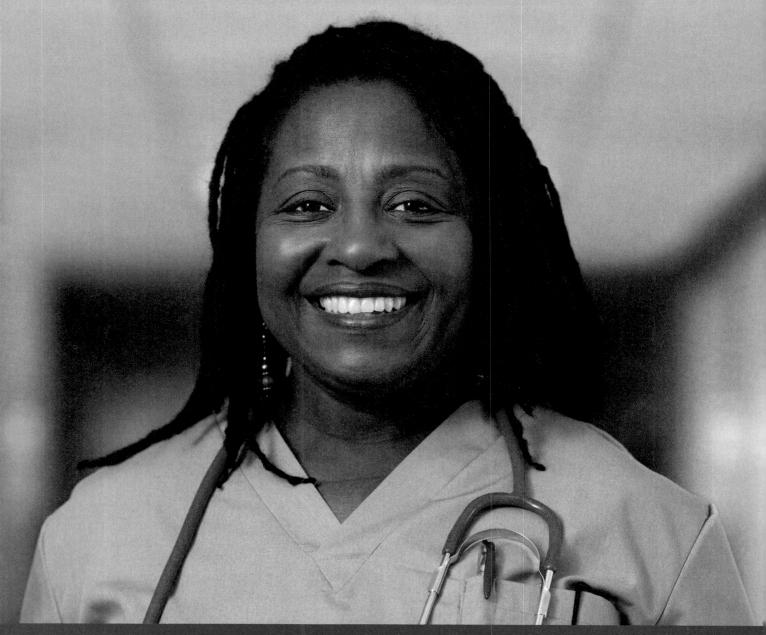

CHAPTER 1

OBJECTIVES

- Describe the basic duties of a nursing assistant.
- Define *scope of practice* as it relates to nursing assistants.
- Explain the six basic principles of patient care.
- Describe the personal qualities of an effective nursing assistant.
- Identify ways to maintain your personal health, hygiene, and appearance.
- Identify OBRA (Omnibus Budget Reconciliation Act of 1987) requirements.
- Identify the members of the health care team.
- Describe the chain of command.

The Nursing Assistant

caregiver A person who provides direct care for someone who is in need.

chain of command A "ladder" of responsibility that defines who can assign tasks to whom.

charge nurse A nurse who supervises other nurses or who is in charge of a department.

conscientiousness Being careful, thorough, and accurate when you complete assignments.

delegation The process of assigning tasks to other trained or qualified people.

empathy Being able to understand or imagine how it would feel to be in someone else's situation.

head nurse The nurse who supervises the nurses and nursing assistants on each shift.

health care team Everyone involved in making and carrying out health care decisions. The patient is the center of the health care team.

hygiene A condition of cleanliness and health.

licensed practical nurse (LPN) A nurse who has completed a one- to two-year training program and has passed a state licensing exam. LPNs work under the supervision of an RN, a doctor, or a dentist.

licensed vocational nurse (LVN) A nurse who has completed a practical nursing program taught either in public vocational high schools or other state-approved programs. LVNs work under the supervision of an RN, a doctor, or a dentist.

nursing assistant A person who is trained and state-approved to give basic personal care to patients in a health care facility, especially one that provides long-term care. Nursing assistants work under the supervision of an RN, an LPN, or an LVN.

objectivity The ability to see and accept facts or conditions as they are, without personal interpretation or bias.

Omnibus Budget Reconciliation Act of 1987 (OBRA) A congressional act that established the minimum federal training requirements for nursing assistants working in long-term care facilities.

perseverance Sticking to a task until it has been completed, no matter how many obstacles you meet.

procedures Established methods of doing patient care tasks.

professionalism Conduct that meets the standards of a profession.

reciprocity The recognition by one state of another state's certification, licensing, or registration.

registered nurse (RN) A trained health care provider with a nursing degree or certificate who carries out the orders of doctors, gives medications, performs some treatments and therapies, and sets up care plans. A registered nurse has passed a licensing exam given by a state board of nursing.

registry An official record or listing of people who have successfully completed a state-approved nursing assistant training and evaluation program.

rehabilitation The process of restoring patients to their highest possible physical, psychological, and social functioning after an injury or illness.

restorative care The everyday process of restoring patients to their highest possible physical, psychological, and social functioning on a long-term basis.

scope of practice The things a health care worker can and cannot do by law.

shift report A summary of what went on during the previous shift that may affect patient care techniques and decisions.

stress The body's response to any emotional, social, or economic factor that produces tension or anxiety.

The Nursing Assistant and Caregiving

A **nursing assistant** is a person who is trained and state-certified to give basic personal care in a health care facility. Nursing assistants help care for people who are physically or mentally ill or disabled. Under the supervision of nursing and medical staff, they perform the following patient care tasks:

- Answer patient's call lights
- Deliver messages
- Serve meals
- Make beds
- Help patients eat, dress, and bathe
- Provide basic skin care for patients
- Check patients' temperature, pulse rate, breathing rate, and blood pressure
- Help patients get in and out of bed and walk
- Assist with certain **procedures** (established methods of doing patient care tasks)

They also keep patients' rooms neat, help set up equipment, and organize supplies. Nursing assistants have more contact with patients than any other kind of health care provider. For this reason, nursing and medical staff rely on nursing assistants to observe the physical, mental, and emotional condition of their patients and report changes.

These tasks are all part of caregiving. **See Figure 1-1.** A **caregiver** is a person who provides direct care for someone who is in need. Most of the tasks nursing assistants perform help people who need some kind of direct care. By performing their work well, nursing assistants make life safer, easier, and more comfortable for the people they serve.

The New Nursing Assistant

Suppose you have recently completed your state-approved training program and passed the state test. Today is your first day on the job. It might go something like this:

When you arrive on the unit, you meet the head nurse, your supervisor, your team leader, and the rest of the health care team. (You will learn more about the members of the health care team later in this chapter.) Some team members are new, and some are experienced. Soon after you arrive on the unit, you will receive a **shift report** that tells you what went on during the previous shift. Your supervisor will give you your assignment for the day. She may assign you to tasks and patients, or she may delegate (pass on) specific duties to you. She will also tell you which tasks you can perform on your own and those for which you need help.

Your assignment includes the names of the people you will care for and their care needs today. You will need to know how to perform various tasks and procedures of care to fit the needs of individual patients. One person may need a complete bath, and another may need to be taken to the shower. Another person may need to be put on the commode every two hours, and still another may be able to walk to the bathroom when you prompt her.

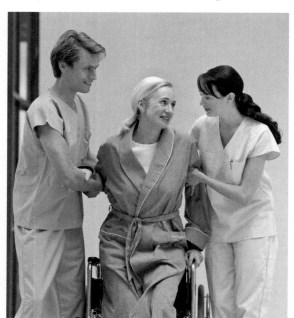

○ **Figure 1-1.** Nursing assistants help people who need care.

You will need to make a list of all of the tasks you are to perform. Organize your day and supplies so that you can complete each task efficiently. Because this is your first day, you may have questions about many things. Don't be afraid to ask other nursing assistants, your team leader, or the supervisor for guidance when necessary. Remember, they were new on the job once, too.

What Nursing Assistants Do

As a nursing assistant, you may work in many different kinds of places, or *facilities*. Wherever you work, you will follow the same basic steps to provide patient care. Throughout this text, you will learn the procedures performed by nursing assistants. The tasks listed below are a brief introduction to what you will learn and what you will do as a nursing assistant.

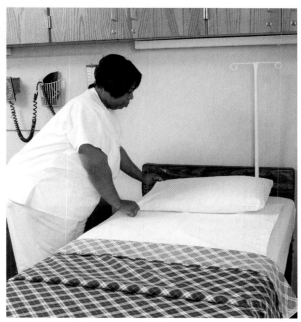

O Figure 1-2. **A well-made bed provides comfort for patients.**

Clean and Organize the Patient's Living Area. You will need to follow the facility's procedures for cleaning rooms. That may mean changing linens and sorting dirty linens. It may include cleaning patients' closets and drawers regularly, with their permission. It includes making beds so that the patients will be in a safe, clean, comfortable environment. **See Figure 1-2.** In all these tasks, you will follow the rules of patient privacy. You may also be asked to dust and organize much of the equipment used in patient care.

Assist Patients with Personal Care. The term *personal care* includes the things we all do every day to care for our bodies. We feed ourselves, bathe, dress and groom ourselves, toilet, move about, and get in and out of chairs. Patients differ in the amount of help they need with their personal care. Some patients are able to provide their own personal care. They may need your help only in setting up the items they will use. Others need extensive help. The needs of most patients will fall somewhere in between.

Keep Patients Safe. Some patients need help to walk. Some may fall out of bed or wander off into dangerous situations. As a nursing assistant, you will make sure that a patient walks safely and uses the proper walking aid, if necessary. Every facility has rules for protecting patients' safety. You will help apply many of these rules for each patient.

Help Patients Receive Nutrition. As a nursing assistant, you will serve patients foods and liquids. In some cases, you may also prepare the meals. Some patients are on special diets. You will make sure these patients receive the correct diet. In some cases, patients are fed by certain kinds of tubes or lines. In these cases, you will follow your supervisor's orders and rules for this type of feeding.

Help Patients with Elimination. Patients require various levels of help with eliminating waste (urine and feces). Some may be able to handle their own elimination needs. Patients who have recently had surgery or who are bedridden usually need your assistance. Other patients may have medical conditions that result in a temporary inability to care for their own elimination needs. You will help them with a bedpan, urinal, commode, or toilet and clean them after elimination has taken place. **See Figure 1-3.**

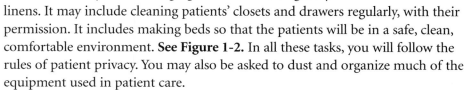

SAFETY FIRST

One of the many environments a nursing assistant may work in is the patient's home. Slips and falls cause many serious injuries in the home. When evaluating the safety of a patient's home, look for potential areas where the patient could fall. Remove throw rugs and anything that blocks hallways and doors. Make sure that items the patient uses often, such as a pitcher of drinking water, are nearby and easily accessible.

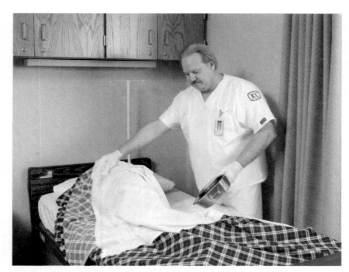

○ **Figure 1-3.** Patients who are bedridden need help with their elimination needs. This nursing assistant is helping a bedridden patient by providing a bedpan.

Assist in Rehabilitation and Therapy Programs. Your work may include providing rehabilitative care. **Rehabilitation** is the process of restoring patients to their highest possible physical, psychological, and social functioning after an injury or illness. A patient in rehabilitation has to learn or relearn activities, such as walking, dressing, speaking, or swallowing. The patient may also need to relearn to use muscles.

When the relearning or restoring process happens on a daily basis, it is called **restorative care**. If you work in a long-term care facility or nursing home, you may be asked to help with some of these procedures under the direction of a supervisor, therapist, or doctor. Many long-term care facilities are developing programs for rehabilitation aides that require nursing assistants to receive additional training and certification.

Handle Emergencies. Unforeseen emergencies do occur in health care facilities. When they do, you will follow the facility's emergency procedures. These procedures are designed to evacuate the patients as safely as possible. They are also designed to avoid dangerous situations for you and other staff members. No matter what the situation, using common sense is always the best first step.

Report and Record Observations. As a nursing assistant, you are an important "reporter" to the health care team. You will share information that is used in planning decisions about the patient's care, and you will record information as requested. You may also be the first to notice a change in a patient's condition. You are uniquely qualified to do this, because you see patients more often and for longer periods of time than other health care staff.

Measure Vital Signs. A person's vital signs include temperature, pulse rate, respirations, blood pressure, height and weight, and pain level. **See Figure 1-4.** When reporting vital signs to the nurse, you will be accurate and concise. If a reading is abnormal, it must be reported at once.

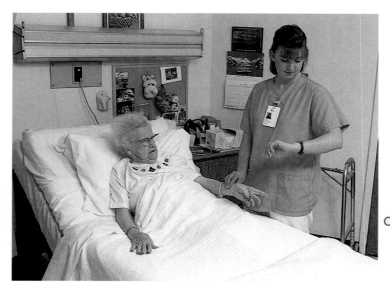

○ **Figure 1-4.** Nursing assistants measure and record the vital signs of people in their care.

Doing the Job Well

As you perform your duties, there are several general things you can do to help you provide quality care to your patients. Following these guidelines will also help keep you and your patients safe.

Communicate Clearly. When people are ill, they often experience emotions more intensely than they normally would. Patients may be afraid, or they may be angry. Nursing assistants learn to communicate clearly and accurately with people who are ill, confused, happy, or sad, and even with people who are dying. **See Figure 1-5.**

The other members of the health care team also depend on your input. As a nursing assistant, you are an important member of the health care team. You will communicate clearly and accurately with others in the team so there will be no misunderstandings about patient care.

Patients often have friends and family who want to know exactly what is going on. You can answer general questions in a clear manner. Refer them to the right person for questions that you are not allowed to answer specifically.

Follow Legal and Ethical Guidelines. States have laws and regulations for care in long-term care facilities. You will follow all regulations that apply to you. In addition to legal guidelines, ethical guidelines ensure that you are doing a fair and honest job and that no patient is being harmed.

Work Within the Scope of Practice. What you can and cannot do in your job is defined by law. This is called your **scope of practice**. Staying within your scope of practice helps keep both you and your patients safe.

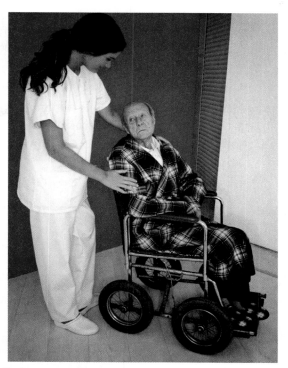

O **Figure 1-5.** Effective caregiving includes good communication with the person receiving care. Here, a resident is enjoying a talk with a nursing assistant.

Principles of Care

There are six basic principles of care to follow when you work with patients. **See Table 1-1.** As you read about each principle of care, think about it as it applies to you. For example, how do you think people should treat you if they are treating you "with dignity"? By understanding how you would like to be treated, you can better understand how patients will want to be treated.

O **Table 1-1. Six Basic Principles of Care**

1. Dignity	Show respect for patients and for yourself.
2. Privacy	Respect the privacy and confidentiality of all patients.
3. Communication	Maintain clear and accurate communication with patients, family members, visitors, and coworkers.
4. Safety	Practice common-sense safety measures at all times.
5. Independence	Show your ability to work on your own by following the techniques you have learned carefully and thoughtfully.
6. Infection Control	Follow all guidelines to prevent the spread of infection.

Characteristics of a Good Communicator

Good communication skills are important for all nursing assistants. Characteristics of a person who communicates successfully include:

- Being a good listener
- Trying to see the other person's point of view
- Expressing needs and concerns honestly
- Speaking in terms the listener can understand
- Using positive body language
- Being nonjudgmental

Practice

1. What characteristics might be a barrier to (prevent) good communication? (Keep in mind the characteristics of a successful communicator.)

2. Find a partner in your class. Take turns playing the role of a patient and a nursing assistant. Role-play the following scenarios. Then discuss how to communicate effectively in these situations.

    a. Gina, the nursing assistant, arrives at the patient's room with a severe headache. Mrs. Blackwell, the patient, is lonely and wants to talk. She has a very loud, grating voice that makes Gina's headache even worse.

    b. Mr. Williams, a long-term care patient, is a picky eater. Vanessa, the nursing assistant, asks him what he wants for lunch, and he decides on a grilled cheese sandwich and fruit. When Vanessa brings him the lunch, he frowns and tells her he hates grilled cheese.

Qualities of an Effective Nursing Assistant

The nursing assistant is one of the caregivers on the health care team. A **health care team** includes everyone involved in making and carrying out health care decisions. In some cases, such as in home health care, nursing assistants are the only people who see a client every day. In other situations, such as in a hospital, the nursing assistant is one member of a large health care team. No matter what the situation, basic caregiving is the nursing assistant's most important skill.

Nursing assistants have certain qualities, or characteristics, that help them do their job well. The characteristics of a good nursing assistant are described below.

Honesty. The characteristics of honesty include fair and straightforward conduct and telling the truth. They know right from wrong and act accordingly. They report any errors immediately.

Dependability. The ability to be trusted or relied upon is an important quality for all health care workers. A nursing assistant shows dependability by arriving on time, performing all tasks carefully, and not leaving until the patient has been cared for properly. For example, if the next shift's worker does not arrive, a dependable caregiver makes other arrangements before leaving.

Vital Skills `WRITING`

Main Idea and Supporting Details

As a nursing assistant, you are expected to be able to write chart notes and record other observations in writing. The key to any well-written paragraph is good organization. First, decide on the topic your paragraph will cover. This will be your main idea. Write a sentence that describes your main idea.

Example:

> **Main Idea:** helping patients receive nutrition
> **Sentence About Main Idea:** One of a nursing assistant's duties is to help patients receive nutrition.

Next, jot down what you plan to say about your main idea. What points do you want to make in your paragraph? These points are called *supporting details*. Arrange your supporting details in a logical order.

Finally, write your paragraph. Because of the thought you put into the paragraph in the preceding steps, your paragraph will be organized and easy to follow.

Practice

Review the six basic principles of care in Table 1-1. Choose one of the six principles and write a paragraph about it. Use the procedure outlined here to create a well-written paragraph.

Conscientiousness. Being careful, thorough, and accurate when you follow orders or complete assignments is **conscientiousness**. A conscientious worker manages time wisely, prioritizes responsibilities, and meets completion dates set by employers and clients. Being conscientious also involves taking responsibility for your own actions. A conscientious nursing assistant reports errors and accidents promptly to the charge nurse or supervisor.

Perseverance. Closely related to conscientiousness, **perseverance** means sticking to a task until it has been completed, no matter how many obstacles you meet.

Empathy. Being able to understand or imagine how it would feel to be in someone else's situation is known as **empathy**. Realizing how others might feel can help you comfort and care for patients with patience and kindness. Recognizing patients' feelings helps you achieve better outcomes.

Patience. The ability to remain calm in a stressful situation without becoming annoyed or impatient is a valuable asset. Some patients have slow reactions or are not able to do what is asked. For example, some patients with mental illness may not be able to understand what is said to them. Babies cannot explain when they do not feel well and may cry for long periods of time. These situations require caregivers to have patience and take the time to understand each person's needs.

Helpfulness. Giving assistance with an attitude that shows concern for others is the mark of an excellent nursing assistant. Doing this job well requires more than just performing basic tasks. For example, if you are bringing a meal to a patient, ask if there is anything else the patient needs. A little extra effort on your part may make a patient more comfortable or ease the burden of a coworker.

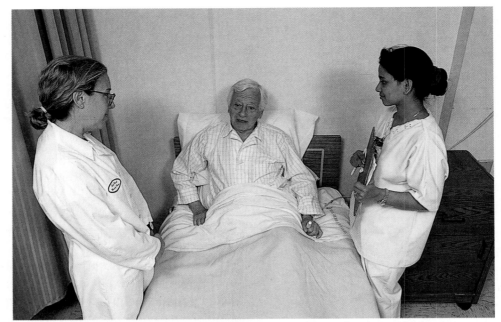

○ Figure 1-6. A nurse and a nursing assistant discussing care with a patient in a professional manner.

Professionalism. Displaying conduct that meets the standards of a profession is called **professionalism**. An effective nursing assistant acts in a professional manner toward coworkers, patients, visitors, and family members. **See Figure 1-6.** Being professional means not gossiping. It also means behaving in a businesslike way and obeying all of the standards for a nursing assistant in your state.

Objectivity. The ability to see and accept facts or conditions as they are, without a personal interpretation, is known as **objectivity**. As a nursing assistant, you may come across situations that seem wrong to you. It is important to learn the facts before judging these situations. If you are objective, you do not allow your emotions or personal opinion to overtake good judgment.

Positive Attitude. You display a positive attitude when you enjoy and show a genuine interest in your work and in the well-being of those around you. You respect each person, no matter how ill or disabled that person may be.

Personal Health and Wellness

Because nursing assistants often work in environments where patients are ill, they need to take extra care to stay healthy. They must not bring illness or germs to the facility. In addition, they need the energy to complete the day's activities.

Illnesses and infections are transmitted in several ways. Germs can be passed by touching or are carried in the air. Handwashing is a major preventive measure in the spread of germs. Even touching your own eyes with hands that have not been washed can spread illness from a patient to you.

Airborne germs may be harder to control. Some simple measures, however, offer some protection for both you and the patient. Always cover your mouth when coughing, and use a tissue when sneezing. Make sure that patients do the same if they are able. Wear a mouth mask in a room where a patient is on respiratory isolation.

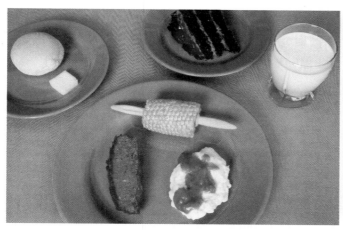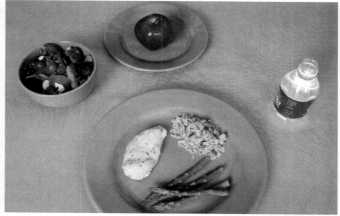

○ **Figure 1-7.** Which of the meals shown here is more likely to help you stay healthy on the job?

The best disease prevention measure is to maintain your own good health. A healthy body and mind will help you perform your job well and also give you a sense of well-being. The keys to good health are a balanced diet, adequate sleep and rest, exercise, avoiding unsafe behaviors, practicing safe behaviors, and managing stress.

Diet. The first step to good health is a good diet. What you eat and drink can determine the health of your mind as well as your body. Foods contain vitamins that are important to health. Water is a vital part of your daily diet. A balanced diet contains a certain amount of each type of nutrient.

Improper diet is the cause of many illnesses. For example, lack of iron may result in anemia, and too much sugar can cause irritability. Many conditions can be caused by poor nutrition. **See Figure 1-7.**

Sleep and Rest. Your body needs a period of rest after expending energy all day. The ideal rest for most adults is eight hours of sleep per night, although busy schedules often make it hard to get enough sleep. Lack of rest can make you irritable, careless, and forgetful, or may impair your judgment. Rest is an important part of maintaining good health. Even if you work an evening or night shift, you still need to plan sufficient time to rest each day.

Exercise. During the day, nursing assistants perform many physical tasks. They may make many beds, and they may walk long distances. For some, this may serve as enough exercise in a daily routine. For most people, however, a separate exercise routine three or four times a week is healthful. Exercise does not have to take place in a gym or in a structured setting. It may be as simple as stretching, as walking up and down the stairs to your apartment twice a day instead of taking an elevator, or walking to work instead of riding the bus or driving.

Exercise benefits your body in a number of ways. It helps control your weight and your blood pressure. During exercise, your brain releases substances called *endorphins* that make you feel good and that have been shown to relieve stress. **See Figure 1-8.** For women, exercise can help prevent the brittle bones and bent posture that often come with aging.

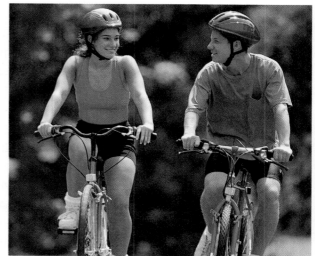

○ **Figure 1-8.** Exercise makes you feel good and helps relieve stress.

Vital Skills — MATH

Calculating Calorie Requirements

Diet plus exercise equals good health. As a working professional, you will want to maintain your good health and maintain a healthy body weight. The fact is, if you eat more calories than you use, you will gain weight. If you use more than you eat, you will lose weight. To maintain your weight, you should eat about as many calories as you use.

To calculate the number of calories you need to maintain your current weight, follow these steps:

1. Calculate your basal metabolic rate. This is the rate at which your body uses calories when you are at rest. It equals your body weight multiplied by 11 (for females) or 12 (for males).
2. Record your current weight.
3. Multiply your body weight (in pounds) $\times$ $\frac{1}{3}$ $\times$ the number of hours you are awake each day.
4. Add your results from steps 1 and 3 to find the number of calories you need each day to maintain your current weight.

Practice

Use the steps shown above to calculate the daily calorie requirement for a 160-pound male. Show your work on a separate piece of paper.

$\frac{1}{3}$

Avoiding Unsafe Behaviors

Your behavior can affect the way you think and feel. It can also affect the way you perform your job. For instance, a nursing assistant who works under the influence of drugs or alcohol puts patients at risk for harm.

- Smoking can lead to respiratory problems, heart disease, and cancer. Smoking while pregnant can harm an unborn child.
- Drinking excessive amounts of alcohol can cause disease and can lead to a lowered ability to think clearly and act properly.
- Illegal drugs or the illegal use of prescription drugs can also alter thinking and cause foolish actions. Nursing assistants who work in hospitals see the harmful effects of the misuse of certain drugs. Pediatric wards care for many "crack babies." Many people every year are injured in accidents caused by alcohol- or drug-impaired drivers. Drug abuse can also get you into serious trouble with the law.

Practicing Safe Behaviors. To prevent injuries and protect your health, practice the following safe behaviors:

- Wear a seat belt every time you are in a car, whether or not you are driving.
- Wear a helmet when you ride a motorcycle, a bicycle, or a skateboard.
- Use good body mechanics when you lift or transfer patients.

Managing Stress. Stress is your body's response to any emotional, social, or economic factor that produces tension. Long-term stress can harm your health. Stress in your personal life can affect your work. Learn to deal with stress by exercising, eating well, and getting plenty of rest and sleep. Take time for yourself and develop a support system of people you can talk to about what is causing you to feel stress.

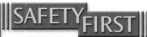

SAFETY FIRST

Smoking creates a fire hazard. If you work in a home care environment, never smoke in a client's home—doing so puts your client at risk. Never smoke in an area where oxygen is being administered or stored.

Hygiene

Neat, clean people practice good hygiene. **Hygiene** is a condition of cleanliness and health. Patients, their family members, and your coworkers expect you to look clean and healthy. If you do not, they may question the type of care you give.

Cleanliness. Cleanliness is important in avoiding infection. Frequent handwashing slows the transfer of bacteria. Cleanliness is also a major factor in your appearance. If patients see that you are clean and that your clothes are clean, they will feel more comfortable with you. The personal care you take in washing, bathing, or showering is your responsibility. Because the work is strenuous, you need to wear underarm deodorant to control perspiration odors. You should also shower or bathe at the end of each workday. Remember to change undergarments every day to avoid unpleasant odors.

Oral Hygiene. Taking care of your teeth and gums helps keep your mouth healthy. Mouth care is an important part of your daily personal hygiene. Brush your teeth after every meal if possible. Flossing your teeth daily will help avoid gum disease. You may also wish to rinse your mouth with mouthwash at least once a day to help avoid bad breath. This is important, because you will work closely with staff and patients.

Professional Appearance. Besides being clean, you should be sure to present a professional appearance when on the job. Most health care facilities and home care agencies have dress code policies. These policies provide guidelines about the types of clothing that are acceptable at work. Some places require nursing assistants to wear certain colors. Others require a specific uniform with the facility's name on it. Still others may accept any clothing that is of a certain color, neat, and professional looking. A uniform or professional-looking clothing signals that you are a competent health care worker. **Figure 1-9** shows nursing assistants dressed appropriately for work.

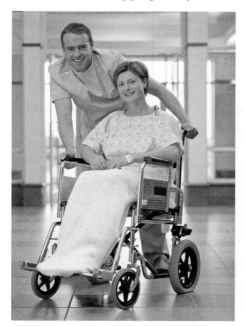 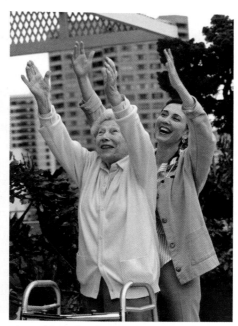

○ **Figure 1-9.** The nursing assistant on the left cares for residents in a long-term care facility. The nursing assistant on the right is taking a home health care client for a walk. Both nursing assistants are neat and dressed appropriately for their jobs.

The following guidelines are necessary to present a professional appearance and to keep yourself and patients safe from harm:

- **Keep jewelry to a minimum.** Large rings or rings with sharp edges can scratch patients and tear gloves. Necklaces, bracelets, and large earrings can catch on patients' clothing. Confused patients may grab at them.
- **Keep fingernails clean, short, and filed.** Long or ragged fingernails can scratch patients and tear gloves. Most facilities prefer unpolished fingernails, because chipped nail polish is a place for germs to grow, and it can look dirty and unprofessional.
- **Use cosmetics in moderation.** Too much makeup looks unprofessional. Perfumes from makeup, colognes, or body powders may nauseate or cause allergic reactions in some patients.
- **Wear clean, comfortable shoes and socks or hose.** Because nursing assistants stand on their feet much of every day, comfortable, professional-looking shoes are important. Wear only low-heeled shoes for comfort and safety.
- **Avoid tattoos and body piercings.** They are unsafe practices. Besides not looking professional, they can spread germs to you and others.

OBRA and State Testing

In the past, nurses provided on-the-job training to nursing assistants. There was no formal education or training until the federal government passed the **Omnibus Budget Reconciliation Act of 1987**, or **OBRA**. OBRA's purpose is to improve the quality of life for residents in long-term care facilities.

OBRA was passed after many complaints were received about long-term care facilities. Inspections showed that the complaints were justified. The federal government responded with a national standard for any facility that receives funds under Medicare.

The minimum federal requirement for nursing assistants under OBRA is 75 hours of specified training. In addition, all nursing assistants must demonstrate knowledge of the basic skills and procedures outlined in OBRA. Each state has developed a competency (skills) test based on OBRA requirements. Nursing assistants must pass a state-approved test in order to work in the state. Some states issue *certification* to nursing assistants who pass the test. In other states, nursing assistants are *licensed* or *registered*. Check with your instructor or search the Internet for more information about your state.

Many states have reciprocity agreements. **Reciprocity** means that the states recognize each other's certification, licensure, or registration. If you are certified by one state and move to another, your certification may be valid in the second state if the two states have a reciprocity agreement.

OBRA competencies are described in **Table 1-2**. Individual states may have additional required skills or may not allow nursing assistants to perform some tasks.

A criminal background check is done before you can start to work as a nursing assistant. Your employer is also required to consult the nursing assistant registry that is maintained in each state. This **registry** is an official listing of people who have successfully completed a state-approved nursing assistant program.

○Table 1-2. OBRA Competencies*

States vary in which OBRA tasks and objectives nursing assistants may perform.

OBRA Tasks and Objectives	Specific Objectives	Procedures
Care for the resident's environment	Keep resident's area safe and neat Make sure linens are clean	Bedmaking
Use standard precautions	Prevent the spread of infection Collect samples in an isolation unit	Handwashing; gloving; gowning and masking Isolation technique Sample collection in isolation
Apply proper body mechanics in moving or helping patients move Follow safety measures in moving, transferring, or assisting residents	Turn the patient or resident Move the resident in bed Use a transfer belt Help resident into a chair or wheelchair Transfer unconscious residents Assist residents in ambulation Help a falling resident Transport residents Help a resident using a walking aid Help a resident with range-of-motion exercises	Turning a resident toward and away from you Moving and transferring a resident by yourself and with a coworker Using a transfer belt Transferring from bed to wheelchair or chair Transporting unconscious residents by stretcher or wheelchair Helping a falling patient Assisting the independent resident Performing range-of-motion exercises with a resident
Understand and measure vital signs	Check temperature by various methods Measure pulses and respirations Measure and weigh the resident by various methods Check blood pressure	Checking temperature orally; apically; and rectally Checking a tympanic temperature Measuring a radial and an apical pulse Counting respirations Checking blood pressure Weighing and measuring on an upright scale and on a wheelchair scale Weighing and measuring while in bed
Use proper bedmaking techniques	Make a bed for a new resident, a current resident, a surgical patient, and making a bed while occupied	Making a closed bed, an open bed, a surgical bed, and an occupied bed

○**Table 1-2.** OBRA Competencies continued

OBRA Tasks and Objectives	Specific Objectives	Procedures
Provide personal care	Help residents bathe or shower Provide perineal care Provide hand and foot care Dress and undress the resident Provide or assist with oral hygiene Care for dentures, hearing aids, and eyeglasses Give a back rub Shave the resident Assist with elimination Collect urinary drainage Assist with nutrition	Assisting with a bath or shower Giving a partial bath and a bed bath or shampoo Giving perineal care to a female resident and to a male resident Caring for fingernails Giving foot and toenail care (except for diabetics) Dressing and undressing a resident Caring for dentures and eyeglasses Providing a bedpan and a urinal Assisting with a bedside commode Emptying and cleaning a catheter or drainage unit Collecting urinary drainage Serving the resident who can eat and drink unaided Assist with feeding Feeding the resident who cannot eat or drink unaided
Record intake and output	Measure and record intake and output	Measuring and recording fluid intake and output
Provide postmortem care	Care for the body of a resident after death	Providing postmortem care
Provide emergency care	Help patients who are choking	Performing the Heimlich maneuver Helping an unconscious adult who cannot breathe
Demonstrate proper response to the resident's behavior	Relate Maslow's hierarchy of basic human needs to individual residents Observe and report any cases in which resident's basic human needs are not being met Learn the skills needed in verbal, nonverbal, written, and electronic communication Communicate effectively with patients who are disoriented, depressed, angry, apathetic, or who have physical communication barriers such as poor hearing or eyesight	

○ Table 1-2. OBRA Competencies continued

OBRA Tasks and Objectives	Specific Objectives
Demonstrate proper response to the resident's behavior (continued)	Use effective communication skills with residents, their guests, and coworkers; understand family interactions and the nursing assistant's role in them
	Know how to use touch and other forms of body language effectively
	Identify the basic psychological reactions to illness, disability, and life changes and how they affect the resident's ability to function in a long-term care environment
	Understand the role the resident's self-esteem plays in the program of care
Understand developmental changes associated with the aging process	Describe physical, social, and psychological changes that take place during the aging process
	Know the interventions necessary to help the elderly resident function physically, spiritually, psychologically, socially, and recreationally
	Communicate effectively with aging residents
Care for cognitively impaired residents	Understand the behavior of cognitively impaired residents
	Know how to communicate and respond to cognitively impaired residents
	Help in reducing the effects of cognitive impairments
Care for residents' psychological and social needs	Help the grieving resident
	Help resolve disputes
	Encourage resident participation in social activities

Understanding the Health Care Team

The health care team always consists of at least two people—you and the person receiving care. In many states, nursing assistants are hired directly by clients or clients' families for home health care. They report only to these clients, and each pair works as a team. In most situations, however, nursing assistants are part of a larger team that provides care for the patient, client, or resident. **Figure 1-10** shows the health care team structure in a large nursing home.

Nursing Staff

A nurse carries out the orders of doctors. Nurses can give medications, perform treatments, administer some therapies, and assign care. Some nurses are in positions of great responsibility. They may manage and train others, direct a facility's department or unit, and have overall responsibility for patient care. Nurses see patients much more often than doctors do. As a result, doctors depend on nurses' observations. In some workplaces, a number of nurses are on the premises at all times. Other facilities have only one **head nurse** who supervises the nurses and nursing assistants on each shift. A nurse who supervises other nurses or who is in charge of a department may be called a **charge nurse**.

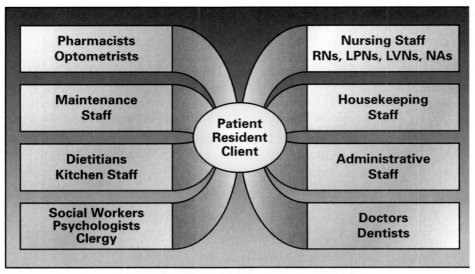

O **Figure 1-10.** The health care team structure in a large nursing home. The person receiving care is always at the center of the health care team.

Registered Nurses. A **registered nurse (RN)** has a nursing degree or diploma, has passed an examination given by a state board of nursing, and has a license to practice in a particular state. The associate degree of nursing (A.D.N.) may follow completion of a two-year program at a community college, or it may be a diploma from a two- to three-year hospital program. The nursing degree may also be a four-year university bachelor of science in nursing (B.S.N.). It may include further education, such as that required for a *nurse practitioner* (a nurse licensed to perform some tasks formerly done only by physicians). Registered nurses plan, set policies, and administer procedures. They also do assessments, apply and evaluate care, develop a plan of care, and assign personal care tasks.

Licensed Practical Nurses. A **licensed practical nurse (LPN)** completes a one- to two-year program in a vocational school, in a hospital program, or at a community college. LPNs take a licensing exam from a state board of nursing and receive a license once they pass. LPNs do not take as many courses as do RNs. They work under the supervision of an RN, a doctor, or a dentist. They work on assigned tasks (give medication, change bandages, and so on) under the direction of an RN or physician. They make observations but do not plan care for patients.

Licensed Vocational Nurses. A **licensed vocational nurse (LVN)** completes a practical nursing program. In most states, it is the same as an LPN program and is offered at community colleges or state-approved facilities. In some states, however, LVN programs are taught only in public vocational high schools.

Nursing Assistants. A nursing assistant may be called a nurse's aide, CNA (certified nursing assistant), nursing technician, health care assistant, geriatric assistant, patient care assistant, or some other title. Nursing assistants give basic personal care to patients, residents, and clients either in a facility or in a home. Each

Summarizing Information

One way you can help yourself remember what you read is to create a summary of the information. A *summary* contains only the major points of a passage. Writing a summary of each section of a chapter as you read it can also help you study for tests.

For example, suppose you were asked to summarize the "What Nursing Assistants Do" section of this chapter (pages 21-22). Your summary might look something like that in **Figure A**. Notice that it contains only the main points, without any details. By jotting down the main points, you can more easily remember the details related to each point.

What Nursing Assistants Do
- clean and organize patient's room
- assist patients with personal care
- keep patients safe
- help patients receive nutrition (eating, drinking, tube or line care with supervision)
- help patients with elimination of urine and feces
- assist in rehabilitation and restorative care
- handle emergencies
- report and record observations about patients
- measure vital signs

○Figure A

Practice

1. Read or reread the "Nursing Staff" section of this chapter (pages 33-35). Summarize the information. Remember to include only the main points or ideas.
2. Read your summary after you have finished it. Will it help you remember the main points later? If not, revise your summary to make it more useful.

task must be performed according to the criteria of the occupation. Nursing assistants must pass an examination and receive a state approval before being hired as permanent employees. Nursing assistants work under the supervision of an RN, an LPN, or an LVN.

Other Professional Staff

Doctors provide medical services to patients. Laws in most states require that only licensed doctors diagnose illness, prescribe medications and therapies, and perform most kinds of surgery. General practitioners (GPs) provide a range of medical services. Doctors who work in a single area of medicine are called *specialists*. For example, psychiatrists are medical doctors who work with patients who have mental illness. Dentists care for patients' teeth and gums.

In large facilities, many professional staff people are needed to provide patient care. Pharmacists fill the prescriptions for medicines prescribed by doctors. Optometrists fill prescriptions for eyeglasses. Dietitians order meal plans and special diets for patients and residents and teach proper nutrition. Psychologists provide mental and emotional therapy for patients.

Other professional staff members work directly with the patient or with the patient's family or friends. Some provide social services (activities that promote social well-being). Social workers may help coordinate family needs and work on insurance problems. Some social workers are trained to give psychological counseling. Most facilities have regular visits by clergy for patients who wish to discuss spiritual matters.

Other people serve as consultants and help with problem solving or educational seminars for staff. Activity directors plan and implement daily activities. Physical, occupational, and speech therapists work with patients needing help in such tasks as speaking or swallowing. X-ray and laboratory technicians perform various medical tests.

As you can see, there are many resources available for people living in health care facilities. You may report to the nurse if a patient or resident is in need of these services. If family members ask you questions about these services, direct them to speak with the nurse.

Support Services

There are many people who provide support to the professional staff and patients. They include:
- Administrative staff members, such as receptionists, ward clerks, secretaries, and other office staff who handle clerical and administrative duties.
- Kitchen staff members, who plan and cook meals.
- Maintenance staff members, who run and clean the buildings and equipment.
- Housekeeping staff members, who clean rooms and maintain facilities.
- Laundry services and supply companies. They usually come to the facility as needed.
- Volunteer staff members, who deliver mail and flowers, sit with patients, and help with administrative tasks.

Chain of Command

Within the nursing staff, tasks often need to be assigned to various employees. These assignments follow a chain of command. A **chain of command** is a "ladder" that defines who can assign tasks to whom. **See Figure 1-11.** The process of assigning tasks to other trained or qualified people is known as **delegation**. A registered nurse may delegate tasks to another registered nurse, LPN, LVN, or nursing assistant. The LPN and the LVN can delegate tasks to another LPN, LVN, or nursing assistant. The nursing assistant cannot assign tasks to others.

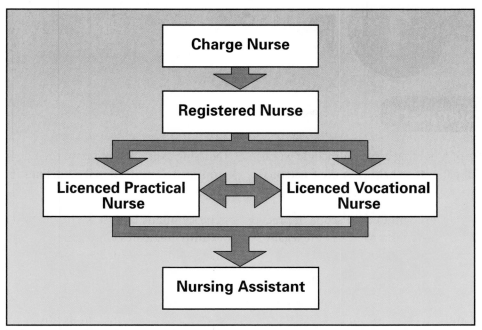

O **Figure 1-11.** Chain of command for a nursing assistant. Any person on the chart can assign tasks to others at the same level or on a lower level.

The nurses and supervisors who assign tasks follow five "rights," or rules for delegating tasks to others. Although nursing assistants cannot assign tasks, you should know what the five "rights" are, because they affect your work.

- **The right task.** Is the task within the nursing assistant's scope of practice?
- **The right circumstance.** What are the patient's physical, mental, emotional, and spiritual needs at this time?
- **The right person.** Does the nursing assistant have the training and experience to safely perform the task?
- **The right directions and communication.** The nurse must give clear and concise directions. The nursing assistant makes certain that he or she understands them.
- **The right supervision.** The nurse guides, directs, and evaluates the care given by nursing assistants.

Choosing a Career as a Nursing Assistant

Deciding that you want to be a nursing assistant is the first step to beginning a rewarding career. The demand for nursing assistants is increasing, and their role in health care is an important one. There are many opportunities and many ways that you can study even further if you wish to advance your education. The next chapter discusses the types of workplaces that employ nursing assistants. The types of jobs available differ greatly, but all require certain personal characteristics and all require attention to the six basic principles of care.

FOCUS ON

Networking

Certified nursing assistants can join state and national professional associations to network with others. Through membership, you can gain leadership skills and support and recognition for your work. The National Network of Career Nursing Assistants (NNCNA) and the National Association of Geriatric Nursing Assistants (NAGNA) focus on improving quality of care by elevating the professional standards of practice for nursing assistants.

Chapter Summary

- The basic tasks of a nursing assistant include working closely with patients to help with their personal care and safety.

- Nursing assistants work within their scope of practice, performing only the tasks that they are legally allowed to do.

- Nursing assistants follow six basic principles of care based on dignity, privacy, communication, safety, independence, and infection control.

- Nursing assistants possess certain basic personal qualities that enable them to work well with patients, family members, and other staff members.

- Nursing assistants maintain their good health and conform to professional guidelines for hygiene and appearance.

- The Omnibus Budget Reconciliation Act of 1987 (OBRA) regulates long-term care facilities and outlines minimum federal competencies and training requirements for nursing assistants.

- The health care team includes everyone involved in making and carrying out health care decisions. The patient is the center of the health care team.

- The chain of command determines who can delegate tasks to whom in a health care setting.

VOCABULARY REVIEW

Directions: Match the letter of each definition in the second column with the correct vocabulary term in the first column. Write your answers on a separate sheet of paper.

Vocabulary

1. caregiver
2. charge nurse
3. conscientiousness
4. health care team
5. licensed practical nurse
6. nursing assistant
7. objectivity
8. professionalism
9. reciprocity
10. registered nurse
11. registry
12. scope of practice

Definitions

A. The ability to see and accept facts or conditions as they are, without a personal interpretation.

B. The things a health care worker can and cannot do by law.

C. A nurse who has completed a one- to two-year training program and has passed a state licensing exam.

D. Conduct that meets the standards of a profession.

E. An official record or listing of people who have successfully completed a state-approved nursing assistant training and competency evaluation program.

F. A nurse who supervises other nurses or who is in charge of a department.

G. The recognition by one state of another state's certification, licensing, or registration.

H. A trained health care provider with a nursing degree or certificate who carries out the orders of doctors, gives medications, performs some treatments and therapies, and sets up care plans.

I. Everyone involved in making and carrying out health care decisions.

J. A person who provides direct care for someone who is in need.

K. Being careful, thorough, and accurate.

L. A person who is trained and state-approved to give basic personal care in a health care facility, especially one that provides long-term care.

Check Your Knowledge

Review Questions: Answer each of the following questions on a separate sheet of paper.

1. Name five basic tasks that nursing assistants perform routinely.

2. Briefly explain how nursing assistants help patients receive nutrition.

3. Describe the six basic principles of care.

4. Why is empathy an important personal quality for a nursing assistant?

5. Identify two reasons nursing assistants should maintain their own good health.

6. Why should nursing assistants avoid unsafe behaviors?

7. Why should nursing assistants keep jewelry to a minimum when at work?

8. How does the Omnibus Budget Reconciliation Act of 1987 affect nursing assistants?

9. What is reciprocity, and how does it affect nursing assistants?

10. Briefly describe the nursing chain of command in a health care setting.

True or False: Read each statement carefully. Then write *True* or *False* by the statement number on a separate sheet of paper.

1. The six principles of care apply only to nursing assistants who work in long-term care facilities.

2. Objectivity means you can understand how a patient feels.

3. Nursing assistants must meet all of OBRA's minimum requirements to be certified.

4. Registered nurses may prescribe treatment for illness.

5. A nursing assistant might receive assignments from an RN or from an LPN.

Think and Decide

Directions: Think about each of the following scenarios. Answer each question on a separate sheet of paper.

1. You have passed your state-approved test to become a nursing assistant, and today is your first day on the job. In your training, you learned all of the proper procedures and did all of your clinical work, but you have not had any experience with shift reports. When your supervisor hands you the shift report from the previous shift, you are unsure what to do with it. What should you do?

2. Mrs. G. is a hospital patient who had abdominal surgery yesterday. She insists that she can use the toilet if you will just help her get into a wheelchair and take her to the bathroom area. According to her chart, she is on complete bed rest. However, she appears very embarrassed about needing help and wants to care for herself. What should you do?

3. Mr. B. is an 84-year-old hospital patient who was admitted through the emergency room last night after being involved in a traffic accident. This morning, his 80-year-old wife has come to visit. She is extremely upset and asks you again and again, "What's wrong with him?" How should you answer?

4. As you are walking down the hall, you see Mr. R. try to stand up from his wheelchair during an argument with another patient. He falls. He is not injured, but the other patient begins laughing, and Mr. R. is embarrassed. What should you do?

5. You are working 30 hours per week at a local long-term care facility while attending classes at a community college to become an LPN. Lately, you have been feeling tired all the time, and some of the residents have complained to your supervisor that you seem cross with them and have a short temper. Your supervisor calls you into her office to discuss the complaints. What might be causing this problem? How can you correct it?

6. You have been working at a long-term care facility for more than a year now. You like your work, but you tend to become very stressed when a resident under your care dies. Four residents have died since you have been working here. Although all of the deaths were expected, the stress tends to affect your work for days afterward. What might you do to relieve the stress?

7. Lisa, who is one of your coworkers at a long-term care facility, often comes to work in rumpled clothes. Her hair is often dirty. One of the residents you care for mentions to you that she feels uncomfortable when Lisa is caring for her because Lisa "smells bad." What should you tell the resident? What other measures might you take?

8. One of the rules at your facility is to keep jewelry to a minimum. Usually, you obey that rule. However, you received a beautiful necklace for your birthday. It is short, so you do not think it will be a safety hazard to wear it just once to work. As you are caring for a slightly confused resident, she grabs the necklace and pulls hard. What should you do?

CNA Certification Exam Prep

Directions: This practice test contains ten questions. Each question has four suggested answers. For each question, choose the ONE that best answers the question or completes the statement. Write your answers on a separate sheet of paper.

1. The document that tells you what went on during the previous shift in a health care facility is the
   A. I&O report.
   B. shift report.
   C. assignment list.
   D. duty roster.

2. You are a nursing assistant at a long-term care facility. Which of the following tasks might you do on a daily basis?
   A. Cook meals for patients.
   B. Give patients medications.
   C. Help your patients bathe.
   D. Create care plans for patients.

3. A patient at a long-term care facility had a stroke. For the last several months, you have been working on a daily basis to help him relearn how to feed himself. This process is
   A. rehabilitation.
   B. safety training.
   C. enrichment.
   D. restorative care.

4. Which of the following is one of the six basic principles of care?
   A. safety
   B. conscientiousness
   C. professionalism
   D. objectivity

5. Professional appearance for a nursing assistant includes
   A. wearing jewelry.
   B. having visible piercings and tattoos.
   C. wearing a clean, neat uniform.
   D. using perfume to cover bad odors.

6. You are scheduled to report to your home-bound client's home at 8:00 AM. You are having car trouble and cannot arrive on time. You should
   A. notify your supervisor.
   B. call the client and say you'll be late.
   C. get there as quickly as you can without calling anyone.
   D. take your car to be fixed immediately.

7. Formal education and training for nursing assistants was first offered as a result of
   A. OSHA.
   B. JCAHO.
   C. NCHSTE.
   D. OBRA.

8. To be eligible to sit for a state-approved nursing assistant test, you must
   A. receive a high school diploma or GED.
   B. have at least 40 hours of training.
   C. have at least 75 hours of training.
   D. complete the paperwork and pay a fee.

9. Creating patient care plans is within the scope of practice of
   A. registered nurses.
   B. licensed practical nurses.
   C. licensed vocational nurses.
   D. nursing assistants.

10. The chain of command for a nursing assistant begins with
    A. answering to family members.
    B. following orders from a physician.
    C. communicating with the charge nurse.
    D. arguing with the patient.

CHAPTER 2

St. Elizabeth's Medical Center

EMERGENCY Center ↗
Enter from Washington Street

↖ **To Main Entrance and Parking**

OBJECTIVES

- Describe systems theory and its components.
- List trends affecting the delivery of health care.
- Identify the major types of health care facilities.
- Identify the patients served by each type of health care facility.
- Explain the nursing assistant's role in each type of health care facility.
- Describe private and group health care financing.
- Describe government-sponsored health care programs.
- Identify organizations that regulate health care.

Workplaces in the Health Care Industry

VOCABULARY

adult day-care center A facility that provides care for adult clients during the day.

assisted-living facility A residential complex in which residents live in their own units but where health care services are provided as necessary.

bioethics The study of the ethical questions and problems associated with medical research and delivery of health care.

client A person receiving service from a health care provider.

clinic A facility for the diagnosis and treatment of outpatients.

continuum of care A system that provides health care for people throughout their life span.

group home A small facility that serves as a residence for several people with long-term physical or mental disabilities.

Health Insurance Portability and Accountability Act (HIPAA) A federal regulation protecting the security of medical records and patients' privacy.

home health aide A person who provides basic personal care and health-related services for a client in the client's home.

hospice A facility or program that provides physical and emotional care and support for terminally ill patients and their families.

hospital A facility that provides medical or surgical care to sick or injured people who stay overnight or longer. Many hospitals also provide outpatient services.

Joint Commission on Accreditation of Healthcare Organizations (JCAHO) An independent, not-for-profit organization that sets the standards by which health care quality is measured.

long-term care facility A residential facility that provides care for people with chronic disorders or disabilities who need assistance with daily care.

Medicaid Federal and state health care funding for people who meet certain guidelines.

Medicare Federal health care funding for people over age 65 and for people under 65 with certain disabilities.

Occupational Safety and Health Administration (OSHA) The federal government agency that protects the health and safety of employees.

patient A person receiving health care services in a health care provider's office, a clinic, or a hospital.

rehabilitation center A hospital or other facility devoted to retraining patients to enable them to function as fully as possible.

resident A person who lives in a long-term care facility.

subacute care unit An area in a long-term care facility that provides care for patients who are too ill to be in the general population but who have been released from the acute care of a hospital.

The Health Care Delivery System

A *system* is a group of components that work together to solve a problem or achieve a goal. A health care delivery system examines the health needs of a community and determines how to solve problems of illness, disease, and injury. The goal of a health care delivery system is to provide timely access to cost-effective health care that meets quality standards. All systems are composed of four broad parts: inputs, processes, outcomes, and feedback. A health care delivery system might function according to the model shown in **Figure 2-1**.

- **Inputs.** This includes human resources—all of the health care personnel who bring their skills and expertise to provide health care to people. It also includes other resources, such as medical technology, equipment, supplies, and drugs. Less tangible resources include financing, time, energy, and information.
- **Processes.** Generally, the processes are the activities needed to solve the problem or meet the goal. This includes all of the services provided to patients at health care facilities, as well as education and research.
- **Outcomes.** The combination of inputs and processes leads to outcomes—what the health care delivery system has been able to achieve. Outcomes include patient wellness, client satisfaction, team productivity, cost-effectiveness, and efficiency.
- **Feedback.** The outcomes must be evaluated to determine if the system is working. This evaluation creates a feedback loop, leading to improvements in resources and processes and to still better outcomes.

Trends Affecting the Delivery of Health Care

Over time, community needs change, and health care delivery systems must adapt. In this challenging environment, it's important for employees to be aware of trends that affect the delivery of health care. Think about how each of the following trends affects health care in your area.

- Rapidly rising costs
- Managed care
- Use of advanced technology
- Aging population
- Use of new drugs and treatments
- Use of alternative therapies and complementary medicine
- General lifestyle and behavioral trends
- Rapidly spreading and emerging diseases

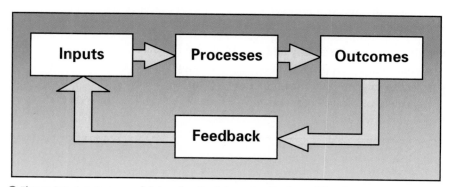

O **Figure 2-1.** A systems model. In a feedback loop, feedback modifies the input continually to achieve better results.

- Rising liability costs for health care providers and facilities
- Changes in government and other regulatory agencies

For example, at one time, doctor's offices and hospitals were the primary sites for patients to receive care. However, technology, medical advances, and rising costs in health care have led to the following cost-cutting measures.

- Hospitals discharge patients earlier.
- More patients receive care at home or in skilled-care units.
- Many diagnostic tests and procedures, including some surgeries, are performed at outpatient facilities.
- Illnesses or injuries that are not life threatening are treated at urgent care facilities or community health centers rather than hospital emergency rooms.
- Health care providers other than doctors are trained to provide care.

Other Factors That Affect Health Care Systems

Health care systems must also be sensitive to other current issues and factors. For example, medical and scientific researchers are constantly trying to develop improved medicines and medical devices. As these medicines and devices are approved, health care systems generally incorporate them. However, some advances bring up ethical questions. These are questions about what people consider right and wrong. **Bioethics** is the study of the ethical questions and problems associated with medical research.

Differences in education, occupation, and income also affect the health care system. How should a community deal with these differences? Also, as more and more communities become multicultural, differences in cultural beliefs and values become important.

Continuum of Care

A health care delivery system strives to meet the needs of the community it serves. In most cases, the system provides a **continuum of care** that meets a person's health care needs throughout the life span. **See Figure 2-2.** For example, a newborn's health care really begins months before birth, as the mother receives prenatal care. On the other end of the continuum, caregivers help people who are terminally ill make the transition from life to death.

Health Care Facilities

As a nursing assistant, you will have many kinds of workplaces to choose from during the course of your career. You will care for many different kinds of people. Some people receive care at home, while others travel to day-care centers.

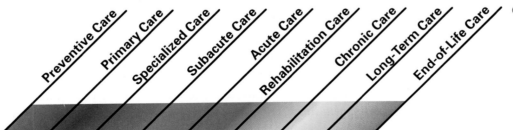

O Figure 2-2. Health care delivery systems provide a continuum of care to the community and to people across the life span.

Vital Skills — WRITING

Idea Maps

Before you begin to write a paragraph, it is a good idea to organize your thoughts. What kinds of things do you want to say? How do they relate to each other? One way to organize your thoughts is to create an idea map. On a blank sheet of paper, write your main idea or topic and circle it. In the space around the circle, write each thought you want to include. Circle these as well. Then draw lines from circle to circle to show how the ideas relate to each other. The example in **Figure A** shows an idea map for a paragraph about factors that affect health care systems. By showing how your ideas relate to each other, you can get a better idea of how to present your thoughts in writing.

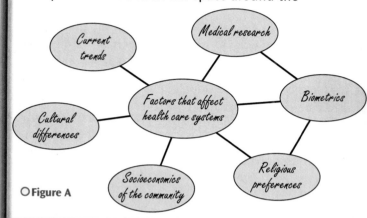

Current trends

Medical research

Cultural differences

Factors that affect health care systems

Biometrics

Socioeconomics of the community

Religious preferences

○ Figure A

Practice

Choose one of the current trends listed in this section. Write a paragraph about how that trend affects health care in the United States. Before you begin the paragraph, create an idea map to organize your ideas. Hand in both your idea map and your paragraph to your instructor.

Others may be recovering from acute illnesses in subacute care or short-term care facilities. (An *acute* illness is short-term and is often intense. Subacute care is care needed after an acute illness begins to subside.) Many are residents in a variety of long-term care facilities. Each place employs health care workers to care for its clients, residents, or patients.

The words *client*, *resident*, and *patient* are often used interchangeably. In this text:

- A **client** is any person receiving service from a health care provider. This includes people being cared for in a home or day-care setting, as well as healthy people receiving periodic wellness exams or blood pressure checks.
- A **resident** is a person living in a long-term care facility.
- A **patient** is a person receiving health care services in a health care provider's office, a clinic, or a hospital. *Outpatients* receive diagnosis or treatment at a hospital or clinic but are not hospitalized overnight. *Inpatients* are admitted to a hospital overnight for diagnosis or treatment. Some inpatients stay at the hospital for an extended time.

In some cases, these terms overlap. For example, a client who goes to a health care provider's office for a wellness exam is also considered a patient. In all cases, the client, patient, or resident is the central person on the health care team.

There are also many terms for the facilities that give care. Some terms, such as *hospital* and *health care provider's office*, are specific. Others, such as *adult home*, *nursing home*, *retirement living*, and *assisted-living facility*, might overlap. The following are general descriptions of the most common types of facilities.

Hospitals

Traditionally, a **hospital** is a facility that provides medical or surgical care to sick or injured people who stay overnight or longer. Many hospitals also provide outpatient services, such as diagnostic tests and surgical procedures. Most provide emergency or trauma care. Hospitals are sometimes called *medical centers*. They may serve as rehabilitation centers, and some, such as psychiatric hospitals, include residential or outpatient programs.

Hospitals can be either public or private. Public hospitals are not-for-profit and are overseen by city, state, or federal agencies. Private hospitals are generally for-profit businesses. They are also regulated by the government, although they have more control over how they provide services.

Some hospitals specialize in certain kinds of care. Veterans Administration hospitals treat current and former members of the armed forces. Cancer care hospitals specialize in cancer treatment. Maternity hospitals serve women who are giving birth and their newborn babies.

Hospitals that have educational programs for doctors and nurses are called *teaching hospitals*. At teaching hospitals, medical students, nursing students, and other health care providers gain clinical experience by working with patients. **See Figure 2-3.** Such hospitals sometimes include a program for nursing assistants. Most employ nursing assistants in the same capacity as nonteaching hospitals.

Nursing assistants use their caregiving skills working in a hospital. They measure vital signs, assist with activities of daily living, and assist with nutrition and elimination. They receive instructions from a charge nurse and sometimes from a licensed nurse.

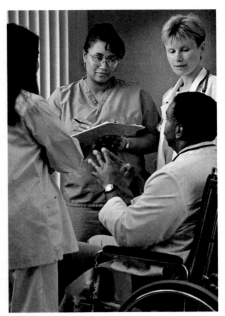

O **Figure 2-3. The medical students and interns shown here are going on rounds with their instructor, the doctor who is discussing the patient's diagnosis.**

Rehabilitation Centers

A **rehabilitation center** is a hospital or other facility devoted to retraining patients to enable them to function as fully as possible. Patients who have had accidents, strokes, or physical trauma that affect their abilities may be sent to rehabilitation centers. Rehabilitation doctors and therapists train or retrain patients using physical and mental exercises to increase their level of independence. Nursing assistants work in residential rehabilitation centers in much the same way as in hospitals. They may also assist therapists in working with patients. However, they may only do this under the direct supervision of therapists. **See Figure 2-4.**

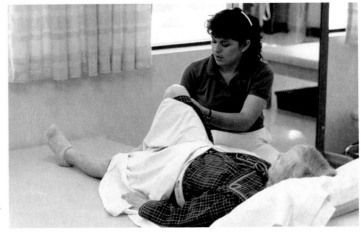

O **Figure 2-4. Nursing assistants work under the direction of physical therapists to help residents gain more mobility through retraining.**

Health Care Providers' Offices and Clinics

Patients visit a health care provider's office or a clinic for examinations, preventive health care, and treatment of specific health problems. A **clinic** is a facility for the diagnosis and treatment of outpatients. Nursing assistants can assist licensed nurses in such facilities. They may help set up patient examination rooms by disposing of or cleaning used materials and putting clean paper on examination tables. They may also greet and escort patients from the waiting room to the examination room and measure their vital signs. They make sure the patient is ready to see the health care provider. **See Figure 2-5.**

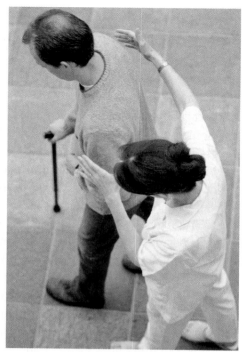

O **Figure 2-5.** This nursing assistant is escorting a patient at a medical clinic to an examination room. After she checks his vital signs and records basic information, she will notify the doctor that the patient is ready.

Long-Term Care Facilities

A **long-term care facility** is a residential facility that provides care for people with chronic disorders or disabilities who need assistance with daily care. These facilities are sometimes called *nursing homes* or *skilled nursing facilities*. Many residents are elderly. Others have disabilities. They usually require some help with daily activities. **See Figure 2-6.** They may also require some level of medical care. Long-term care facilities have many nursing assistants on staff, because most residents require the kind of caregiving that nursing assistants provide.

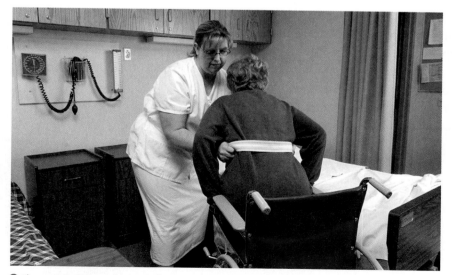

O **Figure 2-6.** Most residents in long-term care facilities need some help with daily activities. This nursing assistant is transferring the resident to a wheelchair to go to the dining room.

Subacute Care Units

Patients released from hospitals may need further medical care during a recovery period. Insurance plans seldom allow for this follow-up care in a general hospital setting. A **subacute care unit** is an area in a long-term care facility that provides care for patients who are too ill to be in the general population, but who have been released from the acute care of a hospital. **See Figure 2-7.** Patients are usually in the subacute care unit temporarily to recover from an illness, accident, or other trauma.

Nursing assistants in these settings provide much the same services that they do in hospitals or long-term care facilities. Patients, many of whom require partial or complete bed rest, often need assistance with the activities of daily living. More nursing assistants are assigned to these areas because of the acute nature of the patients' problems. Nursing assistants are usually supervised by a licensed nurse in these facilities.

Assisted-Living Facilities

An **assisted-living facility** is a residential complex, usually for the elderly or people with disabilities. Residents live in their own units, but health care services are provided as necessary. It is a type of long-term care facility. A large assisted-living complex may, however, include a unit for residents requiring more direct care. Assisted-living facilities provide residents with a house, apartment, condominium, or room. **See Figure 2-8.** Residents pay a fixed monthly fee for all services. Some facilities require residents to purchase a unit. Some make provisions for residents who cannot afford to pay.

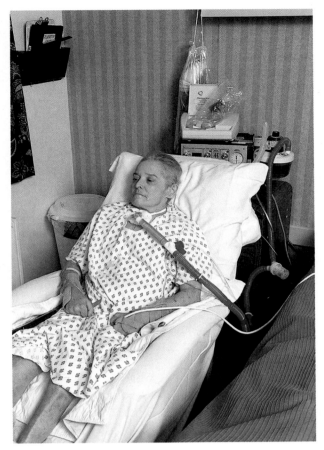

O **Figure 2-7.** The patient shown here was released from the hospital to a subacute care unit a week ago. She is learning to rely on the respirator less and less.

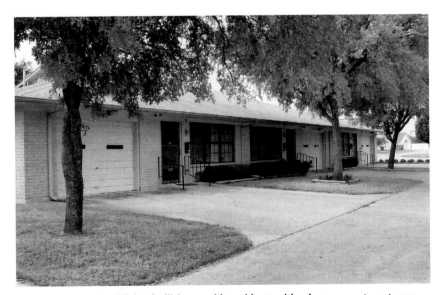

O **Figure 2-8.** Assisted-living facilities provide residents with a house, apartment, condominium, or room. Residents receive varying levels of care.

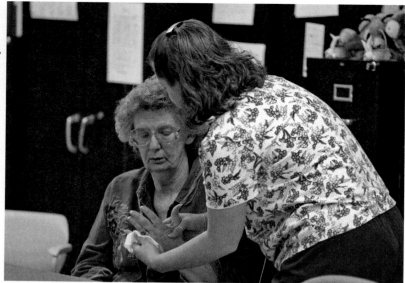

○ **Figure 2-9.** Escorting a client into a day-care facility where her medication is monitored. The client eats two meals a day, participates in planned activities, and socializes with other day-care clients at the facility.

People move to assisted-living facilities for a variety of reasons. Some are planning for a future time when they may need care. Others need some level of care and prefer to be in a simpler environment. Once they enter a facility, they may stay for the rest of their lives, no matter what level of care they eventually need. Some assisted-living facilities, however, do not provide this guarantee. In this case, residents who can no longer care for themselves may move to a different long-term care facility.

Adult Day-Care Centers

An **adult day-care center** is a facility that provides care for adult (usually elderly) clients during the day. Adult day-care centers have been created in response to a growing need in society. **See Figure 2-9.** Traditionally, families provided the daily care needed by older people and by people with disabilities. Now that most men and women work outside the home, they seek alternatives to care for family members.

Adult day-care centers provide meals, activities, and social interaction for adults who need supervision and/or minimal care. For example, clients with Alzheimer's disease may need to be watched so they do not wander off and possibly get lost or hurt. Many of these people need help with meals or using the toilet. Others need guidance to participate in exercise and activities. Nursing assistants who work in such facilities help with many of these tasks.

Home Health Care Agencies

Some people prefer to stay at home even when they need help with the activities of daily living. These clients feel most comfortable in their own homes, so they hire nursing assistants or home health aides to provide assistance. A **home health aide** is a person who provides basic personal care and health-related services for a client in the client's home. Home health care can be an effective alternative to more expensive residential care. **See Figure 2-10.** Nursing assistants perform a variety of important tasks in home care. Home health aides may also provide light housekeeping, laundry, shopping, and meal preparation in addition to assisting the client with the activities of daily living.

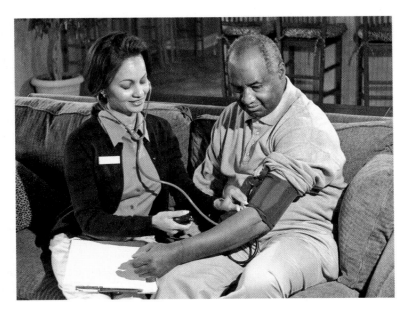

Figure 2-10. This nursing assistant comes to the client's home each day to measure his vital signs and to make sure he is getting sufficient nutrition.

Group Homes

A **group home** serves as a residence for several people with long-term physical or mental disabilities. It is a small, assisted-living arrangement in which residents are supervised while they live in the general community. **See Figure 2-11.** The supervisor may be a social worker. Nursing assistants are employed to provide care for residents who need some level of daily assistance. Some group homes contract with a home health agency or a public health nurse to serve as a consultant for the residents.

Hospice

A **hospice** is a facility or program that provides physical and emotional care and support for terminally ill patients and their families. *Hospice* can refer to:
- A facility that offers certain services to terminally ill people.
- A service that provides in-home care for terminally ill people.
- An association that supports the rights of people who are dying and serves them with compassion.

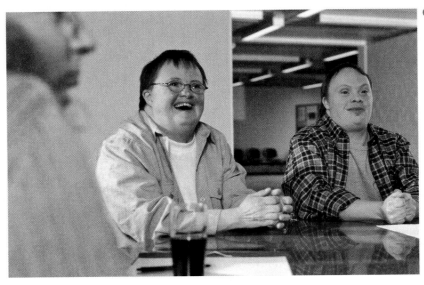

Figure 2-11. These residents of a group home enjoy each other's company at mealtime. The nursing assistant helps some of the residents with activities of daily living.

Hospice work involves many of the same tasks as long-term care facilities for nursing assistants. Hospices, in general, do not give medical care other than that necessary to keep a person comfortable and as free of pain as possible.

Nursing assistants also provide hospice care in the home. This care is usually under the supervision of a hospice nurse who is an RN. The hospice nurse visits a home hospice client regularly to adjust or administer medication. The nurse also instructs nursing assistants in how to keep the patient's environment clean, odor-free, and comfortable. Nursing assistants in home hospice situations often work closely with family and friends who visit or live in the home. **See Figure 2-12.**

Workplace Management

The organizational structure of health care facilities generally includes various levels of management staff, depending on the size of the facility. Some supervisors or managers have medical training. Some have other types of training or preparation for their position.

Hospital Staff

Hospitals usually have an administrative director who oversees the facility. The administrator may or may not be a licensed medical doctor and is likely to have a financial background. Department heads report to the administrator. They have specialized professional training and experience. The head of the surgery department is a surgeon. The head of pediatrics (care of children) is a pediatrician. The head of social services is a social worker. The head of nursing or director of nursing is a registered nurse with a college degree and experience. **See Figure 2-13.**

The nursing staff is a major department in health care facilities. The nursing staff includes registered nurses (RNs), licensed practical nurses (LPNs), licensed vocational nurses (LVNs), and nursing assistants. It also includes advanced practice nurses (APNs), who are RNs with additional education in certain clinical areas, such as midwifery or anesthetics. The entire nursing staff reports to the director of nursing.

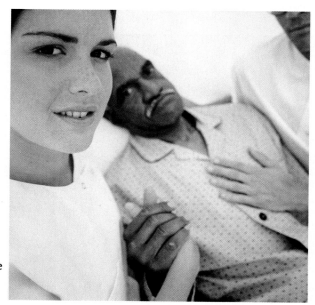

○ **Figure 2-12. Providing hospice care in the home of a terminally ill client.**

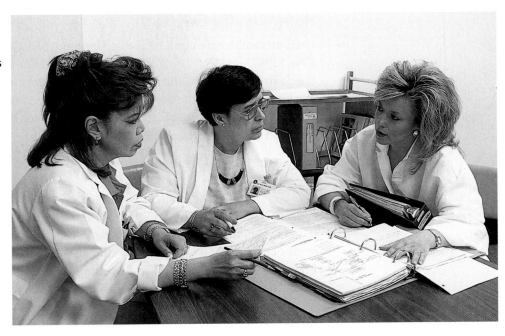

○ Figure 2-13. A staff meeting of health care workers in a hospital. The dietitian, nurse, and social worker discuss care plans for new patients.

Nursing supervisors are usually RNs who supervise a facility or unit. A head nurse directs a ward or unit, such as an intensive care unit. Each unit also has a shift charge nurse who supervises the nursing staff in that area during a specific time (day, evening, or night shift). Charge nurses are usually RNs. RNs, LPNs, or LVNs are assigned to each nursing unit and report to the charge nurse. The LPNs or LVNs also supervise the work of the nursing assistants.

Long-Term Care Staff

A nursing home or long-term care facility is run by a business owner, administrator, or director who is not necessarily a medical doctor. It is not as highly structured as a hospital, but there is usually a director of nursing. Large facilities have many other supervisory nurses. Nursing assistants report directly to nurses. In small facilities, they may report directly to a nurse or the business owner. State law dictates staffing requirements. **Figure 2-14** shows an organizational chart of the management of a nursing home.

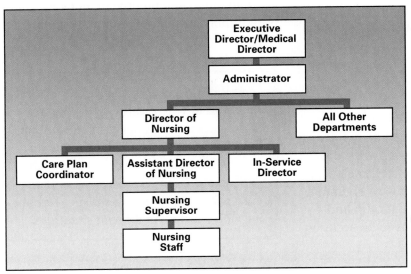

○ Figure 2-14. A management organization chart for a large long-term care facility that employs more than 300 people.

Home Health Care Staff

Home health care agencies are run by supervisors, at least some of whom are RNs, LPNs, or LVNs. The nursing assistants and home health aides who provide the daily care report to the nurses. In home situations, nursing assistants generally work alone with the client. A nurse may visit to dispense medication, adjust ordered changes in prescribed medication, assess or evaluate care, or observe an infection or change a bandage.

Paying for Health Care

One factor driving the delivery of health care is cost. The organizations that pay for most health care—for example, private insurance and government-sponsored programs—work to develop ways of keeping costs under control. Preventive health programs are an example. The theory is that they save money in the long run by keeping people healthy longer. Another example is the increasing use of nursing assistants in health care facilities. By employing trained nursing assistants to assist the nursing staff, health care facilities can deliver quality health care in a cost-effective way.

As a nursing assistant, you will hear about health care costs and the development of new programs. In general, the developments in the last few years have been good for nursing assistant employment. Since most facilities are trying to cut costs, they may employ fewer higher-level professionals and hire more nursing assistants. The outlook for job growth for nursing assistants is excellent.

Vital Skills   COMMUNICATION

Courtesy

In any health care environment, you are likely to hear many complaints about the complications of dealing with medical insurance claims and payment issues. For most people, health and treatment are the most important issues. They are reluctant to bother with money matters. How can you best handle the situation when a patient or the patient's family begins to complain to you about these and other problems?

One of the most effective tools you can use is common courtesy. Courtesy can be defined as well-mannered, polite behavior with consideration for others. When others become angry, do not let yourself be pulled into an argument or confrontation. Instead, remain calm and polite, even if the person seems to be accusing you of things that are completely beyond your control. Find out if there is anything you can do to improve the situation. In some cases, you may be able to tell the person who to contact for help. In others, you may not be able to do anything but listen quietly. In all cases, courtesy is an important tool for communicating with others.

Practice

In groups of two or three, role-play scenarios that involve angry patients or families. One person should play the nursing assistant, and the others should play the patient and family. Switch roles so that everyone has a chance to practice responding with courtesy in difficult situations.

Health care is paid for in various ways. Some people purchase individual health insurance, and some participate in a group insurance plan, usually through their employers. The government also provides health coverage for both the elderly and people who meet eligibility guidelines. Out-of-pocket expenses are those paid directly by people who have no insurance coverage. They also include paying for expenses not covered by an insurance plan, such as a co-payment or a deductible.

Private and Group Insurance

Most people who are employed full-time can get private or group insurance through their employer. These types of insurance include:

- **Fee-for-service plans.** These plans generally cost the consumer the most but provide the widest range of choices of health care providers, facilities, and services. People generally pay out-of-pocket expenses, including an annual deductible fee and a percentage of health care costs.
- **Managed care plans.** These plans are group health plans that provide care from a pool of providers and facilities. They are designed to lower costs for the insurer and the insured. They generally involve a network of physicians and health care facilities, often associated with a particular hospital. Each health care provider is paid a set dollar amount monthly for the care of each patient. Costs tend to be lower, but people may have fewer health care choices. Managed care plans generally emphasize wellness and preventive care.
- **Long-term care insurance.** This insurance can be purchased to cover the costs of an extended stay in a long-term care facility. Sometimes, home health care is also covered.

Government-Sponsored Programs

Medicare is federal health care funding for people over age 65 and for people under 65 with certain disabilities. Supplemental insurance policies are available to pay for expenses that Medicare does not cover. **Medicaid** is federal and state health care funding for people who meet certain guidelines. **See Figure 2-15.**

Regulating Health Care

Health care involves people and their wellness, so the health care industry tries to balance human needs with the need to control costs. Government agencies and other organizations have created regulations and standards to govern health care facilities. Facilities are required by law to meet certain health and safety regulations and quality standards to retain their licenses, certification, and accreditation. They are subject to inspections by state and federal government agencies as well as other organizations.

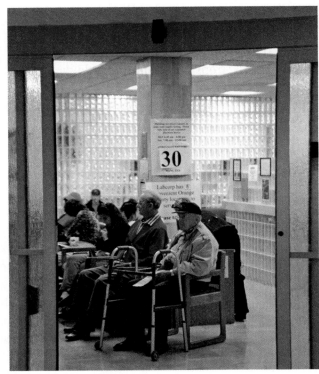

○ **Figure 2-15.** Many people qualify for Medicaid. In this program, their medical expenses are paid by the state.

Calculating Insurance Payments

One example of private insurance is the 80/20 plan. In this plan, the patient pays a predetermined deductible amount toward a medical bill. The insurance company pays 80% of the remaining amount due, and the patient pays the other 20%. As an informed consumer of health care services, you should be able to calculate how much you owe on a given bill.

As an example, let's say that Ani's hospital bill is $10,820.00. She has an 80/20 insurance plan with a $500.00 deductible. How much of this amount will she pay? How much will the insurance company pay? Follow the steps below to find out. Write your calculations on a separate sheet of paper.

1. Subtract the insurance deductible from the total bill: $10,820.00 − $500.00 = $10,320.00

2. Calculate 80% of the new amount after the deductible is removed. To do this, multiply your answer from step 1 by .80: $10,320.00 × .80 = $8,256.00. This is the amount the insurance company will pay.

3. Find out how much Ani must pay in addition to the deductible. To do this, subtract the amount the insurance company will pay (step 2) from the amount remaining after the deductible is paid (step 1): $10,320.00 − $8,256.00 = $2,064.00

4. Find the total amount Ani owes by adding the deductible and the amount she must pay of the remaining bill (step 3): $500.00 + $2,064.00 = $2,564.00

5. Check your work by adding the deductible, the amount the insurance will pay, and the amount Ani will pay in addition to the deductible: $500.00 + $8,256.00 + $2,064.00 = $10,820.00

If the answer in step 5 matches the full amount of the original hospital bill, you know that you have done the math correctly.

Practice

For each of the following bills, calculate how much the patient must pay and how much the insurance company will pay. Be sure to check your work. Write your calculations and answers on a separate sheet of paper.

1. Jeremy has an 80/20 insurance policy with a $250.00 deductible. His recent outpatient surgical bill totaled $5,412.00.

2. Kathi has an 80/20 insurance policy with a $1,000.00 deductible. Her recent hospital bill was $17,980.00.

- The **Occupational Safety and Health Administration (OSHA)** is the federal government agency that protects the health and safety of employees. When inspecting a health care facility, OSHA reviews policies and procedures, such as those governing infection control and contamination by hazardous materials.
- The **Joint Commission on Accreditation of Healthcare Organizations (JCAHO)** is an independent, not-for-profit organization that sets the standards by which health care quality is measured. JCAHO reviews and evaluates the performance of health care facilities and awards accreditation to facilities that meet or exceed its standards for quality. **See Figure 2-16.**
- The **Health Insurance Portability and Accountability Act (HIPAA)** is a federal regulation protecting the security of medical records and patients' privacy. HIPAA standardizes the electronic transfer of medical information. It should result in significant savings to the health care industry and the government.

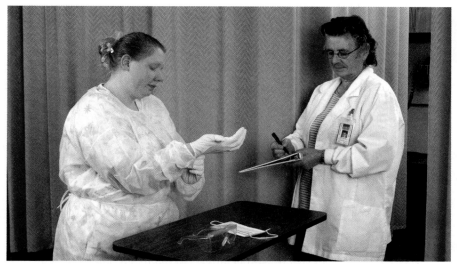

○ **Figure 2-16. A JCAHO surveyor evaluates a nursing assistant performing a procedure.**

- The Omnibus Budget Reconciliation Act (OBRA) of 1987 protects residents in long-term care facilities and ensures their quality of care. See Chapter 1 for more information.
- State laws regulate staffing, levels of care, training, the environment, and other concerns.

Vital Skills   READING

Determining What Is Important

As a nursing assistant, you will encounter and perhaps give to patients documents such as those explaining their rights and responsibilities in health care situations. Some of these documents will be clearer and easier to read than others. When you find a document or paragraph that is unclear, take a few moments to determine what the most important points are. This may make the rest of the document easier to understand. Then, if you still do not understand, ask someone for assistance.

Practice

The paragraph in **Figure A** is part of the HIPAA statement used by a doctor's office in accordance with federal law. Read the text and determine the important points. List these points on a separate sheet of paper. If there are any you do not understand, ask your instructor to explain them. Then reread the paragraph. Is it easier to understand this time?

We are required by law to maintain the privacy of your individually identifiable health information and to provide you with this notice, which describes our legal duties and privacy practices with respect to your individually identifiable health information. This information is created or obtained by health care personnel in this office and may consist of information about your past, present, or future physical and/or mental health condition, the provision of medical services to you, or with respect to which there is a reasonable basis to believe the information can be used to identify you. When we use or share your individually identifiable health information with others, we are required to abide by the terms of this notice.

○ **Figure A**

Chapter Summary

- A system is a group of components working together to solve a problem or achieve a goal.

- Health care systems must adapt to changes that affect the delivery of health care.

- Clients, patients, and residents are served by various types of health care facilities.

- Trained nursing assistants participate on health care teams in all types of health care facilities.

- Fee-for-service plans, managed care, and long-term care insurance are some of the types of private and group plans that pay for health care services.

- Medicare and Medicaid are government-sponsored plans that pay for some health care services.

- Health care facilities are regulated and evaluated by a number of government and other agencies that set safety and quality standards.

VOCABULARY REVIEW

Directions: Match the letter of each definition in the second column with the correct vocabulary term in the first column. Write your answers on a separate sheet of paper.

Vocabulary

1. adult day-care center
2. assisted-living facility
3. client
4. clinic
5. group home
6. hospice
7. hospital
8. long-term care facility
9. patient
10. rehabilitation center
11. resident
12. subacute care unit

Definitions

A. A facility or a program that provides physical and emotional care and support for terminally ill patients and their families.

B. A small facility that serves as a residence for several people with long-term physical or mental disabilities.

C. A residential facility that provides care for people with chronic disorders or disabilities who need assistance with daily care.

D. A residential complex, usually for the elderly or people with disabilities, where residents live in their own units but where health care services are provided as necessary.

E. A person receiving health care services in a health care provider's office, a clinic, or a hospital.

F. A facility for the diagnosis and treatment of outpatients.

G. A person who lives in a long-term care facility.

H. An area in a long-term care facility that provides care for patients who are too ill to be in the general population but who have been released from the acute care of a hospital.

I. A facility that provides care for adult (usually elderly) clients during the day.

J. A person receiving service from a health care provider, usually at home or in a day-care setting.

K. A hospital or other facility devoted to retraining patients to enable them to function as fully as possible.

L. A facility that provides medical or surgical care to sick or injured people who stay overnight or longer.

Check Your Knowledge

Review Questions: Answer each of the following questions on a separate sheet of paper.

1. Explain the purpose of each component of a system.
2. What are the processes in a health care delivery system?
3. Name four trends that can affect the delivery of health care.
4. What is an outpatient?
5. Explain the difference between a hospital and a long-term care facility.
6. Why might a person choose to live in an assisted-living facility?
7. Who supervises nursing assistants in a long-term care facility?
8. Why do people have fewer health care choices when using a managed care plan?
9. Explain the difference between Medicare and Medicaid.
10. What is OSHA?

True or False: Read each statement carefully. Then write *True* or *False* by the statement number on a separate sheet of paper.

1. Rising costs in health care have led to patients being discharged earlier from the hospital.
2. An acute illness is one that is short-term.
3. People with injuries typically recover in hospice care.
4. A hospice is a place, a belief in a type of care, and a service to provide home care for the terminally ill.
5. JCAHO is a government agency that sets standards for health care facilities.

Think and Decide

Directions: Think about each of the following scenarios. Answer each question on a separate sheet of paper.

1. Rosa works in a large subacute care facility. Communication among the nursing staff is an ongoing problem. A crisis occurs when Rosa does not get the news about a new policy regarding new admissions to the facility. When the supervisor asks her why she is still following the old policy, Rosa explains that she didn't know about the new policy. She tells her supervisor that this is not the first time information has failed to reach her. The supervisor asks Rosa to draw up a plan to help ensure that everyone is informed of new policies and procedures. Using the systems model, develop a plan that Rosa might propose to her supervisor.

2. Mr. R. was laid off work several months ago when the company he worked for downsized. His wife works part-time, but her salary alone is not enough to pay all of the bills, and she does not have health insurance. Unable to find another job in his field, Mr. R. begins doing odd jobs and "handyman" work. One day, he slips off a roof he is repairing and injures his back and ankle. The property owner does not have liability insurance, so Mr. R. refuses to go to a hospital or even see a doctor. What alternatives might you recommend to Mr. R.?

3. Janice is a nursing assistant in a clinic that sees many elderly patients. When 83-year-old Mrs. P. arrives for her appointment, Janice hands her a HIPAA statement to read. Mrs. P. says, "Not another form to read! I get so tired of reading forms, and besides, I didn't bring my reading glasses. What is this one for?" How should Janice respond?

4. Ed is a nursing assistant in a rehabilitation center. Many of the nursing assistants in this center have been trained to help the therapists with physical rehabilitation, but Ed has not. When a coworker calls in sick, the supervisor asks Ed to take over some of the coworker's patients for the day. Two of these patients require physical therapy, but Ed does not feel comfortable helping the therapist because he has not received training. What should he do?

5. As a nursing assistant in a subacute care facility, Jenette works closely with several patients. One of her patients is J.W., an elderly man who is in the facility while he recovers from heart surgery. He has recently taken a turn for the worse. He confides to Jenette, "I just know they're not going to let me go home. They're going to stick me into one of those assisted-living places. I don't want to live there! I want to go home." What should Jenette do?

6. JoElyn, a student who is currently enrolled in a CNA course, asks her friend Miguel how his family is doing. She knows that his mother is dying of lung cancer. Miguel replies that his mother wants to die at home, but it is becoming harder and harder for his family to care for her. What options might JoElyn mention to Miguel?

CNA Certification Exam Prep

Directions: This practice test contains ten questions. Each question has four suggested answers. For each question, choose the ONE that best answers the question or completes the statement. Write your answers on a separate sheet of paper.

1. One of your patients states that she believes women have the right to choose whether they want to keep a pregnancy or not. Your response is to:
   A. explain your religious beliefs.
   B. argue with her.
   C. listen.
   D. do nothing.

2. People cared for at a long-term care facility are called
   A. clients.
   B. residents.
   C. patients.
   D. elderly people.

3. Medicare is government-sponsored health care funding for
   A. people at or below poverty level.
   B. children.
   C. people over age 65.
   D. teenagers.

4. The federal agency that inspects facilities for safety and infection control is
   A. JCAHO.
   B. HIPAA.
   C. OBRA.
   D. OSHA.

5. The agency that protects patient privacy is
   A. OSHA.
   B. HIPAA.
   C. OBRA.
   D. JCAHO.

6. A long-term care facility is for people who need
   A. care for acute illnesses.
   B. day care only.
   C. care for chronic disorders or disabilities.
   D. end-of-life care.

7. Hospice is a facility or program that serves
   A. people who need retraining.
   B. people with disabilities.
   C. terminally ill patients.
   D. emergency or acute care patients.

8. Managed care is
   A. health care funding for people over age 65.
   B. a plan that uses a pre-screened pool of providers and facilities.
   C. health care funding for children.
   D. a long-term health care plan.

9. You are caring for Mr. Shinto, who has a sore on his right heel, but he won't let you touch his foot. Your first action is to
   A. tell him you have to care for his foot.
   B. ask the nurse about his cultural needs.
   C. avoid caring for his foot.
   D. ask someone else to perform the care.

10. A rehabilitation center is a facility for
    A. treating outpatients.
    B. retraining patients to enable them to function as fully as possible.
    C. providing acute medical or surgical care to sick or injured people.
    D. terminally ill patients.

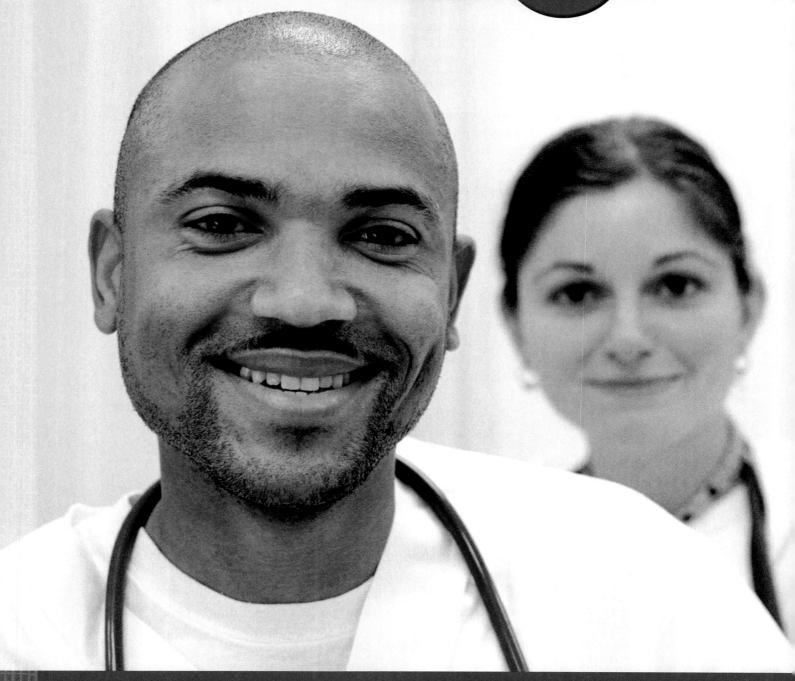

CHAPTER 3

OBJECTIVES

- Explain how to organize a job search.
- Identify documents to prepare before applying for jobs.
- Prepare a résumé and a cover letter.

- Prepare a personal data sheet and correctly fill out an application form.
- Identify sources of job leads.
- Prepare for and participate in a job interview.

- Describe aspects of starting a new job.
- Describe methods of personal and professional growth.

Getting a Job as a Nursing Assistant

VOCABULARY

application form A questionnaire filled out by a job applicant that summarizes the person's qualifications.

career portfolio A collection of a person's educational and professional achievements.

continuing education Programs for adult learners at high schools, colleges, and universities.

cover letter A short letter that introduces you to an employer. It explains why you are sending your résumé and why you are the right person for the job.

entrepreneur A person who plans, organizes, and runs a business.

job interview A formal meeting between a job candidate and an employer.

job shadowing Following another employee on the job to learn the routine.

networking Communicating with people you know to share information.

orientation A program that explains an employer's policies, procedures, and benefits to a new employee.

personal data sheet A document containing the personal information likely to be needed when applying for a job.

reference A person who knows you well and is willing to recommend you for a job.

résumé A written summary of job qualifications, including education, skills, and work experience.

work ethic A positive attitude about your work, including honesty, trustworthiness, reliability, and responsibility.

Organizing Your Job Search

This is an exciting time to plan a health care career. There are more jobs for nursing assistants than ever before. According to the U.S. Department of Labor, nursing assistants have held almost 1.5 million jobs in recent years. At least through the year 2012, overall employment of nursing assistants will grow faster than the average for all occupations.

Organizing your job search and finding a job is a full-time job itself. Even though the number of opportunities is growing, you will want to find the best situation for yourself. You should plan to invest as much time as possible in your job search. Your investment of time and effort will pay off when you find an excellent, rewarding position. **See Figure 3-1.**

Determining Priorities

You will need to determine priorities when searching for the right job. Create a list of important job features to help you narrow your search. Think about the following:

- **What type of facility would you prefer?** Would you rather work with a variety of patients in a hospital setting? Perhaps you would prefer working with elderly residents in a long-term care facility or an assisted-living facility. You might enjoy working in a small group home where you can really get to know the residents.
- **How far can you travel to get to work?** Whether you use public transportation, drive your own car, or ride a bike, you will need to make sure that work is a reasonable distance from where you live. Will you have another way to get to work if your car breaks down? Your transportation must be reliable so you can get to work on time.
- **What hours would you like to work?** If you have children, will you have child care available during your work shifts? Most nursing assistants work full-time—about 40 hours per week on a day, evening, or night shift. Some of these shifts overlap, and others require a reduced staff. All facilities have some level of around-the-clock care, so there are opportunities for part-time work. Nursing assistants may work only nights, weekends, or evenings, or on a rotating shift. Some have jobs that require living in a patient's home.

Preparing Documents

Potential employers will need information about you to determine whether to hire you. You can help yourself be organized and present a professional appearance by preparing this information in advance. To do this, you will need to prepare several types of documents and materials before applying for jobs.

Résumé. A **résumé** (pronounced REH-zoom-ay) is a written summary of job qualifications, including education, skills, and work experience. Your résumé should be professional—neat, organized, and concise. It should be one to two pages long, and never longer than two pages.

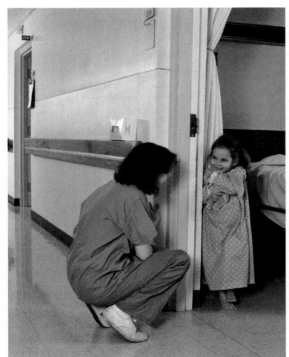

O **Figure 3-1. Investing time and energy in a job search will help ensure a rewarding position.**

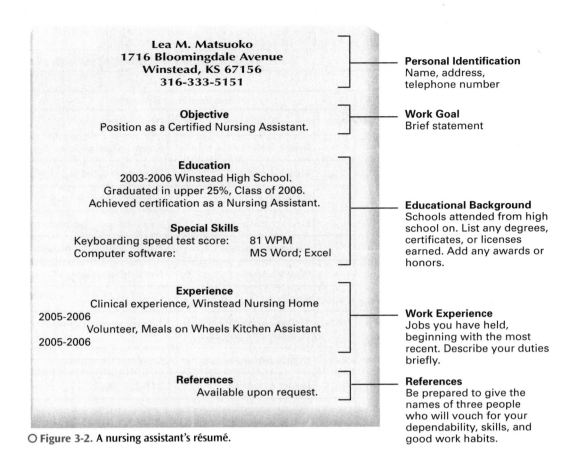

Lea M. Matsuoko
1716 Bloomingdale Avenue
Winstead, KS 67156
316-333-5151

Personal Identification
Name, address, telephone number

Objective
Position as a Certified Nursing Assistant.

Work Goal
Brief statement

Education
2003-2006 Winstead High School.
Graduated in upper 25%, Class of 2006.
Achieved certification as a Nursing Assistant.

Special Skills
Keyboarding speed test score: 81 WPM
Computer software: MS Word; Excel

Educational Background
Schools attended from high school on. List any degrees, certificates, or licenses earned. Add any awards or honors.

Experience
Clinical experience, Winstead Nursing Home
2005-2006
Volunteer, Meals on Wheels Kitchen Assistant
2005-2006

Work Experience
Jobs you have held, beginning with the most recent. Describe your duties briefly.

References
Available upon request.

References
Be prepared to give the names of three people who will vouch for your dependability, skills, and good work habits.

○ **Figure 3-2. A nursing assistant's résumé.**

There are a number of ways to format a résumé. A chronological format often works best. In this format, list your most recent work experience first, then your previous job, and so on. Do the same with your educational experience. **Figure 3-2** shows a sample. Your school and the public library have resources that provide other examples of effective résumés.

Be sure to include other experiences you've had, such as volunteer work and community service. Include honors and awards that you have received. Prepare your résumé on a computer and print it on white or off-white paper. If you do not have a computer or printer, you can use the public library's equipment or a résumé service.

References. Create a list of three or four references. A **reference** is a person who knows you well and is willing to recommend you for a job. You should ask people ahead of time if you may list their names. Teachers, coworkers, and former employers are the best references to use. If your résumé is short (less than a page), include the list. Otherwise, write "Available upon request" under the heading "References." Provide current contact information for your references, including name, job title, address, and phone number. Also include your e-mail address, if you have one.

Cover Letter. When you send your résumé to potential employers, include a cover letter. A **cover letter** is a short letter that introduces you to an employer. In the letter, explain why you are sending your résumé and why you are the right person for the job. The cover letter should address aspects of a specific job, but you can create a general letter that you can modify for each job application.

Vital Skills ⟨ WRITING ⟩

Proofreading

When writing your résumé, you'll concentrate on organizing your information and making sure your facts are accurate. When you're finished, however, you'll need to proofread your work. Submitting a résumé full of errors will not impress a potential employer. When you proofread, check for errors in capitalization, punctuation, and spelling.

Proofreading Symbols		
⊙	Insert a period.	Dr⊙Brown
∧	Insert letters or words.	Reported Director of Nursing
⋀	Insert a comma.	Volunteer Concord Hospital
≡	Capitalize a letter.	Willow manor Home
/	Lowercase a letter.	Available on Request
◡	Close up a space.	Gradu ated with honors
#	Insert a space.	NursingAssistant
ⓢⓟ	Spell out.	Concord, (H.S.) ⓢⓟ
∼	Transpose the position of letters or words.	Acheived certification
℘	Delete letters or words.	Clinnical Experience
/=/	Insert a hyphen.	316-333 1551

○ Figure A

Practice

Working in teams, write a fictitious résumé for a nursing assistant who is applying for jobs for the first time. Trade résumés with another team and proofread each other's work. Use the proofreading symbols in Figure A to show the corrections that must be made to create an error-free résumé.

Personal Data Sheet. Your **personal data sheet** contains all of the personal information you may need as you apply for jobs. Include dates and phone numbers, for example, that you might otherwise forget. An example is shown in **Figure 3-3.**

Official Documents. You may not need to use the following documents to apply for jobs, but you will need them after you have been hired. It is important to have them ready ahead of time.

- Social Security card and number.
- Certified Nursing Assistant diploma or certificate. You may also need to provide proof that you are on the state's registry.
- A driver's license or some other valid form of identification.

If you apply for a job that requires you to drive to clients at their homes every day, you may need to show a driver's license and proof of automobile insurance.

Identifying Job Leads

About one-half of nursing assistant jobs are found in long-term care facilities. **See Figure 3-4.** Another one-fourth of nursing assistants work in hospitals. Additional new jobs will be in rehabilitation, home care, and other services. Jobs can be found in residential care facilities, mental health settings, and private households. Possible positions include:

- Geriatric aide
- Geriatric technician
- Personal care technician
- Hospital attendant
- Mental health assistant
- Nursing assistant
- Rehabilitation or restorative nursing assistant
- Child care attendant
- Companion and homemaker
- Home health aide
- Occupational therapy aide
- Physical therapy aide

How do you find job leads for these positions?

Networking. Communicating with people you know to share information is called **networking**. In this process, you develop relationships that will help you locate other contacts to assist you with job goals. As you network, you also help the other person or group accomplish their goals. Networking is considered the best way to find a job.

Instructors, friends who are working, and other health care professionals you know can put you in touch with people who know of job openings. Consider

Personal Data Sheet

Name ———————————— Social Security Number ——————
Address ——————————————————————————————
Date of Birth ———————————— Place of Birth ——————————
Telephone ——————————————————————————————
Awards/Honors/Offices ——————————————————————————
Other ————————————————————————————————

Educational Background

	Name	Address	Dates Attended From	To
Junior High School				
High School				
Course of Study				
Favorite Subject(s)				

Employment History (Begin with current or most recent.)
Company ———————————— Telephone ——————————
Address ——————————————————————————————
Dates of Employment: From ———————————— To ——————
Job Title and Duties ————————————————————————————
Supervisor ————————————————————————————
Last Wage ———————— Reason for Leaving ————————————

Company ———————————— Telephone ——————————
Address ——————————————————————————————
Dates of Employment: From ———————————— To ——————
Job Title and Duties ————————————————————————————
Supervisor ————————————————————————————
Last Wage ———————— Reason for Leaving ————————————

Company ———————————— Telephone ——————————
Address ——————————————————————————————
Dates of Employment: From ———————————— To ——————
Job Title and Duties ————————————————————————————
Supervisor ————————————————————————————
Last Wage ———————— Reason for Leaving ————————————

References (Names of people who can provide information about your personal, school, or work background.)

	Name	Address	Telephone Home	Work	Relationship
1.					
2.					
3.					

○ **Figure 3-3.** Take a personal data sheet to remind you of phone numbers and other details when filling out application forms.

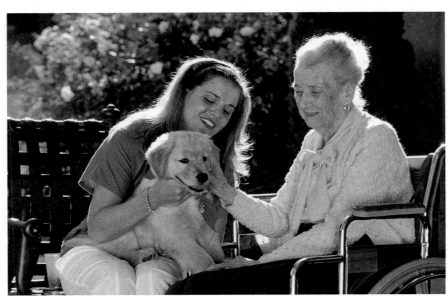

○ **Figure 3-4.** Many nursing assistants find employment in long-term care facilities.

joining a professional association for nursing assistants. Such associations provide information and help with job hunts. They distribute career guides, directories of members, and newsletters. They may hold job fairs in your area. In turn, your membership fee and involvement help the association with its goals of furthering professional recognition.

Classified Ads. Many available jobs are listed in classified ads in the local newspaper. **See Figure 3-5**. They may also be available in the online edition of the newspaper. Some papers separate jobs according to type, such as technicians, nurses, and so on. Others group jobs under a heading such as "medical employment." Ads generally provide detailed information about hours, qualifications needed, and who to contact. Follow up promptly on every ad that might lead to a job you want. If you wait, you may be too late.

Employment Agencies. Many jobs are offered through employment agencies, which match workers with jobs. Employers contact the agency with their requirements for filling a particular position. The agency then contacts qualified people who have applied to the agency.

For the best results, contact agencies that specialize in health care employment. Make an appointment to fill out an application form. The agency will contact you when an employer has a suitable job opening. The agency will set up an appointment for an interview with the employer.

Health Care Facilities. Many larger health care facilities, such as hospitals, provide a job line. The job line is a telephone recording that is updated daily. It lists job openings and also explains how to contact the human resources department. You can also call the facility's human resources department for job information.

Online Searches. There are two ways to search for a nursing assistant job online. First, many health care facilities maintain an online job listing. If you would like to work at a certain facility, you can go to its Web site to find any posted job openings. In many cases, you can apply by submitting your résumé online.

The second way to find a job online is to use a search engine such as Google® or Yahoo® to search for openings in your area. Use search terms including "nursing assistant," "job," and the name of your city or county. The search engine will list Web sites that match your search terms. You may even find an organization that specializes in posting health care jobs on the Internet.

Other Sources. Associations, directories, and magazines in the health care field often provide job leads. Associations may have job listings. Directories provide lists of employers, such as hospitals or government agencies, that are hiring health care workers. Magazines and periodicals available at school or the public library may list possible leads.

Even if you are not applying for a specific job opening, you may call or write to an employer directly. You can ask if there are any openings or if you may submit your résumé for future consideration. Ask to speak to the director of nursing or the human resources director. If you are writing a letter to find out if there are jobs, call first to get the name of the contact person. Then you can send the letter directly to that person.

HOME HEALTH AIDES
NURSING ASSISTANTS

Help us to help others! We have openings for nursing assistants to provide personal care and perform light housekeeping duties for our patients in their homes. Positions are part time, morning and/or evening hours available, including weekends. A car and a telephone are required. We pay competitive wages and mileage for your car. For more information, call:

860-482-6419

THE SMITH HOME HEALTH SERVICES, INC.
62 Commercial Blvd.
Torrington, CT 06790
EOE

Figure 3-5. A classified ad for nursing assistants and home health aides.

Staying Organized

Keep track of all of your contacts with employers by using index cards or creating a computer file. Include the name of the facility, the contact person's name and title, the phone number, the address, and where you got the lead. Jot down notes, such as directions to the facility. Note the date that you contacted the employer.

Enter the appointments you make for job interviews in a calendar or date book. Coordinate these appointments with your other daily activities so that you do not schedule two at once.

Applying for Jobs

Employers are looking for the best person to fill each job. They decide whom to hire based on the person's qualifications, the impression each person makes, and how well they think the person will fit in with their health care team. During your job search, remember that first impressions count the most. The way you speak, the way you are groomed and dressed, and the attitude and confidence you demonstrate are as important as your specific skills.

How do employers begin to gather information about job candidates? Employers usually ask you to complete an **application form**. This is a questionnaire filled out by a job applicant that summarizes the person's qualifications. The application form gives employers a quick summary of each person who is applying for a job, so they can decide whom to interview. These forms vary from one to four pages. **See Figure 3-6.** You will also need to provide your résumé.

Follow these guidelines when completing an application form:

- Complete the application form neatly. Spell all words correctly. Print, if that is what the form requests.
- Use a pen rather than a pencil.
- Do not skip any questions. If a question does not apply to you, write "Not Applicable" (or "NA") on the line.
- Use your correct, complete name and address.
- Some applications ask for your date of birth or marital status. Employers cannot legally require you to answer these questions. Leave them blank.
- If asked for a job preference, be specific.
- Most application forms ask for a list of schools you have attended. Using your personal data sheet, include all schools and the dates you attended.
- The application form also asks about previous jobs. Fill out this section in reverse order. Begin with your most recent job and end with the first job you had.
- The application form often asks for references. Use your personal data sheet to provide accurate names and contact information.
- On the signature line, be sure to write, not print, your full name.

Application for Employment

All qualified applicants will receive consideration for employment and promotion without regard to race, creed, religion, color, age, sex, national origin, handicap, or marital status. This application is effective for 90 days. If you wish to be considered for employment thereafter, you must complete a new application.

Date _____

Name _____ Telephone (___) _____
          Last   First   Middle Initial   Area Code

Address _____
          Number & Street   Apt. #   City   State   Zip

Length of time at that address _____ Previous address _____

Position you are applying for_____ Rate of pay expected _____ per month

Were you previously employed by us?_____ If yes, when?_____

State any other experiences, skills, or qualifications which you feel would especially fit you for work with us:_____

Applying for: Full-time _____ Part-time _____ Days _____ Evenings _____ Midnight _____ Alternating _____ Any_____

Location preferred: Downtown St. Paul _____ Eagan_____ Westbury _____ Other_____

Are you at least 18 years of age?_____ Will you take a physical examination?_____

List any friends or relatives working for us _____
                                                          Name   Relationship
          _____
                                                          Name   Relationship

Referred to our facility by_____

School	Name and Location	Course of Major	Graduated
Elementary	_____	_____	☐ yes ☐ no
High School	_____	_____	☐ yes ☐ no
College	_____	_____	☐ yes ☐ no
Other (specify)	_____	_____	☐ yes ☐ no

Do you plan any additional education?_____ If yes, describe _____
_____

List in order all employers, beginning with your most recent employment:

Name & Location of Company	From Mo Yr	To Mo Yr	Salary	Supervisor	Reason for Leaving
1)					
2)					
3)					
4)					

Describe the work you did with:

Company #1._____

Company #2._____

Company #3._____

Company #4._____

May we contact the employers listed above?_____ If not, indicate by number which one(s) you do not wish us to contact _____

CERTIFICATION OF APPLICANT

I hereby certify that the facts set forth in the above employment application are true and complete to the best of my knowledge. I understand that if I am employed, falsified statements on this application shall be considered sufficient cause for dismissal, and that no contractual rights or obligations are created by said employment application.

Signature of Applicant _____

○ **Figure 3-6.** An employment application form for a nursing assistant position.

Interviewing

A **job interview** is a formal meeting between a job candidate and an employer. If your application form or résumé is selected, the employer will call you to set up an interview. An interview is your best chance to convince the employer that you are the best candidate for the job. It also gives the employer a way to evaluate you. Most interviews are fairly short, lasting from a few minutes to under an hour. Some are longer. Some interviews are conducted by more than one person.

Preparing for the Interview

How can you increase your chances of success? Take time to organize your thoughts and think about the type of impression you want to make before going to an interview.

Find Out About the Employer and the Job. Do some research about the employer. Do you know anyone who works there, or who used to work there? Learn the types of health care services that are offered. Find out the size and type of facility. For example, is it a public or private hospital, a rehabilitation center, an office or clinic, or a long-term care or day-care facility?

Show that you are knowledgeable about the facility to make a good impression at the interview. For example, in a long-term care facility, you might ask about how the health care team is organized. You could also ask if there is a subacute care unit or an Alzheimer's unit. If possible, ask to review the job description, too. Check that the requirements match the skills and procedures for which you have been trained.

Practice Answering and Asking Questions. You can expect to be a little nervous at the beginning of an interview. Practice answering typical questions with another student beforehand. **See Figure 3-7.** The following questions are often asked during an interview:

- How do you get along with other team members?
- What are your greatest strengths?
- What are your greatest weaknesses?
- Can you take criticism without feeling hurt or upset?
- How well do you work under stress?
- What type of patients do you find most difficult to work with?
- What did you like least and best about your last job?
- What are your career goals?

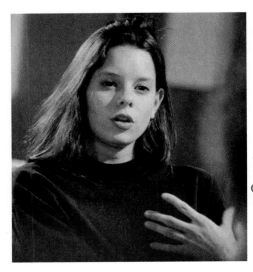

○ **Figure 3-7.** Practice asking and answering interview questions with friends to develop a confident manner and smooth responses.

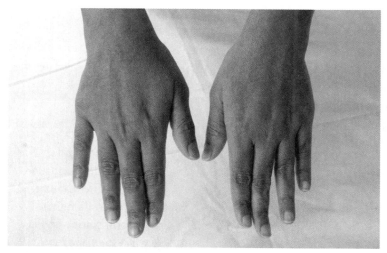

Plan Your Appearance. Make sure you look neat and well-groomed for a job interview. Bathe, wear deodorant, and brush your teeth. Your fingernails should be short and clean. Wear clean business attire. This can include a shirt, tie, and trousers for men. It can include a blouse and skirt or trousers, or a dress for women. **See Figure 3-8.**

○ **Figure 3-8.** Many interviewers look closely at the applicant's nails. Short, clean nails reduce the risk of picking up germs under the nails and transmitting infections to patients.

Vital Skills (MATH)

Calculating Time

Your job interview with the human resources representative at a rehabilitation center is scheduled for Tuesday morning at 10:00. You want to arrive 15 minutes before your appointment time.

- Driving to the rehabilitation center will take 20 minutes.
- Sometimes parking is hard to find, so you will park 5 minutes walking distance away.
- It takes about 7 minutes to get from the main entrance to the elevators and to the 6th floor, Room 601.
- You want to arrive 15 minutes early.
1. Calculate how much time it will take you to arrive for the interview.

   ADD 20 + 5 + 7 + 15 = 47 minutes

   You need to allow 47 minutes from the time you leave home to arrive 15 minutes early at Room 601.
2. What time should you leave?

   Your appointment is at 10:00.

CONVERT hour to minutes: 1 hour = 60 minutes
SUBTRACT 47 minutes
60 − 47 = 13

You would need to leave your home at 9:13.

To check your answer, add 47 minutes to 9:13 = 10:00.

Practice

1. You have an appointment for an interview at a local hospital at 2:30 PM. It will take you 15 minutes to drive to the hospital and another 10 to park in the parking garage and walk to the human resources department on the third floor. You want to arrive 10 minutes early. How much time should you allow to arrive for the interview?
2. You have an appointment for an interview at a subacute care facility at 4:00 PM. It will take you 18 minutes to drive to the facility, but parking will not be a problem. You can park and walk to the nursing director's office in about 8 minutes. At what time should you leave home to arrive 15 minutes early?

Allow Enough Time. If it has been more than a week since you made the interview appointment, call ahead to confirm the date and time. Give yourself plenty of time to get ready and get to the interview. Plan on arriving about 15 minutes early. Take a practice trip ahead of time to find out how long it takes to get to the facility and to check parking availability and other details.

In addition to these preparations, make sure you bring your résumé, legal documents, and any notes you have made with you. Also bring a pencil or pen and blank paper for taking notes.

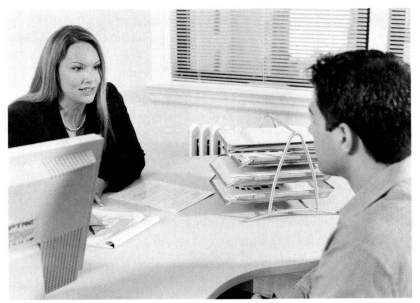

O **Figure 3-9.** During your interview, sit up straight and maintain eye contact with the interviewer.

A Successful Interview

Remember, you want to make a good first impression. It is important to project confidence, enthusiasm, and a positive attitude. Smile when you meet the person or people who will interview you. If the interviewer offers to shake hands, grasp the person's hand firmly.

Do not sit down until asked. Take the chair the interviewer points out, or take a seat next to the interviewer. Never put your papers, briefcase, or purse on the interviewer's desk. Look directly at the interviewer when you are being asked or are answering questions. **See Figure 3-9.**

As you respond, speak clearly and listen closely. Use body language to show that you understand the interviewer. As you sit, lean slightly forward to indicate interest. Smile or nod to show agreement. Follow the tone and pace the interviewer establishes. If the interviewer is serious, be serious. If the person is informal, you may be somewhat informal, too.

When the interviewer asks about your background, you can provide more information than you gave on your application form or résumé. In general, avoid one-word or one-line answers, but do answer concisely. Try to match your skills and experience with those required by the position. If you are asked about a task you have not done, say that you are eager to learn and to become part of the team. It is important to explain honestly why you left another job. However, do not speak negatively about former employers. If you are asked a question you cannot answer, be honest in saying so.

Plan to ask some questions, too. Make a list of topics before the interview. After the interviewer has finished, ask if you may ask some questions. If you sense that the interviewer is impatient or on a tight schedule, be brief. Ask only the most important questions.

Here are a few more tips:
- Do not bite your nails, chew gum, or smoke during the interview.
- Do not bring children or friends to the interview.
- Do not use your cell phone or pager during the interview. Turn them off before you arrive.

FOCUS ON

Leadership

Leadership is one of the characteristics employers look for when they interview job applicants. Remember that a good leader knows how to follow as well as how to lead. You can demonstrate leadership by asking well-chosen questions related to the job (leading) and by responding to verbal and nonverbal cues given by the interviewer (following).

Sender-Receiver Model

Communication is based on a simple model. One person is the sender, and one is the receiver. The sender sends a message. The receiver receives the message and then provides feedback—a response to the message sent. Communication is successful only when the receiver understands the message that is sent. **Figure A** shows the basic sender-receiver model.

The medium is the method of sending the message. A job interview is a type of medium. It's a face-to-face method of sending and receiving messages.

Practice

With a partner, role-play a job interview. One person will be the employer and one the job applicant. Ask questions clearly. Provide simple, straightforward answers. When you are the receiver and do not understand the message that is sent, politely ask the sender to clarify the message. Trade roles so that each person can practice being the sender and the receiver.

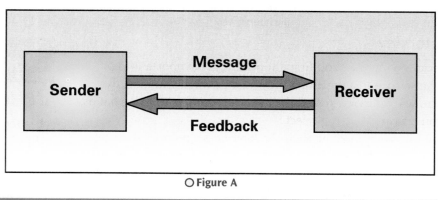

○ Figure A

Following Up

It is good practice to send a letter to the interviewer a day or so after an interview. In this follow-up letter, thank the interviewer and explain again why you are especially qualified for the position. State how much you would like to become part of the health care team in that facility.

If you have not heard from the employer after a week, call the interviewer. Explain that you were interviewed for the particular job, and then ask if a hiring decision has been made. If the answer is "no," show your interest by saying that you would very much like to be selected for this job. If the answer is "yes," thank the interviewer for taking the time to speak with you. Ask to be considered for other positions that become available. Leaving an interviewer with a positive impression is important in case you apply there again.

Getting a Job Offer

If you receive a job offer, you can ask for a day or two to think about it. Take this time to think about the pros and cons of taking the job. If you decide to accept, you can phone the employer and also send a letter of acceptance.

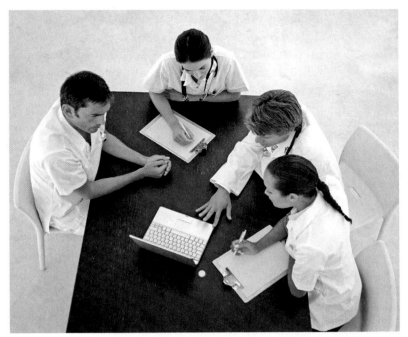

O **Figure 3-10.** Some large facilities conduct formal orientation meetings for new employees.

What if you do not want to accept the offer? Maybe the salary is too low or the job was not what you expected. Do not reject the offer right away. Again, take a day or two to consider in case you change your mind. When you call back, thank the employer for the opportunity and give a brief reason for rejecting the offer. Be courteous and remember that you might want to apply for a different position later.

Starting Your New Job

Your first few days on the job may be confusing, but they will also be exciting. You will meet your supervisors and coworkers. You may also meet the patients you will be assisting. First, though, you will probably need to fill out paperwork and learn your way around the workplace.

Orientation

Many workplaces provide an orientation for new employees on the first day or over several days. An **orientation** is a program that explains the employer's policies, procedures, and benefits. It often includes a tour of the facility and an introduction to coworkers. Orientation can be formal or informal. A larger facility might have a more formal program, with a presentation lasting the entire day. **See Figure 3-10.** An informal way of learning about the workplace is job shadowing. In **job shadowing**, you follow another employee on the job to learn the routine.

You will likely receive a job description, an employee handbook, and other agency information. You will also learn about the facility's dress code and appearance standards. For instance, you may be required to wear a specific color and style of uniform. You may have to wear a certain type of shoes.

During orientation, or sometime on your first day, the human resources department will ask you to complete some paperwork. For example, you will need to complete an Employee's Withholding Allowance Certificate. It is also called a Form W-4. You need to fill out the form so your employer can withhold (take out) the correct amount of federal income tax from your pay. **See Figure 3-11.** There may be other forms to fill out, such as health insurance applications.

The human resources department or personnel director will copy your driver's license or photo ID for your personnel file. Your personnel file began when the facility offered you a job. It contains your application form and résumé, your certification, a criminal background check, and the results of your interview. Other documents are added to your personnel file during the course of your employment, including performance reviews. It is your employer's responsibility to maintain your file and provide an orientation to the facility.

Personal Allowances Worksheet (Keep for your records.)

A Enter "1" for **yourself** if no one else can claim you as a dependent . . . . **A** _____

B Enter "1" if:
- You are single and have only one job; or
- You are married, have only one job, and your spouse does not work; or
- Your wages from a second job or your spouse's wages (or the total of both) are $1,000 or less.

. . **B** _____

C Enter "1" for your **spouse.** But, you may choose to enter "-0-" if you are married and have either a working spouse or more than one job. (Entering "-0-" may help you avoid having too little tax withheld.) . . . . **C** _____

D Enter number of **dependents** (other than your spouse or yourself) you will claim on your tax return . . . . . **D** _____

E Enter "1" if you will file as **head of household** on your tax return (see conditions under **Head of household** above) . **E** _____

F Enter "1" if you have at least $1,500 of **child or dependent care expenses** for which you plan to claim a credit . . **F** _____
(**Note.** Do **not** include child support payments. See **Pub. 503,** Child and Dependent Care Expenses, for details.)

G **Child Tax Credit** (including additional child tax credit):
- If your total income will be less than $54,000 ($79,000 if married), enter "2" for each eligible child.
- If your total income will be between $54,000 and $84,000 ($79,000 and $119,000 if married), enter "1" for each eligible child plus "1" **additional** if you have four or more eligible children. **G** _____

H Add lines A through G and enter total here. (**Note.** This may be different from the number of exemptions you claim on your tax return.) ▶ **H** _____

For accuracy, complete all worksheets that apply.	• If you plan to **itemize or claim adjustments to income** and want to reduce your withholding, see the **Deductions and Adjustments Worksheet** on page 2.
	• If you have **more than one job** or are **married and you and your spouse both work** and the combined earnings from all jobs exceed $35,000 ($25,000 if married) see the **Two-Earner/Two-Job Worksheet** on page 2 to avoid having too little tax withheld.
	• If **neither** of the above situations applies, **stop here** and enter the number from line H on line 5 of Form W-4 below.

----------------------- **Cut here and give Form W-4 to your employer. Keep the top part for your records.** -----------------------

| Form **W-4** | **Employee's Withholding Allowance Certificate** | OMB No. 1545-0010 |
| Department of the Treasury Internal Revenue Service | ▶ Whether you are entitled to claim a certain number of allowances or exemption from withholding is subject to review by the IRS. Your employer may be required to send a copy of this form to the IRS. | 2_____ |

| 1 Type or print your first name and middle initial | Last name | 2 Your social security number |
| Louise C. | Hogan | 000 : 00 : 0000 |

Home address (number and street or rural route)	3 ☒ Single ☐ Married ☐ Married, but withhold at higher Single rate.
1841 W. Palo Verde	Note. If married, but legally separated, or spouse is a nonresident alien, check the "Single" box.
City or town, state, and ZIP code	4 If your last name differs from that shown on your social security card, check here. You must call 1-800-772-1213 for a new card. ▶ ☐
Gallup , NM 00000	

5 Total number of allowances you are claiming (from line H above **or** from the applicable worksheet on page 2) **5** | O

6 Additional amount, if any, you want withheld from each paycheck . . . . **6** $

7 I claim exemption from withholding for 2___, and I certify that I meet **both** of the following conditions for exemption.
- Last year I had a right to a refund of **all** federal income tax withheld because I had **no** tax liability **and**
- This year I expect a refund of **all** federal income tax withheld because I expect to have **no** tax liability.
If you meet both conditions, write "Exempt" here . . . . ▶ | **7**

Under penalties of perjury, I declare that I have examined this certificate and to the best of my knowledge and belief, it is true, correct, and complete.

Employee's signature
(Form is not valid unless you sign it.) ▶ *Louise C. Hogan* | Date ▶ **3/15**

| 8 Employer's name and address (Employer: Complete lines 8 and 10 only if sending to the IRS.) | 9 Office code (optional) | 10 Employer identification number (EIN) |

For **Privacy Act and Paperwork Reduction Act Notice, see page 2.** | Cat. No. 10220Q | Form **W-4**

○ **Figure 3-11.** Employee's Withholding Allowance Certificate Form W-4.

Collaborative Questions

Collaborating with someone means that you work together on a project or problem. By asking each other questions about a text, a group of people can increase their understanding of the text's meaning. Questions can be asked to comprehend, analyze, and then apply the meaning.

Practice

Tax forms can be confusing. Read the "Personal Allowances Worksheet" directions in Form W-4 in Figure 3-11. As you read, write questions about any of the steps you do not understand. Share your questions with a partner and try to answer each other's questions.

Health and Safety

It is the responsibility of the employer to provide a safe working environment. The employer must ensure that employees are healthy. State and federal laws require workers in health care facilities to undergo certain tests, either before work begins or within a certain amount of time after starting the job. They include:

- A physical examination to certify that you are healthy.
- A tuberculosis (TB) skin test to find out if you have an active infection or have been exposed to tuberculosis. *Note:* If you have had a positive TB skin test in the past, provide proof of the previous test results. Do not repeat the TB skin test.

You will also be asked whether you want to receive a vaccination for Hepatitis B virus. Although the employer must by law provide the vaccination, you may decline to take it. If you decline, you will need to sign a waiver. Most employers will pay for the tests and vaccines. The employer might also require a drug test and a criminal background check. Home health care agencies are very likely to require the criminal background check.

Personal and Professional Growth

Now that you have a job, you must work hard to keep it. You will need to continue developing your skills and education for the following reasons:

- To keep up-to-date in a rapidly changing job market.
- To keep your job in the face of job reductions, such as lay-offs.
- To advance in your career path.

SAFETY FIRST

Working in a health care facility, especially a hospital, you could come in contact with someone with active Hepatitis B virus. Hepatitis B is a highly contagious, sometimes fatal disease. A vaccination is available and is recommended for all health care workers. Before making a decision, discuss the benefits and possible side effects of the vaccine with your primary care physician.

Work Ethic

To keep your job, you must have a good **work ethic**. This means that you have a positive attitude about your work and that you are honest, trustworthy, reliable, and responsible. It means that you respect others' privacy and always observe confidentiality. You must show up to work on time and work all of your scheduled hours. Make arrangements ahead of time for child care and transportation.

Working when scheduled, being cheerful and friendly, performing delegated tasks to the best of your ability, helping others, and being kind are all part of a good work ethic. The work you do is very important. Nurses, patients, and family members rely on you to give good care. **See Figure 3-12.**

Career Advancement

There can be many opportunities for advancement as a nursing assistant. You will need to think about your career path. Planning ahead and setting goals for yourself can help you obtain what you want in your professional career. It is important to:

- Establish short-term career goals.
- Develop long-term career planning strategies.
- Construct a career portfolio. A **career portfolio** is a collection of educational and professional achievements. Keep it up-to-date, adding new certificates, honors, awards, and a list of professional courses you have taken. You will have a record of your success to show when seeking a promotion or when applying for another job.

Federal law requires that you take a certain number of in-service hours each year to maintain your skills. You will have many opportunities to meet this requirement. Many employers provide staff development programs. These programs include seminars and in-services that teach new procedures and skills. Many facilities offer financial assistance for continuing education. **Continuing education** includes programs for adult learners at high schools, colleges, and universities. Some continuing education courses are also offered online.

You may see other opportunities that you want to pursue on your own. Networking is a

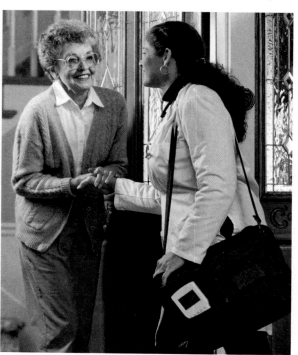

O **Figure 3-12.** Arriving at work on time or a few minutes early is an important part of a good work ethic.

great tool for career advancement. People you know may be aware of an open position in another facility and can put you in touch with the right contact.

Making Transitions

Recognizing when you need to change jobs is important. You may find a new job closer to home. You may find a job with higher pay or with a greater chance of advancement. Going to school, child care, and illness can create reasons for finding another job. It is important, though, that you do not just hop from job to job. Always keep your career in mind when you change jobs. Evaluate the new job to make sure that it is better than your current job.

Changing from one job to another can be smooth if you plan carefully. If you do decide to accept another job, notify your current employer in writing. Prepare a letter of resignation or complete a form in the human resources office. **See Figure 3-13.** Give at least two weeks notice so your employer can find someone to replace you. Include the following in your written notice:

- Your reason for leaving
- The last day you will work
- Comments thanking the employer for the opportunity to work in the facility

The human resources department may ask you to participate in an exit interview. They will ask questions about your work experience there. Answer honestly but do not be negative. They are trying to learn how they can make working at their facility better for their employees.

FOCUS ON

Entrepreneurship

What would it take to run your own home health care agency? You would need to have certain entrepreneurial skills. An **entrepreneur** is a person who plans, organizes, and then runs a business. Successful entrepreneurs are good decision makers. They are self-motivated, hard-working, and willing to take some risks. How would you get started? First, you need an idea. Then research and plan by asking and answering the following questions.

- What need will you fill or what service will you provide?
- Where will you locate your business?
- How will you hire employees?
- How will you obtain financing?
- What is your competition?
- Who will benefit?

Mrs. Janet Sullivan
Director of Nursing
Willow Manor Care
2332 N. Prospect
Smithtown, IL 60600

July 2, 2007

Dear Mrs. Sullivan:

This letter is to inform you that I will be resigning my position as 2nd shift Nursing Assistant, effective July 18. Due to family obligations, we are moving away from the area.

At this time, I want to thank you for giving me the opportunity to be a part of the health care team at Willow Manor.

Sincerely,

Debra Scott

Debra Scott

○ **Figure 3-13.** A resignation letter.

Chapter Summary

- Organizing a job search includes determining priorities, preparing documents, identifying job leads, and staying organized.

- It is important to have a number of documents prepared before beginning a job search. They include a résumé, a reference list, a cover letter, a personal data sheet, and certain official documents.

- A résumé and cover letter introduce the job applicant to the employer.

- Keeping a personal data sheet helps the job applicant complete the application form when applying for a job. The application form must be filled out completely and accurately.

- When seeking a job, all sources of job leads should be tried. They include networking, classified ads, employment agencies, and health care facilities.

- Preparing ahead of time helps ensure that a job interview will be successful.

- During an interview, good communication and body language convey confidence and enthusiasm.

- New employees usually participate in orientation, completing paperwork and certain health and safety tests.

- Methods of personal and professional growth include developing a good work ethic, working on career advancement, and planning for change.

VOCABULARY REVIEW

Directions: Match the letter of each definition in the second column with the correct vocabulary term in the first column. Write your answers on a separate sheet of paper.

Vocabulary

1. application form
2. continuing education
3. cover letter
4. job interview
5. job shadowing
6. networking
7. orientation
8. personal data sheet
9. reference
10. résumé

Definitions

A. A program that explains an employer's policies, procedures, and benefits to a new employee.
B. Following another employee on the job to learn the routine.
C. A document containing the personal information likely to be needed when applying for a job.
D. Programs for adult learners at high schools, colleges, and universities.
E. A written summary of job qualifications, including education, skills, and work experience.
F. A short letter that introduces you to an employer. It explains why you are sending your résumé and why you are the right person for the job.
G. A formal meeting between a job candidate and an employer.
H. A questionnaire filled out by a job applicant that summarizes the person's qualifications.
I. A person who knows you well and is willing to recommend you for a job.
J. Communicating with people you know to share information.

Check Your Knowledge

Review Questions: Answer each of the following questions on a separate sheet of paper.

1. Explain how to organize a job search.

2. What information should be included in a résumé?

3. What documents should you prepare before applying for a job?

4. Name four ways to find job leads.

5. How can you keep track of your job applications and appointments?

6. How can you prepare for an interview?

7. What should be included in a follow-up letter after an interview?

8. Once you begin a new job, how will you learn about the policies and procedures?

9. Name three reasons you should continue to develop your skills after getting a job.

10. Why is it important to keep a career portfolio?

True or False: Read each statement carefully. Then write *True* or *False* by the statement number on a separate sheet of paper.

1. Friends and relatives are the best people to use for references.

2. When signing an application form, write your full name rather than printing it.

3. Your résumé should include your birth date and marital status.

4. Saying something negative about a former employer during an interview is acceptable if you are being honest.

5. Filling out a Form W-4 is important, so your employer can withhold the correct amount of federal income tax from your pay.

Think and Decide

Directions: Think about each of the following scenarios. Answer each question on a separate sheet of paper.

1. Helen and Maria each apply for the same position at Grovenor Hospital. Helen answers all the questions the interviewer asks but acts withdrawn. The interviewer has difficulty hearing her answers. Maria asks several questions about the hospital's new wing. Even though they are equally qualified, Maria gets the job. Why do you think Maria was chosen?

2. Celina is at a job interview at a local long-term care facility. Her interviewer states that the facility has had a rapid turnover in the last several months because several of the nursing assistants have decided to get married. Soon after they marry, they leave their jobs. The interviewer asks Celina whether she is married. What should Celina say?

3. Ethan is on his way to a job interview at a hospital across town. He is well-prepared for the interview and has dressed appropriately. He has allowed time on his way to the interview to stop for a quick lunch at a deli counter. While eating his lunch, he accidentally spills some of his soft drink on his shirt. By this time, he has 20 minutes to get to the interview, and the hospital is still about 15 minutes away. What should he do?

4. Calla is looking for her first job. She has not worked even part-time while she completed her schooling, so she has no professional references. What can Calla say or write when asked for references?

5. Shalonda has been hired as a nursing assistant at a subacute care facility. She shows up each day on time and dressed appropriately, with a positive attitude toward her work. By the middle of her first week, however, she finds that most of her coworkers are overworked, stressed out, and short of temper. She becomes discouraged and decides she really doesn't like the job very much. What should Shalonda do?

6. Gene has worked two days at his new job as geriatric aide at an assisted-living facility. This morning, his car wouldn't start. A neighbor provided jumper cables and tried to start the car, but it still wouldn't start. The neighbor offers to take Gene to work, but can't guarantee that he'll be available to bring Gene home after work. Gene realizes that this would not solve the problem permanently. What should he do?

7. Ann has applied to several different facilities for work as a nursing assistant. She has received offers of employment from two of them: Starlight Retirement Center and Mayview General Hospital. Starlight offers better pay, but is 35 miles from Ann's home. Mayview is only 5 miles from Ann's home, but they want her to work the night shift, and Ann would prefer to work either a day shift or an evening shift. Make a list of the advantages and disadvantages of each job. Which offer do you think Ann should accept? Why?

CNA Certification Exam Prep

Directions: This practice test contains ten questions. Each question has four suggested answers. For each question, choose the ONE that best answers the question or completes the statement. Write your answers on a separate sheet of paper.

1. For which of the following positions might a certified nursing assistant apply?
   A. geriatric aide
   B. mental health assistant
   C. nursing assistant
   D. all of the above

2. According to the sender-receiver model, which of the following must be true for successful communication?
   A. A sender sends a message to a receiver.
   B. The receiver understands the message.
   C. The receiver sends feedback to the sender.
   D. The sender sends feedback to the receiver.

3. To prepare for an interview, you should
   A. dress in your oldest clothes to show that you need the job.
   B. practice answering questions.
   C. buy minted gum to chew during the interview to avoid bad breath.
   D. all of the above.

4. Which type of facility hires the majority of nursing assistants?
   A. hospitals
   B. home care agencies
   C. long-term care facilities
   D. rehabilitation centers

5. What is the most important thing to consider before you attend a job interview?
   A. personal appearance
   B. portfolio on hand
   C. making a good first impression
   D. all of the above

6. For a successful job interview,
   A. prepare for the interview by researching the position and the company.
   B. talk for at least 30 minutes to show off your knowledge.
   C. send an e-mail message of your intention to come for an interview.
   D. call just before your scheduled interview to say you can't make it.

7. Which of the following should you do if you have to leave a job?
   A. give your employer a day's notice
   B. not show up for work
   C. use up all of your vacation
   D. give your employer two weeks' notice

8. Which of the following documents will you need before you begin looking for a job?
   A. school transcripts
   B. an updated résumé
   C. a letter of interest in the job
   D. Social Security card

9. For a job interview, you should
   A. wear clean, neat clothing.
   B. use your best jewelry.
   C. wear blue jeans.
   D. both A and B.

10. If you have not heard from a potential employer after an interview, you should
    A. decide that you won't get the job.
    B. call the interviewer next month.
    C. call the interviewer after a week.
    D. send a letter to the interviewer.

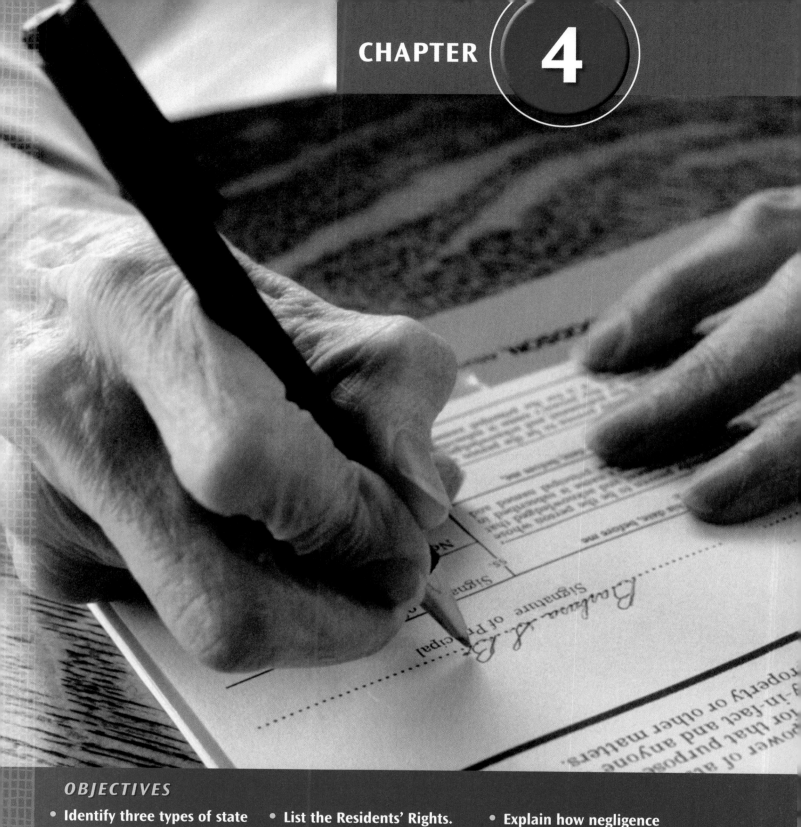

CHAPTER 4

OBJECTIVES

- **Identify three types of state and federal protection that protect patients' and residents' legal rights.**
- **List rights provided by the Patient's Bill of Rights.**

- **List the Residents' Rights.**
- **Explain the nursing assistant's role in protecting patients' and residents' rights.**

- **Explain how negligence and malpractice can harm patients.**

Legal Rights and Ethics

VOCABULARY

abuse The willful mistreatment of someone.

advance directive A legal document that specifies how medical decisions should be made in the future if a person becomes unable to make them.

assault The attempt or threat to touch another person's body without the person's consent.

battery Touching another person's body without the person's consent.

coercion An attempt to force someone to do something against his or her will.

confidentiality Keeping information about a patient private.

discrimination Treating a patient unfairly because of race, religion, sex, ethnic origin, age, or physical disability.

do not resuscitate (DNR) order A medical treatment order that tells health care providers not to use cardiopulmonary resuscitation (CPR) on a person if the person's heart or breathing stops.

ethical standards The set of rules for proper personal and professional conduct.

exploitation Taking advantage of someone financially, physically, or in any other manner.

grievance A formal complaint.

harassment Troubling, tormenting, offending, or worrying a person by one's behavior or speech.

health care proxy A legal document appointing someone, often a friend or family member, to make health care decisions on your behalf.

informed consent A patient's understanding and agreement to an action or procedure that has been explained.

intentional tort Causing harm or injury to a person or property on purpose.

invasion of privacy A violation of law that occurs when a patient is not protected from unwanted visitors or from unwanted release of confidential information.

legal rights The rights of all people under the law.

liability Legal responsibility for what someone does or fails to do.

living will A legal document stating how a person wishes to be treated in the event of serious or catastrophic illness.

malpractice The act or conduct of a trained health care provider that does not meet established standards or that goes beyond the provider's skill or scope of practice and results in harm.

negligence The failure of a trained health care provider to perform in a reasonable, careful manner and according to established standards, which results in unintentionally causing harm.

ombudsman A person who supports the health, welfare, safety, and rights of residents in long-term care facilities.

organ donation form A legal document that states a person's wish to donate all or some organs or tissues to people who need them or to train health care workers.

Patient's Bill of Rights The guidelines that health care staff must follow to ensure that patients are protected in the hospital.

privacy Freedom from intrusion of any kind.

protocols Specific rules for how to do tasks at a health care facility.

Residents' Rights Rights for home health care clients and residents of long-term care facilities provided by OBRA regulations.

tort A wrongful act that causes injury to another person or the person's property.

unintentional tort The act of causing harm or injury to a person or property without meaning to.

unlawful restraint Restraining or restricting the movements of another person without consent.

Protecting Patients' Legal Rights

In the United States, all citizens have **legal rights**—rights that are protected by law. People receiving health care have additional specific legal rights. The health care team protects these rights by following professional, legal standards of care. They also follow ethical standards. **Ethical standards** are the accepted set of rules for proper personal and professional conduct. That means doing the right thing for the patient when providing care.

Federal Protection

The federal government provides protection for people who need health care in a variety of settings. For example, the **Patient's Bill of Rights** consists of guidelines that health care staff must follow to ensure that patients are protected in the hospital. According to the Patient's Bill of Rights, all hospital activities should be carried out with concern for the values and dignity of patients. Most hospitals provide a brochure to their patients explaining these rights. **See Figure 4-1.**

——— Patient's Bill of Rights ———

1. The right to considerate and respectful care.
2. The right to complete, up-to-date, and understandable information about their diagnosis, treatments, how long it will take to recover, and other possible ways to handle the condition.
3. The right to make decisions about their planned care and the right to refuse care.
4. The right to name someone to make health care decisions for them if they become unable to make decisions for themselves.
5. The right to privacy in all procedures, examinations, and discussions of treatment.
6. The right to confidential handling of all information and records about their care.
7. The right to look over and have all records about their care explained.
8. The right to suggest changes in planned care or to transfer to another facility.
9. The right to be informed about the business relationships among the hospital and other facilities that are part of the treatment and care.
10. The right to decide whether to take part in experimental treatments.
11. The right to understand their care options after a hospital stay.
12. The right to know about the hospital's policies for settling disputes and to examine and receive an explanation of all charges.

○ **Figure 4-1.** A Patient's Bill of Rights.

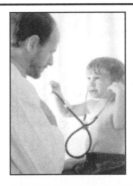

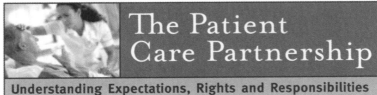

The Patient Care Partnership

Understanding Expectations, Rights and Responsibilities

What to expect during your hospital stay:

- High quality hospital care.

- A clean and safe environment.

- Involvement in your care.

- Protection of your privacy.

- Help when leaving the hospital.

- Help with your billing claims.

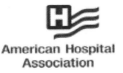

American Hospital Association

○ **Figure 4-2.** Many hospitals provide this brochure to patients when they are admitted or when they arrive for a medical procedure.

The American Hospital Association (AHA) has created a brochure titled "The Patient Care Partnership." **See Figure 4-2.** This brochure explains what patients can expect during a stay in a hospital. It also explains patients' rights and responsibilities while in the hospital.

Federal OBRA regulations provide additional rights for home health care clients and residents of long-term care facilities. These rights are called the **Residents' Rights. See Figure 4-3.** By protecting these rights, the staff help ensure that residents have a good quality of life. They also ensure dignity, choice, and self-determination. Nursing facilities must inform residents of the Residents' Rights orally and in writing before or during admission to the facility.

Residents' Rights

1. **The right to free choice**—to choose a doctor, to be told ahead of time about changes in care or treatment, to take part in planning their care and treatment, to refuse treatment, to give themselves their medications (if the nurse approves), and to make choices about all aspects of life that are important to them, such as who their visitors are.

2. **The right to freedom from restraints and abuse**—to be free from physical, verbal, sexual, chemical, or mental abuse, from being neglected, and from seclusion that is not chosen.

3. **The right to privacy and confidentiality** regarding all parts of their treatment, their records, and their communications and meetings with visitors and other residents. Residents also have the right not to have their bodies exposed unnecessarily.

4. **The right to file complaints**, voice grievances, form groups (such as a residents' council), and work with a long-term care ombudsman, a person who supports the rights and welfare of residents. The ombudsman is usually a volunteer who has been trained in advocacy work.

5. **The right to manage their own funds**, to receive their government benefits, to know the findings of state inspections of their facility, and to choose whether to perform or not perform work for the facility.

6. **The right to take part in activities**, such as social or religious services, to use their personal possessions and clothing, and to share a room with their spouse.

7. **The right to be told in writing** if care is going to be denied, changed, or ended, and to appeal to the facility's managers when this situation occurs.

○ **Figure 4-3.** The main points of the Residents' Rights provided by OBRA regulations.

The federal Health Insurance Portability and Accountability Act (HIPAA) includes a privacy rule to protect personal health information. **Privacy** is freedom from intrusion of any kind. The privacy rule also gives patients the right to see their medical records. It gives them more control over how their health information is used and who can see it. As a nursing assistant, you may not reveal or discuss information in a patient's chart or record with anyone other than members of the patient's health care team.

Another federal protection is the Older Americans Act. This act ensures that communities will provide services to older people. One service is the ombudsman program. A long-term care **ombudsman** is a person with legal training who supports the health, welfare, safety, and rights of residents in long-term care facilities. Ombudsmen usually have the power to investigate complaints and resolve the issue or take legal action when needed. The purpose of the ombudsman program is to protect the rights of frail, elderly, and disabled citizens who may not be able to speak for themselves. The ombudsman's name, address, and phone number must be posted in the facility where everyone can see it. If a resident has a **grievance** (a formal complaint) about care, the ombudsman can try to resolve the problem with the facility staff. In some cases, the nursing assistant is responsible for contacting the ombudsman. **See Figure 4-4.**

All states have adopted these rights. It is your responsibility to learn these rights, as well as additional laws and rights in your state.

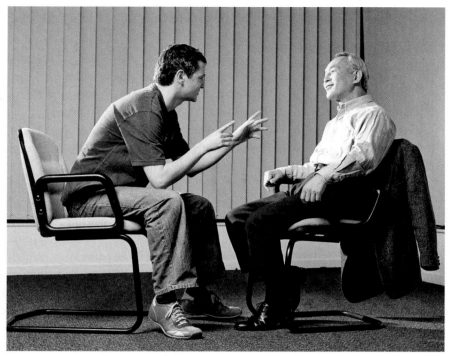

O **Figure 4-4.** A long-term care ombudsman works with a resident to resolve a grievance with the facility staff.

Vital Skills (COMMUNICATION)

Active Listening

As a caregiver, you should listen carefully when the patient speaks. *Active listening* is a good way to make sure you understand the patient's point. An active listener uses the following techniques:

- Reflection: Listen not only to the words the person is saying, but how he or she is saying it. How does the person feel about this topic?
- Restatement: Restate what the person said in your own words. You don't have to agree with the statement. You only need to make sure that you understand it.
- Clarification: Ask questions as necessary to clarify the person's point.

Practice

In teams of two, practice active listening techniques using the following scenarios. One person should play the role of a patient or resident who is upset. The other should play a nursing assistant using active listening techniques. Trade roles frequently.

- The patient complains that the nursing assistant never answers his call light.
- The patient wants to be taken outside for a walk even though it's 20 degrees outside and snowing.
- The resident no longer likes her room and wants to be moved to another one.

A *dilemma* is a situation in which it is hard to decide the right thing to do. You will face ethical dilemmas many times in your career. For instance, you might see another nursing assistant—a friend of yours—cause a patient to fall by making her walk too fast. The nursing assistant helps her up but does not report the incident. Should you report the incident? You have an ethical duty to report any incident in which a patient is or might be injured, no matter how slightly. You should do so even if the assistant involved is a friend. *Always* do what is best for the people in your care.

Ethical Behavior

Nursing assistants, like all health care professionals, must comply with the Patient's Bill of Rights and Residents' Rights. They follow all legal and ethical standards when caring for patients. As a nursing assistant, you must maintain a high standard of ethics. You must follow the rules of conduct for nursing assistants. **See Figure 4-5.** This includes helping those in your care and doing no harm.

Any behavior that might harm a patient is unethical and may also be illegal. It is also unethical to try to influence any patient's health care or financial decisions or the terms of a will. Taking advantage of patients is **exploitation**. For instance, accepting or demanding a tip for your services is a form of exploitation.

Trying to force patients to do something against their will is **coercion**. For example, suppose your duties today include taking a wheelchair-bound patient around the grounds of the long-term care facility so that she can get some fresh air, as recommended by her specialist. When you approach the patient, she is interested in a television program and does not want to go. Forcing her to go anyway by moving her wheelchair out to the garden would be coercion. A better way to handle this situation is to agree with her on a different time for the outing, if possible. If your schedule does not permit this, report to your supervisor.

Rules of Conduct for Nursing Assistants

- **Put your patients' needs before your own.**
- **Respect the privacy of all people in your care.**
- **Keep patients' and residents' rights in mind as you care for them.**
- **Practice confidentiality regarding all patients and residents.**
- **Respect every person—patients, their family members, your coworkers, and other staff members.**
- **Perform every task and procedure safely and conscientiously.**
- **Do not perform any tasks or procedures for which you have not been trained.**
- **Follow the orders given by the nurse or supervisor to the best of your ability.**
- **Stay within your scope of practice.**
- **Act professionally at all times.**
- **Do not use any drugs that have not been prescribed by a health care professional.**
- **Be a loyal employee and coworker.**
- **Be a responsible citizen of your community.**

○ Figure 4-5. The nursing assistant's rules of conduct.

Vital Skills — MATH

Using 24-Hour Time

Client records are legal documents that contain documentation of the care clients have received. A client's record can be used to help prove or disprove a claim. For this reason, entries in client records must be clearly written. A chart note that says simply "8:00—Mrs. Blackwell reported feeling dizzy and nauseated" is not clear. Did the writer mean 8:00 AM or 8:00 PM? If Mrs. Blackwell later has a heart attack, the answer might be very important.

To resolve issues like this one, health care facilities generally use the 24-hour clock. It is also called *international time* or *military time*. The 24-hour period starts after midnight, which is 2400 hours. The first hour (1:00 AM) is 0100 hours. This time system continues through 12:00 noon, which is 1200 hours. Then, instead of saying 1:00 PM, you say 1300 hours and so on, as shown in **Figure A**. The last hour noted is 11:00 PM, which is 2300 hours. The very last minute before midnight is 23:59. This system is used to avoid confusion when speaking or writing the time. When you say or write 1900 hours, you always mean 7:00 at night. There is no confusion about whether you mean 7:00 in the morning.

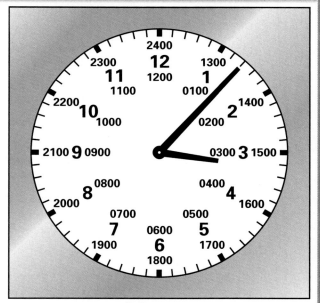

○ Figure A

Practice

Mrs. Jones suffered a stroke. She cannot always use her call light. Her care plan states that she is to be checked every two hours. Your shift begins at 2:30 PM. According to her chart, the last time Mrs. Jones was checked before your shift started was 1400 hours. Using the 24-hour clock, what is the first time you would check on Mrs. Jones? Write your answer on a separate piece of paper.

Advance Directives

Everyone has the right to make health care decisions in advance. An **advance directive** is a legal document that specifies how medical decisions should be made in the future if you become unable to make them yourself. There are several types of advance directives.

- A **health care proxy** appoints someone, often a friend or family member, to make health care decisions for you. In some states, a health care proxy may be called a health care power of attorney, medical power of attorney, or health care surrogate designation.

- A **living will** states how you wish to be treated in the event of a serious illness. See Figure 4-6. It may state, for example, that no life support systems are to be used.
- A **do not resuscitate (DNR) order** is a medical treatment order that tells health care providers not to use cardiopulmonary resuscitation (CPR) on you if your heart or breathing stops. Some hospice organizations require a DNR for all of their patients.
- An **organ donation form** is also a legal document. It states your wish to donate all or some of your organs and tissues to people who need them. You may also specify that your body may be used for training health care workers.

Federal law requires that everyone who is admitted to a health care facility be told about their right to make an advance directive. Many people, especially those entering long-term care facilities, have completed one or more of these forms. All of these are legal documents that must be obeyed by health care workers. Even if you do not agree with a patient's wishes, you must abide by them.

Living Will

Declaration made this day by:

_____
Name (please print)

_____ , 2 _____

Being of sound mind, I willfully and voluntarily make known my desire that my moment of death shall not be postponed under the circumstances set forth below and that I do hereby declare:

If, at any time, I should have an incurable injury, disease, or illness judged to be a terminal condition by my attending physician who has personally examined me, and has determined that my death is imminent except for life-sustaining procedures, I direct that such procedures be withheld or withdrawn and that I be permitted to die naturally with only the administration of medication, sustenance, or the performance of any medical procedure deemed necessary to provide me with comfort care.

In the absence of my ability to give directions regarding the use of such life-sustaining procedures, it is my intention that my family and physician shall honor this declaration as the final expression of my legal right to refuse medical or surgical treatment.

I understand the full import of this declaration, and I am emotionally and mentally competent to make this declaration.

_____
Signature of Applicant

_____
Address

_____
City, County, State, Country

The declarant has been personally known to me and I believe him/her to be of sound mind. I further certify that the above instrument was made on the date thereof, signed and declared by the declarant and myself.

WITNESS (Other than a relative)

_____
Name (please print)

_____
Signature

_____
Address

_____
City, County, State, Country

○ **Figure 4-6.** A living will can help ensure that the wishes of a dying patient are honored.

Violations of the Law

As a nursing assistant, you are in a good position to protect patients from violations of the law. Like all other health care professionals, however, if you commit any of these violations, you can be sued or charged with a crime. Also, if you do not protect patients from violations of the law, you can be sued or charged with a crime. It is therefore important to understand patient or resident rights. By understanding the law, you can avoid making mistakes and being held responsible for them.

Most of the legal rules that guide your caregiving are civil laws. Torts are part of civil law. The word *tort* comes from the French word meaning "wrong." A **tort** is a wrongful act that causes injury to another person or the person's property. Torts may be intentional or unintentional. A person who commits a tort can be sued for damages. Some torts are also crimes.

Liability is the legal responsibility for what someone does or fails to do. A nursing assistant's liability involves taking responsibility for his or her own actions in patient care. It involves obeying the law.

Intentional Torts

An **intentional tort** is the act of causing harm or injury to a person or property on purpose. The following are intentional torts that nursing assistants must guard against committing.

Assault and Battery. The attempt or threat to touch another person's body without the person's consent is called **assault**. **Battery** is touching another's body without the person's consent.

• Before providing care to a patient, explain what you are going to do. Encourage the patient to ask questions. Then get the patient's permission to provide the care that has been ordered. You can then give the care with the patient's **informed consent**. This term means that the action has been explained and that the patient understands and agrees to it. **See Figure 4-7.**

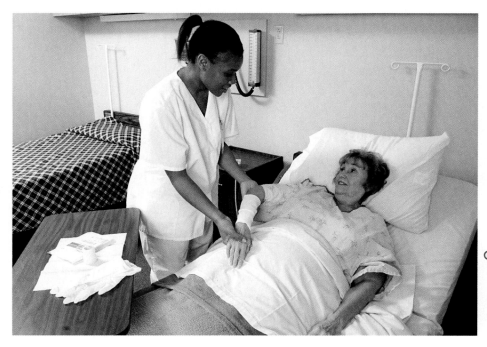

○ Figure 4-7. The nursing assistant explains an ordered procedure to the patient before beginning so that the patient can give informed consent for the procedure.

- Do not provide the care if the patient refuses. Instead, report the situation immediately to the supervisor or nurse.

Theft. Taking the personal property of another person without his or her consent is theft. It is a crime even if the item has little value. Stealing or helping someone else steal is a crime. Guilty people may be imprisoned. They can also be sued for damages.

- You are responsible for respecting a patient's personal possessions.
- You are responsible for reporting theft that you know about.

Unlawful Restraint. In some cases, restraints may be needed to protect a patient from harming himself or others. *Physical restraints* prevent a person's natural movements. Physical restraints include tying a patient to a chair or locking a patient in a room. *Chemical restraints* are medications that change a person's behavior by making them drowsy or dulling the senses to reduce their movements. Doctors may order restraints (and document the need for them) only if a patient has a medical condition requiring such treatment. Restraining a person without such an order is **unlawful restraint** or false imprisonment.

- Unless you have been instructed to use protective devices, which are designed to keep patients from harming themselves or others, never do anything that would keep people from moving freely.
- If you have been instructed to use protective devices, be sure to explain the procedure to the patient. You will learn more about when to use restraints legally in Chapter 6.

Discrimination. Treating a patient unfairly because of race, religion, sex, ethnic origin, age, or physical disability is **discrimination**. For example, not allowing patients to display religious articles in their rooms is religious discrimination.

- Show respect for each person.
- Do not allow your feelings or beliefs to stand in the way of protecting the rights of those in your care. **See Figure 4-8.**

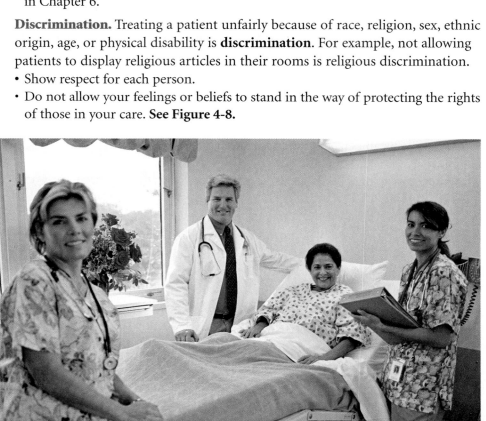

○ **Figure 4-8.** Treat all patients equally and with respect.

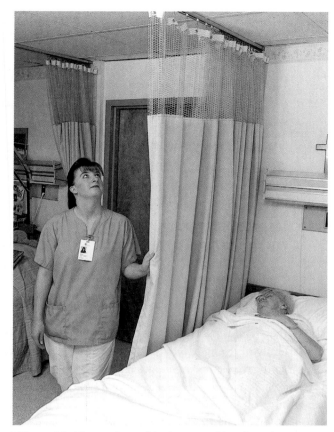

○ **Figure 4-9.** The nursing assistant can provide privacy for a patient by pulling the curtain around the bed area.

Invasion of Privacy. You should protect your patients from unwanted visitors. You should also provide privacy during any kind of procedure. Not providing this protection is a form of **invasion of privacy**. You should also keep information about the patient's treatment confidential. **Confidentiality** means keeping information about a patient private. It can be shared only with other health care team members. Specifically, you can do these things to protect a patient against invasion of privacy:

• Provide privacy to the patient during procedures. **See Figure 4-9.**

• Keep all information about the patient's condition, treatment, and all medical records confidential.

• Do not discuss the patient in public places within the facility, such as a lounge, or outside the facility.

• If visitors other than family or friends ask questions about the patient, suggest that they speak with the supervisor or nurse.

Harassment. You should also protect your patients from harassment. **Harassment** is troubling, tormenting, offending, or worrying a person by one's behavior or speech. Harassment can be sexual, or it can be based on discrimination or even simple dislike.

• If you see a patient being harassed, remove the source of harassment. For example, if another patient is picking on one of your patients, gently lead your patient away or politely ask the other patient to stop.

• In your personal conduct, stay away from jokes, pictures, or remarks that might offend other people.

Signs of Abuse
• Unexplained bruises, cuts, scratches, or swellings
• Unexplained burns or broken bones
• Poor personal hygiene, dirty clothes, no oral hygiene
• Bed sores
• Unexplained venereal disease or genital infections
• Weight loss or dehydration
• Limited movements
• Depression or withdrawal
• Agitation or anxiety
• Fear of being touched

○ **Figure 4-10.** Nursing assistants must learn to recognize signs of abuse so that they can report suspected abuse.

FOCUS ON

A Safe Working Environment

Just as patients have a right to be safe from abuse, nursing assistants have a right to a safe working environment. Some patients may become abusive toward you. If this happens, report it to your supervisor immediately. Respecting the patient's rights does not mean that you should accept abusive behavior.

Abuse. The willful mistreatment of someone is called **abuse**. *Physical abuse* is purposefully harming a patient's body. It can involve hitting, slapping, kicking, pinching, or depriving a patient of needed care. *Verbal abuse* is threatening or yelling at a patient. *Emotional abuse* involves threatening a patient or doing something you know will upset the patient. Unkind gestures are also abusive. *Sexual abuse* is harming a patient's body in a sexual way or performing sexual acts with a patient. It also includes sexual harassment and touching a patient on the breasts, buttocks, or genitals unnecessarily.

• Do not allow anyone to abuse your patients in any way.
• Many cases of abuse go unnoticed. Learn to recognize the signs of abuse. **See Figure 4-10.**
• You have a legal responsibility to report abuse to a supervisor, local social services department, or facility advocate if you see abuse or signs of abuse.
• In your own conduct, never treat a patient roughly. Avoid swearing at or teasing patients.

Unintentional Torts

An **unintentional tort** is the act of causing harm or injury to a person or property without meaning to. You must always be aware of what you are doing and be responsible for your actions.

Negligence. **Negligence** is the failure of a trained care provider to perform in a reasonable, careful manner and according to established standards, which results in harm. It means acting with neglect. Giving poor personal care and ignoring a patient are negligent acts.

• Perform all work and procedures conscientiously.
• Learn to recognize when someone in your care is being neglected by another health care team member. Follow the rules for reporting neglect.

Fact vs. Opinion

Occasionally, a resident makes a complaint regarding an intentional tort such as theft or abuse. When this happens, it becomes very important for everyone involved to be able to distinguish fact from opinion. A *fact* is anything that can be proved. For example, the statement "The blankets in this facility are blue" is a fact. *Opinion* is what people think about a subject or their interpretation of it. The statement "Blue blankets are pretty" is an opinion. Only facts can be used to decide lawsuits and resident complaints.

> **Practice**
>
> Mr. D'ha is accusing the nursing assistant on the night shift, Jesse Streeter, of abusing him physically. Read each of the following statements about this case and decide which involve facts and which are statements of opinion. Then make a two-column list. List the facts in one column and the opinions in the other. (Note: Some of the statements may have some elements of fact and some of opinion.)
>
> - Mr. D'ha: "Jesse doesn't like me."
> - Jesse Streeter: "Mr. D'ha needs help getting to the bathroom two or three times every night."
> - Mr. D'ha: "Look! You can see the bruises on my arms from where she handles me roughly!"
> - Jesse Streeter: "Mr. D'ha is taking Warfarin, a blood thinner that increases the possibility of bruising."
> - Mr. D'ha: "Jesse bruises me on purpose because she doesn't like having to help me to the bathroom so often."
> - Jesse Streeter: "Mr. D'ha is complaining just because he likes the attention it brings him."

Malpractice. Any act or conduct of a trained care provider that does not meet established standards or that goes beyond the provider's skill or scope of practice and results in harm is considered **malpractice**. Malpractice sometimes occurs as a result of negligence.
- Do only those things that you have been taught to do and that are within your scope of practice. No one can force you to perform a procedure that is beyond your training. In the view of the law, you are responsible for your own actions.
- Perform your work carefully.
- Tell the supervisor or nurse if you are asked to do something for which you are not trained.

Clear, Concise Writing

Patient charts and other paperwork are legal documents. It is your responsibility to write in a clear manner that cannot be misunderstood. Keep these rules in mind whenever you write:

- Stick to the subject. Do not "wander" onto other topics.
- Never use ten words if two words will do. Long, "flowery" sentences are more difficult to read and understand.
- Choose the right words. Use a dictionary or thesaurus if necessary to find exactly the right word. This is especially important in health care documents.

Practice

Telemedicine is a broad term that is used for health care facilities in different locations sharing information using telephones, video, off-site databases, and so on. As telemedicine has matured, it has raised many legal questions regarding liability, privacy, and malpractice. The paragraph shown below is a poorly written chart note about a resident's complaint regarding telemedicine practices. Analyze the paragraph and then rewrite it. Make your paragraph clear, precise, and easy to read and understand. Remove any information that does not belong. Use the vocabulary presented in this chapter whenever possible.

Patient: T. W. Simmon

Patient ID: 555-55-55

Admission: 8/10/20--

Date: *8/16/20--*   **Time:** *14:20*

Notes: *Mr. Simmons was agitated today. He claims they keep running tests on him but won't give him his test results. The nurses keep telling him he has to wait until the results are entered into a database that's kept way down in Atlanta somewhere. They have this telemedicine thing where everybody's results are stored in a single electronic database. Mr. Simmons has had several blood tests, an EKG, and I don't remember what else. He claims they took seven tubes of blood! Anyway, they keep putting him off about the results. He is accusing the staff at this facility of failing to perform their duties in a reasonable manner according to established standards. He believes he is suffering as a result. He says that yesterday he asked who all has access to his test results. You know what they told him? They said that every physician and therapist in all of the hospitals in the whole area have access to that database that contains his test results. That upset him even more because he believes that is a violation of his confidential information. I informed the nurse of this complaint.*

Protecting Yourself

After reading this chapter, it may seem to you that there are many legal pitfalls in being a nursing assistant, but that is not necessarily true. Health care facilities use **protocols** (specific rules for how to do tasks at a health care facility) to help protect all health care workers, including nursing assistants. Your first task when you accept a job at a health care facility is to become familiar with its protocols. By following facility protocol and staying within your scope of practice, you can enjoy your job without having to worry about legal issues.

The law itself helps protect you by requiring that you not perform certain tasks that are not within your scope of practice. These are some of the tasks you must not do:

Do Not Administer Medication. Nursing assistants are not allowed to give medication to patients. Some states even prohibit nursing assistants from feeding a client food that contains medicine. This is because giving medication is beyond the nursing assistant's training and scope of practice. Oxygen is treated as a form of medication. You may assist a patient in taking medicine by bringing the container and water to him or her, but you may never actually give medication.

Do Not Discuss a Patient's Diagnosis or Treatment. Patients have a right to privacy. You must not communicate any information you have to someone who is not on the staff. Patients' privacy rights include confidentiality regarding their illness, treatment, and wishes. It is the role of the doctor to discuss the patient's condition. Nurses can further clarify what a doctor has already told the patient or family member, but nursing assistants are not allowed to do so.

If family or friends pressure you for medical information, simply refer them to the licensed nurse or doctor. You can always comfort a patient in general terms, but never discuss actual personal or medical issues.

Do Not Diagnose a Patient. Nursing assistants are not trained to give a diagnosis. Even if a patient asks what you think, do not give an opinion. This includes questions about test results, what you think about a condition, or any similar question. Sometimes you may think your own family member has had the same condition, but you should not discuss this with the patient. No two people react the same way to the same condition. Often, one condition looks like another, but tests may prove that it is something entirely different. When a patient inquires about a diagnosis, be courteous and refer the patient to the doctor or nurse.

Do Not Prescribe Treatment or Medication. Only doctors can legally prescribe medications. Also, only a licensed medical doctor can prescribe certain courses of treatment.

Do Not Perform Sterile Procedures. Some procedures require the use of sterile technique. This means that everything that comes in contact with the patient's body must be free of microorganisms. This is particularly true in surgery, but it is also true in a number of other procedures, such as changing a sterile dressing.

As you work, most of these things will become second nature—you won't even have to think about them. If you follow these rules, along with facility protocols, you will be well on your way to a fun, rewarding career as a nursing assistant.

4 Review

Chapter Summary

- State and federal laws protect the legal rights of patients and residents.

- The Patient's Bill of Rights protects the legal rights of patients in hospitals.

- Residents' Rights protect the legal rights of residents in long-term care facilities and clients in home care.

- Nursing assistants, like all health care professionals, must follow ethical standards and rules of conduct to protect the people in their care.

- Nursing assistants must protect the people in their care from violations of the law that can harm them.

- Negligence and malpractice are acts that unintentionally or intentionally harm patients.

VOCABULARY REVIEW

Directions: Match the letter of each definition in the second column with the correct vocabulary term in the first column. Write your answers on a separate sheet of paper.

Vocabulary

1. abuse
2. assault
3. battery
4. coercion
5. confidentiality
6. exploitation
7. harassment
8. health care proxy
9. informed consent
10. intentional tort
11. liability
12. living will
13. malpractice
14. unintentional tort

Definitions

A. Keeping information about a patient private
B. Taking advantage of someone
C. A legal document appointing someone, often a friend or family member, to make health care decisions on a patient's behalf
D. A legal document stating how a person wishes to be treated in the event of serious or catastrophic illness
E. A patient's understanding and agreement to an action or procedure that has been explained
F. The attempt or threat to touch another person's body without the person's consent
G. The act of causing harm or injury to a person or property on purpose
H. Touching another person's body without the person's consent
I. Legal responsibility for what someone does or fails to do
J. The act or conduct of a trained care provider that does not meet established standards or that goes beyond the provider's skill or scope of practice and results in harm
K. An attempt to force someone to do something against his or her will
L. The willful mistreatment of someone
M. The act of causing harm or injury to a person or property without meaning to
N. Troubling, tormenting, offending, or worrying a person by one's behavior or speech

Check Your Knowledge

Review Questions: Answer each of the following questions on a separate sheet of paper.

1. List five of the rights in the Patient's Bill of Rights.

2. How can an ombudsman help a resident of a long-term care facility?

3. If you see another nursing assistant harm a patient, what should you do?

4. What is theft?

5. Describe two types of unlawful restraint.

6. Give an example of discrimination against a patient.

7. What is harassment?

8. List four signs of abuse.

9. What is an advance directive?

10. How can you help protect people in your care from malpractice?

True or False: Read each statement carefully. Then write *True* or *False* by the statement number on a separate sheet of paper.

1. Residents' Rights were developed by the federal government as part of OBRA 87 regulations.

2. An ombudsman cannot help a resident of a long-term care facility take legal action.

3. Nursing assistants can be charged with a crime if they threaten to touch a patient without the patient's informed consent.

4. Locking a patient in a room is invasion of privacy.

5. Making fun of a patient is emotional abuse.

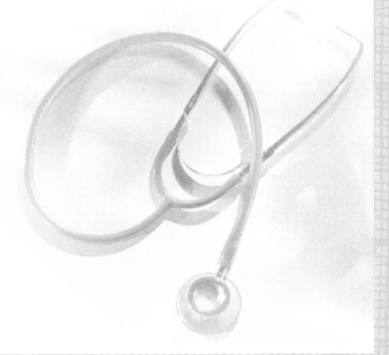

Think and Decide

Directions: Think about each of the following scenarios. Answer each question on a separate sheet of paper.

1. Mrs. Tyler is admitted to a long-term care facility. She is given paperwork, including the Residents' Rights. After Mrs. Tyler is settled in her new room, the nursing assistant caring for her assists her to the bathroom. The nursing assistant leaves and does not shut the door or draw the curtain to provide a barrier. What right is being violated?

2. Amy is a nursing assistant who is taking care of Mrs. Olson. After getting Mrs. Olson ready for lunch and taking her to the dining room, she returns to Mrs. Olson's room. Amy makes the bed and straightens the room. Later, on her own lunch break, Amy confides to her best friend Jan that she has found the perfect birthday present for her nephew: a Beanie Baby that she found on Mrs. Olson's night stand. Amy says she removed the Beanie Baby and put it in her locker. She will take it home after her shift. Which kind of law is broken by removing the Beanie Baby? What are the consequences? What should Jan do?

3. Mr. Jones has his call light on. It has been on for more than 30 minutes. It goes unanswered. Mr. Jones gets up and tries to go to the bathroom. When the nursing assistant arrives 10 minutes later, she discovers that he has fallen and broken his left hip. What legal term defines what happened to Mr. Jones? What must the nursing assistant do now?

4. Mrs. Lopez is a long-term care resident who has been under your care for several months now. One day, her son takes you aside privately and hands you a $20 bill. He says, "Here is a little gift for you for being so kind to my mother." How would you handle this situation?

5. You are a nursing assistant working the day shift at Whitefield Nursing Home. You have been caring for Mr. Lee since his admission three weeks ago. This morning, his daughter, Kwan Lee, approaches you with a deep concern about the care her father is receiving. What should you do?

6. Mrs. Smith keeps getting out of her wheelchair. She is at risk for falls. The nursing assistant caring for her on this shift is Sue Ann. Sue Ann reminds her repeatedly not to get out of the chair without assistance, but Mrs. Smith keeps getting up anyway. Sue Ann is very concerned that Mrs. Smith will fall and be hurt. However, she cannot remain in the room with Mrs. Smith because she has other residents to see to also. At her wit's end, Sue Ann finally gets a restraint and ties it around Mrs. Smith's waist and then to the wheelchair. What would you have done if you were in this situation? Use problem-solving techniques to solve the problem without violating Mrs. Smith's rights. Identify the problem, brainstorm possible solutions, choose the best solution to the problem, and implement the solution.

CNA Certification Exam Prep

Directions: This practice test contains ten questions. Each question has four suggested answers. For each question, choose the ONE that best answers the question or completes the statement. Write your answers on a separate sheet of paper.

1. A resident gives the nursing assistant $50 as a thank-you for her work. The nursing assistant should
   A. take the money and purchase something for the unit.
   B. politely refuse the money.
   C. ask the nurse in charge what to do.
   D. take the money with appropriate thanks.

2. Mr. Jolsen, a resident in your care, has a terminal illness. The legal document used to appoint a family member to make health care decisions for him if he becomes unable to make these decisions is called a
   A. living will.
   B. legal rights document.
   C. health care proxy.
   D. legal issues document.

3. Residents have the right to
   A. smoke in any area of a nursing home facility.
   B. have access to a telephone.
   C. look at other residents' medical charts.
   D. go anywhere in the facility.

4. Harming a person's reputation by writing untrue things is called
   A. slander.
   B. libel.
   C. battery.
   D. invasion of privacy.

5. After caring for a resident, which of the following items should the nursing assistant make sure is within the resident's reach?
   A. intercom
   B. light
   C. call light
   D. terminal

6. A nursing assistant bathes a paralyzed patient without first obtaining the patient's consent. This is considered
   A. negligence.
   B. malpractice.
   C. battery.
   D. invasion of privacy.

7. All of the following are examples of abuse or neglect **except**
   A. leaving a resident in a wet, soiled bed.
   B. leaving a resident alone in a bathtub.
   C. restraining a resident according to a physician's order.
   D. threatening to withhold a resident's meal.

8. To best communicate with a resident who is totally deaf, the nursing assistant should
   A. avoid eye contact.
   B. write out information.
   C. smile and talk fast.
   D. smile and talk loudly.

9. A resident refuses to wear a clothing protector at dinner. The nursing assistant should
   A. put it on the resident anyway.
   B. respect the resident's wishes.
   C. tell the resident she has to wear it.
   D. report the resident's wishes to the charge nurse.

10. When a patient is scheduled to have an invasive procedure, what must the health care professional obtain from the patient?
    A. restraint order
    B. privacy statement
    C. living will
    D. informed consent

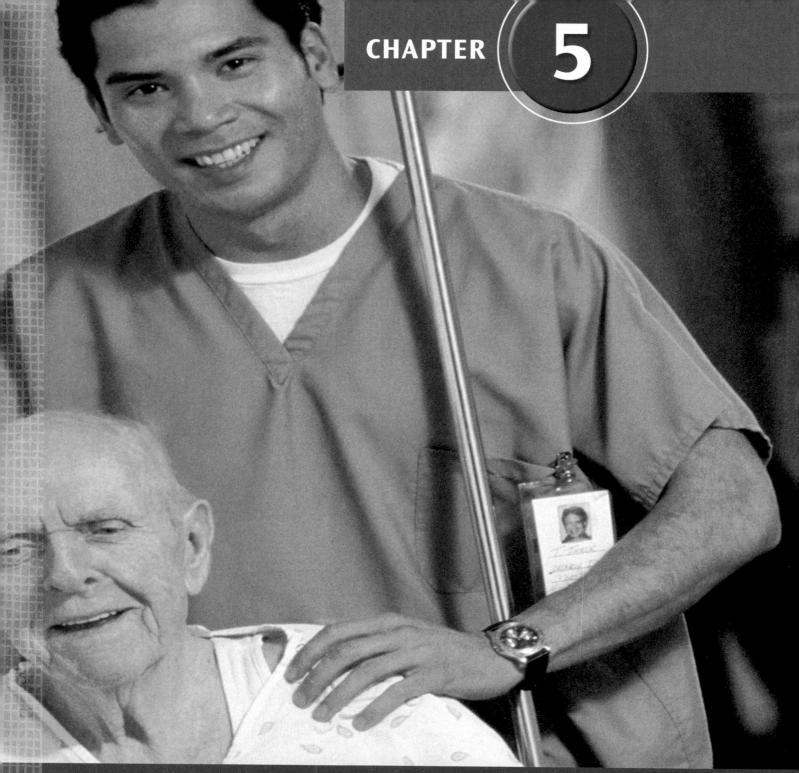

CHAPTER 5

OBJECTIVES

- Identify the basic needs that all people have.
- Explain ways to meet patients' physical, security, social, and esteem needs.

- Recognize psychological reactions to illness.
- Discuss the importance of valuing diversity among patients.

- Explain how to respond appropriately to visitors.

Patient Needs

activities of daily living (ADLs) The physical tasks necessary to maintain oneself. They include eating, self-care, grooming, dressing, and mobility.

culture The accumulation of customs, values, and beliefs shared by a people.

defense mechanisms Unconscious ways of protecting oneself from bad feelings such as shame, anxiety, fear, or loss of self-esteem.

emotional well-being A state of feeling contented and happy.

esteem needs Those needs that must be met to have a feeling of self-worth.

health A state of complete physical, mental, emotional, and social well-being.

illness Sickness, disease, or ailment.

need Anything that is necessary to maintain life and well-being.

physical needs The basic human needs for oxygen, food, water, sleep, elimination, and shelter.

security needs The group of needs that, when met, make one feel safe.

self-actualization needs The psychological needs that, when met, enable a person to reach his or her highest potential.

social needs The group of needs that, when met, make a person feel accepted and loved.

social well-being A feeling of being able to form and maintain relationships with family and friends.

Basic Human Needs

All people have basic physical and psychological needs. A **need** is anything that is necessary to maintain life and well-being. Basic needs must be met for a person to keep well physically, socially, psychologically, spiritually, and emotionally.

Abraham Maslow, a psychologist, organized basic human needs into five levels. The levels are ranked in a *hierarchy* according to their importance. **See Figure 5-1.** According to Maslow, lower level needs must be met before higher level needs can be met.

Physical Needs

At the first level are **physical needs**. These are the needs for oxygen, food, water, sleep, elimination, and shelter. Until these needs are met, it is difficult for a person to think of anything else. We tend to take meeting physical needs for granted. Most of us have enough food and water, and we can breathe freely and sleep regularly. Remember, though, that when these basic needs are *not* met, life itself may be threatened. For example, not getting enough sleep can make driving a car unsafe. Not getting enough sleep when you are ill can slow the body's healing process.

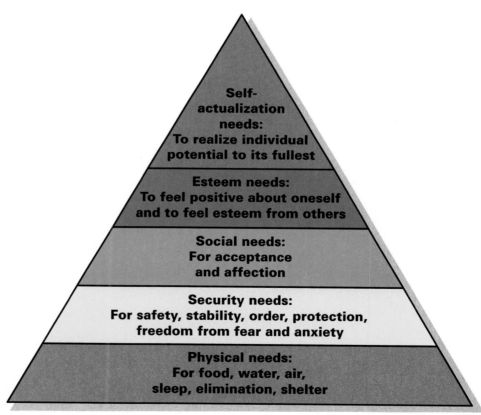

○ **Figure 5-1. Maslow's hierarchy of needs.**

Security Needs

The second level covers **security needs**. They include safety, stability, order, protection, and freedom from fear and anxiety. People need to feel *secure*—to feel that they have enough resources and that they are safe. A small child may feel secure when being held. An adult may feel secure by having enough savings for future needs. A hospital patient may feel secure after an upcoming procedure is explained. A long-term care resident may feel secure when the environment is clean and safe. **See Figure 5-2.**

Social Needs

The group of needs that, when met, make a person feel accepted and loved are called **social needs**. Whether in a formal group, such as with coworkers, or in a family setting, meaningful relationships with others are vital.

Esteem Needs

At the fourth level are **esteem needs**—those that must be met to have a feeling of self-worth. People need to feel good about themselves, to feel useful, and to be respected by others. Children need praise from their families and teachers. Adolescents want to be admired by their peer group. Adults need recognition from others about their success at work and in family life.

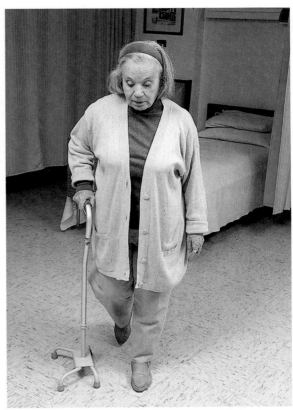

O **Figure 5-2.** The nursing assistant keeps the environment free of obstacles to help meet the patient's security needs.

Self-Actualization Needs

At the highest level are **self-actualization needs**. These are the psychological needs that, when met, enable a person to reach his or her highest potential. Most people try to learn and grow throughout their lives. At this level, people are creative. They are confident and want to help others. Generally, all of the other basic needs must be met before a person can meet these needs.

Meeting Patient Needs

Health is a state of physical, mental, emotional, and social well-being. People in good health have bodies that function properly to eat and digest food, eliminate wastes, use the senses, think, feel, move, sleep, rest, breathe, and defend against disease. Healthy people have a sense of **emotional well-being**, which is a state of feeling contented and happy. They have a sense of **social well-being**, which is a feeling of being able to form and maintain relationships with family and friends. They can cope with stresses and problems. They can make reasonable decisions about their lives.

Vital Skills READING

Make Personal Connections

It is often easier to understand and remember what you read if you make personal connections while you read. For example, you might be reading about something that reminds you of a vacation you took last summer. Should you push the thought of vacation out of your mind so that you can read the article? Not necessarily.

Instead, take a few moments to remember the vacation and think about how it connects with the article. Why did the article make you think of that particular vacation? You won't want to spend hours daydreaming, of course. However, taking a little time to make connections between what you read and your personal experiences can be very helpful. You may find that you remember more clearly both the vacation and the article you have read.

Practice

Search through the local newspaper or on the Internet to find a public interest article about someone whose social needs have been met in some way. Take the time to make personal connections: Does it remind you of an experience you have had in the past, or something a friend has experienced?

Put the article away for a week. Then, without looking at the article, try to remember what it was about. Write down the key points you remember. Then look at the article to see how well you remembered the content. Did making personal connections help you remember the article?

Illness is sickness, disease, or ailment. Patients' illnesses cover a wide range. Patients can be ill in different ways, too. For instance, a mentally ill patient may be physically strong but unable to make good decisions about what to eat or how to behave.

People suffering from illnesses have the same basic needs as everyone else. As a nursing assistant, you can help patients meet these needs by making them feel relaxed, comfortable, and safe in the health care facility. You can show a caring attitude for each patient by being eager to help and by behaving ethically and with courtesy. This includes:

- Maintaining the patient's privacy.
- Knocking before you enter the room.
- Introducing yourself.
- Explaining what you are going to do.
- Encouraging the patient to be part of the decision-making process when possible.

Meeting Physical Needs

People who are ill may not be able to meet some or all of their physical needs. For example, some patients may need help with the **activities of daily living (ADLs)**. These are the physical tasks necessary to maintain oneself. They include everyday routines, such as eating, bathing, dressing, grooming, bowel and bladder elimination, and movement. **See Figure 5-3.**

Some patients need just a little help with these activities, such as assistance steadying a fork as they eat. Other patients depend on you for all of their personal care and grooming needs. As a nursing assistant, you help meet each patient's physical needs. You provide assistance with breathing, receiving nutrition, elimination, sleep, and physical movement. There are procedures and ways to help patients in every type of situation.

Oxygen. Some patients have difficulty breathing for a number of reasons. This condition is serious, because death can follow in minutes when a person is deprived of air. Breathing may be improved by adjusting the patient's position in the hospital bed. In other cases, oxygen—the part of the air that we must breathe in to live—must be ordered by a doctor and supplied carefully.

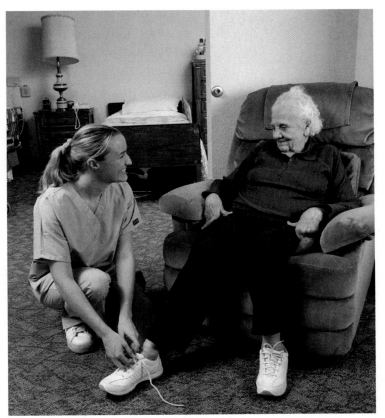

○ **Figure 5-3.** Nursing assistants help patients with activities of daily living (ADLs) to meet their physical needs.

Vital Skills WRITING

Creative Writing

Self-actualization activities are the "fun" activities. They are the ones you can only get to after all of your other needs have been met. You can express your own feelings and try new things. One possible way to express yourself is to use *creative writing*. In creative writing, you can choose your own topic and decide what you want to say about it. You can even decide what form it should take. Will you write a story, perhaps? A factual report? A poem?

Practice

Writing creatively requires that you think creatively—and that takes a little practice. For this activity, let's say you want to create something for children who are in the hospital for the first time. You want to set their minds at ease about their surroundings and make them feel safe and secure.

Use your imagination and any experience you may have with children. What format should you use? Would a "pretend" story be best? Should you include pictures? Plan your creative writing carefully. First, write a few sentences to outline your topic and what you will say about it. Then develop the project using as much creativity as possible. Be prepared to read and/or show the finished activity to the class.

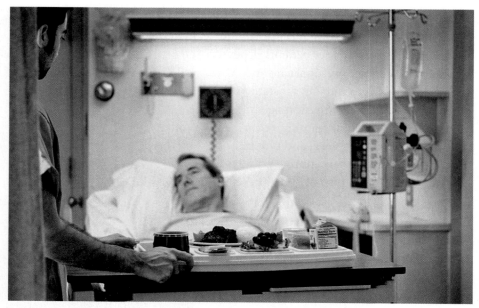

○ **Figure 5-4.** The nursing assistant serves food to a bedridden patient to help meet his need for proper nutrition.

Water and Food. We need water almost as much as we need oxygen to survive. Water is supplied to the body in both fluids and foods. To avoid *dehydration* (a dangerous lack of fluid in the body), a proper amount of water must be consumed every day. When the weather is warm or a patient has fever or illness, the need for water is greater. The basic minimum daily water requirement to survive is 1500 cubic centimeters (cc). The ideal amount is 2000 to 2500 cc.

However, certain chronic illnesses, such as kidney failure and congestive heart failure, cause patients to retain fluid abnormally. (See Chapter 26, "Nutrition.") In these cases, a fluid restriction and 24-hour intake monitoring may be ordered.

As a nursing assistant, you will assist patients in receiving proper nutrition. You will give patients a chance to prepare for mealtimes by washing their hands and face. To make mealtimes more pleasant and food more appealing, you can remove unneeded equipment and close bathroom doors. Make the patient comfortable in the bed or chair. Serving food at the proper temperature will avoid burns or difficulty in eating. **See Figure 5-4.**

Some patients may need your help to eat, or may need to be prompted to eat. Some may be on special diets. Others cannot eat food by mouth and must be nourished using different methods. A tube through the nose to the stomach may be used. Fluids may be replaced through a tube into the veins.

Elimination. Elimination must function properly to rid the body of liquid and solid wastes. You may assist in the elimination of wastes from the patient's body in a number of ways. Bathing the patient removes perspiration and helps keep skin healthy. Patients may need help moving to and from the bathroom. For those who cannot use the toilet, you may provide commodes, bedpans, urinals, or other aids. Other procedures, such as enemas, may need to be used in some cases to remove wastes. In all these activities, respect the patient's right to privacy. Always remember the person's dignity.

Sleep. Adequate rest is critical for recovery and well-being. Noise or pain may keep patients from sleeping. You can help control the environment by lowering your voice, keeping the light in the patient's room low, and moving quietly. You

Vital Skills MATH

Calculating Distance

Mr. Estevez has been admitted to a rehabilitation hospital. A stroke has left him unable to walk without assistance. His goal is to regain the ability to walk enough so that he can return home.

You will be caring for Mr. Estevez. The rehabilitation team tells you to record on the flow sheet the number of feet Mr. Estevez is able to walk every day. When Mr. Estevez meets his goal, a total of 800 feet, he may return home.

Practice

On a separate sheet of paper, total the figures in the flow sheet in Figure A to determine if Mr. Estevez has met his goal at the end of four weeks.

1. Add the figures for days 1 through 7 for each week.
2. Add the daily totals for weeks 1 through 4 to find the total number of feet Mr. Estevez has walked.
3. Has Mr. Estevez achieved his goal? What other information might need to be taken into account?

○ Figure A

	Week 1	Week 2	Week 3	Week 4
Day 1	10 feet	20 feet	32 feet	20 feet
Day 2	15 feet	28 feet	28 feet	26 feet
Day 3	15 feet	20 feet	30 feet	30 feet
Day 4	22 feet	26 feet	30 feet	28 feet
Day 5	18 feet	30 feet	36 feet	18 feet
Day 6	24 feet	18 feet	38 feet	23 feet
Day 7	15 feet	24 feet	32 feet	22 feet
Totals	___?___ Feet	___?___ Feet	___?___ Feet	___?___ Feet

can calm a restless patient with a soothing back rub, soft music, or quietly listening to the patient's conversation. Medication should be used as a last resort. The type of medication, dosage, and frequency of medication can be ordered only by a doctor.

Physical Movement. Healthy people may take physical movement for granted. Patients with restricted mobility, however, have special problems meeting their basic needs. For example, bedridden patients are subject to a number of problems. They lose muscle tone and strength. They may develop blood clots, muscle spasms, or skin problems. Patients may lose their appetites or become unable to eliminate wastes. Difficulty in breathing is common. Bones may weaken and become brittle because of a loss of calcium.

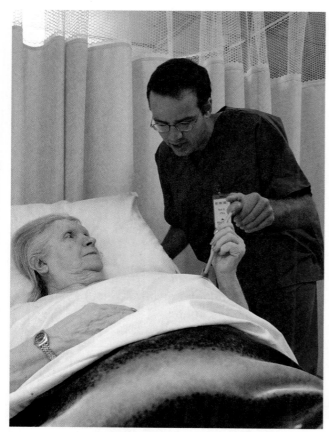

○ **Figure 5-5.** The nursing assistant places the call light within the patient's reach for safety and to help relieve the patient's anxiety.

If patients are able to move around by themselves, encourage regular activities. When patients need help standing, walking, or getting in or out of bed, you may provide help. If patients cannot move at all without assistance, follow procedures to help avoid the types of problems bedridden people are likely to have. For example, bathing, applying lotion, and changing the patient's position help avoid skin problems. In other cases, you will learn how to turn and reposition a person in bed. You will help patients with other movements to prevent loss of mobility and physical injury.

Meeting Security Needs

Part of making patients feel secure is keeping them safe and warm. You should always follow safety precautions. The patient's bed or room should be safe, and side rails should be up when needed. Patients should know how to get help when needed. The call signal must be within easy reach. The room should be kept uncluttered to avoid hazards. Also, patients feel more secure when they understand what is going on around them. It is important to take time to explain a procedure to the patient. Communication is the key to meeting most security needs. **See Figure 5-5.**

If you are working on a pediatric ward, you will be caring for children and their families. It may be hard sometimes to understand children's needs. Keep in mind that parents can often help explain their children's needs. Children may be fearful when they are away from home and in a strange place. Their parents' presence can calm their fears. For these reasons, parents are commonly asked to visit and to stay overnight with their children.

Meeting Social and Esteem Needs

Helping meet patients' needs for a sense of belonging, love, human contact, and self-esteem is extremely important. Healthy people are used to thinking of themselves as competent, active adults in charge of their lives. Entering a health care facility or having an illness can make people feel dependent and lose their self-esteem.

Aging can bring severe blows to self-esteem—loss of physical control, lessening of mental acuity, and changes in life situations. Nursing assistants can bolster the self-esteem of ailing or aging patients by treating them with respect and trying to get them to recount their experiences. Many people who work with the elderly find listening to their life stories enriching and intellectually stimulating.

Illness may cause *psychological reactions*. This means that a patient might react to the illness in ways that are not directly caused by the illness itself. At times, patients may feel helpless because they are too weak or ill to take care of themselves. They may be in pain. They may worry about hospital bills, caring for their family, or being dependent on others. Patients may be concerned about their illness, disability, or death. They may become frightened or sad. **See Figure 5-6.**

Some people react by using defense mechanisms. **Defense mechanisms** are unconscious ways of protecting oneself from bad feelings such as shame, anxiety, fear, or loss of self-esteem. Some defense mechanisms are anger, denial, sadness, withdrawal, and depression.

For example, sometimes anger is the patient's defense mechanism, and you are the closest target. The angry patient may find fault with whatever you do. It may be difficult to avoid taking the criticism personally. Try to understand the patient's feelings and to realize that the anger is the real cause, not your actions. Remember that the patient may not realize the underlying reasons for the anger. Show an understanding of the stresses on patients by offering emotional support. Think about how you might feel in a similar situation so that you can have empathy for the patient, family, and friends. Be a good listener, even when the patient is angry. Treat the patient as an individual who needs your help.

Some illnesses are *chronic* (long-term). Chronic illnesses can make a patient feel very discouraged. Act in ways that give patients a sense of independence. Encourage their attempts to do as much for themselves as they are able. Be patient and do not rush patients who are attempting to keep control over their own lives. Always treat patients with dignity and respect.

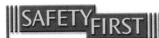

SAFETY FIRST

If a patient becomes disruptive or violent, remain calm and speak quietly to the patient. Try to keep the patient—and other patients—safe. Do not question or argue with the person, but instead show understanding. Call for help if you cannot help the person bring his or her behavior under control or if your own safety is at risk.

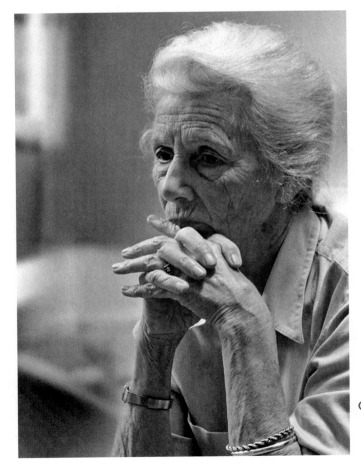

○ **Figure 5-6.** Patients may feel worried, frightened, or sad. Nursing assistants can reach out to them to provide emotional support.

Religious Practices

Religion relates to a person's spiritual beliefs, needs, and practices. Like culture, a person's religion influences health and illness practices. In some religions, people use rituals for healing, support, or comfort during illness. Some may want to pray and observe certain religious practices. Always be respectful of these practices even if they differ from your own. If a member of the clergy visits the patient, make sure the room is orderly. Provide a chair and make sure that there is privacy.

The need for human touch is important, too. Children need to be held and touched by their caregivers. As people grow older, touching may be reserved for close family or friends, but their contact is often not available to them in health care facilities. A friendly hug and smile from a nursing assistant, or a pat on the back, can help reduce loneliness. *Always ask first* if you can hug or touch a patient.

Encourage patients who feel lonely to get involved with others. Many health care facilities provide social activities so that patients can get to know each other. **See Figure 5-7.** Patients who feel alone or isolated from others may need extra attention, such as:

- Asking how they feel.
- Listening to their concerns and fears.
- Laughing together about something.
- Being nonjudgmental.

Valuing Diversity

Each patient has a unique cultural background. **Culture** is the accumulation of customs, values, and beliefs shared by a people. For example, the Native American culture has its own set of rituals, stories, beliefs, and items held in high regard, such as special headgear made of feathers or beadwork. As a nursing assistant, you will help care for people from different countries, ethnic backgrounds, and religions. **See Figure 5-8.**

A patient's culture often affects his or her beliefs, practices, and behavior concerning health and treatment. These beliefs, traditions, and values may be different from yours. For example, some cultures believe in the practice of "folk medicine." The patient's family or friends may wish to bring a healer to see the patient.

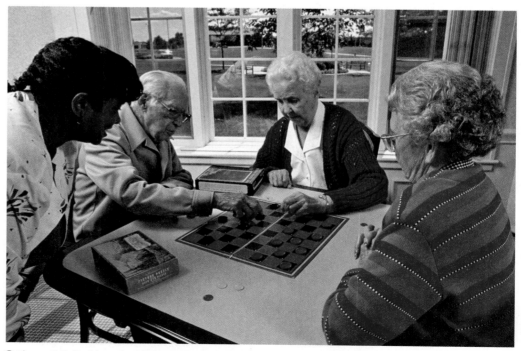

○ **Figure 5-7.** Residents in this long-term care facility enjoy social activities. These opportunities to socialize reduce feelings of loneliness and help meet the residents' social needs.

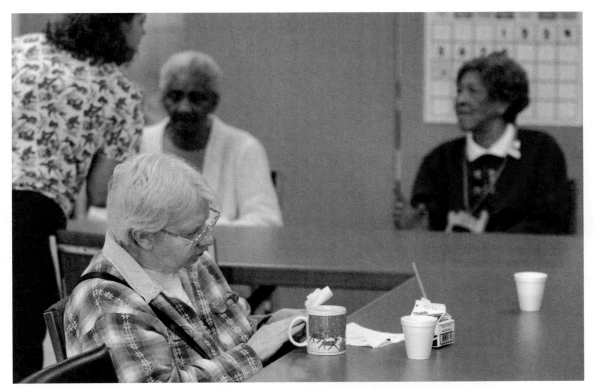

O **Figure 5-8.** Nursing assistants care for people from many different cultures and social backgrounds.

These differences in customs can seem strange to you, but you must learn to respect them. Be tolerant and accept patients as they are. Understand your own feelings and how they may affect patients. For example, think about your own views of what defines good medical care. You may think that people should never refuse medical care under any circumstances. However, others may think differently on this point.

Remember that your job is to help make the patient comfortable. Learn about religions and customs that differ from your own. For example, in some cultures, it is embarrassing for people to have their legs, head, or arms uncovered when strangers are present. Some cultures prohibit various foods. By trying to understand differences, you can help protect each patient's sense of privacy and meet his or her individual needs.

Interacting with Visitors

Patients' families and friends are also part of patient care. They are concerned about their loved ones in a health care facility. Their visits are important emotionally to patients and can help them cope with their illness or condition. Visitors sometimes help provide support and care for the patient. For example, they may help with grooming. **See Figure 5-9.** It is important for you to be helpful and sensitive to their needs, as long as they do not interfere with your patient's needs or medical treatment.

Family and friends should have privacy during visits. **See Figure 5-10.** If you must give the patient care during a visit, treat the visitors with courtesy. Ask the visitors to wait outside the patient's area and let them know when they can return.

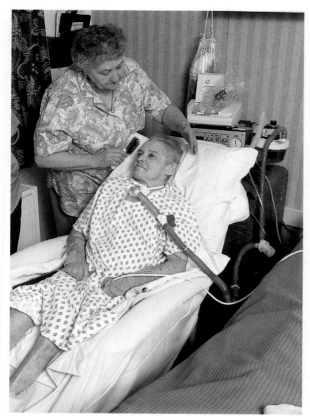

○ **Figure 5-9. This patient's sister visits daily and helps her with grooming.**

Keeping Visitors Informed

Learn the rules about visiting in your health care facility. Visitors often ask questions about scheduled hours and which family members can visit. Some facilities restrict visits to adults. Others also permit children to visit. Be prepared to tell visitors about other areas of the facility, such as the cafeteria or gift shop. Let them know where and when they can make telephone calls. When visiting hours are over, courteously inform visitors that it is time to leave.

Responding to Challenging Visitors

Sometimes visitors are demanding and anxious. They may have psychological reactions to their loved one's illness. Some visitors are depressed or feel guilty about the patient's condition. Others are angry and want to blame someone—the doctor, the hospital, or perhaps the nursing assistant. Communicate with visitors with courtesy, empathy, tact, and emotional control.

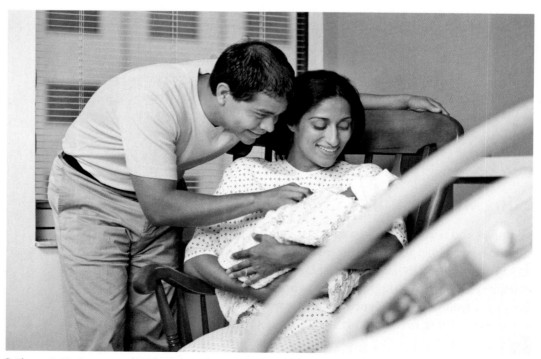

○ **Figure 5-10. Respect patients' privacy when they visit with family and friends.**

Vital Skills (COMMUNICATION)

Language Barriers

Occasionally, you may need to work with patients who either do not speak English at all or speak it poorly. This presents a language barrier that affects the way you work with the patient. It can also be frustrating for you as you try to complete your duties.

If the health care facility does not have a translator, you may have to rely on family members to translate for you. You should also learn to adapt. For example, you can point to objects, write notes, and listen to what the person calls each object. Make a storyboard of pictures of common words. Ask questions of family and friends. In fact, you can turn the situation into a positive one in which you begin to learn a new language. Communicate with the person both verbally and nonverbally.

As you work with patients who have trouble understanding you, be sure to demonstrate patience and understanding. Remember that if they do not understand what you say, your use of positive body language is critical.

Practice

In teams of two, practice overcoming language barriers. One student should pretend to be a resident who does not understand English. The other should play a nursing assistant trying to communicate with the resident. Try to communicate the following ideas:

- It's a beautiful day. Would you like to go for a walk outside?
- It's time for dinner. May I help you into your wheelchair?
- Would you like to brush your teeth?

Be alert for visitors who seem to tire or upset the patient. Report these situations to your supervisor. Remember to listen courteously to visitors' remarks, even when they complain. If you are accused of treating the patient poorly, respond by saying, "I understand that you are upset." Report these situations to your supervisor, but do not become involved in the family's disagreements. It is important to keep your own thoughts or opinions about patients and visitors to yourself. Always show respect for the family's feelings. Remember that they are dealing with a difficult situation.

Working with Families at Home

Home health aides may interact in other ways with family members. You may care for an elderly parent of adults who work all day. When your shift ends, you will need to give a full progress report. The person you care for may become sad and feel helpless and a burden to his or her children. On the other hand, the adult children may feel they are letting their parent down for not being there all the time. Be a good listener and offer emotional support to both. Do not, however, become involved in family difficulties.

Chapter Summary

- All people have the same basic physical, security, social, esteem, and self-actualization needs.

- Nursing assistants help meet patients' physical, security, social, and esteem needs.

- Nursing assistants can help patients by recognizing their psychological reactions to illness and loss.

- Valuing diversity among patients means respecting their differences and treating them fairly and equally.

- Interacting with visitors includes respecting their concerns while protecting the patient's needs.

VOCABULARY REVIEW

Directions: Match the letter of each definition in the second column with the correct vocabulary term in the first column. Write your answers on a separate sheet of paper.

Vocabulary

1. activities of daily living (ADLs)
2. defense mechanisms
3. emotional well-being
4. esteem needs
5. health
6. physical needs
7. security needs
8. self-actualization needs
9. social needs
10. social well-being

Definitions

A. Unconscious ways of protecting the self from bad feelings, such as shame, anxiety, fear, or loss of self-esteem.

B. A state of complete physical, mental, emotional, and social well-being.

C. The basic human needs for oxygen, food, water, sleep, elimination, and shelter.

D. The group of needs that, when met, make one feel safe.

E. The group of needs that, when met, make a person feel accepted and loved.

F. The psychological needs that, when met, enable a person to reach his or her highest potential.

G. Those needs that must be met to have a feeling of self-worth.

H. The physical tasks necessary to maintain oneself.

I. A feeling of being able to form and maintain relationships with family and friends.

J. A state of feeling contented and happy.

Check Your Knowledge

Review Questions: Answer each of the following questions on a separate sheet of paper.

1. What is a need?

2. List the basic human needs according to Maslow's hierarchy of needs.

3. List four security needs.

4. What are the five physical needs that nursing assistants help patients meet?

5. How can a nursing assistant help meet a patient's security needs?

6. What are some defense mechanisms that nursing assistants should be aware of?

7. How can you provide extra attention to patients who seem lonely and withdrawn?

8. What is culture?

9. What should you do if you need to provide care to a patient who has visitors?

10. If you notice that a certain visitor tires or upsets your patient, what should you do?

True or False: Read each statement carefully. Then write *True* or *False* by the statement number on a separate sheet of paper.

1. There is a wide range between complete health and illness.

2. People who are ill do not have the same basic needs as healthy people.

3. Thinking about the stresses that patients might have helps you understand their psychological reactions.

4. Respecting a patient's traditions is a way of valuing diversity.

5. It is correct to argue with an angry or disruptive visitor.

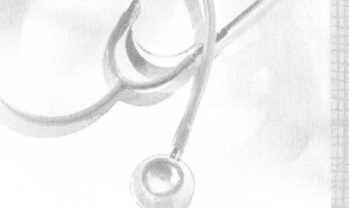

Think and Decide

Directions: Think about each of the following scenarios. Answer each question on a separate sheet of paper.

1. You are making rounds and you come upon Mr. Caine's room. He is sitting in a chair. He is looking out the window with tears coming down his face. How would you approach Mr. Caine?

2. Mrs. Scott is an 81-year-old resident. Usually, she looks forward to Tuesday mornings because she enjoys participating in the pottery class. This morning, as you wheel her to the common area for the class, you notice that she is lacking her usual enthusiasm. She doesn't appear to be depressed, but she looks ready to fall asleep. What, if anything, should you do?

3. Molly Schwartz is expected to be in Pace Convalescent Center for another three to four weeks while she recovers from a broken hip. Several times when you have entered her room, you have found her looking sad. When you ask if anything is wrong, she explains. Passover, a Jewish holiday with dietary restrictions, starts next week. She doesn't want to cause problems, but she would really like to observe Passover in the traditional manner. She has no local family or friends. What can you do to help her?

4. Mr. Benedetto is a new resident at the long-term care facility who speaks very little English. Mr. Gardener has been a resident at the facility for almost a year. As you push Mr. Benedetto's wheelchair past Mr. Gardener's room, Mr. Gardener starts shouting insults at Mr. Benedetto, Italians, and foreigners in general. What should you do?

5. Anne Sherman is an elderly hospital patient who underwent triple cardiac bypass surgery a week ago. She wants to go home. Her physician says she can go home when she succeeds in walking the length of the surgical ward twice a day, with assistance. You are to help her walk as far as possible once during each shift. For the first few days, she is eager to walk, even though she is obviously in pain and doesn't get very far. Then she begins to make excuses not to walk. Each time you approach her, she has a different excuse. She is too tired, or she is dizzy, or she is expecting visitors. What should you do?

6. At the local hospital, volunteers regularly visit patient rooms to talk with patients and try to cheer them up or interest them in activities such as puzzles and games. Jill is a 16-year-old who was involved in a car accident and has several broken bones. Today a volunteer comes to visit Jill. Jill reacts angrily and rudely, telling the volunteer to leave immediately and not come back with "those silly games." What, if anything, should you do?

7. Ben is a five-year-old who has been admitted to the pediatric ward after a severe asthma attack. While his father is at the hospital with him, Ben seems fine. Then his father leaves, promising to come back in a few hours. As soon as the father leaves, Ben becomes very upset. He won't stop crying, and he is starting to wheeze again. What should you do?

CNA Certification Exam Prep

Directions: This practice test contains ten questions. Each question has four suggested answers. For each question, choose the ONE that best answers the question or completes the statement. Write your answers on a separate sheet of paper.

1. Which of the following is **not** a basic human need?
   - A. security needs
   - B. esteem needs
   - C. social needs
   - D. property needs

2. Which of the following is a physical need of patients?
   - A. activities
   - B. food
   - C. friendship
   - D. security

3. As a nursing assistant, which of the following measures can you take to provide patient safety?
   - A. ensure that side rails are up as needed
   - B. spend time talking with the patient
   - C. give medicine for pain as needed
   - D. lock the patient's door when you leave

4. What populations are most often provided care in a long-term care facility?
   - A. geriatric population (over 65)
   - B. pediatric population (under 18)
   - C. middle-aged population (19 to 64)
   - D. pediatric and middle-aged populations

5. Which of the following is an example of a defense mechanism?
   - A. sadness
   - B. fear
   - C. denial
   - D. shame

6. What can a nursing assistant do to assist a patient who is having trouble breathing?
   - A. administer oxygen
   - B. adjust the patient's position in bed
   - C. encourage the person to walk around
   - D. offer water to prevent dehydration

7. You should understand cultural beliefs, practices, and behaviors so that you can
   - A. explain to patients how they must change their behaviors.
   - B. identify and respect your patient's needs.
   - C. warn visitors not to bring in cultural items to avoid upsetting the patient.
   - D. None of the above.

8. An example of an ADL is
   - A. laughing.
   - B. reading.
   - C. crying.
   - D. dressing.

9. What is the first (lowest) level in Maslow's hierarchy of needs?
   - A. self-actualization
   - B. security
   - C. social needs
   - D. physical needs

10. The group of needs that, when met, make people feel safe are called
    - A. social needs.
    - B. social well-being.
    - C. security needs.
    - D. self-actualization needs.

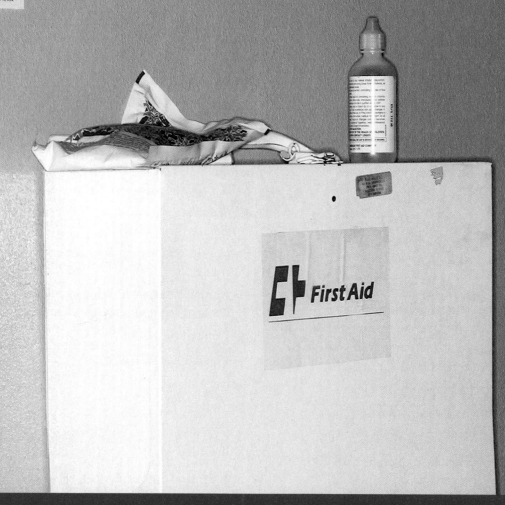

CHAPTER 6

OBJECTIVES

- Identify the nursing assistant's role in keeping patients safe.
- Identify and report environmental and equipment hazards.
- Describe safety guidelines to follow when working with hazardous materials.
- Explain how to prevent fires and what to do in a fire emergency.

- Demonstrate the use of a fire extinguisher and fire blanket.
- Describe the nursing assistant's role in disaster preparedness and what to do if a disaster happens.
- Explain why verifying a patient's identity is important.
- List fall prevention techniques.

- Describe the safe use of oxygen.
- Identify alternatives to the use of physical and chemical restraints.
- Apply physical restraints correctly.
- Explain the purpose of an incident report.

Safety

ABC Class (All Class) fire extinguisher An extinguisher used for all types of fires.

aerosol therapy Moisture and/or medication inhaled into the lungs.

ambulatory Able to walk with or without the help of a walking aid.

chemical restraints Medications given to decrease activity and control behavior.

Class A fire extinguisher An extinguisher used for fires involving combustibles.

Class B fire extinguisher An extinguisher used for fires involving grease.

Class C fire extinguisher An extinguisher for electrical fires and flammable gases.

croupette A small portable oxygen device that resembles a tent, used for infants and young children.

disaster A sudden event that injures many people and causes major damage.

emergency An event calling for immediate action.

face mask An oxygen delivery device that covers the nose and mouth.

fire blanket A blanket made of strong material that does not burn easily. Used to smother small fires and sometimes to transport patients.

hand rail A rail that is placed along a hallway, in a bathroom, or in a stairway to steady ambulatory patients and prevent falls.

hazardous material Any agent that has the potential to cause harm.

incident An accident, error, or unusual event.

incident report A form used to report accidents, errors, or unusual events.

material safety data sheet (MSDS) A document that provides information about the potential hazards associated with a particular substance.

nasal cannula An oxygen delivery device made of plastic tubing with two prongs that are inserted into the nostrils.

nasal catheter An oxygen delivery device made of a small plastic or rubber tube that is inserted into a patient's nose.

oxygen A colorless, odorless, tasteless gas that is essential for life.

oxygen tent A plastic covering on a frame that is placed over a patient's upper body. It delivers a higher percentage of oxygen than is available in air.

P.A.S.S. The sequence of critical steps when using a fire extinguisher.

personal protective equipment (PPE) Special clothing or gear worn to protect against different types of hazards.

physical restraints Protective devices that limit movement and keep patients from harming themselves or others.

R.A.C.E. The sequence of critical steps in a fire emergency.

side rail A rail attached to the side of a bed that can be raised to prevent falling out of bed.

walking aids Devices such as walkers, canes, and crutches used by patients who need assistance to walk.

Creating a Safe Environment

Part of a nursing assistant's job is to ensure patients' safety. Patients can be injured in an accident or **emergency** (an event calling for immediate action). Even if they are not injured, they may be anxious or frightened about what is happening. Most patients need assistance when accidents and emergencies occur. Many are bedridden and cannot help themselves. Those who are able to walk may not be able to react quickly. They may be confused or afraid. A safe environment keeps accidents and emergencies to a minimum. It also makes patients feel secure.

Environmental Safety Measures

Many safety precautions are based on common sense. Watch for the following types of environmental hazards. They can cause fires, electrocution, falls, burns, and other serious injuries. Report these hazards to your supervisor in a health care facility or to the client's family in a home care setting.

- **Damaged or frayed wiring on electrical appliances.**
- **Extension cords.** Do not use extension cords. Never run wiring under carpets or across floors.
- **Improper plugs.** Do not use a three-pronged plug if one of the prongs is missing. Never try to force a three-pronged plug into a two-pronged outlet. If necessary, use a three-pronged adapter to connect the plug. Never pull on a cord to unplug an outlet. Always grasp the plug.
- **Overloaded outlets.** Do not plug too many items into a wall outlet. Using adapters that provide more outlets can cause fire or electrical problems by overloading circuits. **See Figure 6-1.**
- **Electrical cords near water.** Make sure hands are dry before inserting a plug into or removing from an electrical outlet. Keep electrical equipment away from sinks, bathtubs, showers, or other wet areas.

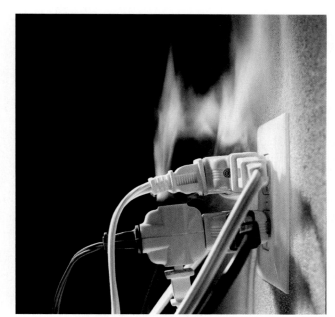

○ **Figure 6-1.** Overloaded circuits are a fire hazard.

- **Flammable materials.** When in a client's home, remind families to keep all flammable materials away from stoves, heaters, and fireplaces.
- **Missing or malfunctioning smoke detectors.** Make sure that all in-home smoke detectors are in good working order. Check the batteries regularly.
- **Throw rugs and mats that can slip.** Use nonskid rubber backing or adhesive strips on all rugs, or remove the rugs, if the patient agrees.
- **Poisons, such as household cleaners, and medications within easy reach.** Keep all poisonous materials out of reach of the patient. If there is a child in the home, lock up these items. Label all medications as needed and keep out of children's reach.
- **Pieces of glass or debris on the floor.** Do not clean up glass with your bare hands. Put on gloves. Use wet paper towels to pick up the pieces. Then vacuum and mop the floor.

- **Scalding hot water.** Always check the temperature of showers and bath water. Dip your elbow or wrist into the water to make sure the temperature is safe. Use a bath thermometer if one is available. **See Figure 6-2.** Bath water should be 100° to 115° Fahrenheit.

Equipment Safety Measures

Caring for equipment may be part of your responsibility in a health care facility or in a home care environment. Equipment includes beds and wheelchairs, as well as electrical or electronic devices and appliances. Follow these guidelines for safe use and care of equipment.

- Make sure you understand how to operate equipment. If you are unsure of a procedure, ask your supervisor.
- If you notice that equipment is faulty in any way, report it to your supervisor. Tape a note to the equipment stating the problem and that it should not be used until repaired.
- Make sure that bed rails lock in place.
- Check a wheelchair to make sure the wheels lock properly before assisting a patient into the chair.
- Make sure there are no loose screws, wheels, or control knobs on all types of equipment.
- Check call lights and signals to make sure they are working properly.
- Store equipment according to the facility's policies and procedures.

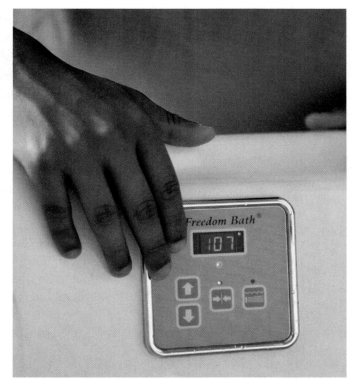

○ **Figure 6-2.** Bath water must be checked to ensure that the patient will not be burned.

Hazardous Materials

A **hazardous material** is any agent that has the potential to cause harm. Many hazardous materials can be found in the home and the workplace. Examples of hazardous materials include paint removers, acetone, cleaning fluids, chlorine bleach, medications, lead, and mercury. **See Figure 6-3.**

Hazardous materials are defined and regulated by the Occupational Safety and Health Administration (OSHA). They may be flammable, corrosive, air or water reactive, or toxic. It is the responsibility of all employers to provide employees with warnings and safeguards to protect them from hazardous materials.

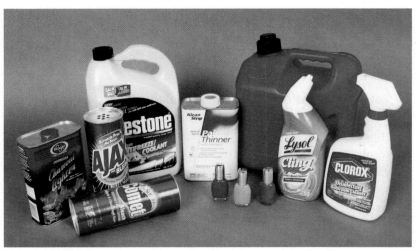

○ **Figure 6-3.** Many chemicals that are found in the home may be considered hazardous materials.

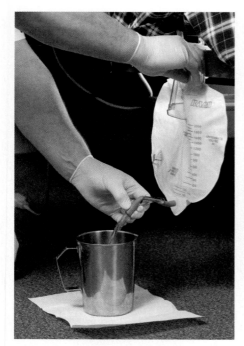

○ **Figure 6-4.** This nursing assistant wears disposable gloves to help protect himself from disease.

Warnings, Signs, and Labels. All hazardous materials must be clearly labeled to warn everyone of their contents. Labels also address immediate and long-term effects if the chemicals are mishandled.

Personal Protective Equipment. Special clothing or gear worn to protect against different types of hazards is called **personal protective equipment (PPE).** For instance, disposable gloves are a type of PPE. **See Figure 6-4.**

Material Safety Data Sheets. A document that provides information about the potential hazards associated with a particular substance is called a **material safety data sheet (MSDS).** Information found on an MSDS includes:
- A description of the product.
- Physical and health hazards.
- Safe handling, storage, and disposal techniques.
- What to do in case of a spill.
- First-aid interventions.
- PPE required to be worn.

All health care workers must know how to work safely with hazardous chemicals and other materials that may pose a health hazard. Know the location of MSDS. Always read the MSDS before using any hazardous material for the first time. Answer questions or concerns about necessary precautions before you begin working with a new material or substance. **See Figure 6-5.**

Material Safety Guidelines. Follow these hazardous material safety guidelines in the health care facility and in the home:
- Read and follow instructions for use, storage, and disposal of all hazardous materials.
- Wear recommended PPE.
- Use care to avoid spills.
- Store chemicals in their original containers.
- Never mix substances.

Vital Skills (READING)

MSDS: Using the Dictionary

Material data safety sheets often contain chemical or scientific vocabulary that is difficult to understand. If you run across a word you don't know, look it up in the dictionary. Guessing what a word might mean is okay in some situations, but not when safety is involved. An MSDS always involves safety, so take the time to look up unfamiliar words.

Practice

Find an MSDS online or use one provided by your instructor. Read the MSDS carefully. On a sheet of paper, make a list of the words you do not understand. Use a dictionary (or use an online dictionary) to find the meaning of each word on your list. Write down the meaning of each word. Then reread the MSDS. Consult your list of definitions as necessary.

Material Safety Data Sheet (MSDS)

MSDS #: 46.00
Revision Date:

Section 1 — Chemical Product and Company Identification

Ammonia

Flinn Scientific, Inc. P.O. Box 219 Batavia, IL 60510 (800) 452-1261

CHEMTREC Emergency Phone Number: (800) 424-9300

Section 2 — Composition, Information on Ingredients

Ammonium Hydroxide (1336-21-6) 8-10%, Water (7732-18-5) 90-92%
Synonym: household ammonia, ammonia solution, aqueous ammonia
CAS#: 7664-41-7

Section 3 — Hazards Identification

White cloudy liquid with strong ammonia odor .
Mildly toxic by ingestion and inhalation. Irritating to body tissues. Lachrymator.
Avoid all body tissue contact.

Health-2
Flammability-0
Reactivity-1
Exposure-2
Storage-3

0 is low hazard, 3 is high hazard

Section 4 — First Aid Measures

Call a physician, seek medical attention for further treatment, observation and support after first aid.
Inhalation: Remove to fresh air at once. If breathing has stopped give artificial respiration immediately.
Eye: Immediately flush with fresh water for 15 minutes.
External: Wash continuously with fresh water for 15 minutes.
Internal: Give large quantities of water. Call a physician or poison control at once.

Section 5 — Exposure Controls , Personal Protection

Avoid contact with eyes, skin and clothing. Wear chemical splash goggles, chemical-resistant gloves and chemical-resistant apron.
Use exhaust ventilation to keep airborne concentrations low.

○ **Figure 6-5.** Material safety data sheets for potentially harmful substances must be posted in health care facilities.

- Do not use any substance that does not have a label.
- Do not use aerosol products around open flames.
- Store all flammable materials in well-ventilated areas.
- Keep the Poison Control phone number near the phone or in an easy-to-locate area. **See Figure 6-6.**
- Report any incident involving hazardous materials to a supervisor.

Personal Safety on the Job

Your personal safety is your first and foremost responsibility. You must keep yourself safe so that you can care for your patients. Follow these personal safety guidelines:

- Always be aware of your environment. Watch out for hazards and accidents in the making. Report hazards immediately.

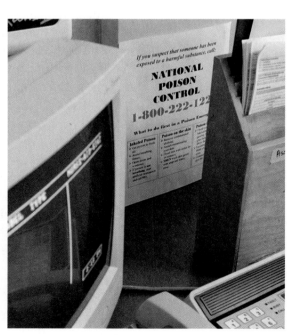

○ **Figure 6-6.** Locate the Poison Control phone number and other emergency numbers in your facility.

- Know the fire safety precautions for your facility. Know what to do in a fire emergency.
- Always walk in the halls and on stairs—never run. Use the hand rails on stairways. Be especially careful at intersections and when carrying equipment or walking with patients.
- Do not horse around. It is inappropriate and dangerous.
- Use proper body mechanics to avoid personal injury. Chapter 16 covers correct body mechanics.
- Report to the supervisor anything that you think could be harmful to you or your patients.
- Follow general safety guidelines for handling hazardous materials.
- Know all the ways to control infection. Use handwashing and other standard precautions whenever necessary. Chapter 11 covers standard precautions and infection control.

Fire Safety

Fire in a health care facility can quickly become a tragedy. Lives can be lost in a fire due to both flames and smoke inhalation. Property can be damaged or lost. Like all health care employees, nursing assistants are responsible for keeping the environment safe from fire.

Fire Prevention

The best defense against fire is fire prevention. Part of your training when working in a health care facility will include fire prevention training.

The number-one fire hazard is smoking. Most health care facilities now prohibit all smoking, though some long-term facilities permit smoking in authorized areas. If patients do smoke, they must be supervised and smoke only in designated areas. Smokers should use deep metal ashtrays that are emptied into metal containers. Make sure all ashes are extinguished.

Follow these guidelines to prevent fires:
- Keep areas uncluttered and free of debris.
- Always empty waste into appropriate containers.
- Keep all flammable materials away from heat sources.
- Make sure that smoke detectors are in good working order. **See Figure 6-7.**
- Never allow a patient to smoke in bed.
- Never allow smoking in areas where oxygen is in use, because oxygen is highly flammable.
- Keep matches and other flammable materials out of reach of patients and children. All smoking materials should be locked up in a designated area. Only employees should be able to access the materials.
- Always supervise patients when they smoke.
- Always be aware of potential fire hazards and report them immediately.

Fire Emergencies

Even though every effort is made to prevent a fire, you must be prepared in case a fire does occur. You must remain calm. Although this may be difficult, it is essential so that you can assess the situation quickly and act appropriately.

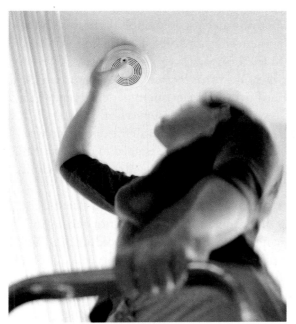

○ **Figure 6-7.** Smoke detectors should be tested periodically to make sure they work properly. This nursing assistant is testing a bedroom smoke detector for her home health client.

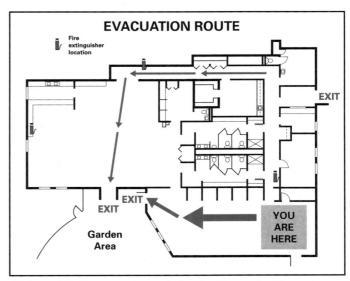

○ **Figure 6-8.** Everyone who works in a health care facility must understand the evacuation plan.

Patients may panic and become confused and disoriented, so you need to know the evacuation procedures and to be in control. Give directions in a firm, clear, calm voice. Explain what you are doing and reassure patients that they will be safe.

During emergency training, you will learn how to use the facility's fire equipment, how to evacuate patients, and how to keep yourself safe. You should:

- Learn evacuation routes and practice them until you know them well. **See Figure 6-8.** Be aware of secondary escape routes in case the main routes are unsafe or blocked. You will not be able to use elevators unless directed by emergency workers.
- Be aware of your surroundings in case a safe situation becomes unsafe and you suddenly need to change your exit plan. Learn and use alternative exit routes.
- Know the location of fire equipment and fire call boxes. Know how to operate fire alarms, fire doors and escapes, fire extinguishers, and sprinklers.
- Participate in fire drills. State laws require health facilities to conduct fire drills on a regular basis. These drills are important because patients may become confused and disoriented during an emergency. They may be unable to help themselves. You will be taught how to help them in case of a fire emergency.
- When in a client's home, work with families to help them develop their own evacuation plan.

If a fire does occur at a health care facility, keep your body low when moving through a smoke-filled room. Warm air rises. If a room is filled with smoke, the cleanest air is nearest to the floor. Remember **R.A.C.E.**, the sequence of critical steps in a fire emergency.

- **Remove patients.** Move patients who are in immediate danger to safety. Escort patients who are ambulatory. Move bedridden patients by using a fire blanket or by rolling the beds to a safe area.

SAFETY FIRST

When working in a client's home, place emergency phone numbers near the telephone. In many communities "9-1-1" is called for all emergencies. Make a list of phone numbers for the patient's doctors, family members, and poison control, if this has not been done by the RN. To report an emergency in a home without a phone, go to the nearest neighbor or pay phone and dial 9-1-1.

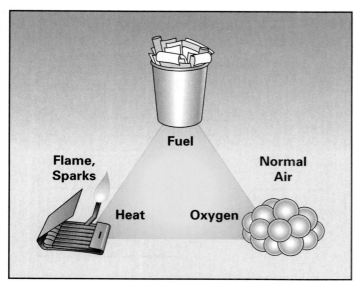

○ **Figure 6-9.** The three elements that must be present to sustain a fire.

• **A**ctivate alarms. Sound the alarm to alert the entire facility that there is a fire. You may need to tell the operator or switchboard exactly where the fire is located. The operator can alert the fire department and other emergency help, as well as the facility supervisor.

• **C**ontain the fire. Close all fire doors and windows. Fire doors are designed to contain a fire. You should close doors and windows to eliminate drafts that could fuel the fire.

• **E**xtinguish the fire *or* **E**vacuate patients. Use a fire extinguisher on a small fire only if you can manage it safely. (See Procedure 6-1.) You will be trained to assess which types of fires can be put out with a fire extinguisher. If you are unsure of your ability to extinguish a fire, leave the area and wait for trained firefighters to arrive.

A fire needs three elements to sustain itself: fuel (anything that is able to burn), heat, and oxygen. **See Figure 6-9.** The most effective method for putting out a fire is to cut off the fire's oxygen and/or remove its fuel source. If a fire starts in a pan on the stove, you can put a lid on the pan to shut off the oxygen. This contains and extinguishes the fire. You can also turn off the stove to remove the heat source.

Several types of tools can be used to fight fires. Health care facilities are required to keep fire extinguishers. They are usually in clearly marked boxes in hallways and stairwells. Some facilities have additional firefighting equipment, such as axes for breaking into or out of a room. They may also have fire blankets for protecting and transporting patients. Some facilities also keep water hoses in hall closets.

Fire Extinguishers. A fire extinguisher can be used to put out a small fire. All health facility employees are required to learn how to use a fire extinguisher. Courses are usually given a few times each year at the workplace by local firefighters. **See Figure 6-10.**

Fire extinguishers are labeled by class to indicate which kinds of fires they can extinguish. **Class A fire extinguishers** are used for fires involving common combustibles such as paper, wood, and plastics. **Class B**

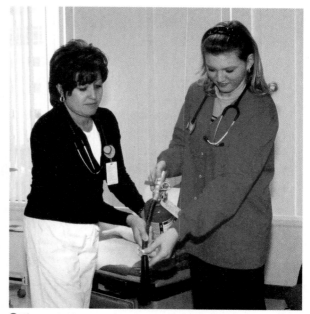

○ **Figure 6-10. Learn how to use a fire extinguisher properly.**

fire extinguishers** are used for grease fires. **Class C fire extinguishers** are used for electrical fires and flammable gases. **ABC Class (All Class) fire extinguishers** can be used for any type of fire. Most health facilities have ABC fire extinguishers. You should know where the fire extinguishers are in your facility.

Remember **P.A.S.S.**, the sequence of critical steps when using a fire extinguisher.

- **P**ull the pin. The safety pin keeps the fire extinguisher from being activated accidentally. The pin must be removed before the extinguisher can be used.
- **A**im the nozzle at the base of the fire.
- **S**queeze the handle to extinguish the flames.
- **S**weep the nozzle back and forth along the base of the fire.

Procedure 6-1

Using a Fire Extinguisher

Equipment: fire extinguisher

1. Hold the fire extinguisher upright. **See Figure 6-11A.**
2. Remove the safety pin as shown in **Figure 6-11B.**
3. Direct the hose at the base of the fire. **See Figure 6-11C.**
4. Push or squeeze the top handle down to close as shown in **Figure 6-11D.**

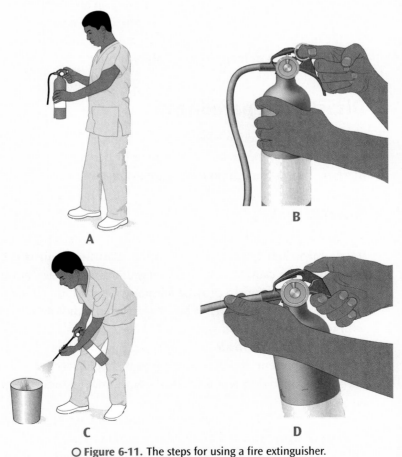

○ **Figure 6-11.** The steps for using a fire extinguisher.

Procedure 6-2

Using a Fire Blanket to Move a Patient

Equipment: fire blanket • helper

1. Roll the patient onto his or her side, facing away from you. Be sure to tell the patient what you are doing.
2. Place the fire blanket diagonally under the patient. Roll the patient onto his or her back.
3. Wrap the patient in the blanket. Wrap as you would wrap a blanket around a baby.
4. Lower the bed to the lowest position. Loosen the bottom bed sheet and use it as a sling to gently lower the patient to the floor.
5. Grasp the edge of the blanket at the patient's head and shoulders. Get into a crawling position and pull the patient along the floor. Stay as low as possible when smoke is present.

Note: This procedure can also be used to move a patient down a staircase. Be sure to grasp the blanket at the head of the patient and protect the head by lifting the blanket as you go slowly down the stairs.

Fire Blankets. One way to put out a small fire is to cut off the oxygen supply by covering it with something that is nonflammable. A **fire blanket** is a blanket made of strong material that doesn't burn easily. Fire blankets are kept with the fire extinguishers in many health care facilities.

Fire blankets (and other strong blankets) can also help you remove weak or disabled patients from a smoky area if you are the only rescuer available. You can use the blanket to protect and pull the patient to safety. Fire blankets can also be used to transport as many as four babies at once.

Disaster Preparedness

A **disaster** is a sudden event that injures many people and causes major damage. Disasters can be caused by nature or by people. For every type of disaster, there are things you can do to prepare in advance.

Natural Disasters

Many types of extreme weather conditions can cause disasters. They include floods, tornadoes, hurricanes, and earthquakes. **See Figure 6-12.** Natural disasters of all kinds can cause power failures. Health care facilities, however, usually have emergency generators to provide temporary electricity in the most critical areas. Facilities also keep a supply of battery-powered radios and flashlights. Be familiar with where they are kept.

Hurricanes and tornadoes are often accompanied by a lightning hazard. When lightning is present, you and your patients should stay away from metal objects, telephones, open doors, and windows. Since water conducts electricity, avoid tubs and shower stalls.

Wind is the highest risk in a tornado. Seek shelter in a basement, if possible, and avoid standing near windows. They can blow out in a tornado, and flying glass can cause severe injuries. If you are in a building without a basement, seek shelter in an interior room on the lowest level.

When a hurricane is approaching, you will usually have adequate warning. Follow the directions of emergency workers if they are present. Otherwise, follow the safety procedures you have learned. If you and your patients are trapped in a flooded area as a result of a hurricane or any other disaster, follow your facility's protocol and the instructions of emergency workers.

Disasters Caused by People

Not all disasters are caused by nature. Many disasters in the world today are caused by people. These include bombings, sniper attacks, riots, explosions, chemical spills or leaks, and chemical and germ warfare. Unlike most natural disasters, disasters that are caused by people often happen with no warning at all. In most cases, the most you can do to prepare for them in advance is to participate in disaster preparedness drills and know the procedures to be followed. Have an emergency plan in mind for various types of disasters.

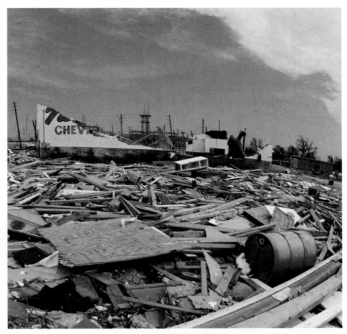

○ **Figure 6-12.** Hurricanes can cause the total destruction of anything in their path.

Disaster Guidelines

Your supervisor will train you in emergency and disaster procedures for the facility. Knowing what to do will give you confidence in your ability to help yourself and your patients. General guidelines for preparing for and acting in a disaster include:

- **Be prepared.** Know the emergency procedures for the facility. Know the fire and disaster evacuation plans and all emergency exits. Know where fire extinguishers are located.
- **Call for help.** Do not act beyond your level of knowledge or skill. If you call to report a disaster situation, be sure to include information about the type of disaster, its location, and the number of injured people, if any. You may also need to give information about the best door or parking lot to gain access.
- **Move patients who are in immediate danger.** Do not leave patients alone.
- **Speak calmly in short, concise sentences.** Keep the patient as calm and comfortable as possible.
- **Follow the directions of emergency workers.**

When major natural or people-caused disasters happen, military and/or emergency teams are usually called in to direct rescue efforts. **See Figure 6-13.** Depending on the scope of the disaster, they may set up zones or areas for different types of patients. For example, all critically ill or injured people may be placed in a "red zone." Do your part to help by following the instructions of the team in charge.

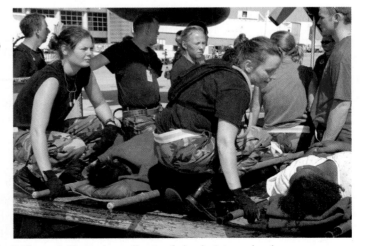

○ **Figure 6-13.** During a disaster, federal, state, or local emergency authorities take charge of the affected area to coordinate and direct rescue efforts.

Routine Patient Safety

So far, this chapter has discussed preparations you should make to protect yourself and your patients from environmental hazards and what to do in case of fire or disaster. However, you are also responsible for patient safety on a more routine basis. The rest of this chapter explains how you can protect the safety of your patients every day.

Verifying Patient Identity

Properly identifying patients is one of the most basic, yet most important, steps in keeping them safe. Many facilities place identification (ID) bracelets

Vital Skills COMMUNICATION

Communicating in Emergencies

When a disaster or emergency happens, it is often important to move patients or residents to safety quickly. It is easy to forget good communication techniques in these stressful situations. Remember that patients will be frightened and confused. Some will seem uncooperative. Others may insist on asking endless questions.

The best way to ensure patient cooperation is often to provide a quick explanation in terms the patients can understand. Use simple words that will not require further discussion. Remain calm, but stress to patients the need to move quickly.

As an example, suppose a major river in your area is expected to rise well beyond its banks. It is expected to flood the rehabilitation center, and you have been asked to begin moving patients to safety. You might provide the following information:

Information	Example
The nature of the emergency	The river is rising and is expected to flood this facility.
A brief explanation of why you need to move the patient	Flood water is rising quickly, so we need to move you to higher ground.
Where you will move the patient	General hospital has agreed to provide temporary food, shelter, and medical treatment for our patients.
How you intend to move the patient	Let me help you into the wheelchair so that I can take you to the bus waiting outside.

Now the patient has enough information to feel more in control and less apprehensive about what is happening. In many cases, this is enough to ensure the patient's cooperation.

Practice

Use role-playing techniques to practice communicating with uncooperative, frantic, or scared patients in an emergency situation. Possible scenarios include: flood (any health care facility), tornado warning at a long-term care facility, hurricane preparation, major power outage in a home care environment. Take turns playing the patient and the nursing assistant so that everyone can practice.

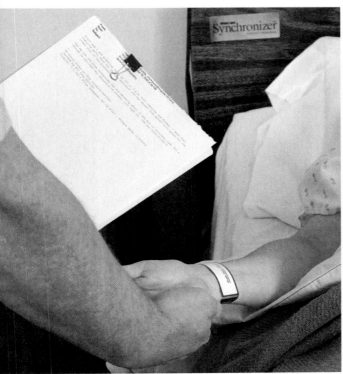

○ **Figure 6-14.** The nursing assistant verifies the patient's identity before giving care.

on patients when they are admitted for care. Mistakes can occur in health care when caregivers do not properly check a patient's ID. This can result in the wrong care being given to a patient. Before caring for any patient, always check the patient's name on the ID bracelet. **See Figure 6-14.**

Many facilities now require a second identification to be checked, such as the patient's birth date. Long-term care facilities may use photographs to identify patients instead of ID bracelets. No matter what system is being used, make sure the right care is given to the right person.

SAFETY FIRST

Inform patients about the safety measures available to them. Point out the signal cords or call lights in their rooms and in their bathrooms. Reinforce safety measures that patients can take themselves.

Fall Prevention

Falls are the most common type of accident, especially for older patients. However, any patient can fall. A patient may be confused because of hearing or vision problems or impaired by illness or by medications. A surgical patient may be weak and unsteady. Some people may become dizzy or lightheaded when moving from lying to sitting or from sitting to standing. These people may need extra time for these activities.

Several devices can be used to help prevent patients from falling. Some of the most common devices include:

- **Walking aids.** An **ambulatory** patient is one who is able to walk with or without the help of a walking aid. Doctors order **walking aids**—walkers, canes, or crutches—for patients who need assistance to walk. Each piece of equipment must be fitted to the patient by a physical therapist. Walking aids should have nonskid tips to prevent slipping.

- **Side rails.** A rail attached to the side of a bed that can be raised to prevent falling out of bed is called a **side rail**, or bed rail. **See Figure 6-15.** Side rails lock into place. They are regarded as a type of restraint and may require a doctor's order.

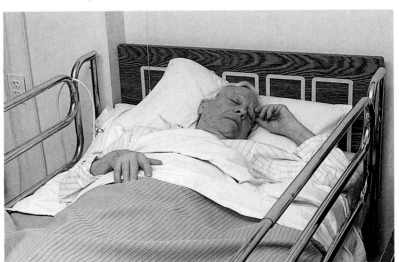

○ **Figure 6-15.** A resident with a history of falling rests in bed with the side rails up, as his doctor ordered.

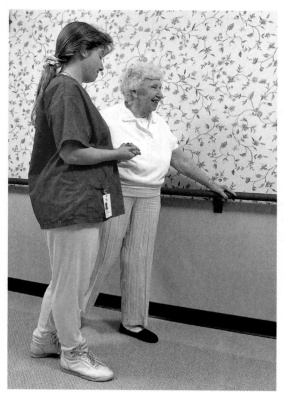

○ **Figure 6-16.** Hand rails enable this resident to walk in the hallways with the help of a nursing assistant.

- **Hand rails.** A rail that is placed along a hallway, in a bathroom, or in a stairway to steady ambulatory patients and prevent falls is called a **hand rail**. Encourage your patients to use hand rails. **See Figure 6-16.**

Follow these guidelines to help prevent falls in the health care facility and in the home:

- Always walk with an unsteady patient.
- Be sure the patient wears nonskid footwear to avoid slipping. Shoes that slip on without ties or Velcro closures are dangerous.
- Help unsteady patients in and out of bed and allow them to stand for a brief time if they feel lightheaded.
- Encourage the patient to grasp hand rails in hallways and stairways.
- Be alert for signs of dizziness or unsteadiness. If a patient complains of dizziness, check the pulse and notify the nurse immediately.
- Keep the signal cord or call light within the patient's reach at all times. Answer the signal within 3 to 5 minutes.
- Keep the patient's bed in its lowest position. For bedridden patients, make sure the side rails are in the *up* position and securely locked.
- As a patient sits down, lock the wheels of a chair or place it against a wall to brace it.
- Keep a night-light in the patient's room.
- Maintain good lighting in rooms and hallways.
- Create a safe walking environment. Keep floors and hallways clear of clutter. Make sure there are clear, unobstructed paths for the patient to move around safely. **See Figure 6-17.**
- Discuss the removal of throw rugs in a home care situation with the client and/or the client's family.
- Wipe up spills immediately. Steer patients away from wet floors.
- To minimize confusion, avoid rearranging furniture.
- Keep electrical cords and extension cords out of the way.

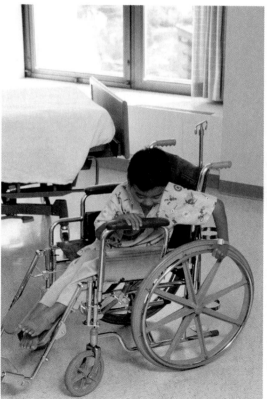

○ **Figure 6-17.** The floor must be clear to enable this patient to be moved around in the room.

Oxygen Therapy Safety

Oxygen is a colorless, odorless, tasteless gas that is essential for breathing. The air we breathe is 21% oxygen. However, some patients need more oxygen than normal air contains. Doctors may order oxygen for patients who are not getting enough oxygen in their blood.

Oxygen is considered a medication. As a nursing assistant, you are therefore not responsible for administering oxygen. This is done by a respiratory therapist or a nurse. You may, however, be caring for a patient who is receiving oxygen therapy. You need to know how to give safe care to these patients. **See Figure 6-18.**

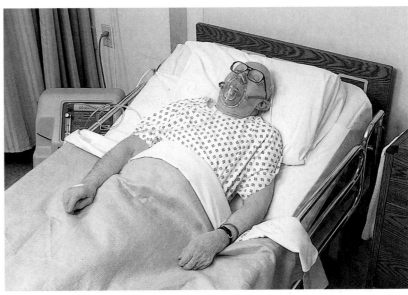

O **Figure 6-18.** A resident receives oxygen in bed. The nursing assistant checks the tubing for kinks or other obstructions.

Doctors prescribe a specific rate of oxygen flow for a specific amount of time. Some patients receive oxygen continuously. Others receive it on an as-needed basis, usually determined by the nurse or doctor. You should be aware of the amount of oxygen your patient is receiving and the type of equipment being used.

Oxygen Delivery Devices. Oxygen is delivered to the patient from compressed oxygen tanks, portable liquid oxygen, or oxygen concentrators. Some portable oxygen tanks are on wheels. Some are small enough and light enough to be carried. They allow an ambulatory patient to be mobile. **See Figure 6-19.** Portable tanks are connected to a nasal catheter, nasal cannula, or face mask. Portable

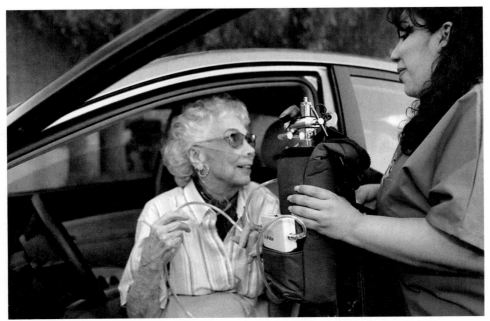

O **Figure 6-19.** People who need to use oxygen can carry small portable devices easily in the car. This gives them the freedom to run errands such as shopping and going to the doctor's office.

○ **Figure 6-20.** The type of oxygen delivery device used depends on the patient's oxygen needs.

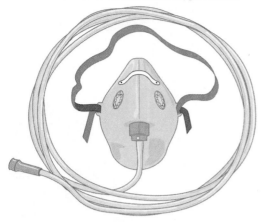

Oxygen mask

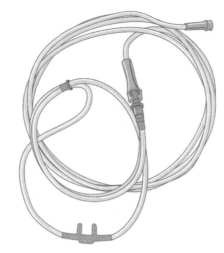

Nasal cannula

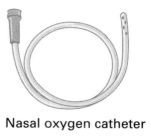

Nasal oxygen catheter

tanks are under pressure and must be handled carefully to avoid leaks or damage to the tank. They are strapped into place when stored. Some facilities use large oxygen tanks strapped to the wall or a carrier if they do not have wall units. A special device called a *flowmeter* is used with oxygen to control the flow. It regulates the amount of oxygen a patient receives. The doctor orders one of several delivery devices based on the flow rate needed and the patient's circumstances. **See Figure 6-20.**

Vital Skills MATH

Reading an Oxygen Pressure Gauge

Although you cannot give oxygen therapy to patients, you should understand how to read the gauges on an oxygen tank. The pressure gauge shows how much oxygen is left in the tank. If the tank runs low, you may be the first to notice.

Pressure gauges show the amount of oxygen left in psi (pressure per square inch). For most oxygen tanks, the gauge on a full tank shows 2000 psi. If the gauge reads 1500 psi, the tank is three-quarters full. If the gauge reads 1000 psi, it is half full, and so on.

Because oxygen tanks or cylinders are available in many different sizes and capacities, they empty at different rates. The prescribed rate of flow also affects how quickly a tank empties. You do not need to be able to calculate how much time a cylinder has left before it is empty. However, you do need to realize that a small, portable tank with a gauge reading of 500 psi will be empty much sooner than a large, floorstanding oxygen cylinder. For example, a portable, backpack-style oxygen tank with a pressure of 500 psi may only have 15 minutes of oxygen left at a flow rate of 2 liters per minute.

Practice

With other students, practice reading the pressure gauge on oxygen tanks in your school lab or, if possible, in a clinical setting. At what point on each size tank would you consider notifying your supervisor that the tank is low? For what size tank would a low reading be most critical?

- A **nasal cannula** is made of plastic tubing with two prongs that are inserted into the patient's nostrils. The tubing fits around the patient's ears and connects to the oxygen source. You must check the patient's skin around the ears, on the cheeks, and under the nose for irritation.
- A **nasal catheter** is a small plastic or rubber tube that is inserted into the patient's nose. The tubing is taped to the nose and temples. Check the patient's skin around the nose for evidence of irritation or skin encrustation.
- A **face mask** covers the nose and mouth. It is held in place with straps that go around the head. The mask is removed periodically for eating and drinking, and to wash and dry the patient's face. While removed, it is replaced with a nasal cannula. Some patients feel frightened or *claustrophobic* (closed in) when wearing a face mask and need reassurance.
- An **oxygen tent** is a plastic covering on a frame that is placed over a patient's upper body. The oxygen circulates throughout. The tent is tucked under the mattress to prevent leakage. Oxygen tents are rarely used today because other methods are considered more reliable.
- A **croupette** is a small portable oxygen device that resembles a tent and provides cool, humid air to infants and young children. It may cover the entire child or be placed just over the child's upper body.

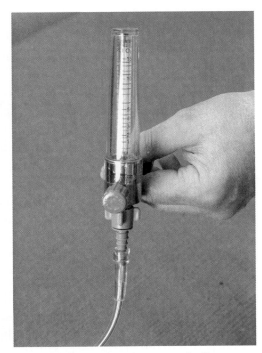

○ **Figure 6-21.** Learning how to read a flowmeter allows you to check the patient's oxygen flow rate.

Aerosol Therapy. Along with the delivery of oxygen, patients may receive **aerosol therapy**, in which moisture and/or medication is delivered into the lungs. The purpose of this therapy is to loosen mucus in the lungs or open passageways to ease breathing. Aerosol therapy can be delivered along with oxygen in an IPPR (intermittent positive pressure respiration) machine. Patients may use a *nebulizer*, which changes liquids into a fine mist to be breathed into the lungs. The nursing assistant never decides to give aerosol therapy, but may be instructed to help a patient who is receiving such therapy.

Oxygen Safety Guidelines. To make sure patients receive a safe amount of oxygen:
- Know the rate of oxygen flow the doctor has ordered.
- Learn how to read the flowmeter so you can check the rate each time you attend to the patient. **See Figure 6-21.**
- Notify your supervisor if there is any change in the rate of oxygen flow or in the patient's breathing.
- Make sure the tubes going to the oxygen source are free of kinks or obstructions.
- Never remove the device unless a nurse or supervisor instructs you to.

Concentrated oxygen helps fuel fires and makes things burn much more rapidly than they would in normal air. Oxygen is flammable, so you must be especially careful about fire safety in an area where patients receive oxygen. Sparks and static present extreme hazards around pure oxygen. When oxygen is in use, special precautions must be taken to prevent fires and to administer the oxygen safely.
- Smoking is *never* allowed in an area where oxygen is being administered or stored.

- Remove all smoking materials, including cigarettes and matches, from the room if visitors have brought any. Patients' smoking materials either are not allowed, or they are stored with medication to be handed out on a supervised basis.
- Turn off electrical equipment before unplugging it. Remove any unnecessary electrical equipment from the room.
- Dress the patient in cotton clothing. Use all-cotton linens, including blankets. Synthetic fabrics and wool can cause static electricity.
- Do not operate electrical equipment unnecessarily.
- Remove any materials that could ignite easily, including alcohol, cleaning products, and nail polish remover.
- Post warning signs such as "No Flammable Materials" to help ensure patient safety.

Using Restraints Safely

Maintaining safety for patients may involve the application of restraints. **Physical restraints** are protective devices that limit movement and keep patients from harming themselves or others. They prevent patients from falling out of beds, chairs, stretchers, and wheelchairs. They can also prevent a patient from scratching a wound or pulling at tubing or dressings. **Chemical restraints** are medications given to decrease activity and control behavior.

Long ago, patients who were agitated were either physically restrained or chemically restrained. It is now understood that many of these patients respond better to gentle handling and care. The latest OBRA guidelines call for minimizing the use of restraints. The goal is to provide patient *care*, not patient restraint. Restraints should be used only when necessary to prevent patients from hurting themselves or others. It is important that the *least restrictive* type of restraint be used that will accomplish the intended purpose.

Restraints contribute to complications such as depression and pressure ulcers. Alternatives to restraints should be used whenever possible. Alternatives include:
- Moving the patient near the nursing station.
- Following a consistent toileting schedule.
- Offering a variety of activities.
- Enlisting family members to stay with the patient.
- Watching for and reporting signs of pain.
- Providing adequate nutrition.
- Using bed and chair alarms.
- Changing the patient's environment. **See Figure 6-22.**

After all other care options have been tried and have failed, the patient's doctor issues an order for a restraint. The doctor's written order specifies:
- The type of restraint.
- The purpose of the restraint.
- The length of time the patient is to be restrained.
- The frequency of removal or release and reapplication.

States have rules about what types of restraints may be used and which facilities have the authority to use them. In some states, family consent is also required. Explain the type and the purpose of the restraints to the patient and family members. There may be a meeting with all interested people before

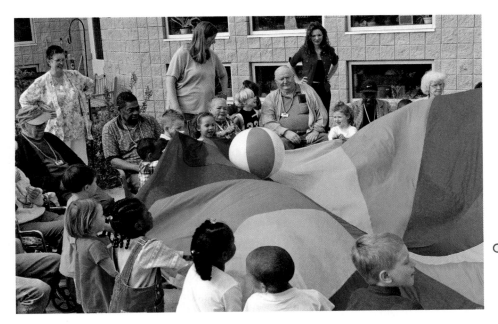

○ **Figure 6-22.** Pleasant alternatives to restraints include changing the patient's environment and offering a variety of activities.

restraints are used. Some facilities allow restraints to be removed when a visitor or family member is present and can take responsibility for monitoring the patient.

It is a patient's right not to be restrained unnecessarily or for the convenience of the staff. If you are in doubt as to why the patient needs a restraint, ask your supervisor. It is the responsibility of everyone involved in caring for patients to respect their dignity and to uphold their basic human rights. Unnecessary restraint of a patient could constitute false imprisonment. (See Chapter 4.)

Guidelines for Applying Restraints. Restraints can be applied to the upper body, waist, elbows, wrists, or ankles. When you apply a restraint, you need to allow the patient some movement in the restrained area. You must also check the patient's skin every 15 to 30 minutes, depending on the type of restraint and the facility's policies. Check for circulation, swelling, color, and temperature. Make sure the restraint is not too tight. Restraints are generally removed every 2 hours for movement and for activities of daily living. They must be off for a minimum of 15 minutes.

Follow these guidelines to apply restraints safely:

- Use the correct size and type of restraint. Before applying a restraint, check that it is clean and in good repair. Always apply restraints according to the manufacturer's directions. If you have questions, ask your supervisor. **See Figure 6-23.**
- Make sure the patient is in correct body alignment before and after applying the restraint. Pad any bony areas that could be bruised by a restraint. Always place the restraint over clothing or padding, not over bare skin.

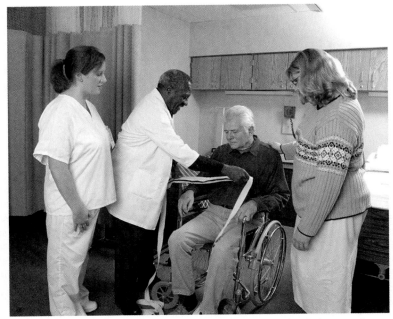

○ **Figure 6-23.** This RN is demonstrating how to apply a safety belt correctly.

- The restraint should not be too tight. A tight restraint can affect breathing and circulation. Make sure the patient can breathe naturally in a chest restraint.
- Immediately notify your supervisor if you find the fingers or toes cold or blue in color, if you cannot locate a pulse, if the patient complains about tingling or numbness in the restrained area, or if the patient is in an unsafe position.
- Provide appropriate patient care, ensuring that all the patient's needs are met while in a restraint.
- Remove restraints every 2 hours. At this time, check the patient and record information in the patient's record. Keep the restraints off for a minimum of 15 minutes.
- If you are using restraints on a bedridden patient, secure the restraint to the bed frame. Do not secure the restraint to the side rail. Keep the bow or tie out of the patient's reach and keep the side rails locked in the *up* position. Position the patient in the center of the mattress in correct body alignment.
- Use a quick-release tie, such as a clove hitch, so you can quickly release the knot in case of emergency. **See Figure 6-24.** Health facilities usually have a policy about what tie to use.
- Keep a pair of scissors within the staff's easy reach, though out of reach of the patient. In an emergency, you can cut the ties to release the patient quickly.
- If a patient becomes angry and tries to fight the restraint, provide reassurance and support to the patient and the family. Report the situation to your supervisor.

Wrist and Ankle Restraints. A wrist restraint limits the movement of a patient's arm. An ankle restraint limits the movement of the leg.

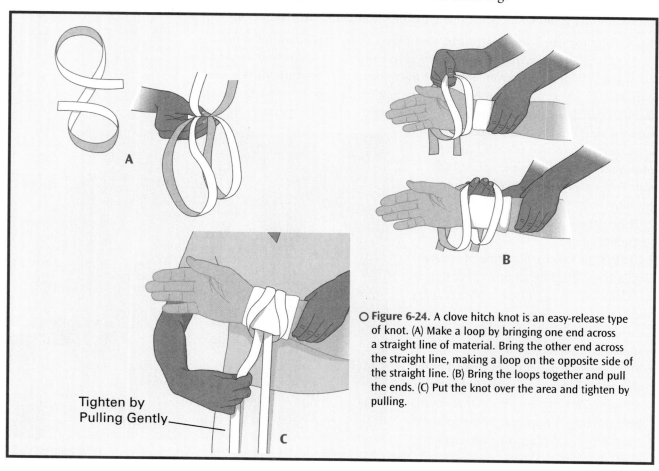

Tighten by Pulling Gently

○ **Figure 6-24.** A clove hitch knot is an easy-release type of knot. (A) Make a loop by bringing one end across a straight line of material. Bring the other end across the straight line, making a loop on the opposite side of the straight line. (B) Bring the loops together and pull the ends. (C) Put the knot over the area and tighten by pulling.

Procedure 6-3

Applying a Wrist or Ankle Restraint

Equipment: padding • wrist or ankle restraint

1. Make sure there is a written order for the restraint before you begin the procedure.
2. Wash your hands.
3. Check the patient's ID bracelet and call the patient by name. Introduce yourself to the patient.
4. Roll the curtains around the bed for privacy. If the patient has visitors, try to avoid putting the restraints on until they leave. Ask the visitors to let you know when they are leaving so you can put on the safety restraints as soon as the patient is alone. If the visitors are close family or friends who are supportive of the restraints, however, you can describe the restraints to them as well as to the patient.
5. Explain to the patient that you are about to apply a restraint.
6. Provide an opportunity for the patient to use the bathroom, if necessary.
7. Position the bed to a comfortable working height.
8. Place the patient in a comfortable position in correct body alignment.
9. Place the soft edge of the restraint against the patient after checking the condition of the skin. (Do not apply a restraint over inflamed or broken skin.) Place it over clothing or padding. Wrap the restraint around the wrist or ankle, and smooth the fabric of the restraint. Make sure there are no wrinkles to cause skin irritation.
10. Gently pull the ends of the straps through the fastening ring. Make sure the restraint is secure but not tight.
11. Test for proper fit by putting two of your fingers between the restraint and the patient. If your fingers do not fit, loosen the restraint. **See Figure 6-25.**
12. Move the arm or leg into a comfortable position.
13. Tie the ends of the strap to the bed frame with a tie according to the facility's policies and procedures.
14. Check the pulse, color, and temperature of the patient's wrist or ankle.
15. Put the bed back in its normal position. Raise the side rails if ordered.
16. Give the patient the signal cord. Recheck the patient before leaving the room. Make sure the patient is comfortable and the signal cord is within easy reach.
17. Unscreen the patient.
18. Wash your hands.
19. Remove the restraint every 2 hours to reposition the patient. Provide patient care and exercise.

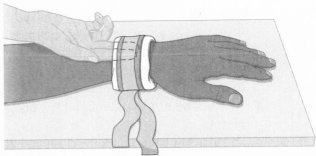

O **Figure 6-25.** Put two fingers between the wrist and the restraint to make sure the fit is correct.

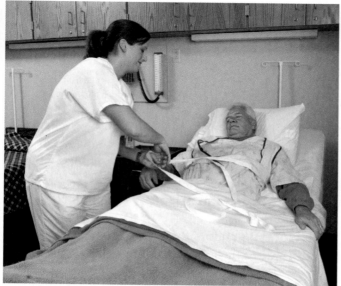

Mitt Restraints. Mitt restraints limit movement of the fingers, but the patient can still move the hand and wrist. A mitt restraint prevents the patient from pulling out tubes, scratching, or touching wounds. Mitt restraints also allow ambulatory Alzheimer's patients to move around freely within the facility while preventing them from taking other patients' belongings.

Jacket or Vest Restraints. A jacket restraint prevents a patient from falling out of bed or a wheelchair. **See Figure 6-26.** The jacket or vest is always worn so that it crosses in the front. It is applied over clothing or pajamas.

○ **Figure 6-26.** A jacket restraint is always applied so that it crosses in the front.

Procedure 6-4

Applying a Mitt Restraint

Equipment: mitt restraint • hand roll (a rolled washcloth or cylinder-shaped object to support the hand in a comfortable position)

1. Make sure there is a written order for the restraint before you begin the procedure.
2. Wash your hands.
3. Check the patient's ID bracelet and call the patient by name. Introduce yourself to the patient.
4. Pull the curtains around the bed for privacy. Ask visitors to step out of the room.
5. Explain to the patient that you are about to apply a restraint and allow the patient to use the bathroom if necessary.
6. Position the bed to a comfortable working height.
7. The patient's hand should be clean and dry.
8. Place a hand roll in the patient's hand so the hand is comfortable. **See Figure 6-27.**
9. Apply the mitt restraint. Tie the straps to the bed frame according to the facility's policies and procedures.
10. Make sure the restraint is secure but not tight. Check the pulse, color, and temperature of the wrist.

11. Put the bed back in its normal position. Raise the side rails if ordered.
12. Check that the patient is comfortably positioned before leaving the room. Make sure the patient is positioned in correct body alignment and the signal cord is within easy reach.
13. Unscreen the patient.
14. Wash your hands.
15. Remove the restraint every 2 hours to reposition the patient. Provide patient care and exercise.

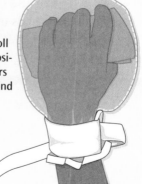

○ **Figure 6-27.** A mitt restraint should be used with a hand roll to ensure proper positioning of the fingers and to make the hand comfortable.

Procedure 6-5

Applying a Jacket or Vest Restraint

Equipment: jacket restraint

1. Make sure you have a written physician's order for the restraint before you begin the procedure.
2. Wash your hands.
3. Check the patient's ID bracelet and call the patient by name. Introduce yourself to the patient.
4. Provide privacy. Ask visitors to step out of the room.
5. Explain to the patient that you are about to apply a restraint and allow the patient to use the bathroom if necessary.
6. Position the bed to a comfortable working height.
7. Assist the patient to a sitting position. Slip the patient's arms into the armholes of the jacket or vest. Cross the straps over the patient's chest. Be sure the restraint is the correct size for the patient.
8. Help the patient lie down.
9. Pull the loose end of the strap through the slot in the jacket, making sure there are no wrinkles in the jacket.
10. Place the patient in a comfortable position.
11. Tie the straps to the bed frame under the mattress.
12. Make sure the restraint is secure but not tight. Test for fit and comfort by inserting two fingers between the restraint and the patient.
13. Put the bed back to its normal position. Raise the side rails if ordered.
14. Give the patient the signal cord. Check the patient's position and comfort before leaving the room and make sure the signal cord is within easy reach.
15. Unscreen the patient.
16. Wash your hands.
17. Remove the restraint every 2 hours to reposition the patient. Provide patient care and exercise.

Safety Belts. A safety belt also prevents a patient from falling out of bed or from a wheelchair or chair. **See Figure 6-28.** The belt wraps around the patient's waist and is tied to a bed frame or to the back frame of a wheelchair or chair. It is applied over clothing or pajamas.

Some safety belt restraints are designed so that they can be used both in a wheelchair and in a bed. The ties can be tied in back of the wheelchair or to the bed frame. This type of restraint may be more cost-effective for home care clients. Remember, however, that restraints may only be used on a physician's order.

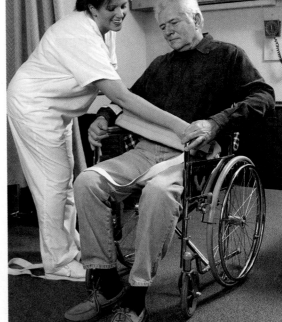

○ **Figure 6-28.** A safety belt used by a resident in a wheelchair can prevent falls.

Procedure 6-6

SP

Applying a Safety Belt Restraint

Equipment: safety belt restraint

1. Make sure you have a written physician's order for the restraint before beginning the procedure.
2. Wash your hands.
3. Check the patient's ID bracelet and call the patient by name. Introduce yourself to the patient.
4. Provide privacy. Ask visitors to step out of the room.
5. Explain to the patient that you are about to apply a restraint and allow the patient to use the bathroom if necessary.
6. Position the bed to a comfortable working height.
7. Assist the patient to a sitting position.
8. Place the safety belt across the front of the patient's waist. Pull the ties to the back.
9. Pull the ties through the slots in the belt. Smooth all the wrinkles from the fabric of the restraint.
10. Help the patient lie down.
11. Place the patient in a comfortable position.
12. Tie the straps to the bed frame under the mattress.
13. Make sure the restraint is secure but not tight. Test for fit and comfort by inserting two fingers between the restraint and the patient.
14. Put the bed back to its normal position. Raise the side rails if ordered.
15. Give the patient the signal cord. Check the patient's position and comfort before leaving the room.
16. Unscreen the patient.
17. Wash your hands.
18. Remove the restraint every 2 hours to reposition the patient. Provide patient care and exercise.

Elbow Restraints. Small children and babies are placed in elbow restraints to prevent them from touching wounds, scratching, and removing tubing. **See Figure 6-29.** You need to restrain both arms to make these restraints effective. They must be removed often to exercise the arms and administer skin care. Small children may be frustrated with the restraints and need your reassurance.

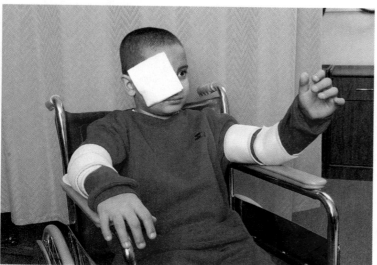

Elbow restraints can also be used to prevent adults from pulling out IVs and other tubing. This protective device prevents patients from bending their arm at the elbow.

An elbow restraint may be disposable, or it may be made of washable fabric. The washable elbow restraint is designed for inserting wooden tongue blades into pockets in the soft fabric. The blades provide extra stability and strength to the elbow area.

○ **Figure 6-29.** Elbow restraints may be used to prevent a young child from scratching a wound.

Procedure 6-7

Applying Elbow Restraints

Equipment: elbow restraints • tongue depressors • safety pins or Velcro straps (whichever is used for securing the restraints)

1. Make sure you have a written order for the restraint before beginning the procedure.
2. Place the tongue depressors in the slots of the elbow restraints.
3. Wash your hands.
4. Check the patient's ID bracelet and call the patient by name. Introduce yourself to the patient.
5. Provide privacy. Ask visitors to step out of the room.
6. Explain to the patient that you are going to apply a restraint.
7. Place the patient in a comfortable position with correct body alignment.
8. Wrap the restraint around the patient's elbow after checking the condition of the skin. (Do not apply a restraint to inflamed or broken skin.) The restraint is placed on top of clothing, pajamas, or padding.
9. Tie the straps around the arm.
10. Secure the restraint to the patient's shirt with the safety pins or Velcro straps.

> **SAFETY FIRST**
>
> Do not use safety pins to secure restraints on small children or babies. If the safety pin accidentally opens, it could puncture the skin. Use Velcro closures only for these patients.

11. Repeat steps 8 through 10 to apply the restraint to the other elbow.
12. Check the restraints for proper fit. They must be secure but not tight.
13. Give the patient the signal cord.
14. Place the patient in a comfortable position.
15. Unscreen the patient.
16. Wash your hands.
17. Check the patient every 15 to 30 minutes.

Reporting Restraint Use. Health facilities have policies and procedures for reporting information about patients' restraints in their medical records. Correct reporting of the use of restraints is essential to meet legal and ethical requirements. At a minimum, you are required to report:

- The type of restraint used.
- How long it was applied.
- How often the patient was checked.

You *may* be required to report:

- The color and condition of the patient's skin when the restraint was removed.
- The type of care given when the restraint was removed.
- The ability of the patient to move when the restraint was removed.

You may also be required to report any patient complaints. For example, a patient might complain about tingling or numbness in the restrained area. Some patients may be confused about or agitated by the restraints, but remember that a restraint is not a punishment. Its purpose is to prevent harm to the patient.

Leadership

An important aspect of leadership is the ability to take necessary actions to ensure patient safety. When an incident occurs, you can demonstrate your leadership skills by reacting calmly and appropriately, within your scope of practice. Take the initiative to make the environment safe for the patient.

Incident Reports

In a health care facility, an **incident** is an accident, error, or unusual event involving a patient or resident. An incident is also called a *variance*. If an incident occurs, you must first take any action needed to secure the safety of the patient or resident. Then verbally report the incident to the nurse or supervisor immediately.

You will also need to file a formal written report within 24 hours. An **incident report**, or variance report, is a form used to report accidents, errors, or unusual events. These reports help employers compile facts and correct problems to prevent future accidents. In most states, they are required and regulated by state law. An incident report should document specific information about the incident, including the date, time, place, names of the patient and staff involved, and a thorough description of the event. **See Figure 6-30.**

INCIDENT REPORT

EMPLOYEE INVOLVED:
Name: _____
Address: _____
Phone: _____
Employee: _____
         (RN, PT, Aide, etc.)

PATIENT INVOLVED:
Name: _____
Address: _____
Phone: _____
FID #: _____

OTHERS INVOLVED: Name: _____ Phone: _____
                Address _____ Relationship: _____

Date of Incident: _____ Time of Incident: _____
Location of Incident:_____
Product/technique involved:_____ Amount: _____ (if applicable)
Incident Reported to: _____ Time: _____ Date: _____

DESCRIPTION OF INCIDENT: (1. Complete Workers Comp. form if on-job injury;
  2. Facts only, no conclusions)

_____
Employee Signature

FOLLOW-UP:
Family aware of incident:_____
Physician aware of incident: _____
Action Taken:

Follow-up/Supervisor's Comments:

Risk Evaluation and Feedback:

○ **Figure 6-30.** Complete incident reports honestly and objectively whenever an incident occurs.

Writing an Incident Report

Before you write an incident report, you must organize your thoughts so that you present a clear and true picture of what actually occurred. Before you begin filling in the actual incident report form, jot down points you need to include on scrap paper. Organize the points into a logical order. Sequential (ordered by time) organization is often best for incident reports. Number the points in the order you want to mention them in the report. Then use your notes to create the actual incident report.

Practice

Using the above suggestions, write an incident report for the following scenario: You work in a long-term care facility. Mrs. G. frequently walks in the hallways to exercise her legs. She is a low risk for falls because she is steady on her feet and has never complained of dizziness, so she walks without the help of a nursing assistant. This morning she is walking as usual. Suddenly, as you watch, an employee with a cart full of laundry supplies comes around the corner and bumps into her. Neither person had time to react to avoid the collision. Write an incident report telling what you saw. Use the format shown in Figure 6-30.

What to Report

Examples of incidents that should be reported include patient falls, all other patient injuries or accidents, violent behavior, and the loss or theft of belongings. Most agencies have specific policies and procedures to follow when filling out incident reports, based on individual state requirements. Check with your supervisor to find out the proper procedures, as well as incidents that require reporting in your state.

When to File the Report

Filing incident reports as soon as possible after the event is part of keeping the workplace safe. Always be completely honest and objective when filling out an incident report. You may feel uncomfortable reporting an incident if it happened because a coworker was irresponsible. However, you must always keep your patients' safety—and your own safety—in mind. By reporting an incident, you can help prevent accidents and other incidents from happening again.

Chapter Summary

- Nursing assistants provide for the safety needs of patients to help prevent accidents and emergencies.

- Hazardous materials have the potential to cause harm and must be handled appropriately following safety guidelines outlined in material safety data sheets.

- A fire emergency requires a nursing assistant to be prepared, remain calm, and understand the proper use of fire extinguishers and fire blankets.

- Nursing assistants should prepare for disasters by learning the procedures established by the community and health care facility for handling each type of disaster.

- The nursing assistant must verify the patient's identity before providing care to ensure that the right care is given to each patient.

- Nursing assistants help identify who is at risk for falls, are aware of hazards leading to falls, and take simple steps to help reduce the risk of falls.

- Patients who are receiving oxygen have special safety needs.

- Restraints are designed to protect the patient from harm and should be used only when all other care options and alternatives have been tried and have failed.

- Nursing assistants file incident reports for legal protection and to reduce the risk of an incident occurring again.

VOCABULARY REVIEW

Directions: Match the letter of each definition in the second column with the correct vocabulary term. Write your answers on a separate sheet of paper.

Vocabulary

1. MSDS
2. ambulatory
3. chemical restraints
4. Class A fire extinguisher
5. Class B fire extinguisher
6. Class C fire extinguisher
7. disaster
8. emergency
9. hazardous material
10. incident report
11. physical restraints

Definitions

A. Any agent that has the potential to cause harm
B. An extinguisher for fires involving grease
C. A form used to report accidents, errors, or unusual events
D. Protective devices that limit movement and keep patients from harming themselves or others
E. Able to walk with or without the help of a walking aid
F. An extinguisher for electrical fires and flammable gases
G. A document that provides information about the potential hazards of a particular substance
H. An extinguisher for fires involving combustibles
I. A sudden catastrophic event that injures many people and causes major damage
J. An event calling for immediate action
K. Medications given to decrease activity and control behavior

Check Your Knowledge

Review Questions: Answer each of the following questions on a separate sheet of paper.

1. What should you do if you find a piece of equipment that is not working properly?

2. Why must you be careful about fire safety in an area where patients receive oxygen?

3. What three elements are required to sustain a fire?

4. What can you do to help families in the home prepare for a possible fire emergency?

5. What are the four critical steps in a fire emergency?

6. When using a fire extinguisher, what are the four critical steps to follow?

7. Name three types of walking aids that are commonly used in hospitals and long-term care facilities.

8. What is a nasal cannula?

9. How often should a physical restraint be removed from a patient? Why?

10. Why is a clove hitch used to tie physical restraints?

True or False: Read each statement carefully. Then write *True* or *False* by the statement number on a separate sheet of paper.

1. Patients are allowed to walk around in their bare feet in hot weather.

2. If the patient's name is posted above the bed in a hospital, it is not necessary to check the patient's identification before providing care.

3. Restraints are used for the convenience of the health care worker.

4. Keep the side rails on an unconscious patient's bed up, unless you are giving patient care or are otherwise instructed by your supervisor.

5. Before applying a restraint, always explain the procedure to the patient and family.

Think and Decide

Directions: Think about each of the following scenarios. Answer each question on a separate sheet of paper.

1. A 45-year-old patient in the hospital is refusing to have his side rails raised because he says he is sure he will not fall out of bed. Should you notify the nurse? Why or why not?

2. You are visiting the home of a 72-year-old client who has a space heater sitting right next to the home's gas stove. What should you do?

3. The doctor has prescribed continuous oxygen by nasal cannula for your home health client. The first day, the client seems to accept the cannula and everything is fine. However, when you arrive the next morning, you find that the client has removed the cannula and turned off the oxygen. When you ask about it, he tells you that the nasal cannula was too limiting. He couldn't get up and move around, and he got tired of sitting in one place all the time, so he just took it off. What should you do?

4. You walk into the room of a long-term resident and notice that the curtain is on fire. What should you do *first*?

5. An 89-year-old long-term care resident is on oxygen therapy continuously with a nasal cannula. When you walk in to help the patient bathe, you notice that the oxygen is turned off, and the patient is acting more confused than usual. Should you notify the nurse? Why or why not?

6. You are working in a facility that emphasizes a restraint-free environment. One patient with Alzheimer's disease is particularly agitated every afternoon at around 4 o'clock. Since the staff knows this is likely to occur, what are some steps they can take to help the patient?

7. The long-term care facility in which you work is participating in a community "Disaster Preparedness" week. Employees have been assigned to teams to create an emergency plan for specific types of disasters. The disaster assigned to your team is flooding. Consider all of the problems a flood can cause for a long-term care facility. Then prepare a draft of an emergency plan for floods that takes those problems into account. Include the entire staff in your plan.

8. Mr. R. has a history of trying to pull out his IV line, and once he actually succeeded. At the beginning of your shift today, you discover that Mr. R. has been placed in mitt restraints. He complains to you that the IV site "really hurts." You look at the site and notice that the area around it is swollen. What should you do?

CNA Certification Exam Prep

Directions: This practice test contains ten questions. Each question has four suggested answers. For each question, choose the ONE that best answers the question or completes the statement. Write your answers on a separate sheet of paper.

1. What type of fire extinguisher should you use for an electrical fire?
   A. Class A
   B. Class B
   C. Class C
   D. Class D

2. What can a nursing assistant do to prevent a resident from falling?
   A. darken the room to prevent glare
   B. clean up spills right away
   C. keep the bed in the highest position
   D. help keep the resident's feet warm

3. Which of the following statements about side rails is true?
   A. In most facilities, side rails are left up on all patient beds to help reduce falls.
   B. If a resident is on bed rest, you can raise the side rails to keep her in bed.
   C. Side rails should be left down if a patient is unconscious.
   D. Some patients consider having the side rails up embarrassing and demeaning.

4. Safety hazards for the elderly may include
   A. frayed electrical cords.
   B. open windows.
   C. rugs with nonskid backing.
   D. all of the above.

5. In the acronym R.A.C.E., what does the A stand for?
   A. answer patients' questions
   B. alert authorities
   C. activate alarms
   D. ask for instructions

6. When using a fire extinguisher, where should you aim the nozzle?
   A. at the top of the fire
   B. at the middle of the fire
   C. at the base of the fire
   D. around the outside of the fire

7. If you have a resident at risk for falls, your action as a nursing assistant is to
   A. apply wrist and ankle restraints.
   B. apply a jacket restraint.
   C. apply a belt restraint.
   D. report to your supervisor.

8. MSDS stands for
   A. Method of Saving Data for Supervisors.
   B. Medical Standards for Data Storage.
   C. Material Standards for Data Safety.
   D. Material Safety Data Sheets.

9. When restraints are removed from a resident, what is the minimum amount of time they should be off before they are reapplied?
   A. 5 minutes
   B. 10 minutes
   C. 15 minutes
   D. 30 minutes

10. Which of the following items is an example of personal protection equipment that is often needed by a nursing assistant?
    A. disposable gloves
    B. steel-toed boots
    C. security needs
    D. gas masks

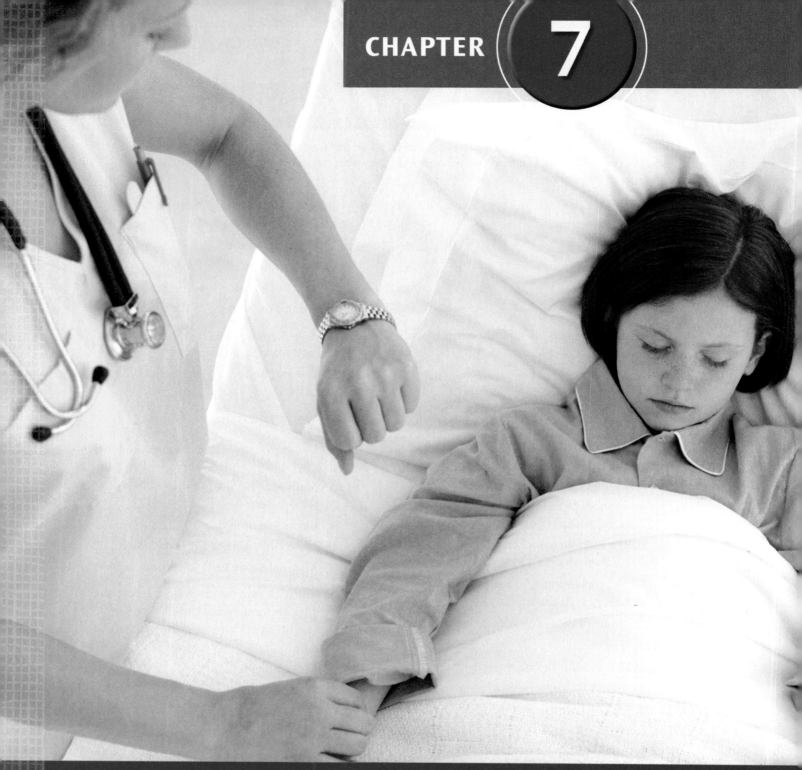

CHAPTER 7

OBJECTIVES

- Explain the importance of measuring the vital signs to patient care.
- Measure and record a person's temperature.
- Measure and record a person's pulse rate.
- Identify normal and abnormal respiration.
- Count a person's rate of respiration.
- Identify normal and abnormal blood pressure values.
- Measure and record a person's blood pressure.
- Explain how to determine a person's pain level.
- Measure a person's height and weight.

Vital Signs

VOCABULARY

apical pulse The pulse heard over the apex of the heart. The apex is the tip of the heart. It is located just below the left nipple.

apical-radial pulse Measurement of the apical and radial pulse at the same time.

apnea The lack of respirations.

blood pressure A measure of the force of the blood flow against artery walls.

body temperature An indicator of the amount of heat in the body. The body temperature equals the amount of heat produced by the body less the amount of heat lost by the body.

bradycardia A slow heart rate; fewer than 60 pulse beats per minute.

bradypnea Slow breathing; fewer than 12 breaths per minute.

Cheyne-Stokes breathing A pattern of breathing in which a series of very deep breaths is followed by very short, shallow breaths.

diastole The period during which the heart muscle relaxes; the heart is at rest.

diastolic pressure A measure of the pressure in the arteries between beats, when the heart is at rest.

dyspnea Difficult, labored, or painful breathing.

hypertension Abnormally high blood pressure.

hypotension Abnormally low blood pressure.

pedal pulse The pulse measured over the dorsalis pedis artery on the top of the foot.

prehypertension Blood pressure that is slightly higher than normal.

pulse deficit The difference between the apical and radial pulses.

pulse oximeter An instrument that measures the percentage of oxygen in the blood.

pulse rate The rate at which the heart beats. The pulse is felt over an artery as waves of blood pass through it.

radial pulse The pulse measured at the wrist.

respiration The process of inhaling (breathing in) and exhaling (breathing out).

shallow breathing Partial breaths that do not fill the lungs with air.

sphygmomanometer A device used to measure blood pressure; often referred to as a *blood pressure cuff*.

stertorous breathing Breaths accompanied by noises.

stethoscope An instrument used to listen to the sounds produced by the heart, lungs, and other body organs.

systole The period during which the heart muscle contracts, pumping blood through the blood vessels.

systolic pressure A measure of the pressure in the arteries when the heart contracts.

tachycardia A rapid heart rate; more than 100 pulse beats per minute.

tachypnea Fast breathing; more than 20 breaths per minute.

thermometer A device used to measure body temperature.

vital signs Important indicators of how body systems are functioning. The basic vital signs include temperature, pulse, respirations, and blood pressure. Pain level is often considered the "fifth" vital sign. In some cases, height and weight are also included.

Working with Vital Signs

An important part of the nursing assistant's job is measuring vital signs. **Vital signs** are important indicators of how well the systems of the body are functioning. The term *vital* means "related to life." The vital signs include body temperature, pulse, respiration, and blood pressure. Some states also include pain level with the vital signs.

Checking a person's vital signs provides a quick summary of three body processes that are essential for life:

- Regulation of body temperature (circulatory system)
- Breathing (respiratory system)
- Heart function (cardiac system)

Vital signs are measured to detect changes in normal body functions. They are affected by sleep, activity, eating, weather, noise, exercise, drugs, anger, fear, anxiety, pain, and illness. They tell about a person's response to treatment.

Accuracy is very important in measuring, recording, and reporting vital signs. If you are unsure of your measurement, *never guess*. Ask your supervisor to check it again and explain why.

Unless otherwise ordered, vital signs are checked with the person lying down or sitting. The person should be at rest when vital signs are measured.

Report the following items to your supervisor at once:

- Changes in vital sign measurement from a previous reading
- Vital signs above the normal range
- Vital signs below the normal range

Vital signs are recorded on graphic sheets or entered into a person's computer record. If the vital signs for a patient are ordered frequently, they are recorded on a flow sheet. **See Figure 7-1.** The doctor and nurse compare the current and past measurements to see how the person is doing.

Measuring Body Temperature

Body temperature is an indicator of the amount of heat in the body. The body is continually making and losing heat. Exercise and other forms of internal and external activity create heat. The body loses heat in a number of ways, including

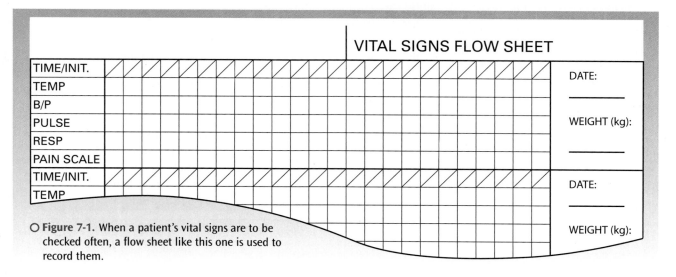

VITAL SIGNS FLOW SHEET

TIME/INIT.																	DATE:
TEMP																	
B/P																	
PULSE																	WEIGHT (kg):
RESP																	
PAIN SCALE																	
TIME/INIT.																	DATE:
TEMP																	

○ **Figure 7-1.** When a patient's vital signs are to be checked often, a flow sheet like this one is used to record them.

WEIGHT (kg):

Vital Skills (WRITING)

Learning Log

The information in a patient's chart is a type of log. As lab tests are performed, their results are added to the chart. The patient's vital signs, consultations by experts, and other medical information are also kept in the chart. Like other logs, a patient's chart allows caregivers to note progress from day to day or even from hour to hour. This makes it easy to review a patient's status at a glance.

Logging can help you learn, too. By writing the information you learn each day, you are at once creating a great study tool and helping yourself remember the information. Studies have shown that when we write something down, we are more likely to remember it later.

O Figure A

Date	What I Learned Today	Follow-Up

Practice

1. Start a learning log for this chapter. Use the log in **Figure A** as a guide. Every day, add the information that you learned.
2. When you have finished the chapter, look through your log. Are your entries helpful? What might you do or write differently to make them more helpful?
3. Use your learning log in this and other chapters to help you study for exams.

perspiration and respiration, and through urine and feces. Body temperature is an important source of information about a person's condition.

In a healthy person, body temperature remains fairly stable. It is normal for it to vary a few degrees up or down during a 24-hour period. Temperature is usually lower in the morning and higher in the afternoon and evening. Temperature can be affected by what is happening inside the body, such as an infection. It can also be affected by external circumstances, such as very cold weather, exercise, and stress.

Normal body temperature also varies slightly depending on how and where it is measured. Common sites for measuring temperature include the mouth, rectum, axilla (armpit), and tympanic membrane (outer ear).

Body temperature is measured using a device called a **thermometer**. Common types of thermometers include glass, disposable, and digital. Most thermometers use either the Fahrenheit (F) or Celsius (C) scale. Normal ranges of body temperature for adults are shown in **Table 7-1**.

Table 7-1. Normal Temperature Ranges

Site of Measurement	Fahrenheit	Celsius
Oral	97.6° F to 99.6° F	36.5° C to 37.5° C
Axillary	96.6° F to 98.6° F	36.0° C to 37.0° C
Rectal	98.6° F to 100.6° F	37.0° C to 38.1° C
Tympanic Membrane	98.6° F	37.0° C

Glass Thermometers

Glass thermometers (clinical thermometers) are hollow tubes with a measurement scale printed on the glass. These thermometers used to contain mercury, which is extremely sensitive to temperature changes. When the temperature went up, the mercury in the glass tube expanded. As it expanded, the mercury flowed up the glass tube, causing the temperature reading on the scale to rise. However, mercury is a highly toxic substance. Glass thermometers today use a nontoxic mercury-like substance such as Galinstan®.

Types of Glass Thermometers. There are several different types of glass thermometers. An oral thermometer measures a patient's temperature in the mouth or under the arm. Oral thermometers generally have a thin, elongated bulb at the end. Rectal thermometers have a stubby, round bulb and are used to measure temperature when inserted in the rectum. A security thermometer also has a round bulb, but is smaller and is used to measure an infant's temperature rectally.

Many facilities use only one type of thermometer for measuring oral, rectal, and axillary temperatures. They use different plastic covers instead of different thermometers. **See Figure 7-2.** Your facility will have specific policies regarding the use and cleaning of thermometers.

Facilities vary widely in the treatment and care of glass thermometers. Some facilities disinfect all thermometers and use them for patients as needed. Others keep a thermometer in each patient's room. That thermometer is cleaned and disinfected right in the room and is used for that patient only. It is best if oral and rectal thermometers are cleaned and stored separately. This is often not possible when facilities use only one type of thermometer for all temperature measurements.

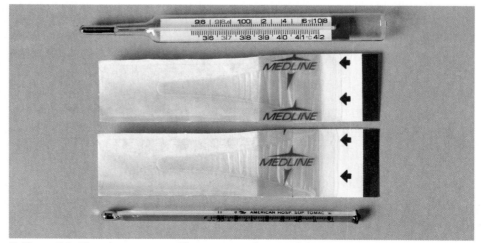

○ **Figure 7-2.** Glass thermometers. The one on top is a rectal thermometer. The one on the bottom is an oral thermometer.

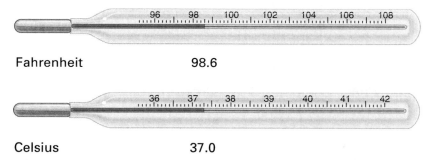

Fahrenheit   98.6

Celsius   37.0

○ **Figure 7-3.** The top thermometer shows a normal reading on a Fahrenheit scale. The bottom thermometer shows a normal reading on a Celsius scale.

Reading a Glass Thermometer. Glass thermometers have a series of long and short lines printed on the side of the tube. On a Fahrenheit thermometer, the long lines indicate whole degrees. The short lines mark two-tenths of a degree. The scale begins at 94° F and goes to 108° F. On a Celsius thermometer, each long line measures one degree. Each short line marks one-tenth of a degree. The scale ranges from 34° C to 42° C. **See Figure 7-3.**

Procedure 7-1   SP OBRA

Reading a Glass Thermometer

Equipment: glass thermometer

1. Pick up the thermometer and hold it at the stem end, using only your thumb and the tips of your fingers. **See Figure 7-4.**
2. Bring the thermometer to eye level and turn it until the side with the printed scale is facing you.
3. Slowly rotate the thermometer until you can see the mercury-like substance inside the tube.

4. Read the measurement. Whether you are using a Fahrenheit or Celsius thermometer, your reading should be to the nearest two-tenths of a degree.
5. Write down the temperature in your notebook or on a form, according to the facility's policy.

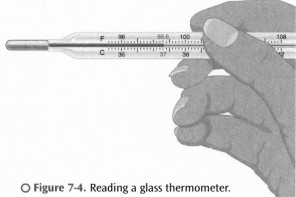

○ **Figure 7-4.** Reading a glass thermometer.

Guidelines for Measuring Temperature Orally

If a patient has had hot or cold food or fluid or has smoked, wait 15 minutes before checking the oral temperature. Temperature should not be measured orally if the patient:

- Is unconscious.
- Has had an injury or surgery to the face, neck, nose, or mouth.
- Is receiving oxygen.
- Breathes through the mouth.
- Has a nasogastric tube.
- Is paralyzed on one side of the body.

Procedure 7-2

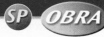

Measuring Oral Temperature with a Glass Thermometer

Equipment: thermometer • tissues • plastic sleeves

1. Identify the patient, check the ID bracelet, and call the patient by name.
2. Introduce yourself.
3. Explain the procedure to the patient.
4. Wash your hands.
5. Provide privacy.
6. Hold the thermometer at the stem end.
7. Run cold water over the thermometer if it has been soaking in a disinfectant.
8. Gently dry the thermometer with tissues, starting at the stem and working toward the bulb.
9. Check the thermometer for cracks or chips.
10. Shake down the thermometer to below 95° F (35° C) by holding it firmly and then snapping your wrist downward.
11. Slide a plastic sleeve over the thermometer. **See Figure 7-5.**
12. Insert the bulb end of the thermometer under the patient's tongue.
13. Have the patient close the lips to help hold the thermometer in place.
14. Wait 3 to 5 minutes.
15. Gently grasp the end of the thermometer and remove it from the patient's mouth.
16. Remove the plastic sleeve and discard in the wastepaper basket. Be careful not to touch the bulb end of the thermometer.
17. Read the thermometer and record the reading according to facility policy.

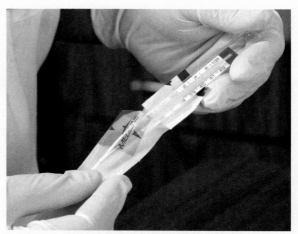

○ **Figure 7-5.** Putting a plastic sleeve on a thermometer.

18. Rinse, wash, and dry the thermometer under cool water.
19. Shake down the thermometer.
20. Soak the thermometer in the thermometer holder with disinfectant solution according to your facility's policy.
21. Check to make sure the patient is comfortable and place the signal light within reach.
22. Unscreen the patient.
23. Wash your hands.
24. Report abnormal temperature readings to the nurse.
25. Record the measurement in your notebook or on a form, according to the facility's policy.

- Has a sore mouth.
- Is combative or disoriented.
- Is an infant or a child younger than five years of age.

Guidelines for Measuring Temperature Rectally

If a patient has just had a bowel movement or has just had the anal area cleaned, wait 15 minutes before measuring the rectal temperature. Temperatures should not be measured rectally if the patient:
- Has had rectal surgery.
- Has a rectal injury or disorder.
- Has diarrhea.
- Has heart disease.
- Is confused or combative.

Procedure 7-3

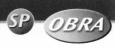

Measuring Rectal Temperature with a Glass Thermometer

Equipment: rectal thermometer • toilet tissue • plastic sleeves • disposable gloves • paper towels • water-soluble lubricant

1. Identify the patient, check the ID bracelet, and call the patient by name.
2. Introduce yourself.
3. Explain the procedure to the patient.
4. Wash your hands. Put on disposable gloves.
5. Provide privacy.
6. Hold the thermometer at the stem end.
7. Run cold water over the thermometer if it has been soaking in a disinfectant.
8. Gently dry the thermometer with tissues, starting at the stem and working toward the bulb.
9. Check the thermometer for cracks or chips.
10. Shake down the thermometer to below 95° F (35° C) by holding it firmly and then snapping your wrist downward.
11. Cover the thermometer with a plastic sleeve.
12. Place a small amount of water-soluble lubricant on a piece of toilet tissue. Lubricate the bulb end of the thermometer to ease insertion.
13. Ask the patient to lie on his or her side. Help the patient turn, if necessary. (If the patient is apprehensive, suggest he or she take a deep breath and slowly exhale as the thermometer is being inserted.)

14. Fold back just enough of the linens to expose the patient's buttocks.
15. With one hand, raise the upper buttock to expose the anus.
16. Using the other hand, gently insert the thermometer ½ inch into the rectum. **See Figure 7-6.**

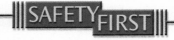

Be very gentle when inserting a rectal thermometer to avoid perforating (puncturing) the rectum.

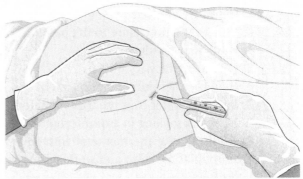

○ **Figure 7-6.** Inserting a rectal thermometer.

17. Hold the thermometer in place for 3 minutes.
18. Remove the thermometer from the patient's rectum.
19. Wipe the patient's anal area with toilet tissue to remove the lubricant. Re-cover the patient's buttocks with the bed linens.
20. Remove the plastic sleeve and discard in the wastepaper basket. Place the used toilet tissue on a paper towel and place the thermometer on a clean paper towel. Discard soiled toilet tissue into the toilet.
21. Read the thermometer and record the reading.
22. Shake down the thermometer.

23. Rinse, wash, and dry the thermometer under cool water. Remove your gloves and discard them.
24. Soak the thermometer in the thermometer holder with disinfectant solution.
25. Wash your hands.
26. Place the signal light within reach and check to make sure the patient is comfortable.
27. Unscreen the patient.
28. Report abnormal temperature readings to the nurse.
29. Record the measurement in the proper place. Place an "R" next to the reading to indicate that it was a rectal reading.

Guidelines for Measuring the Axillary Temperature

If the patient has just cleaned the axilla area or has just applied underarm deodorant or antiperspirant, wait 15 minutes before checking the axillary temperature. The temperature should not be measured on the side of the body that has had recent chest or breast surgery.

Procedure 7-4

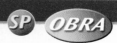

Measuring Axillary Temperature with a Glass Thermometer

Equipment: thermometer • tissues • plastic sleeves

1. Identify the patient and call the patient by name.
2. Introduce yourself.
3. Explain the procedure to the patient.
4. Wash your hands.
5. Provide privacy.
6. Hold the thermometer at the stem end.
7. Run cold water over the thermometer if it has been soaking in a disinfectant.
8. Gently dry the thermometer with tissues, starting at the stem and working toward the bulb.

9. Check the thermometer for cracks or chips.
10. Shake down the thermometer to below 95° F (35° C) by holding it firmly and then snapping your wrist downward.
11. Slide a plastic sleeve over the thermometer.
12. Assist the patient in removing an arm from his or her shirt or gown.
13. Pat the axilla gently with a towel.
14. Position the bulb end of the thermometer in the center of the axilla.

15. Ask the patient to hold the arm close to the body or place the arm over the chest to hold the thermometer in place. **See Figure 7-7.**
16. Wait 10 minutes and then remove the thermometer.
17. Remove the plastic sleeve and discard in the wastepaper basket. Be careful not to touch the bulb end.
18. Read the thermometer and record the reading.
19. Rinse, wash, and dry the thermometer.
20. Shake down the thermometer.
21. Soak the thermometer in the thermometer holder with disinfectant solution.
22. Place the signal light within reach and check to make sure the patient is comfortable.
23. Unscreen the patient.
24. Wash your hands.
25. Report abnormal temperature readings to the nurse.

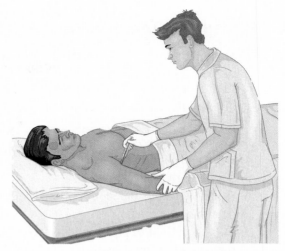

○ **Figure 7-7.** Measuring temperature under the arm using a glass thermometer.

26. Record the measurement in the proper place. Place an "A" next to the reading to indicate that it was an axillary reading.

Disposable Thermometers

Some facilities use disposable paper or plastic thermometers to measure oral temperature. These thermometers are convenient because they measure the temperature in approximately 45 seconds and do not require cleaning. They are used once and then disposed of. Disposable thermometers contain small dots that change color in response to heat.

Electronic Thermometers

Some thermometers are electronic or battery-operated devices that measure body temperature digitally. They are used to measure temperature orally, rectally, and tympanically (in the ear). They measure temperature in approximately 20 to 60 seconds. The handheld unit is kept in a battery charger when not in use. Electronic thermometers meant for oral and rectal use have oral and rectal probes and use a disposable cover or sheath to cover the probe. Tympanic thermometers have a probe designed to fit in the ear and are also used with disposable covers. **See Figure 7-8.**

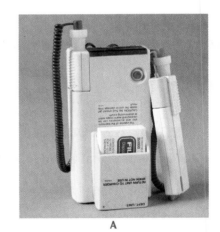

A

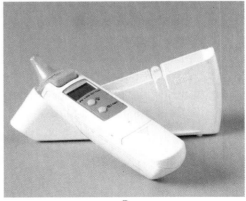

B

○ **Figure 7-8.** The digital thermometer shown in (A) is used to measure oral (blue probe) and rectal (red probe) temperatures. The tympanic thermometer shown in (B) is used to measure temperature in the ear.

Procedure 7-5

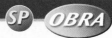

Measuring Temperature with a Tympanic Thermometer

Equipment: tympanic thermometer • probe cover

1. Identify the patient, check the ID bracelet, and call the patient by name.
2. Introduce yourself.
3. Explain the procedure to the patient.
4. Wash your hands.
5. Provide privacy.
6. Place the cone-shaped end of the thermometer into a probe cover.
7. Ask the patient to position his or her head so the ear is in front of you.
8. Gently grasp the outer portion of the patient's earlobe and pull it up and back to allow easier access to the ear canal.
9. Insert the covered probe into the patient's ear canal, pointing the probe down and toward the front of the canal. Press the button to start the reading.
10. Hold the probe in place until you hear or see a signal from the probe. Some models flash a light when the measurement is finished. Other models sound a tone.
11. Remove the probe from the ear canal.
12. Read the probe and record the reading. Place a "T" next to the reading to indicate that it was a tympanic reading.
13. Remove and discard the probe cover.
14. Place the thermometer back in its battery charger.
15. Place the signal light within reach and check to make sure the patient is comfortable.
16. Unscreen the patient.
17. Wash your hands.
18. Report abnormal temperature readings to the nurse.
19. Record the measurement in the proper place.

Procedure 7-6

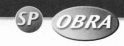

Measuring Temperature with a Digital Thermometer

Equipment: digital thermometer • oral probe • disposable probe sleeves

1. Identify the patient, check the ID bracelet, and call the patient by name.
2. Introduce yourself.
3. Explain the procedure to the patient.
4. Wash your hands.
5. Provide privacy.
6. Place a probe cover over the probe.
7. Ask the patient to wet his or her lips.
8. Insert the probe under the patient's tongue.
9. Hold the probe in place. **See Figure 7-9.**

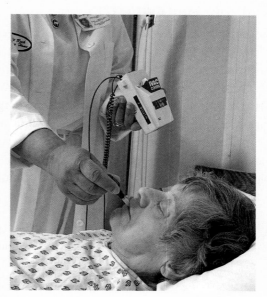

O **Figure 7-9.** Using a digital thermometer.

10. When the temperature measurement is complete, the probe will emit a tone, or a light will flash or stay on continuously. When you hear or see the signal, gently grasp the end of the thermometer and remove it from the patient's mouth.
11. Read and record the patient's temperature.
12. Press the button that ejects the probe cover. Discard the cover into the wastebasket.
13. Place the probe back in the probe holder.
14. Place the signal light within reach and check to make sure the patient is comfortable.
15. Place the thermometer in the charging unit.
16. Unscreen the patient.
17. Wash your hands.
18. Report abnormal temperature readings to the nurse.
19. Record the measurement in the proper place.

Vital Skills   READING

Reading Strategy

Readers generally understand what they read and remember it longer if they have a strategy for reading. One such strategy is to follow specific steps such as these:

- **Pre-Reading:** Preview the text and predict what it will be about. Based on your prediction, establish a purpose for reading.
- **Reading:** Read the text. As you read, connect what you are reading with your own ideas and prior knowledge. Think about how the text fits in with what you already know.
- **Looking Back:** After you read the passage, think about the purpose you established in the Pre-Reading step. Did you achieve your goal? Write down any questions you have about the material.
- **Re-Reading:** Read any parts or sentences you do not understand again. If you still have trouble, ask someone to explain it to you.
- **Remembering:** Discuss what you read and your ideas about it with other people. Summarize the information in the text and list your reactions to it.

Thermometer Handles and Probes

Often you will see variations in the color of thermometer handles and probes. A blue probe indicates that the thermometer should be used for oral and axillary temperatures. A red probe indicates that it should be used for rectal temperatures. Some digital thermometers have two probes: one blue and one red. The color helps in maintaining infection control. There is no difference in their measuring capabilities.

○ Figure A

Practice

Read the text in Figure A. Use the reading strategy discussed here. Write your predictions, purpose, questions, summary, and reactions to the text on a separate sheet of paper or in your learning log.

Measuring a Patient's Pulse Rate

When the heart beats, it pumps blood out to the body through the arteries. This pumping causes the arteries to expand. When the heart rests between beats, the arteries contract. The **pulse rate** is the pressure that can be felt in the artery every time the heart beats.

Pulse measurements provide an overall indication of how well a patient's cardiovascular system is functioning. The pulse rate is affected by many different factors. Emotions such as anger, anxiety, and fear can cause the pulse rate to increase. Exercise, body temperature, air temperature, body position, pain, and certain medications can also cause a higher pulse rate. Other medications can slow the pulse rate. The normal adult pulse rate is between 60 and 100 beats a minute. **See Table 7-2.** Higher or lower readings are abnormal and need to be reported to your supervisor right away.

Table 7-2. Normal Pulse Rates for Various Age Groups

Age	Range
Newborn	120–160
1 month–1 year	80–140
1–6 years	80–120
6 years–adolescence	75–110
Adulthood	60–100
Late adulthood	60–80

When measuring a pulse, also observe the following:
- Pulse rhythm is the contraction and expansion of an artery as the blood passes through the vessel. A normal pulse occurs in a predictable, rhythmic pattern. If a patient has an abnormal pulse rhythm, the time between beats is irregular.
- Pulse force is the amount of force exerted on the arterial walls as the blood is forced through. A strong pulse is easy to feel. Weaker pulses can be hard to find and feel.
- Pulse volume is the amount of blood that is pumped through the arteries.

Abnormal pulse rhythms and weak pulse readings should be reported immediately.

The pulse can be measured at various locations. Most commonly, it is checked at the wrist. Pulse measured at the wrist is called a **radial pulse** because the blood in the wrist flows through the radial artery. *Note:* When checking a radial pulse, never let your thumb touch the patient's wrist, because your thumb has a pulse of its own. Pulse readings can also be checked at the brachial, carotid, dorsalis pedis, femoral, popliteal, posterior tibial, and temporal arteries. **See Figure 7-10.**

The **pedal pulse** is measured over the dorsalis pedis artery on the top of the foot. When measuring the pedal pulse, it is very important not to apply deep pressure. If too much pressure is applied, the pulse will disappear. Place two fingers on the top of the foot and apply gentle pressure. Count the pulse for 1 minute. Then repeat on the other foot. If a pedal pulse is not felt, report it to the nurse at once. An absent pulse can be a sign of peripheral vascular disease (PVD), stroke, or decreased circulation to lower extremities due to diabetes. Pedal pulses are also checked routinely after certain surgeries.

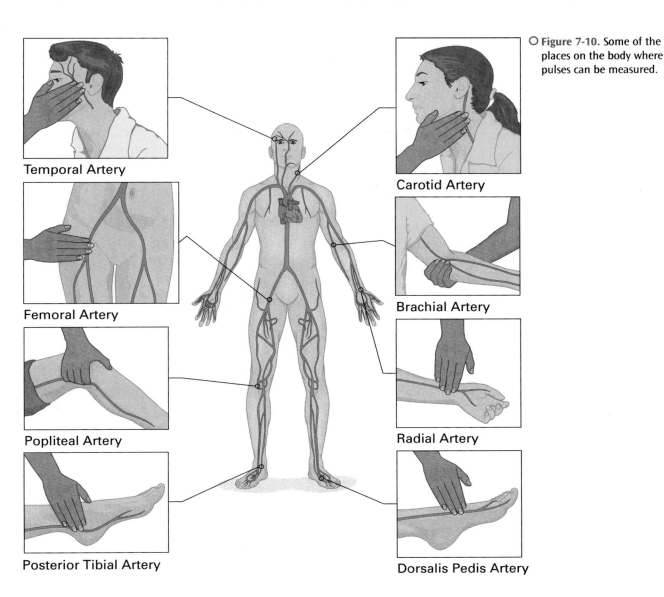

Temporal Artery

Femoral Artery

Popliteal Artery

Posterior Tibial Artery

Carotid Artery

Brachial Artery

Radial Artery

Dorsalis Pedis Artery

○ **Figure** 7-10. Some of the places on the body where pulses can be measured.

The **apical pulse** is located 2 to 3 inches to the left of the sternum (breastbone) and below the left nipple. It is measured with a stethoscope. A **stethoscope** is a device for listening to sounds produced by the heart, lungs, and other body organs. **See Figure 7-11.** By amplifying sounds that occur in the body, a stethoscope makes it easier to hear the sounds clearly and accurately.

The apical and radial pulses should be equal. In some patients, these pulses differ. The difference between the apical and radial pulses is called the **pulse deficit**. *Note:* In some states, nursing assistants are not allowed to measure apical pulses. The apical and radial pulses measured simultaneously are known as the **apical-radial pulse**.

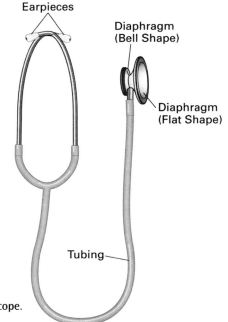

Earpieces

Diaphragm (Bell Shape)

Diaphragm (Flat Shape)

Tubing

○ **Figure 7-11.** The parts of a stethoscope.

Procedure 7-7

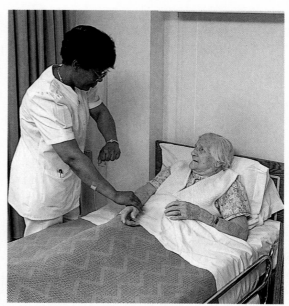

SP OBRA

Measuring a Radial Pulse

Equipment: none

1. Identify the patient, check the ID bracelet, and call the patient by name.
2. Introduce yourself.
3. Explain the procedure to the patient. Ask the patient to sit or lie down and remain quiet and still during the procedure.
4. Wash your hands.
5. Provide privacy.
6. Locate the radial pulse in the patient's wrist using your middle two or three fingers. **See Figure 7-12.**
7. Note the strength and regularity of the pulse.
8. Begin counting the pulse beats and continue counting for 1 minute.
9. Record the pulse rate, force, and rhythm.
10. Place the signal light within reach and check to make sure the patient is comfortable.
11. Unscreen the patient.
12. Wash your hands.
13. Report readings to the nurse immediately if the patient's pulse rate is less than 60 beats per minute or greater than 100 beats per minute, or if any irregularities are heard. **Bradycardia** is a condition with fewer than

○ **Figure 7-12.** Checking a radial pulse.

60 pulse beats per minute. **Tachycardia** is a condition with more than 100 beats per minute.

14. Record the measurement in the proper place.

Procedure 7-8

SP

Measuring an Apical Pulse

Equipment: stethoscope • alcohol wipes

1. Identify the patient, check the ID bracelet, and call the patient by name.
2. Introduce yourself.
3. Explain the procedure to the patient. Ask the patient to be quiet and still during the procedure.
4. Wash your hands.
5. Provide privacy.
6. Using alcohol wipes, clean the diaphragm and earpieces of the stethoscope.
7. Hold the diaphragm in your hand to warm it before placing it on the patient's skin.
8. Position the earpieces in your ears.
9. Place the diaphragm directly over the heart. Keep the diaphragm in position by using the tips of your index and middle fingers.

10. Check to be sure the tubing that connects the diaphragm to the earpieces is free and clear of any objects.
11. Note the strength and regularity of the pulse.
12. Begin counting the pulse beats and continue counting for 1 minute.
13. When you are finished measuring, remove the stethoscope from the patient and then from your ears. Record your measurement.
14. Place the signal light within reach and check to make sure the patient is comfortable.
15. Wipe the earpieces and the diaphragm with alcohol wipes.
16. Store the stethoscope in its appropriate place.
17. Wash your hands.
18. Record the measurement in the proper place.

Measuring Respirations

Respiration is the process of inhaling (breathing in) and exhaling (breathing out). When we inhale, oxygen enters the body and is distributed to the cells. When we exhale, carbon dioxide leaves the body. One inhalation together with one exhalation is considered one respiration.

Respiration Patterns

Normal breathing is quiet and effortless, and follows a regular pattern. Both sides of the chest should rise and fall equally. Respirations are measured in breaths per minute (bpm). Normal rates of respiration are shown in **Table 7-3**.

Table 7-3. Normal Respiration Rates for Various Age Groups

Age Group	Range
Newborns	30–80 bpm
Children	16–30 bpm
Adolescents	15–20 bpm
Adults	12–20 bpm
Older Adults	15–25 bpm

There are a number of abnormal patterns of respiration:
- **Apnea**—the lack of respirations
- **Bradypnea**—fewer than 12 bpm
- **Cheyne-Stokes breathing**—a pattern of breathing in which a series of very deep breaths is followed by very short, shallow breaths. Breathing may stop (apnea) for 10 to 20 seconds.
- **Dyspnea**—difficult, labored, or painful breathing
- **Shallow breathing**—partial breaths that do not fill the lungs with air
- **Stertorous breathing**—breaths accompanied by noises
- **Tachypnea**—more than 20 bpm

Counting Respirations

The patient should be at rest when you measure respirations. You should be able to see the patient's chest rise and fall with each breath. Your measurement of respirations should reflect the patient's relaxed, normal state.

Some patients do not breathe naturally when they are told their breathing is going to be measured. For this reason, you should not tell the patient when you are counting respirations. Respirations are usually measured immediately following a pulse measurement. Keep your fingers in place as if you are still measuring the pulse, so the patient does not know you are counting respirations. **See Figure 7-13.**

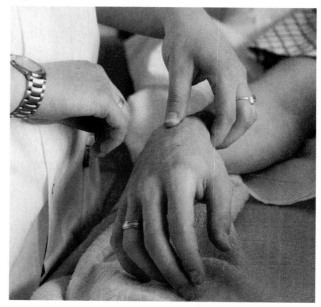

○ **Figure 7-13.** Pretend you are continuing to count a pulse while you actually are counting respirations.

Procedure   7-9

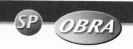

Observing and Measuring Respirations

Equipment: none

1. Identify the patient, check the ID bracelet, and call the patient by name.
2. Introduce yourself.
3. Explain the procedure to the patient. Ask the patient to sit or lie down and remain quiet and still during the procedure.
4. Wash your hands.
5. Provide privacy.
6. Locate the radial pulse in the patient's wrist using your middle two or three fingers.
7. Note the strength and regularity of the pulse.
8. Begin counting the pulse beats and continue counting for 1 minute.
9. Keep your fingers on the patient's wrist. Do not tell the patient that you are now going to measure respirations.
10. When you see the patient's chest rise, begin counting respirations. Each time the chest rises and falls, count one respiration. Continue counting for 1 minute.
11. While you are counting, observe the patient's breathing. Notice whether the patient experiences any difficulty breathing. Check to see whether both sides of the chest rise and fall equally. Observe whether the breaths are regular, and whether they are deep or shallow. Listen for noises while the patient is breathing.
12. After 1 minute has elapsed, stop counting. This is the respiratory rate.
13. Record the respiratory rate and your observations of the patient's breathing.
14. Place the signal light within reach and check to make sure the patient is comfortable.
15. Wash your hands.
16. Report any abnormal reading to the nurse immediately.
17. Record your measurement in the proper place.

Measuring Blood Pressure

Blood pressure is a measure of the force of the blood flow exerted against the walls of an artery. Blood pressure is affected by:

- The strength or force of the heart's pumping.
- The ease with which blood flows through the arteries.
- The amount of blood the heart pumps each time it beats.

A number of factors can influence a blood pressure reading. These include exercise, medications, pain, emotions, age, sex, stress, and the amount of blood in the body at any one time.

Measurement consists of two numbers. The first number represents the pressure of blood flow during **systole**—when the heart contracts. This is known as the **systolic pressure**. This phase is also known as **systole**. The second number represents the pressure of blood flow during **diastole**—when the heart rests between beats. This is called **diastolic pressure**. The blood pressure reading is measured in millimeters (mm) of mercury (Hg). For example, a typical reading might be 120/80 mm Hg.

Because blood pressure readings can vary within the same person from minute to minute, normal values are given in ranges. Abnormal readings are readings outside these ranges that occur consistently. **See Table 7-4.** Abnormally high blood pressure is known as **hypertension**. Blood pressure that is slightly higher than normal is called **prehypertension**. Abnormally low blood pressure is called **hypotension**.

Table 7-4. Blood Pressure Ranges

Classification	Systolic Blood Pressure (mm Hg)		Diastolic Blood Pressure (mm Hg)
Normal	<120	AND	<80
Prehypertension	120–139	OR	80–89
Stage 1 Hypertension	140–159	OR	90–99
Stage 2 Hypertension	≥160	OR	≥100

Blood pressure is measured by an instrument known as a **sphygmomanometer** and a stethoscope. **See Figure 7-14.** The sphygmomanometer consists of a cuff and a measuring device. To measure blood pressure, the cuff is placed around the patient's bare upper arm. Air is then pumped into the cuff by squeezing the bulb on the sphygmomanometer. A numerical scale on the pressure gauge of the sphygmomanometer shows the actual pressure. To measure blood pressure, you also need a stethoscope. The stethoscope is used to obtain the patient's pulse in the brachial artery in the arm.

Note that the exact number given for the systolic and diastolic readings depends to some degree on the type of sphygmomanometer you use. An electronic sphygmomanometer can give an odd-numbered reading such as 85. Mercury and aneroid sphygmomanometers are marked in even measurements of 2, so a reading of 85 is not possible.

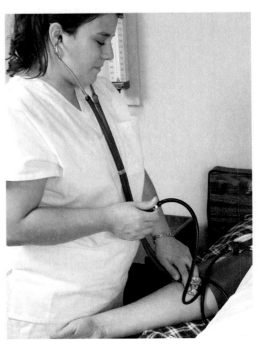

O **Figure 7-14.** Measuring blood pressure with a sphygmomanometer and a stethoscope. This method is considered the most accurate one.

Procedure 7-10

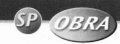

Measuring Blood Pressure

Equipment: sphygmomanometer • stethoscope • alcohol wipes

1. Identify the patient, check the ID bracelet, and call the patient by name.
2. Introduce yourself.
3. Explain the procedure to the patient.
4. Wash your hands.
5. Provide privacy.
6. Using alcohol wipes, clean the diaphragm and the earpieces of the stethoscope.
7. Ask the patient to sit or lie still.
8. Place the patient's arm in a position level with the heart, with the palm of the hand facing up. Make sure the patient is comfortable.
9. Uncover the patient's arm.
10. Squeeze the cuff on the sphygmomanometer to make sure there is no air in the cuff. Close the valve on the bulb.
11. Locate the patient's brachial artery. Place the cuff on the patient's arm, at least 1 inch above the elbow, with the tube over the brachial artery. Make sure the cuff is evenly positioned around the arm and then tighten it so it fits snugly. **See Figure 7-15.**
12. Put the stethoscope around your neck and insert the earpieces in your ears.
13. Find the patient's radial pulse at the wrist.
14. Explain to the patient that as the cuff inflates, he or she will feel a tightness in the arm that may be uncomfortable.
15. Place the diaphragm of the stethoscope over the patient's brachial artery at the inside of the elbow. Begin inflating the cuff by pumping the bulb with your other hand. **See Figure 7-16.**
16. Inflate the cuff an additional 30 mm after you no longer hear the patient's pulse.
17. Keep the stethoscope in place with the index and middle fingers. Do not use your thumb.
18. Turn the valve on the sphygmomanometer counterclockwise and begin to evenly

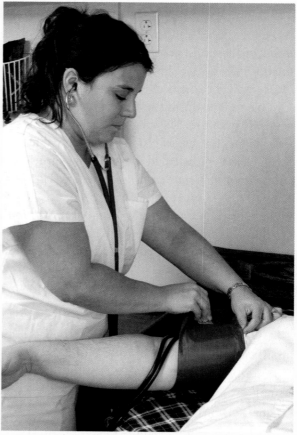

○ **Figure 7-15.** Positioning the cuff on the patient's arm.

deflate the cuff at a rate of 2 to 4 mm per second. **See Figure 7-17.**
19. Notice the reading on the scale when you first hear a sound. This is the patient's systolic reading.
20. As you continue to deflate the cuff, notice the reading on the scale when you no longer hear sound. This is the diastolic reading.
21. Continue letting air out of the cuff until it is completely deflated. Remove the cuff from the patient's arm. Remove the stethoscope.
22. Record the patient's blood pressure reading.
23. Clean the diaphragm and earpieces of the stethoscope with alcohol wipes.

24. Place the signal light within reach and check to make sure the patient is comfortable.
25. Unscreen the patient.
26. Place all equipment back where it belongs.
27. Wash your hands.
28. Report abnormal blood pressure readings to the nurse.
29. Record the measurement in the proper place.

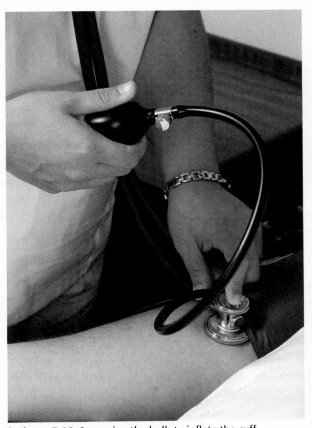

○ **Figure 7-16.** Squeezing the bulb to inflate the cuff.

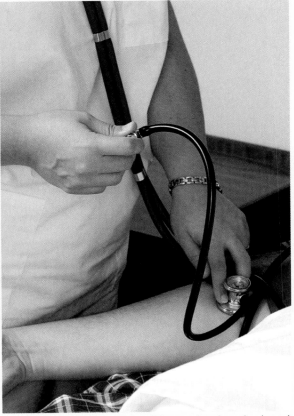

○ **Figure 7-17.** Deflating the cuff by rotating the valve (metal knob).

Pulse Oximetry

Many facilities today include a measure of blood oxygenation as a standard part of measuring vital signs. A **pulse oximeter** is an instrument that measures the percentage of oxygen in the blood. The most common type of pulse oximeter is one that attaches to the patient's finger. **See Figure 7-18.** Pulse oximetry can often detect changes in oxygen levels before other vital signs are affected.

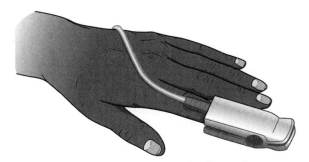

○ **Figure 7-18.** A pulse oximeter with a finger-clip sensor.

Pulse oximeters give readings in percent oxygen saturation. Readings of 95% to 100% are usually considered normal. Lower readings may be present in certain diseases, or they may indicate a new health problem. The nurse will tell you what the minimum percentage should be for a patient. Readings below this level should be reported and recorded. Readings below 70% are life-threatening and should be reported at once.

Determining Pain Level

In both acute and chronic illness, a patient's pain level should be monitored carefully. All pain medications have side effects. Some of those side effects lower a person's ability to function and process information. By knowing a patient's pain level, the doctor can adjust pain medications to keep the patient comfortable with as little loss of function and awareness as possible. If alternative pain management techniques are used, the doctor needs to know which techniques are effective for this patient.

A patient's level of pain also affects the patient in other ways. Intense pain can cause alterations in the patient's blood pressure, respiration, and even level of consciousness. For example, a patient with severe chest pain may breathe shallowly to avoid the intense pain that accompanies normal breathing. A method of determining pain level is therefore needed as a routine part of patient assessment.

Pain is not an easy thing to measure. For one thing, pain perception varies from one person to another. What may seem like intense pain to one person may not seem intense to someone else. People's approach to dealing with or showing pain is different in different cultures. The ability to withstand pain also varies. Some people endure extreme pain without asking for relief. Others find it difficult to endure less severe pain. Only the patient can tell you how much pain he or she is enduring.

Facilities use a pain scale to determine a patient's pain level. There are many different kinds of pain scales. The most commonly used scales are:
- Descriptive scale—Patient is asked to describe the pain as no pain, mild, moderate, or severe.
- Numerical score—Patient is asked to rate the pain on a scale of 1 to 10.
- Visual ("faces") scale—Patient is asked to choose the picture that shows how he or she feels. **See Figure 7-19.** Visual scales are often used for small children and people who are not fluent in a language spoken by the caregiver.

Vital Skills COMMUNICATION

Using Plain Language
Before you check a person's vital signs, be sure to explain the procedure in terms he or she can understand. For example, do not use technical terms when you are talking to a child. Answer any questions about the procedure using clear sentences and language the person will understand.

Practice
You have been assigned to check the blood pressure of a 10-year-old girl. How will you explain the procedure to her? Write your ideas on a separate sheet of paper.

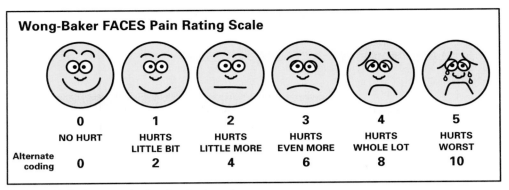

Wong-Baker FACES Pain Rating Scale

	0	1	2	3	4	5
	NO HURT	HURTS LITTLE BIT	HURTS LITTLE MORE	HURTS EVEN MORE	HURTS WHOLE LOT	HURTS WORST
Alternate coding	0	2	4	6	8	10

◯ **Figure 7-19.** An example of a visual pain scale.

Measuring Height and Weight

Significant weight loss or gain can be a sign of a serious health problem or of poor nutrition. Accurate and regular measurements of a patient's weight therefore provide important information to the health care team. In addition, medication dosages are often determined by a patient's weight. Most facilities make a record of the resident's height and weight at the time of admission. Following admission, the frequency of height and weight readings is determined by the health care team.

Height is measured in feet (') and inches (") or centimeters (cm). Weight is measured in pounds (lb) or kilograms (kg). Different types of scales are used, depending on the patient's condition. **See Figure 7-20.** Ambulatory patients are usually weighed on an upright scale. Bedridden patients are weighed with an overbed scale. Patients who cannot stand are weighed in a wheelchair, using a wheelchair scale.

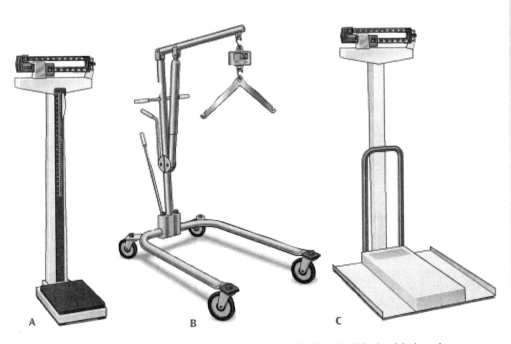

◯ **Figure 7-20.** Different types of scales: (A) upright scale; (B) lift scale; (C) wheelchair scale.

Vital Skills ⬤ MATH

Reading an Upright Scale

To read an upright scale, it is important to know how to read the weight bars correctly. The person's weight equals the sum of the number shown at the upper weight and the number shown at the lower weight.

The lower weight bar is almost always labeled in 50-pound increments: 50, 100, 150, 200, and so on. The labels on the upper weight bar may vary. The one shown in **Figure A** is typical.

Each mark on the upper weight bar means a different number. In **Figure A**, the marks are labeled in increments of 10: 10, 20, 30, 40, and so on. The marks between them divide each 10 pounds into five equal spaces. Therefore, each mark stands for 2 pounds, because 10 pounds divided by 5 equals 2 pounds.

The procedure for reading an upright scale is as follows:

1. Look at the upper weight bar on the scale. Determine what each mark represents.
2. Weigh the person according to the procedure described in this section.
3. Write down the number shown at the lower weight. Note that the correct number to record is the one beneath the arrow on

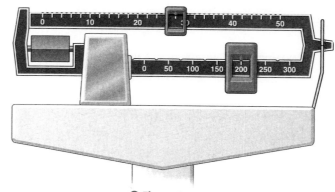

O Figure A

the weight (usually on the right side of the weight). In Figure A, the number is 200.

4. Write down the number shown at the upper weight. In Figure A, the upper weight is set at 28.
5. Add the two numbers together: 200 + 28 = 228. The person in this example weighs 228 lb.

Practice

Find the weight on each scale shown in Figure B. Note: Check the labels on the upper weight bar carefully on each scale. Write your answers on a separate sheet of paper. Show your work.

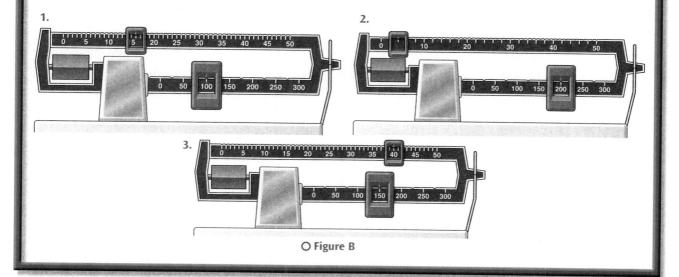

O Figure B

Procedure 7-11

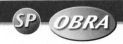

Measuring Height and Weight of an Ambulatory Patient

Equipment: upright scale • paper towels

1. Identify the patient, check the ID bracelet, and call the patient by name.
2. Introduce yourself.
3. Explain the procedure to the patient.
4. Ask the patient if he or she needs to urinate. If the answer is yes, allow the patient to do so before proceeding.
5. Wash your hands.
6. Provide privacy.
7. Place a paper towel over the platform of the scale.
8. Raise the rod that is used to measure height.
9. Check to make sure the weights are set at 0 and that the balance bar moves freely.
10. Ask the patient to remove his or her bathrobe and shoes or slippers. Assist if necessary.
11. Assist the patient to stand on the scale, with good posture and with the arms at the sides. Assist if necessary.
12. Slide the weights on the upper and lower weight bars to positions close to the patient's estimated weight. **See Figure 7-21.**
13. When the balance pointer settles at a position halfway between the upper and lower bar guide, read the scale. To arrive at the patient's weight, add together the numbers where the upper and lower weights are positioned. **See Figure 7-22.** For example, if the large weight is on 150 lb and the small weight is on 24 lb, the patient's weight is 174 lb.
14. Record the patient's weight.
15. Ask the patient to stand very straight facing you.

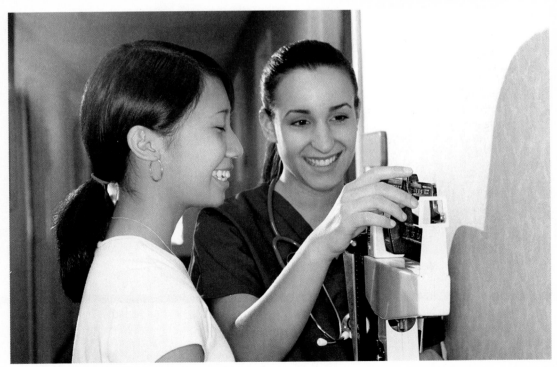

○ **Figure 7-21.** Weighing a patient on an upright scale.

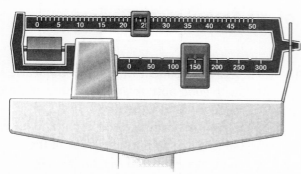

○ **Figure 7-22.** Calculating the weight of the person on the scale.

16. Slide the movable point on the ruler down until it touches the top of the patient's head. This is the patient's height measurement. **See Figure 7-23.**

17. Record the patient's height.
18. Help the patient step off the scale and put on the bathrobe and shoes or slippers. Assist the patient in returning to the chair or bed.
19. Place the signal light within reach and make sure the patient is comfortable.
20. Remove and discard the paper covering the platform of the scale.
21. Wash your hands.
22. Record the measurements in the proper place.

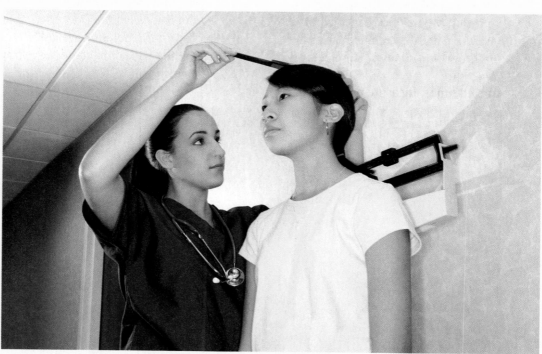

○ **Figure 7-23.** Measuring a patient's height.

Procedure 7-12

SP OBRA

Measuring Height and Weight of a Bedridden Patient

Equipment: overbed scale • tape measure • pencil

1. Identify the patient, check the ID bracelet, and call the patient by name.
2. Introduce yourself.
3. Explain the procedure to the patient.
4. Wash your hands.
5. Provide privacy.
6. Check to be sure the scale is in good condition (no areas of fraying, no straps that do not close properly).
7. Make sure the side rail on the far side of the bed is in the raised and locked position. Lower the side rail on the side of the bed near you.
8. Fanfold the top linens down to the foot of the bed.
9. Assist the patient to lie on his or her back in good body alignment. The arms and legs should be straight. If the patient has contracted limbs, measure each segment (head to shoulder, upper back, lower back, and so on) separately.
10. Using the pencil, make a small mark on the bottom sheet at the top of the patient's head.
11. Make a small pencil mark on the sheet where the patient's feet end.
12. Anchor the tape measure at one end. With the tape measure, measure the distance between the two pencil marks. This is the patient's height. **See Figure 7-24.**
13. Record the patient's height.
14. Remove the overbed scale sling from its suspension straps. Position the sling under the patient as follows:
    a. Ask the patient to turn onto the side facing away from you. Assist if necessary.
    b. Place the sling, folded lengthwise, under the patient.
    c. Ask the patient to turn onto the side facing you. Assist if necessary. Raise the side rail on the side of the bed you have been working on.
    d. Go to the other side of the bed, lower the side rail, and smooth out the sling under the patient.
    e. Assist the patient to resume lying flat on his or her back.
    f. Make sure the patient is positioned securely in the sling.
    g. Hook the sling to the suspension straps. Make sure the sling is securely attached.

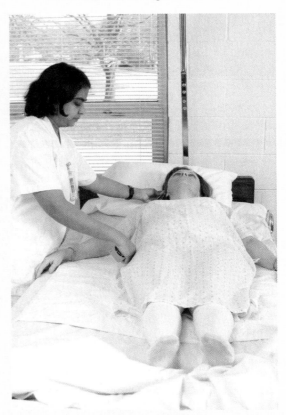

○ **Figure 7-24.** Measuring the height of a bedridden patient.

15. Move the lift frame into position over the bed. Lock the legs of the frame in the maximum open position.
16. Raise the head of the bed until the patient is in a sitting position.
17. Hook the suspension straps to the frame of the scale. Gently place the patient's arms inside the straps.
18. Slowly raise the sling until the patient's body is clear of the bed.
19. Slowly move the lift so that no part of the patient is making contact with the bed. **See Figure 7-25.**
20. Move the weights on the scale until the scale is balanced.
21. Read and record the patient's weight.
22. Slowly move the sling back over the bed until it is centered.

23. Slowly release the sling, while guiding the patient back down toward the bed.
24. Reverse the procedure in Step 14 to remove the sling from underneath the patient.
25. Move the scale away from the bed.
26. Place the signal light within reach and check to make sure the patient is comfortable and in good body alignment.
27. Rearrange the top linens so that they cover the patient appropriately.
28. Raise and lock the side rail on the side of the bed where you have been working.
29. Unscreen the patient.
30. Return the overbed scale to its storage area.
31. Wash your hands.
32. Report and record the measurements.

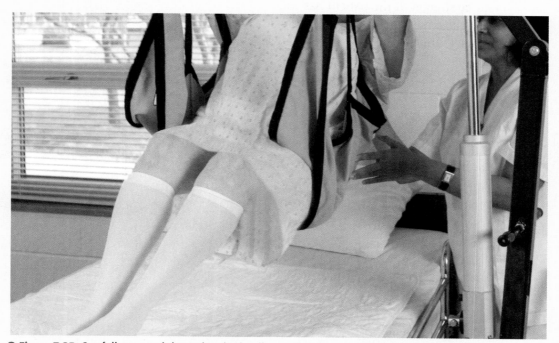

○ **Figure 7-25.** Carefully suspend the patient in the sling so that no part of the patient touches the bed.

Procedure 7-13

Weighing a Patient in a Wheelchair

Equipment: wheelchair scale

1. If the wheelchair has not already been weighed, weigh the wheelchair.
   a. Take the wheelchair to the wheelchair scale. Balance the scale.
   b. Place the ramps of the chair on either side of the scale.
   c. Move the wheelchair onto the platform. Let go of the wheelchair.
   d. Record the wheelchair's weight.
2. Take the wheelchair to the patient's room.
3. Identify the patient, check the ID bracelet, and call the patient by name.
4. Introduce yourself.
5. Explain the procedure to the patient.
6. Wash your hands.
7. Provide privacy.
8. Make sure the bed wheels are locked. Make sure the wheelchair wheels are locked and the footrests are up. **See Figure 7-26.**
9. Transfer the patient into the wheelchair.
10. Wheel the patient to the wheelchair scale, with the wheelchair facing the ramp.
11. Push the wheelchair up the ramp onto the scale platform. Lock the wheels of the wheelchair.
12. Read and record the weight of the wheelchair and the patient.
13. Unlock the wheels and gently pull the wheelchair down the scale platform.

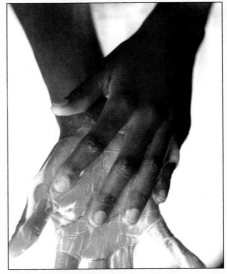

○ **Figure 7-27.** Wash your hands after weighing the patient.

14. Wheel the patient back to his or her room. Return the patient to a chair or to bed.
15. Place the signal light within reach and check to make sure the patient is comfortable and in good body alignment.
16. To arrive at the patient's weight, subtract the weight of the wheelchair alone from the measurement of the wheelchair and patient together. Record the patient's weight.
17. Wash your hands. **See Figure 7-27.**
18. Report and record the measurement.

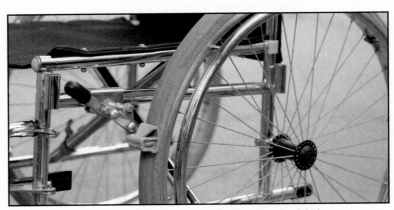

○ **Figure 7-26.** Make sure the wheels are locked on the wheelchair.

Chapter Summary

- Vital signs are important indicators of how well the body is functioning.

- The vital signs include body temperature, pulse, respiration, blood pressure, and pain level. Height and weight are also sometimes included in the vital signs.

- Body temperature is measured with a thermometer. It can be measured orally, rectally, tympanically (in the ears), or under the arms. The range of normal temperature readings varies, depending on where the temperature is measured.

- Pulse measurements provide information on how the cardiovascular system is functioning. Pulse can be measured at various sites throughout the body.

- Respiration is the process of inhaling (breathing in) and exhaling (breathing out). It is measured by counting breaths per minute.

- Blood pressure measures the force of the blood flow exerted against artery walls. Systolic pressure measures the force when blood is pumped out from the heart. Diastolic pressure measures the amount of pressure when the heart is at rest.

- A patient's pain level can be an indication of how well medications are working. Pain influences the other vital signs, so assessment is necessary for both acute and chronic pain.

- Accurate measurements of height and weight provide important information to the health care team, especially for patients with certain diseases and conditions.

VOCABULARY REVIEW

Directions: Match the letter of each definition in the second column with the correct vocabulary term. Write your answers on a separate sheet of paper.

Vocabulary

1. apical pulse
2. blood pressure
3. body temperature
4. bradypnea
5. diastolic pressure
6. dyspnea
7. hypertension
8. hypotension
9. pulse rate
10. radial pulse
11. sphygmomanometer
12. stertorous breathing
13. stethoscope
14. systolic pressure
15. tachycardia

Definitions

A. Abnormally slow breathing
B. Abnormally high blood pressure
C. A measure of the force of the blood flow against the walls of the artery
D. The rate at which the heart beats
E. An instrument used to listen to the sounds produced by the heart, lungs, and other body organs
F. The amount of heat in the body
G. Breaths accompanied by noises
H. The pulse measured at the wrist
I. The pulse felt over the apex of the heart
J. A rapid heart rate
K. A measure of the pressure in the arteries between beats, when the heart is at rest
L. A measuring device used to measure blood pressure
M. A measure of the pressure in the arteries when the heart contracts
N. Abnormally low blood pressure
O. Difficult, labored, or painful breathing

Check Your Knowledge

Review Questions: Answer each of the following questions on a separate sheet of paper.

1. Why are the "vital signs" called *vital* signs? What information do they provide to the health care team?

2. Name four sites at which body temperature can be measured.

3. What is a pulse? Why is a patient's pulse measured?

4. Name at least four places on the body where pulse can be measured and identify the artery at each location.

5. What is pulse deficit?

6. What is the normal range for rate of respiration in a healthy adult?

7. Briefly describe the best way to measure a person's respiration.

8. What do the two numbers in a blood pressure reading measure?

9. What instruments are used to measure blood pressure?

10. Briefly describe how you would obtain the weight of a person in a wheelchair.

True or False: Read each statement carefully. Then write *True* or *False* by the statement number on a separate sheet of paper.

1. A normal body temperature is 99.6° F when measured rectally.

2. A normal adult pulse rate is between 90 and 110 beats per minute.

3. Pulses can be checked at several different pulse points on the body.

4. In an older adult, a normal pulse rate is between 60 and 80 times a minute.

5. The nursing assistant should always inform the patient when measuring respirations.

Think and Decide

Directions: Think about each of the following scenarios. Answer each question on a separate sheet of paper.

1. You have measured 35-year-old M.T.'s temperature using the axillary method. The measurement is 96.7 °F. Should you notify the nurse? Why or why not?

2. Due to another employee's vacation, you have been temporarily reassigned to your facility's neonatal unit. Your supervisor asks you to check the vitals of each infant in the nursery. What method should you use to check the infant's temperature?

3. Mr. B. is one of the patients on whom you routinely check vital signs. He recently had surgery to remove a cancer in his mouth, so you have been measuring his temperature rectally. This morning, Mr. B. has diarrhea. What will you do differently as you check his vital signs?

4. L.G. is a long-term resident who is semiconscious, but generally stable. Today, when you check his respiration, you think he has stopped breathing. You cannot identify any respirations for several seconds. Then, he suddenly starts breathing rapidly. After several seconds, he starts breathing very slowly, at a rate of about 6 respirations per minute. What should you do?

5. Mrs. J. is a long-term resident who has chronic high blood pressure. For the last several weeks, her blood pressure reading has been around 150/90. When you check her vital signs this morning, her blood pressure is 126/70. What action(s) should you take?

6. Mr. P. is a 39-year-old man who had hernia surgery three days ago. His blood pressure on Tuesday was 108/70; on Wednesday, it was 106/74. Today, his blood pressure measures 128/88. What measures, if any, should you take?

7. Six-year-old F.S. has been admitted to your ward after being in the Emergency Room following an automobile accident. As part of your initial assessment, you need to find out how much pain the child is feeling. How should you go about this?

8. Mr. W. is a hospital patient recovering from major abdominal surgery. When you check his vital signs, you ask him how severe his pain is on a scale of 1 to 10, where 1 means no pain at all and 10 means the most severe pain he can imagine. Mr. W. says his pain is at about a level 5. Aside from recording his response, should you take any other action?

CNA Certification Exam Prep

Directions: This practice test contains ten questions. Each question has four suggested answers. For each question, choose the ONE that best answers the question or completes the statement. Write your answers on a separate sheet of paper.

1. The four main vital signs are temperature, pulse, blood pressure, and
   A. weight.
   B. height.
   C. respiration.
   D. agility.

2. Which of the following factors can affect the measurement of vital signs?
   A. exercise
   B. level of consciousness
   C. mental status
   D. hygiene

3. For a resident who has dementia, which site would you use to check temperature?
   A. oral
   B. rectal
   C. axillary
   D. tympanic

4. What safety measures would you take if you broke a mercury thermometer?
   A. ask housekeeping to clean it up
   B. ask the nurse to take care of it
   C. apply PPE and obey facility policy
   D. sweep it up and throw it out

5. Why is it important to obtain pulse and respiration measurements together?
   A. to keep the patient from knowing that you are counting respirations
   B. to obtain a better reading for both pulse and respiration
   C. to check vital signs more quickly
   D. it is more convenient for the patient

6. For a patient with an irregular heartbeat, which site should you use to check a pulse?
   A. pedal
   B. apical
   C. carotid
   D. radial

7. Mrs. Graves' skin is warm and she says she's feeling "achy." What should you do?
   A. give her fluids and assist her to bed
   B. obtain vital signs and report to the nurse
   C. give her Tylenol® and assist her to bed
   D. call EMS; she may be having a stroke

8. You accidentally release the valve too quickly when checking a blood pressure. How long should you wait before retrying?
   A. 15 seconds
   B. 1 to 2 minutes
   C. 5 minutes
   D. 10 minutes

9. A series of deep breaths followed by shallow breaths with periods of no breathing is
   A. stertorous breathing.
   B. tachypnea.
   C. Cheyne-Stokes.
   D. bradypnea.

10. It is important to place a sphygmomanometer correctly
   A. to make the patient more comfortable.
   B. so it looks good on the patient's arm.
   C. to obtain an accurate measurement.
   D. to teach the patient how to do it.

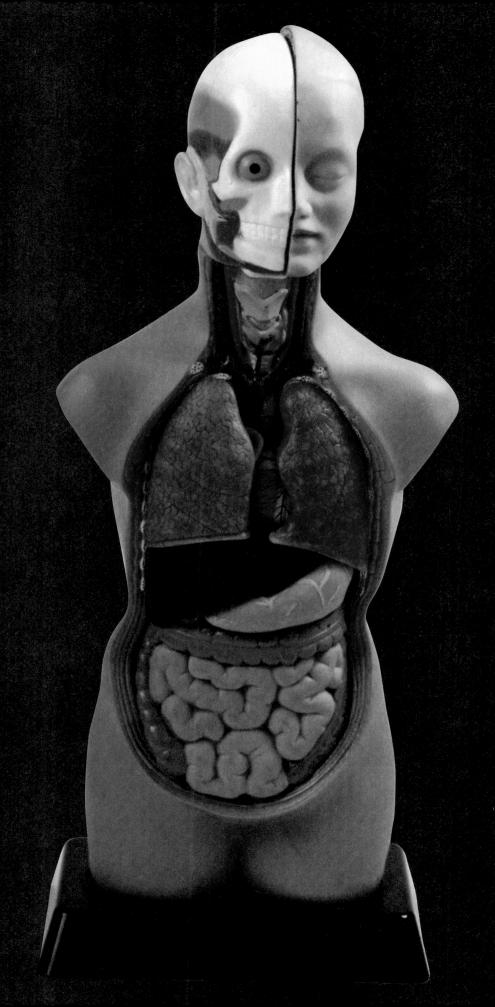

The Human Body

Chapter 8 **Human Growth and Development**

Chapter 9 **Health and the Human Body**

Chapter 10 **Anatomy and Physiology**

Chapter 11 **Infection Control and Standard Precautions**

Unit 2 covers the normal functioning of the human body, as well as what can go wrong with it. This information provides an essential foundation for understanding the needs of people who are ill. Some of the patients you will care for may have infectious diseases. Chapter 11 introduces infection control and the standard precautions you should take when working with those patients.

CHAPTER 8

OBJECTIVES

- Explain the significance of understanding growth and development when caring for individuals of all age groups.

- Describe the growth that takes place during each stage of life.

- Describe the development that takes place during each stage of life.
- Explain how personalities develop and change as we age.

Human Growth and Development

VOCABULARY

development The process of acquiring motor (movement) skills, language skills, social skills, and cognitive (learning) skills.

developmental tasks The set of tasks that must be accomplished to complete a stage of development.

ejaculation The expelling of semen from the body.

growth The process of changing physically in ways that can be measured.

identity An individual's uniqueness and sense of self.

immunization The process of providing protection against specific communicable diseases.

menarche The first menstrual period and the beginning of puberty in girls.

menopause The natural stopping of menstruation that marks the end of the childbearing stage.

neonate A newborn baby in the first 4 weeks after birth.

personality The accumulation of individual traits that distinguish someone.

primary caregiver The person who is mainly responsible for meeting a child's basic needs.

puberty The stage in which the sex organs mature and secondary sex characteristics develop.

reflex An involuntary or automatic physical response.

secondary sex characteristics Gender characteristics such as breasts in females and facial hair in males.

stimulation Activities that excite the senses.

temperament Each person's unique manner of thinking, reacting, and behaving.

well-baby checks Regular visits to a doctor to monitor a baby's progress.

Stages of Growth and Development

From birth to death, people change physically, emotionally, socially, and psychologically. Nursing assistants provide care for both children and adults during all stages of growth and development. Learning how healthy people change during their lives will help you understand your patients' needs.

Growth is the process of changing physically in ways that can be measured. For instance, over the life span, our height and weight change. The process of physical growth occurs in a specific order. The upper body parts develop before the lower body parts. The head and trunk develop before the arms and legs.

Development is the process of acquiring motor (movement) skills, language skills, social skills, and cognitive (learning) skills. Development involves learning simple activities before learning complex activities. For instance, children must learn to walk before they can learn to run. Each stage of development has a set of tasks. These **developmental tasks** must be accomplished to complete the stage of development. Only then can the person move on to the next stage.

Growth and development are woven together. For example, as children become physically stronger and more coordinated, they achieve independence—a developmental stage. They are then able to do things for themselves and rely less on their caregivers.

People grow and develop at their own rates. One child might grow rapidly but develop more slowly than another child. There is a range of ages for normal growth and development. For example, at the age of 6 months, one baby may reach forward and grasp a bottle. Another baby cannot yet control these movements. Both babies may be developing normally. The stages of growth and development occur at approximately the ages that are discussed in the following pages. **See Table 8-1.**

○ **Table 8-1. Stages of Growth and Development**

Neonate and Infancy	Birth to 1 year
Toddler	Ages 1 to 3 years
Preschool	Ages 3 to 5 years
Primary	Ages 6 to 9 years
Preadolescence	Ages 10 to 12 years
Adolescence	Ages 13 to 18 years
Young Adulthood	Ages 19 to 40 years
Middle Adulthood	Ages 41 to 65 years
Late Adulthood and Old Age	Ages 66 and Older

The Neonatal and Infant Periods

The neonatal period consists of the first four weeks after birth. The baby at this stage is called a **neonate**, or newborn. **See Figure 8-1.** At birth, neonates average 20 inches in length and 7 to 8 pounds in weight. Babies grow most rapidly in their first 12 months. At one year of age, the average infant will be 29 to 30 inches in length and weigh 21 to 22 pounds.

Infants usually triple their birth weight by one year of age. The neonate's head makes up about 25 percent of the body length. As the baby grows, the ratio changes. At one year, the head makes up only about 20 percent of the total length.

At birth and for many months, babies depend totally on a caregiver for all their needs. The **primary caregiver** is the person who is mainly responsible for meeting the child's basic needs. That person might be a parent, a grandparent, or another relative or guardian.

When babies are born, some of their body systems are not yet fully functional. For example, the nervous system, sensory system, and musculoskeletal system continue to develop after birth.

The Nervous System. The nervous system is central to infant growth and development. The parts of the brain develop at different rates. The baby has certain unique **reflexes**, or involuntary or automatic physical responses. These reflexes gradually disappear during the first year as the nervous system develops.

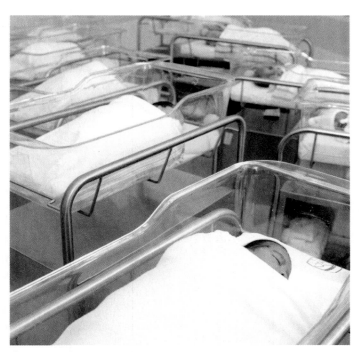

O **Figure 8-1.** Newborn infants, or neonates.

- The *Moro*, or startle, reflex is set off by loud noises. The baby throws the head back and extends the arms and legs.
- The *rooting* reflex is stimulated when the baby's cheek is touched at or near the mouth. The head turns in the direction of the touch. This reflex helps guide the baby's mouth to the nipple for feeding.
- In the *sucking* reflex, the baby sucks automatically when an object is placed in the mouth. **See Figure 8-2.**
- The *grasping* reflex causes the baby to close the fingers around any pressure on the palm of the hand.

O **Figure 8-2.** An infant showing the sucking reflex.

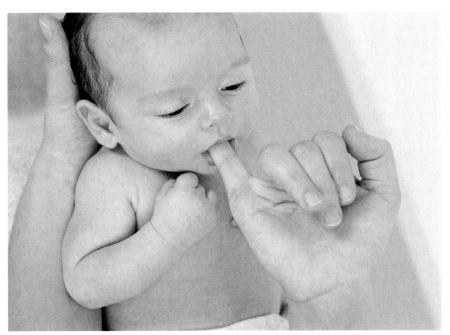

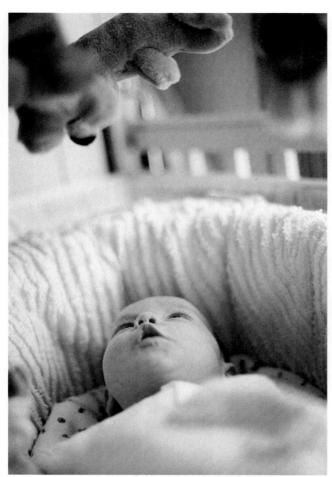

○ **Figure 8-3.** This baby is stimulated by the colors and movement of the mobile.

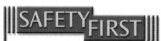

When you care for an infant, be sure to support the head and neck. When lifting an infant, slide one hand under the buttocks and the other under the shoulders and head. Support the neck and head with your forearm as you lift the baby.

The Sensory System. At birth, neonates have all five senses. They can see, hear, taste, smell, and respond to touch. Some senses, however, are more developed than others. Babies need stimulation to grow and develop appropriately. **Stimulation** includes activities that excite the senses and help the baby learn. **See Figure 8-3.**

- **Vision.** Neonates can sense the difference between light and dark. Soon they are able to focus on still objects and then on moving objects. Babies are attracted to bright colors.
- **Hearing.** The sense of hearing is slower to develop. Babies gradually learn to hear where sounds come from. They soon recognize their primary caregiver's voice. Babies also can hear higher frequency sounds than adults and respond better to high-pitched voices.
- **Taste.** Babies react to different tastes, generally preferring sweet flavors.
- **Smell.** Babies also react to odors, especially those that are not pleasant to them.
- **Touch.** Babies become more sensitive to pain and touch as they grow. As their coordination improves, they use this sense to explore the world around them. It is important for babies to be touched. Nurturing touch is important to normal development.

The Musculoskeletal System. A newborn's bones are relatively soft. As babies grow, their bones harden, and muscles gradually become longer and thicker. At first, infants' movements are not under their control. They cannot support their heads, so the head must be well supported. When neck and shoulder muscles are stronger, infants can hold their heads up. For example, most 1-month-old babies can hold their heads up when they are lying on their stomachs.

In three or more months, infants can raise themselves up, lifting their heads and shoulders. They can sit up when supported. The grasping reflex disappears, and they can instead grasp on purpose. They cannot, however, release the grasping motion. Later, they learn to let objects go. At 8 months, infants can generally sit without support. At 9 to 12 months, they can walk while holding onto something or onto someone's hand. Soon after one year of age, most babies can walk on their own. **See Figure 8-4.**

Other Changes. At the same time these physical changes are happening, babies are changing in other important ways. They begin to remember their experiences and to understand cause and effect. Infants also are learning to communicate using language. First, they learn to understand what is being said to them. Gradually, they learn to talk.

Babies also develop emotionally during infancy. In the first few months after birth, they begin to smile in reaction to a caregiver's attention or voice. They develop attachments, first with their primary caregiver and then with other members of the family.

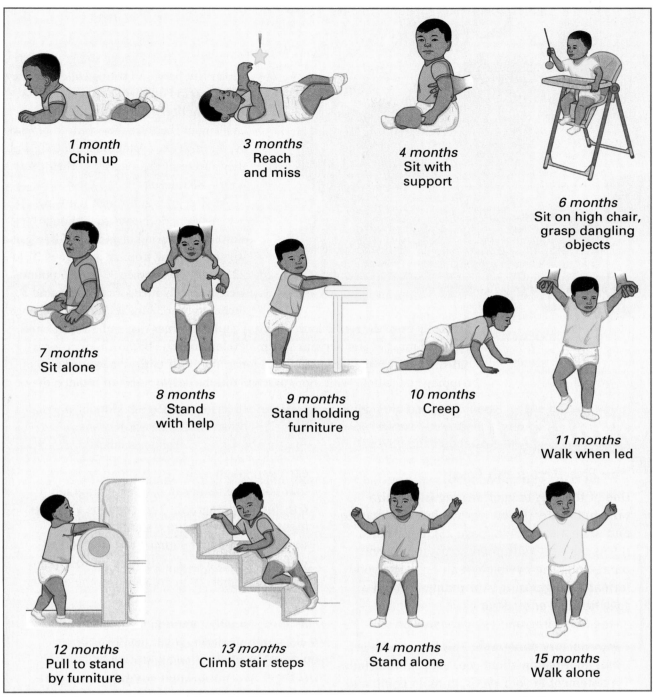

1 month
Chin up

3 months
Reach
and miss

4 months
Sit with
support

6 months
Sit on high chair,
grasp dangling
objects

7 months
Sit alone

8 months
Stand
with help

9 months
Stand holding
furniture

10 months
Creep

11 months
Walk when led

12 months
Pull to stand
by furniture

13 months
Climb stair steps

14 months
Stand alone

15 months
Walk alone

O **Figure 8-4.** The stages of development from 1 to 15 months.

Well-baby checks are critical for monitoring infant growth and development. These checks are regular visits to a health care provider to monitor the baby's progress. **See Figure 8-5.** Another important process for neonates and infants is immunization. **Immunization** is protection against specific communicable diseases. Immunizations are given to babies during their first year to protect them from diseases. Other immunizations are given at several ages through childhood and adolescence.

SAFETY FIRST

Babies can roll over and fall off a bed or table. Never leave or turn your back on a baby that does not have side rails or barriers to keep him or her from falling.

The Toddler Period

During the toddler period (ages 1 to 3 years), children change and grow from dependent babies to young children. They move around on their own and express many emotions. Caring for toddlers is challenging, because they seem to be into everything. They want independence, but they also want the security of their care-givers' attention.

Physical growth through the 1- to 3-year-old period is steady, although slower than during infancy. Children gain weight, growing from an average of 21 to 22 pounds to between 32 and 35 pounds. Height usually increases from around 30 inches to over 38 inches. Children change gradually from the round look of a baby to the slimmer shape of a young child.

As the muscles and nervous system develop, toddlers become more coordinated. At first, as the name *toddler* suggests, they walk with an awkward gait, often tripping and falling. With more practice and the development of balance, they

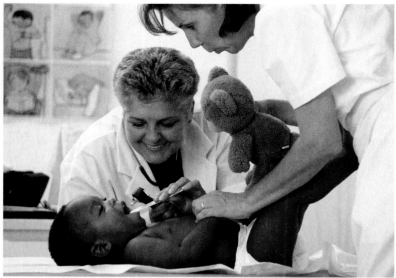

○ Figure 8-5. This baby is getting a well-baby check.

Vital Skills — WRITING

The Five-Paragraph Essay

One of the keys to good writing is organization. In Chapter 1, you learned how to organize and write a paragraph (page 25). But what if you can't get your point across in just one paragraph? The five-paragraph essay is a good format for organizing your thoughts about a specific topic or question.

The five-paragraph essay consists of:

- **Introductory paragraph:** This begins with general information about your subject. It includes a statement of your *thesis*, or main point, and a summary of three ideas or examples that support your main point.
- **Three main body paragraphs:** Each paragraph will focus on one of the ideas or examples you mentioned in the introductory paragraph. (Remember, each paragraph should have its own main idea and supporting details.) End each paragraph with a transitional sentence that takes the reader to the next paragraph.
- **Concluding paragraph:** This contains a restatement of your thesis and a summary of the three examples that support your thesis. End your essay with a final statement on your main topic that signals to the reader that the essay is over.

Before you begin writing, decide on your main point, or thesis. Next, decide on three points or examples that support your thesis. List them in order of their strength in supporting your main topic (strongest to weakest). Plan to address each point in a separate paragraph. Now you are ready to write.

Practice
Write a five-paragraph essay on the importance of well-baby checks.

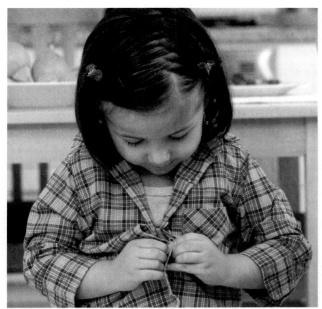

○ **Figure 8-6.** Many toddlers prefer to dress themselves.

learn to walk well. Then they learn to run, climb, and jump. During this time, toilet training takes place. The muscles that operate the bowel and the bladder have developed enough for the child to control them. As their motor skills develop, they become eager to do things for themselves, such as getting dressed. **See Figure 8-6.**

Language skills are also increasing. From age 2 to 3, children can typically use about 200 words and understand about 1,000. Children develop emotionally and socially, too. They begin to understand that there are things they should and should not do. They learn to play alongside other children.

By the end of the toddler period, they begin to recognize themselves as separate individuals. They may develop social skills such as learning to share. However, they are often frustrated by their desire to do things for themselves that they are not yet able to do.

The Preschool Period

During the preschool period (ages 3 to 5 years), growth in height and weight continues. Children grow from an average height of about 38 inches to 44 inches. Weight increases from an average of almost 35 pounds to over 43 pounds. Perhaps the most noticeable change is the shape of the child's body. During the preschool period, children's arms, legs, and torso grow the fastest, so that they start to look more like adults.

Coordination and motor skills improve, and children become stronger. They can do more complicated tasks, such as jump, hop, pedal a tricycle, pour liquids, and print letters and numbers. Language development accelerates, too. By the time children enter first grade, they may recognize between 8,000 and 14,000 words. They also speak in longer sentences.

Preschoolers become less reliant on the primary caregiver. They have definite ideas about how they are alike and how they are different from other children. They also begin to understand the physical differences between boys and girls. They explore their bodies and are curious about gender differences. Socially, they begin to develop friendships with other children. They are more cooperative and begin to care about what others think of them. **See Figure 8-7.**

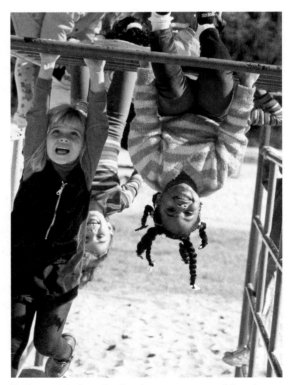

○ **Figure 8-7.** Preschoolers become more social and develop friendships.

Communicating with a Pediatric Patient

In your practice, you may be required to communicate with people of many different age groups and cultures. The way you communicate with a patient depends partly on the patient's age.

How might you have to change the way you communicate when you are caring for a toddler? Toddlers (1 to 3 years) are just beginning to develop their language skills. They have limited vocabulary. Toddlers might not be able to express what they are feeling, or understand what you are telling them. They also might be experiencing fear and anxiety at being in an unfamiliar setting and separated from their family. All of these factors can make communicating with a toddler challenging.

Here are some tips to help you communicate with toddlers:

- Speak in a normal voice.
- Use soothing tones.
- Use a favorite toy or stuffed animal to distract their attention away from the task you are performing.
- Let them touch or hold a safe piece of equipment such as a stethoscope so that it is not frightening to them.
- Explain what you are doing using simple words.

Practice

Think of some of the barriers to communication you might encounter when caring for a toddler. List some ways you might overcome them.

The Primary Period

During the primary period (ages 6 to 9 years), most children begin formal schooling. With exposure to many other children, they learn how to get along with others the same age.

From ages 6 to 9, children grow about 2 inches per year and gain about 6 pounds a year. Their arms and legs grow faster than other parts of their bodies, and their faces change. Growth varies for individual girls and boys. Children of the same age can differ as much as 8 to 10 inches in height.

During this period, motor skills and coordination develop further. They also begin to develop the basic skills of reading, writing, and arithmetic that increase during the rest of the school years. Drawing skills improve, and athletic skills are developed. Social skills develop as well, as children learn to interact with others and understand someone else's point of view. They begin to think logically and to understand the importance of following rules. **See Figure 8-8.** They also begin to develop a moral sense.

The Preadolescent Period

The preadolescent period (ages 10 to 12 years) lasts from childhood to the beginning of adolescence. Girls grow faster than boys during preadolescence. During each year of this period, girls grow an average of 3 inches and gain between 4 and 5 pounds. Boys grow less, about an inch per year, with less weight gain. At age 12, most girls are taller and heavier than most boys the same age. **See Figure 8-9.**

This growth is part of the way the body prepares for **puberty**, the stage in which the sex organs mature and **secondary sex characteristics** develop. These changes include the beginnings of breasts in girls and of facial hair in boys. When puberty is complete, reproduction is possible. Children at this stage need accurate information about sex that is appropriate to their age. Adults should answer questions as completely as possible.

Emotionally and socially, children at this age move beyond the family to peer groups. *Peer groups* consist of children who are about the same age, live in the same neighborhood, or go to the same school. They can help the preadolescent child grow socially by building common experiences and self-esteem. However, the group's values may conflict with the family's. Peer groups may strongly influence what children think and do, both positively and negatively.

The Adolescent Period

During adolescence, every individual experiences great changes. From ages 13 to 18, adolescents usually grow to their adult size, shape, and sexual maturity. However, some people do continue to grow until their early twenties. Girls enter this period generally taller and heavier than boys. Boys begin to grow rapidly between ages 12 and 14.

Puberty causes changes in the skin and sweat glands. Skin may become oilier, and sweat glands produce new body odors. Hair grows on different parts of the body, too. The age at which sexual maturity is reached varies. The first menstrual period, called **menarche**, marks puberty for girls, usually around age 12 or 13. Boys experience puberty about two years later, beginning with the growth of the genitals and the appearance of other secondary sex characteristics. The first **ejaculation**, or the expelling of semen from the body, signals puberty in boys.

Some boys and girls have difficulty accepting these changes. Those who mature earlier or later may feel especially awkward. They may compare themselves to peers and worry about differences. Adolescents are searching for their own **identity**, a uniqueness and a sense of self. During this transition

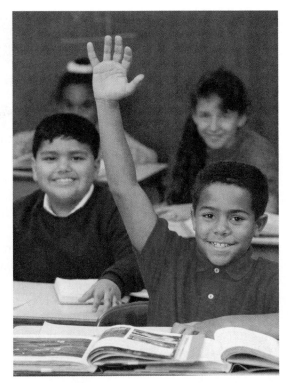

○ **Figure 8-8.** These primary school students have developed the social skills necessary to behave properly in a classroom.

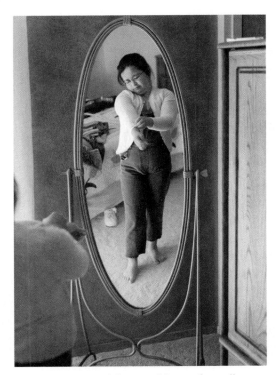

○ **Figure 8-9.** Preadolescent girls are often taller and heavier than boys of the same age.

Converting Inches to Feet and Inches

When you record a patient's height, you will usually record it in inches. For example, you may measure the height of a 7-year-old and record the height as 46 inches. But in casual conversation, we tend to use feet and inches to specify height. For example, you may say that a woman is "five and a half feet tall" or 5 feet, 6 inches.

There are 12 inches in a foot. Therefore, to convert from inches to feet and inches, you divide by 12. For example, if a child's height is 46 inches: $46 \div 12 = 3$, with a remainder of 10. The child is 3 feet, 10 inches tall.

Practice

Find the height of each of the following people in feet and inches.

1. Carlos is 74 inches tall.
2. Beulah is 63 inches tall.
3. Ollie is 55 inches tall.

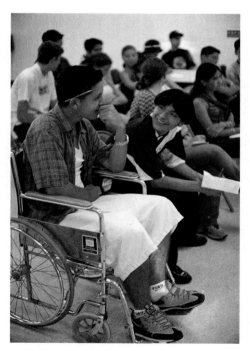

○ **Figure 8-10.** Adolescents often find it easier to communicate with each other than with adults.

period, individuals move from childhood toward adulthood. They begin to understand themselves as emerging adults and as sexual beings.

Early in the adolescent period, teens often find themselves in conflict with their parents. They may disagree on dress, school performance, and rules of dating and sexual behavior. Both parents and teens usually learn to balance the teen's increasing need for independence with family support and values. At this time, peer groups can provide a way for adolescents to talk about topics they feel they cannot discuss with adults. **See Figure 8-10.**

The Young Adulthood Period

During young adulthood (ages 19 to 40 years), adults establish themselves in the areas of work, adult social life, and family life. They make choices and set goals about education and careers. Some people enter the world of work first and take further training to develop skills later. Others pursue a variety of educational experiences before starting their careers.

A major part of young adulthood consists of establishing a family life and a support group of friends. Although some adults remain single, most experience living with another person in marriage.

Couples must develop ways to communicate effectively in order to make good decisions about family planning, finances, and long-term goals. They must learn how to support each other emotionally and psychologically as well. **See Figure 8-11.**

Most couples also make decisions about when or whether to have children. Child-rearing involves a major commitment of the couple's time and resources, so the timing must be carefully planned. Making time for other family members and friends, along with balancing work, family, and outside interests, is also important.

The Middle Adulthood Period

People in middle adulthood (ages 41 to 65 years) move from the peak of careers to approaching retirement. Usually, their children are leaving home and starting their own independent lives. **See Figure 8-12.** Middle-aged adults must adjust to this change while still providing support to their grown children. Also, many adults in this stage have responsibility for an aged parent or parents. They may need to make decisions about their care or cope with the loss of a parent.

Physical changes also occur during middle adulthood. Unlike the changes of childhood, these changes are usually gradual. As people grow older, their muscles become weaker, their bones more brittle, and their lungs and blood vessels less efficient. Women experience **menopause**, the natural stopping of menstruation that marks the end of the childbearing stage. Men may experience hair loss, decreased sexual drive, and decreased muscle tone. Other signs of aging, such as graying hair and the start of wrinkles, become apparent.

The effects of looking older can be more troubling for adults at this stage than the physical effects themselves. Attitudes about aging are as important as the physical changes. As people move into their fifties and sixties, maintaining interest in all aspects of life is very important. People who maintain an active, healthy lifestyle can slow down many of the effects of aging. On the other hand, people who expect to be less healthy as they age often are. Maintaining the proper weight, monitoring diet and basic health, and getting both mental and physical exercise are important ways to remain healthy.

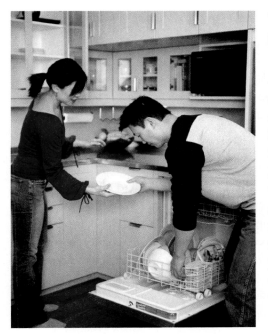

○ Figure 8-11. A young adult couple shares tasks in their first apartment.

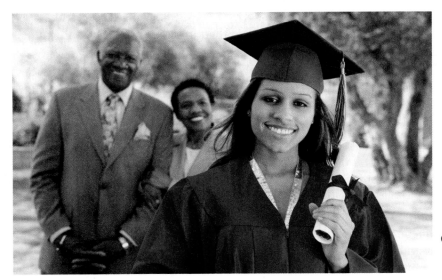

○ Figure 8-12. A couple in the middle adulthood period. Their daughter is graduating from college and leaving home.

Late Adulthood and Old Age

Late adulthood, followed by old age, can be a period of difficulty or enjoyment, depending on a person's physical and mental health. Generally, people ages 66 and older experience a loss of vitality and endurance. The aging process continues, affecting sight, hearing, and other senses. Chronic conditions, such as arthritis and heart disease, may cause loss of strength and the ability to engage in strenuous daily activities.

People in old age face their decline and eventual death. Strength and focus are reduced, and old friends—perhaps one's life partner, too—have died. New friendships and relationships need to be formed. At this stage, people must often deal with loneliness, financial worries, and poor health.

The aging process can affect personality and mental functioning. *Short-term memory* (the ability to remember recent events) may decrease and cause forgetfulness and confusion. Some people experience psychological disorders, declining physical abilities, and a loss of independence. Chapter 24 describes these changes in greater detail and explains how the nursing care team helps aging people to feel more comfortable.

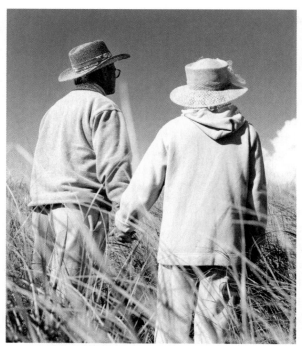

○ **Figure 8-13. People in late adulthood and old age may find travel stimulating.**

Even though aging often includes loss, many people continue to function well. **See Figure 8-13.** If they have a flexible attitude, older people can adapt their interests and activities to these changes. If they are reasonably healthy, they continue enjoying life and being productive. The availability of emotional and physical support is important. Equally important may be the sense of satisfaction with one's life and accomplishments.

Personality Development

From birth, each baby has a different **temperament**, or manner of thinking, reacting, and behaving. For example, some babies are more active than others, some more easygoing, and some more open to new things in their environments. Some children are fairly quiet, and others are noisy.

An individual's unique temperament is the beginning of personality development. The cultural background the family provides is equally important. As we develop, we share family experiences and values. We learn about relating to others through individual trial-and-error experiments. Along the way, we make decisions and solve problems. As we do so, we develop **personality**, which is the accumulation of individual traits that distinguish someone. This process is lifelong. Our personalities are the sum of our behaviors and emotional characteristics.

The psychologist Erik Erikson created a helpful way of looking at the tasks people accomplish as their personalities develop. He believed that we each develop our unique personality as we mature from infancy to old age. According to Erikson, our personalities develop through a number of stages, just as we grow physically from infancy to adulthood. Each stage challenges us to make choices.

Erikson emphasized that, in order to lead a healthy, satisfying life, people must successfully achieve each stage in order to move on to the next. For example, a toddler who does not learn self-control and independence will be dependent on others and may demonstrate a lack of control throughout life. This tendency may make it difficult to accomplish more advanced developmental tasks. **Table 8-2** lists each of these stages and the tasks that must be accomplished to complete each stage successfully.

○ **Table 8-2** Erikson's Stages of Development

Stages	Desired Accomplishments
First year	Hope; trust
Second year	Sense of self-control and self-esteem
Third through fifth years	Able to start activities and enjoy accomplishments
Sixth year through puberty	Sense of being competent; able to use skills and tools to make things
Adolescence	Sense of identity; able to see oneself as a unique person
Early adulthood	Able to love and commit to others
Middle age	Concern for others, for one's children, work, or ideas
Old age	Wisdom—certain of the meaning of one's own life and of personal dignity; acceptance that one will die

Vital Skills — READING

Making Connections

One way to remember what you read is to make connections between the ideas in the text and the people you know. For example, you might be reading about how to care for an older person, and your thoughts keep coming back to your grandmother, who is hearing-impaired. Taking a few minutes to think about her special needs might help you remember what you read about caring for hearing-impaired clients.

The connections you make while reading do not need to be limited to family members. As you are reading about the different age groups for which you will be caring, try to think of people in your community who are members of each group. Making connections to people you know will help you remember what you read. In turn, this will help you better care for people in different age groups.

Practice

Psychologist Erik Erikson outlined eight stages of personality development, and the tasks that are accomplished at each stage. Review Table 8-2 and try to think of a member of your community for each stage of development. Provide an example of how you think that person meets the desired accomplishment for that stage.

Chapter Summary

- Through an understanding of how healthy individuals change during their lives, nursing assistants will be better prepared to care for patient needs at all age levels.

- The neonate and infancy period lasts from birth to one year.

- The stages of childhood include the toddler period, preschool period, primary period, and preadolescent period.

- Adolescence is a transition period in which individuals move from childhood to adulthood.

- A major part of young adulthood consists of establishing a family life, employment, and a social support group of friends.

- Middle adulthood moves the adult through changes in families as children grow and leave home. Gradual physical signs of aging become apparent.

- Changes experienced in late adulthood and old age include psychological changes, declining physical abilities, and sometimes a loss of independence, depending on the person's individual health.

- The psychologist Erik Erikson explored and developed a helpful way of looking at stages of personality development.

VOCABULARY REVIEW

Directions: Match the letter of each definition in the second column with the correct vocabulary term in the first column. Write your answers on a separate sheet of paper.

Vocabulary

1. development
2. developmental tasks
3. ejaculation
4. growth
5. identity
6. immunization
7. menarche
8. menopause
9. neonate
10. personality
11. primary caregiver
12. puberty
13. reflex
14. temperament

Definitions

A. A newborn baby in the first 4 weeks after birth
B. The process of changing physically in ways that can be measured
C. The stage in which the sex organs mature and secondary sex characteristics develop
D. The process of acquiring motor (movement) skills, language skills, social skills, and cognitive (learning) skills
E. Each person's unique manner of thinking, reacting, and behaving
F. An involuntary or automatic physical response
G. The person who is mainly responsible for meeting a child's basic needs
H. The set of tasks that must be accomplished to complete a stage of development
I. An individual's uniqueness and sense of self
J. The first menstrual period and the beginning of puberty in girls
K. The accumulation of individual traits that distinguish someone
L. The ability to expel semen
M. The natural stopping of menstruation that marks the end of the childbearing stage
N. The process of providing protection against specific communicable diseases

Check Your Knowledge

Review Questions: Answer each of the following questions on a separate sheet of paper.

1. List the stages of human growth and development and their time periods.

2. Name the four reflexes of infancy.

3. Give one example of a typical development that occurs during infancy.

4. During what period does toilet training usually occur?

5. Describe the language development by the end of the preschool period.

6. During which stage or stages are children more likely to feel peer pressure?

7. What is puberty?

8. Why is adolescence considered a difficult developmental period?

9. What changes are typical in late adulthood and old age?

10. According to Erikson's stages of development, if a person never successfully accomplishes a sense of identity, what may happen in early adulthood and beyond?

True or False: Read each statement carefully. Then write *True* or *False* by the statement number on a separate sheet of paper.

1. People grow and develop at their own rates.

2. Most people stop developing at age 18.

3. Toddlers may become frustrated because they want to do things for themselves, but cannot always manage them.

4. During adolescence, boys develop more rapidly than girls.

5. Dementia in the elderly may cause short-term memory loss or confusion.

Think and Decide

Directions: Think about each of the following scenarios. Answer each question on a separate sheet of paper.

1. G.T. is a new mother who is worried because she does not know how to hold her neonate. What information about a newborn's growth and development might be helpful for G.T. to know?

2. Your neighbor brought her new infant, Emma, home from the hospital three weeks ago. She tells you that she is worried about Emma. Every time one of the older children slams a door or makes a loud noise, Emma throws her head back and extends her arms and legs. Your neighbor is concerned that this might be an indication of epilepsy. What might really be going on?

3. S.W. is a 2-year-old hospital patient who is refusing to eat. Her mother asks if she should try to feed her daughter. What should you do?

4. H.B. is an 11-year-old male hospital patient whose appendix was removed. He is refusing to wear a hospital gown. He says, "Hospital gowns are for girls. None of my friends would *ever* wear one. I want to wear pajamas!" What should you do?

5. J.C., a hospital patient who is 14, had knee surgery 8 hours ago. She is embarrassed to use the bedside commode, so she has not urinated since surgery. The nurse has instructed you to assist her to the commode at this time. What action(s) should you take?

6. A 50-year-old hospital patient asks you to close the door and leave the room while she bathes. What action(s) should you take?

7. L.V. is a 76-year-old male who has been newly admitted to the nursing home and is in your care. He seems very depressed and is uninterested in any of the activities you mention. He tells you that until recently, his favorite activity was hiking in the mountains. Then he had a stroke and lost much of his mobility. He is now confined to a wheelchair. What might you suggest to decrease his depression and engage his interest?

8. A 90-year-old long-term resident is blind and sometimes forgetful. This resident usually requires assistance with eating, but today she asks if she can feed herself. What should you do?

9. E.L. is a 44-year-old female patient. She has pressed the call button several times in the last half hour, each time requesting a shampoo and help with her makeup. She is scheduled for this care, but you have several other tasks to achieve as well. When you go to her room to explain, she tells you that her son and daughter are flying in and will be coming to see her at 11:30 AM. Why might her personal care seem so important to her? What should you do?

CNA Certification Exam Prep

Directions: This practice test contains ten questions. Each question has four suggested answers. For each question, choose the ONE that best answers the question or completes the statement. Write your answers on a separate sheet of paper.

1. At approximately what age can most infants sit up when supported?
    A. 1 month
    B. 3 months
    C. 6 months
    D. 12 months

2. Which of the following is a developmental task?
    A. playing alongside other children
    B. growing hair
    C. teething
    D. checking a patient's pulse

3. When working with an 18-month-old child, which of the following would the nursing assistant consider *normal*?
    A. the Moro reflex
    B. sharing toys
    C. tying shoelaces
    D. wanting independence

4. A reflex that is set off by loud noises is the
    A. Moro reflex.
    B. rooting reflex.
    C. blink reflex.
    D. grasping reflex.

5. At what age do most children start to gain control over their bowel and bladder functions?
    A. 3 to 6 months
    B. 6 to 8 months
    C. 1 to 3 years
    D. 4 to 5 years

6. An 85-year-old person says "If I die tomorrow, I have no regrets." This person has achieved which accomplishment in Erikson's stages of development?
    A. wisdom and acceptance of death
    B. concern for others, for one's children, work, or ideas
    C. sense of control and self-esteem
    D. hope and trust

7. During which developmental period do females grow noticeably faster than boys?
    A. infant period
    B. toddler period
    C. preschool period
    D. preadolescent period

8. In which developmental period do most children start to communicate with words?
    A. infant period
    B. toddler period
    C. preschool period
    D. preadolescent period

9. Which of the following factors influence personality development?
    A. family experiences and culture
    B. family history and genetics
    C. educational background
    D. ages of the closest friends

10. The first menstrual period and beginning of puberty in girls is called
    A. menopause.
    B. growth reflex.
    C. menarche.
    D. maturity.

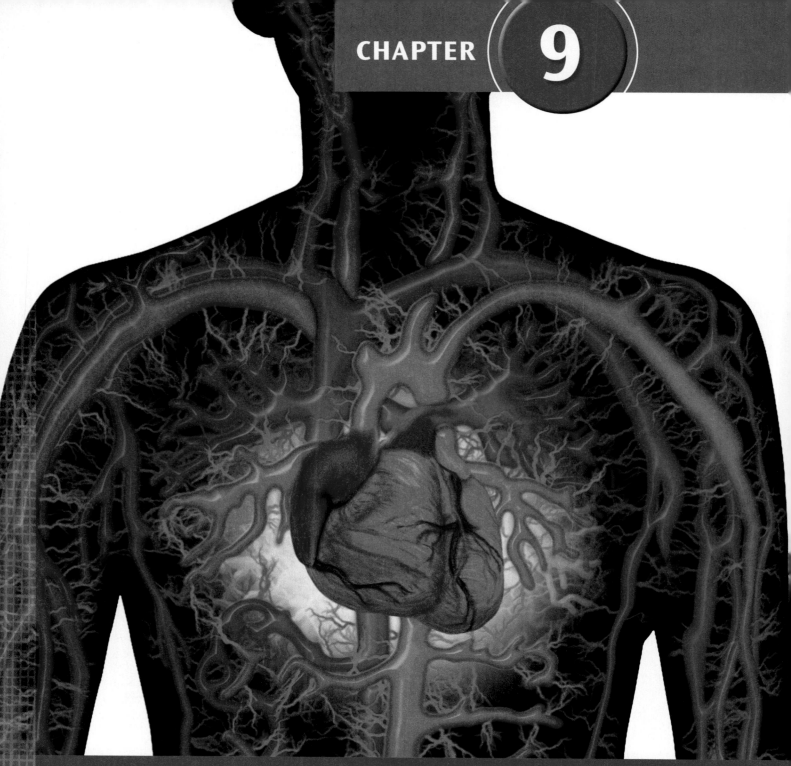

CHAPTER 9

OBJECTIVES

- Identify the four basic structures of the human body.
- Describe the structure and functions of the cell.
- Explain the functions of tissue.

- Describe the four types of tissue in the human body.
- Identify the major cavities within the body.
- Identify ways of explaining locations in the body.

- Explain the structure and functions of major organs of the body.
- Identify common diseases and disorders that affect the major organs.
- Explain how aging affects the senses.

Health and the Human Body

alveoli Tiny air sacs in the lungs.

Alzheimer's disease A degenerative disorder of the brain that affects thinking, memory, judgment, and speech.

anatomical plane An imaginary flat surface that separates two sections of the body or of an organ.

anatomical position The position of the body used in anatomical descriptions: standing upright, facing forward, arms at the side, palms facing forward, feet slightly apart.

atria The two upper chambers of the heart.

brainstem The portion of the brain that houses the control centers for the body's involuntary activities, such as respiration and heartbeat.

cavity A space within the body.

cell The simplest living unit of the body structure.

cerebellum The part of the brain that coordinates activities of the muscles and helps maintain balance.

cerebrum The largest section of the brain. It is responsible for intelligence and thought.

dermis The inner layer of the skin.

diabetes mellitus A disease of the pancreas caused by destruction or damage to the islet cells.

directional terms Words used to describe a body location or direction.

dorsal The back of the body.

epidermis The outer layer of the skin.

hepatitis An inflammatory disease of the liver caused by a virus.

homeostasis The body's state of good health and stability in the face of constant change.

islet cells Cells that produce and secrete the hormone insulin in the pancreas.

myocardial infarction An event in which the blood supply to the myocardium—the heart muscle—is reduced or completely stopped. Also called *heart attack*.

organ Any major body structure made up of two or more tissues working together that performs a specific function.

quadrants A division into four parts, used to describe the areas of the abdomen.

receptor A specialized cell or nerve ending that responds to specific stimuli, such as light, sound, or touch.

system Several organs working together to perform a particular function.

tissue A group of cells with similar structure and function.

ventral The front of the body.

ventricles The two lower chambers of the heart.

Body Structure

As a nursing assistant, everything you do should promote the health and well-being of your patients. In a healthy person, all parts of the body function normally. The body remains stable in the face of constant change, both internal and external. This state of good health is called **homeostasis**. It is important to understand the structure of the human body and how it works when a person is healthy. Then you will more clearly understand what happens when illness or injury occurs, so you can better assist your patients.

The body is a complex structure made up of cells, tissues, organs, and systems. Cells combine to form tissues, tissues combine to form organs, and organs combine to form entire systems. **See Figure 9-1.**

Cells

A **cell** is the simplest living unit of the body. Most cells are so small that they can be seen only with a microscope. The body is made up of millions of cells. They vary in size, shape, and function, but all cells have some needs in common. They need nutrition, water, and oxygen in order to live and function. All cells must also eliminate waste material.

Three basic structures of the cell are the membrane, cytoplasm, and nucleus. **See Figure 9-2.**

- The *cell membrane* is the outer covering of the cell. It holds substances inside the cell and helps the cell maintain its shape. The membrane also allows certain substances to pass through and others not to pass through.
- The *cytoplasm* is a watery substance that surrounds the nucleus. It performs most of the work of the cell.
- The *nucleus* controls the cell's activities, contains the chromosomes, and directs cell reproduction.

Cells do not work alone. Groups of them work together to perform a specific function. For example, blood cells differ from bone cells. Cells have several func-

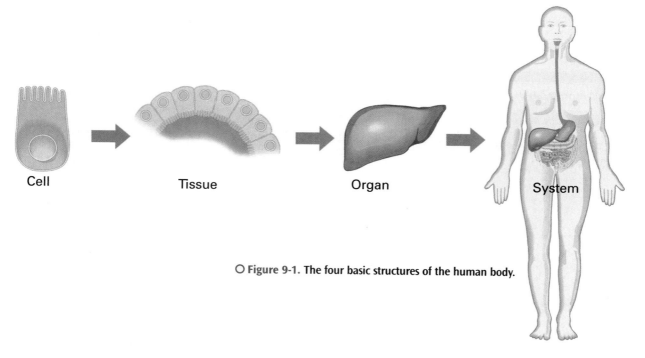

Cell   Tissue   Organ   System

O **Figure 9-1. The four basic structures of the human body.**

tions in the body. They convert substances into energy to stay alive. They grow and can differentiate for varied functions. They reproduce by dividing in half, making exact copies of themselves. They group together with similar cells to become tissue.

Tissues

A **tissue** is a group of cells with similar structure and function working together to perform the same task. Bones, blood, and muscles are tissues. Bones are made up of bone cells, blood is made up of blood cells, and muscles are made up of muscle cells. There are four types of tissue in the body. **See Figure 9-3.**

- *Connective tissues* support and connect parts of the body. Blood, bones, ligaments, and tendons are connective tissues.

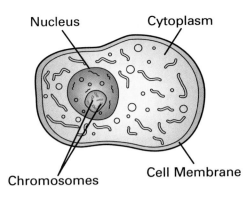

Nucleus   Cytoplasm

Chromosomes   Cell Membrane

○ **Figure 9-2. The structure of a cell.**

Connective Tissue   Epithelial Tissue   Muscle Tissue   Nerve Tissue

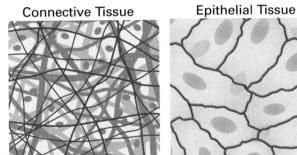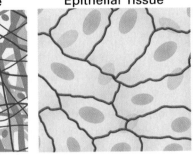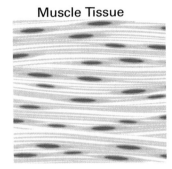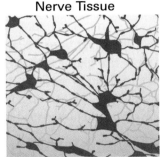

○ **Figure 9-3. The four types of tissues.**

Vital Skills   MATH

Cell Division: Exponential Functions

Cells reproduce themselves by dividing equally. In this way, one cell becomes two, two cells become four, four cells become eight, and so on. This growth rate is said to be *exponential*:

Division 1 (of the original cell) = 2 cells
Division 2 = 2 x 2 = 4 cells
Division 3 = 2 x 2 x 2 = 8 cells
Division 4 = 2 x 2 x 2 x 2 = 16 cells

Do you see a pattern here? You can write these functions more concisely using *exponential notation*:

Division 1 = 2^1 = 2 cells
Division 2 = 2^2 = 4 cells

Division 3 = 2^3 = 8 cells
Division 4 = 2^4 = 16 cells

The superscript number is the number of times the base number (2, in this case) is multiplied by itself.

Practice

1. **How many cells would be present after 8 divisions?**
2. **How many cells would be present after 12 divisions?**
3. **How many cells does the exponential notation 2^{16} represent?**

- *Epithelial tissues* cover the internal and external body surfaces to form a protective covering. The outer layer of skin is an example of epithelial tissue that covers an external surface. The tissue lining the small intestine is an example of internal epithelial tissue.
- *Muscle tissues* allow the body to move by expanding and contracting. Skeletal muscle tissue allows movement of arms, legs, and other parts of the body. Smooth muscle tissue lines the walls of some organs. The heart is made of cardiac muscle tissue.
- *Nerve tissues* create and transmit electrochemical impulses. These impulses carry information throughout the body. For example, the brain sends messages through the nerves to other parts of the body.

Organs and Systems

An **organ** is any major body structure that performs a specific function or functions. Organs are made up of two or more types of tissues that work together. The heart, the lungs, and the brain are organs. Several organs working together to perform a particular function make up a **system**. Examples of systems include the nervous system and the digestive system. You will learn more about systems in Chapter 10.

Body Cavities

A **cavity** is a space within the body. **See Figure 9-4.** Cavities typically contain one or more organs. The body's two major cavities are the dorsal cavity and the ventral cavity. **Dorsal** refers to the back of the body. The dorsal cavity includes:
- The cranial cavity, which contains the brain.
- The spinal cavity, which contains the spinal cord.

Ventral refers to the front of the body. The ventral cavity is divided into the thoracic cavity and the abdominal cavity. These two cavities are separated by a large muscle known as the *diaphragm*.
- The thoracic cavity includes the heart, lungs, and major blood vessels.
- The abdominal cavity contains organs of:
  - The digestive system (stomach, liver, gallbladder, intestines, pancreas, spleen).
  - The reproductive system (in females, the ovaries and uterus; in males, the prostate).
  - The urinary system (kidneys and bladder).

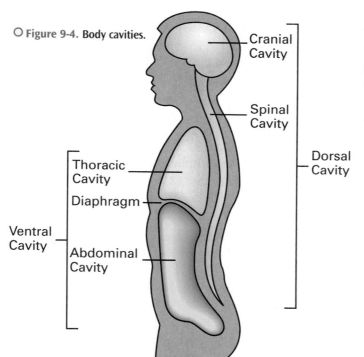

○ Figure 9-4. Body cavities.

Cranial Cavity

Spinal Cavity

Dorsal Cavity

Thoracic Cavity

Diaphragm

Ventral Cavity

Abdominal Cavity

Anatomical Planes and Quadrants

To make structures more easily understandable or "visible," we divide the body into sections. An **anatomical plane** is an imaginary flat surface that separates two sections of the body or of an organ. **See Figure 9-5.**

- The *frontal* or *coronal* plane divides the body into front and back sections.
- The *sagittal* plane divides the body into left and right sections.
- The *horizontal* or *transverse* plane divides the body into upper and lower sections.

The abdomen is a large area of the trunk portion of the body. It can be divided into four smaller **quadrants**, or regions, to better describe the location of pain, scars, or incisions. The divisions occur where a transverse plane and a sagittal plane cross at the navel. **Figure 9-6** illustrates the abdominal quadrants: the right upper quadrant, the right lower quadrant, the left upper quadrant, and the left lower quadrant.

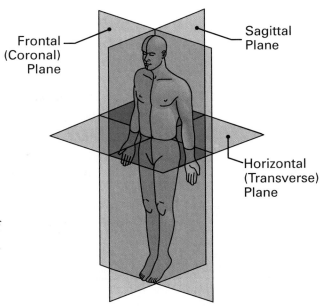

○ **Figure 9-5.** The anatomical planes of the body.

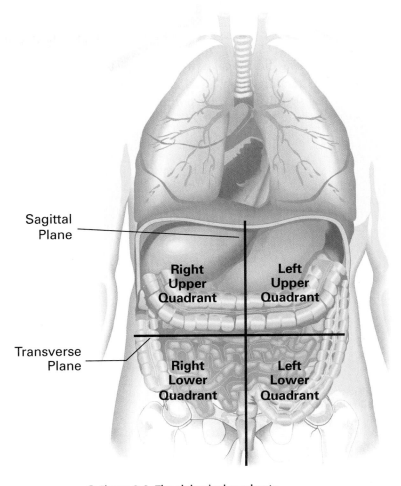

○ **Figure 9-6.** The abdominal quadrants.

Directional Terms

Words used to describe a body location or direction are called **directional terms**. See Table 9-1. Health care professionals use these terms to describe complaints that patients experience in a language that is understood by everyone. For example, if a patient is experiencing pain, the nursing assistant can report the individual's problem more clearly using directional terms.

○ **Table 9-1. Directional Terms**

Term	Direction	Example
superior	above, or higher	The liver is superior to the intestines.
inferior	below, or lower	The liver is inferior to the lungs.
anterior	toward the front	The cornea is on the anterior side of the eyeball.
posterior	toward the back	The iris is posterior to the cornea.
ventral	toward the front	The stomach is on the ventral side of the body.
dorsal	toward the back	The spinal cord is on the dorsal side of the body.
medial	toward the midline	The heart is medial to the lungs.
lateral	away from the midline	The kidneys are lateral to the spinal column.
proximal	closer to the center of the body	The elbow is proximal to the hand.
distal	further from the center of the body	The foot is distal to the knee.

When using directional terms, always picture the body in the **anatomical position**: standing upright, facing forward, arms at the side, palms facing forward, feet slightly apart. This position can be shown in either the anterior or the posterior view. **See Figure 9-7.**

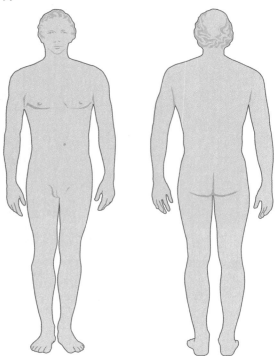

○ **Figure 9-7. The anatomical position. Anterior and posterior views.**

Anterior View   Posterior View

Visualizing Directional Terms

One way to remember the anatomical and directional terms you encountered in this chapter is to visualize them as you read them. When you *visualize*, you create a picture in your mind. These pictures will help you remember new words or concepts that you come across while reading. For example, when you read the directional terms in Table 9-1, try to visualize a human body in your mind. Create a mental picture of a liver above or superior to intestines, or a foot distal to the knee.

While visualizing refers specifically to seeing, you don't have to limit yourself to making pictures in your mind. As you read about the sensory organs later in this chapter, try to think of smells or sounds that might help you remember what you read.

> ### Practice
>
> Working with a partner, review the directional terms in Table 9-1 and the examples given. For each term, write a list of new examples that you can visualize in your mind.

Major Organs of the Body

The human body contains many organs. These organs work together to maintain homeostasis in the body. Learning about the structure and function of some of the body's major organs will help you understand certain diseases.

The Skin

The skin is the largest organ of the human body. It holds the entire body together in one package. It has two layers: the **epidermis**, or outer layer of the skin, and the **dermis**, or inner layer of the skin. **See Figure 9-8.** The skin performs several functions:

- Protects the body from injury and illness
- Regulates body temperature, particularly through sweating
- Maintains fluid balance in the body
- Transmits sensations such as touch, pressure, and pain. It performs this function as a sensory organ, as described later in this chapter.

Part of your job will be to observe signs and symptoms of skin conditions in your patients. Changes in color and texture, as well as open sores and rashes, are clues to a patient's overall health and well-being. You will also care for patients' skin and help skin conditions heal. Skin problems that may be found in patients in health care facilities include pressure ulcers, rashes, lesions, and surgical wounds. These problems should be reported to the nurse.

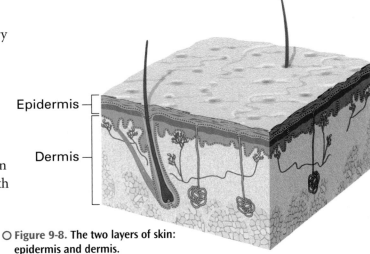

Epidermis —

Dermis —

○ **Figure 9-8.** The two layers of skin: epidermis and dermis.

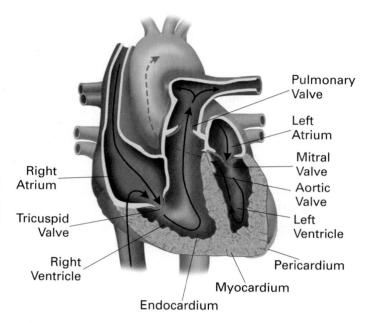

Pulmonary Valve

Left Atrium

Mitral Valve

Aortic Valve

Left Ventricle

Pericardium

Myocardium

Endocardium

Right Atrium

Tricuspid Valve

Right Ventricle

○ **Figure 9-9. The structure of the heart.**

The Heart

The heart is a hollow, fist-sized muscle located in the thoracic cavity, slightly left of the midline and between the lungs. Its primary function is to pump oxygen-rich blood through the body. The heart consists of three layers. **See Figure 9-9.**

- The pericardium is the outer layer. It is the thin sac that encloses the heart.
- The myocardium is the muscular middle layer that makes up the walls of the heart's chambers.
- The endocardium is the lining of the heart's chambers.

The heart is divided into four chambers. The two upper chambers are the **atria** (singular: *atrium*). They receive blood coming in from the body. The two lower chambers are the **ventricles**. They pump blood back to the body. The atria and the ventricles are separated by valves. These four valves are flaps of tissue that allow blood to flow in one direction only as the heart beats. They prevent the blood from the ventricles from backing up into the atria.

- The tricuspid valve is between the right atrium and the right ventricle.
- The pulmonary valve is between the right ventricle and the pulmonary artery. (See Chapter 10 for a discussion of arteries.)
- The mitral valve is between the left atrium and the left ventricle.
- The aortic valve is between the left ventricle and the aorta. (See Chapter 10 for more information about the aorta.)

You will likely care for patients who have experienced myocardial infarction. **Myocardial infarction** occurs when the blood supply to the myocardium—the heart muscle—is reduced or completely stopped. It is also called a *heart attack*. If the blood supply is cut off for more than a few minutes, cells in the heart muscle can die. This causes permanent damage to the heart tissue. The person can become disabled or die, depending on how much and which part of the heart muscle has been damaged.

The Lungs

The lungs are composed of spongy tissues made up of nerves, blood vessels, and tiny air sacs called **alveoli**. The two lungs are located in the thoracic cavity. **See Figure 9-10.** The primary function of the lungs is *respiration*, the process of inhaling and exhaling. When we inhale, the lungs extract oxygen from the air and deliver it to the bloodstream. As we exhale, the lungs expel carbon dioxide, one of the body's waste products.

Each lung is divided into lobes, or parts. The right lung has three lobes, and the left lung has two lobes. The lungs are protected by the ribs and two *pleural membranes*, or sheets of tissue. One lines the inside of the chest cavity. The other covers the lungs. Fluid between these layers cushions the lungs. When the lungs expand upon inhaling, the pleural membranes prevent the lungs from rubbing against the ribs.

Many diseases are associated with the lungs, including lung cancer. Lung cancer occurs when cells in the lungs begin to grow out of control. These cells eventually form tumors that affect the functioning of the lungs. In many lung cancer cases, patients must have all or part of the lung removed surgically. If surgery or other treatment does not stop the cancer's growth, the person can die.

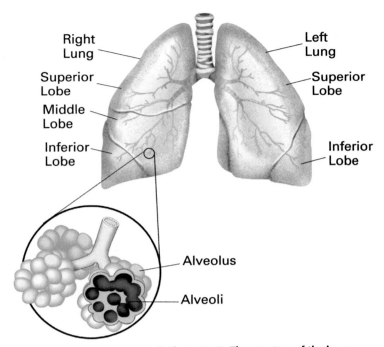

O Figure 9-10. **The structure of the lungs.**

The Liver

The liver is a very large organ weighing about four pounds. At any given time, it contains about 13% of the body's blood supply. It is located in the upper right and center of the abdominal cavity, beneath the diaphragm. It consists of two lobes. **See Figure 9-11.** The liver performs the following important functions:

- Fights infections
- Processes carbohydrates, proteins, and fats to be used by the body for nutrition
- Stores vitamins and minerals for the body's later use
- Changes harmful agents in the body, such as alcohol, into less harmful substances
- Produces blood proteins that help in blood clotting

Hepatitis is an inflammatory disease of the liver caused by a virus. It can be very mild or, at the other extreme, it can sometimes lead to death. There are different types of hepatitis, but the three most common are hepatitis A, B, and C.

Hepatitis A is usually passed from one person to another through the fecal-oral route, particularly in contaminated food or water. Food handlers who do not follow standard food preparation guidelines, such as wearing disposable gloves and using proper handwashing techniques, can place their patrons at risk for hepatitis A.

Hepatitis B is usually transmitted by blood, saliva, contaminated needles, contaminated body fluids, or sexual contact. Vaccines are available for hepatitis A and B. Hepatitis C is also transmitted via the blood and sometimes through sexual contact. This form of hepatitis remains in the blood for years. It can cause serious, and even fatal, liver damage.

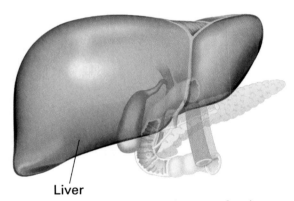

O Figure 9-11. **The liver has many important functions, including helping the body fight infections.**

The Pancreas

The pancreas is located in the left upper abdominal quadrant, behind the stomach. It is about six inches long. **See Figure 9-12.** It manufactures digestive enzymes and juices that break down food into chemicals the body can use. The

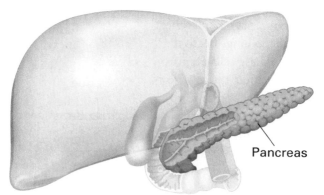
○ **Figure 9-12. The pancreas regulates the body's metabolism of carbohydrates.**

pancreas also contains **islet cells** that produce and secrete the hormone insulin. Insulin is responsible for regulating the body's use of carbohydrates.

The disease most commonly associated with the pancreas is **diabetes mellitus**. It is caused by destruction or damage to the islet cells. Type 1 diabetes is also known as *insulin-dependent diabetes*. It usually begins in childhood. In type 1 diabetes, the pancreas does not produce enough insulin. The patient may need daily insulin injections to supply the insulin that the body is not producing.

In type 2 diabetes (*noninsulin-dependent diabetes*), the pancreas either does not produce enough insulin, or the body has enough insulin but the cells do not respond to the insulin properly. Type 2 diabetes usually occurs in people in middle age. It is usually related to obesity, inactivity, medications, or excessive use of alcohol. In some cases, this type of diabetes may be controlled by diet and exercise alone. Diabetes in general is a major cause of disability and death.

The Brain

The brain is the most complex organ in the body. It regulates the body's activities. Information in the form of impulses is transmitted to the brain from the

Vital Skills   WRITING

Writing Sentences Using New Words

One way to increase your writing skill is to write the new words you encounter in sentences. This chapter contains many new terms, including directional terms and anatomical terms. Try using them in sentences that describe the human body.

Example: The heart, a major organ of the body, is *superior* to the liver.

Practice

In Chapter 1 you learned how to write a paragraph. Remember that you need a main idea and supporting details. Choose three of the major organs (skin, heart, lungs, liver, pancreas, or brain) and write a paragraph about each using the new vocabulary words you learned in this chapter. Try to use at least one new word per sentence and at least one directional term per paragraph.

five senses. The brain processes this information and then activates body organs and systems to perform the appropriate tasks.

The brain weighs about three pounds and is located within the skull. The skull, scalp, fluid, and layers of tissue protect it from injury. For the most part, the brain consists of matter made up of nerve cells.

The largest part of the brain is the **cerebrum. See Figure 9-13.** The cerebrum is responsible for:
• Intelligence, thought, memory, language, and emotion.
• Controlling the body's voluntary muscular movements.
• Processing the information received by the five senses.

The cerebrum is divided into two hemispheres: right and left. These two hemispheres communicate information to each other. The left hemisphere controls movement and activity on the right side of the body. The right hemisphere controls movement and activity on the left side of the body.

The **cerebellum** is the part of the brain that coordinates activities of the muscles and helps maintain balance. It is located inferior to the cerebrum. The **brainstem** is the portion of the brain that houses the control centers for the body's involuntary activities, such as respiration and heartbeat. It also connects the brain to the spinal cord.

Alzheimer's disease is a degenerative (getting worse over time) disorder of the brain that affects thinking, memory, judgment, and speech. Confusion and memory loss are two major signs of the disease. The disease occurs equally in men and women. It is more common in the elderly but can also occur in people in their forties and fifties. It is not, however, part of the normal aging process.

Alzheimer's is a chronic, irreversible disease. As it progresses, individuals may experience changes in personality and behavior, such as anxiety, agitation, or delusions and hallucinations. Its cause is unknown and there is currently no cure. Scientists have discovered, though, that changes have taken place in the structure and functioning of the brain in Alzheimer's patients.

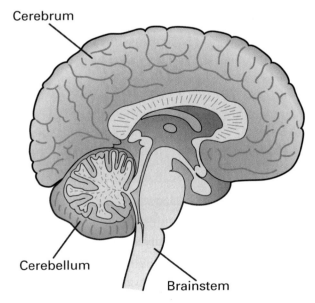

O **Figure 9-13. The major structures of the brain.**

FOCUS ON

Technology
Computed tomography (CT) scanning helps health care professionals "see" the interior of the brain and other parts of the body to diagnose disease and reduce the need for exploratory surgery. The CT scanner sends an extremely thin x-ray beam through a part of the body from many different angles. The computer screen then shows thin slices of the body part. This scan produces more complete and detailed images than conventional x-rays.

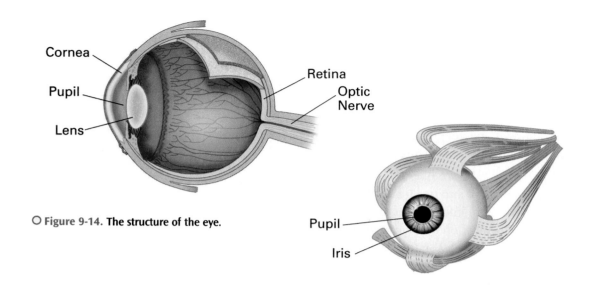

O **Figure 9-14. The structure of the eye.**

The Sensory Organs

Humans receive information about the world around them through the five senses: sight, sound, smell, taste, and touch. The corresponding sensory organs are the eyes, the ears, the nose, the taste buds, and the skin.

All organs have receptors that receive information from the environment. A **receptor** is a specialized cell or nerve ending that responds to specific stimuli, such as light, sound, or touch. Information is sent by the receptors to the brain for processing and interpretation. Then the brain sends back messages to the body, instructing it to perform some movement or activity. If any of the senses are impaired and are not functioning properly, the brain cannot respond appropriately to outside stimuli.

The Eyes. The eyes contain the receptors for vision. **See Figure 9-14.** The eyes are fragile and can be easily injured. They are protected by the bones of the skull, eyelids, eyelashes, and tears. The process of seeing includes these steps:

1. Light enters the eye through the *cornea*, a clear layer around the outside of the eyeball.
2. Light rays pass through the *pupil*, which is the opening in the middle of the *iris* (the colored part of the eye). The pupil changes size to control how much light enters.
3. From the pupil, light passes onto the *lens*.
4. The light is reflected back to the *retina*. The retina lines the posterior portion of the eyeball.
5. From the retina, images received by the eye are sent through the *optic nerve* to the sensory center in the brain. The sensory center interprets the images, so we can recognize and identify objects in our environment.

As people age, their eyes change. The lens becomes less flexible, so the eye loses some ability to focus on objects that are near. Many people over the age of 40 need prescription eyeglasses for reading and other close work. Yellowing of the lens may affect their perception of colors, and many elderly people misread colors as a result.

Another effect of aging is that the iris becomes more rigid, so the eye takes longer to adjust to changes in light. Always turn on the light in a dark room before allowing a patient to enter. This makes it easier for their eyes to adjust, so there is less chance of a fall or injury. Some elderly patients' eyes are sensitive to light and glare. Close blinds and curtains when appropriate to minimize glare. Make sure sunglasses are available for indoor as well as outdoor use.

The Ears. The ears function as the organ for hearing and maintaining balance. When a sound occurs, the ears receive sound waves from outside the body. These waves are then transmitted to the auditory center of the brain for processing.

Figure 9-15 illustrates the three major parts of the ear: the outer ear, the middle ear, and the inner ear.

- The outer ear consists of the auricle and the auditory canal. The *auricle* is the part of the ear that you can see. It is made of cartilage and covered by skin. It directs sound waves to the auditory canal. This canal then directs the sound waves to the middle ear.
- The middle ear is a cavity filled with air in the temporal bone of the skull. The *tympanic membrane* (eardrum) separates the outer and middle ears. Sound waves cause the tympanic membrane to vibrate. The *eustachian tube* connects the middle ear with the throat. It maintains equal amounts of air pressure between the middle ear and the atmosphere, which helps the eardrum vibrate properly. The *ossicles* are three tiny bones that receive vibrations from the eardrum and send them to the inner ear.
- The cochlea and semicircular canals are the major parts of the inner ear. The *cochlea* contains a fluid that transmits sounds to the auditory nerve. This nerve then sends sounds to the brain for processing. The three semicircular canals are important for maintaining balance. They are also filled with fluid. The semicircular canals note when the body is in motion and send this information to the brain. The brain makes adjustments to maintain balance.

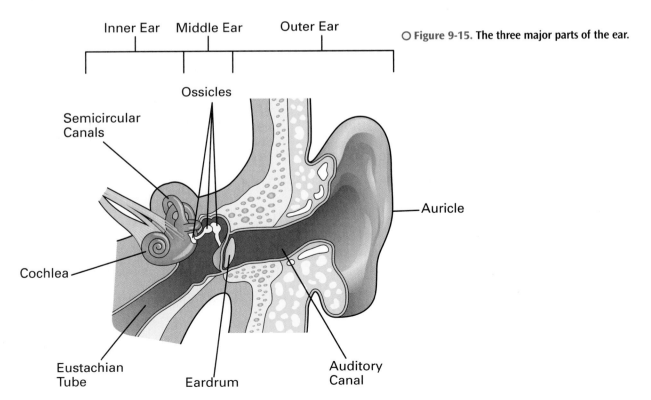

Inner Ear   Middle Ear   Outer Ear

○ **Figure 9-15.** The three major parts of the ear.

Ossicles

Semicircular Canals

Auricle

Cochlea

Eustachian Tube

Eardrum

Auditory Canal

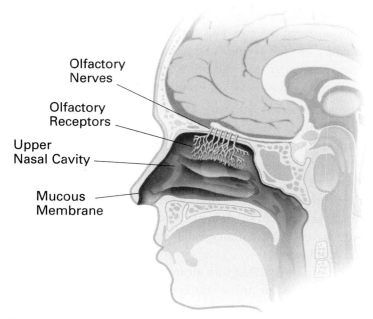

○ **Figure 9-16.** The structure of the nose as a sensory organ.

As people age, the tympanic membrane and ossicles become stiffer. As a result, many older adults lose some capacity for hearing. Low-pitched sounds may become easier for them to hear, but high-pitched sounds may become more difficult. If you are working with a person with hearing loss, face the person when you are speaking. Speak slowly and clearly in a low-pitched tone. You may need to repeat what you say. If so, do not become impatient, raise your voice, or shout.

The Nose. The nose is the sense organ responsible for smell. The upper nasal cavities contain receptors for smell. **See Figure 9-16.** These chemoreceptors detect chemicals that are sniffed into the nose and dissolved in the *mucous membrane* lining the nasal cavity. The receptors cause impulses to be sent to the *olfactory nerves* and into the brain.

As people get older, the number of chemoreceptors decreases. They may lose some of their sense of smell. This can decrease the enjoyment of food, because the food no longer smells the same.

The Taste Buds. The taste buds are the sensory organs of taste located on the surface of the tongue. The taste buds also have chemoreceptors, which detect chemicals from foods when they dissolve in the mouth. When the chemoreceptors send messages to the brain, the brain determines the exact nature of the taste—sweet, sour, salty, or bitter. **See Figure 9-17.**

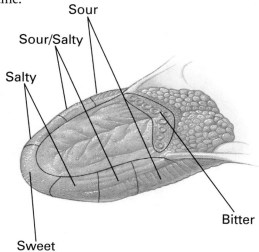

○ **Figure 9-17.** The location of the taste buds on the tongue.

As people age, the number of chemoreceptors in the taste buds decreases. The remaining taste buds become less able to identify tastes. This is especially true for people who are long-term cigarette smokers. Some medications can interfere with the sense of taste. Not being able to taste food can decrease the appetite, which in turn can result in poor nutrition.

The Skin. As a sensory organ, the skin detects hot, cold, touch, pressure, and pain. Tactile receptors and nerve endings are located in the skin all over the body. (*Tactile* means "touch.") They receive stimuli from outside the body and send information to the brain for interpretation. Some parts of the skin contain more tactile receptors than others. The lips and the tips of the fingers and toes are the most sensitive parts of the body to touch.

People with diabetes, peripheral nerve damage due to injury, or multiple sclerosis may have an impaired sense of touch. For example, they may be unable to feel the temperature of bathwater or hot food and beverages. Patients with this type of impairment need special care. You need to make their environment as safe as possible. To prevent burns, check the temperature of food and drinks before serving. If they are too hot, let them cool. Always check the temperature of the water before the patient bathes.

Vital Skills — COMMUNICATION

Feeding a Patient with Sensory Deficits

Sensory impairments can make eating more challenging for patients. Some patients may require extra assistance, and some patients may need to be fed.

For example, a visually impaired person may need your help organizing the tray and opening containers and wrappers. But once she knows where things are on the tray, she may be able to feed herself. What about people with hearing impairment? Might they have any difficulties eating? Perhaps they didn't see the lunch tray being delivered and they aren't aware that their food is waiting for them.

Some sensory deficits might make patients lose interest in eating. For example, as people get older, they may lose some of their sense of smell and taste. Some medications can also interfere with the sense of taste. These factors may decrease a patient's enjoyment of food and decrease his or her appetite, which can result in poor nutrition. Encouraging people to try different foods on their tray and using appropriate seasonings may help patients enjoy their food more.

If you are unsure about feeding a patient with a sensory impairment—or about feeding any patient—be sure to check with your supervisor. Whenever you are feeding patients or helping them to eat, remember to keep the head of the bed up to help swallowing and prevent choking.

Practice

In teams of two, practice feeding patients with sensory impairments. One person can be the patient and the other the nursing assistant. What techniques might you use when you are bringing a lunch tray to a patient who is visually impaired? What about to someone with an impaired sense of touch?

Chapter Summary

- The body is made up of cells, tissues, organs, and systems.
- The cell is the basic building block of the body. Groups of cells form tissues that perform a specific function.
- A tissue is a group of cells that work together to perform a task.
- The four types of tissue are connective, epithelial, muscle, and nerve tissue.
- Cavities are spaces within the body that contain the organs.

- Anatomical planes, quadrants, and directional terms are used to explain the location of body parts and of patient complaints.
- Organs are major structures composed of two or more types of tissue.
- The five sensory organs have receptors that send information to the brain for processing and interpretation.
- As people age, the senses sometimes become diminished. Many elderly people have sensory impairments and may need extra help taking care of themselves.

VOCABULARY REVIEW

Directions: Match the letter of each definition in the second column with the correct vocabulary term in the first column. Write your answers on a separate sheet of paper.

Vocabulary

1. anatomical plane
2. anatomical position
3. atria
4. cavity
5. cell
6. directional term
7. dorsal
8. homeostasis
9. organ
10. quadrants
11. receptor
12. system
13. tissue
14. ventral
15. ventricles

Definitions

A. The two upper chambers of the heart
B. Words used to describe a body location or direction
C. The body's state of good health and stability in the face of constant change
D. A division into four parts, used to describe the areas of the abdomen
E. The back of the body
F. The two lower chambers of the heart
G. An imaginary flat surface that separates two sections of the body or of an organ
H. A group of cells with similar structure and function
I. A space within the body
J. Several organs working together to perform a particular function
K. The simplest living unit of the body structure
L. Any major body structure made up of two or more tissues working together that performs a specific function
M. The front of the body
N. The position of the body used in anatomical descriptions
O. A specialized cell or nerve ending that responds to specific stimuli

Check Your Knowledge

Review Questions: Answer each of the following questions on a separate sheet of paper.

1. What four structures make up the body?
2. What is the function of the cell's nucleus?
3. What are the functions of connective tissue?
4. Which organs are located in the thoracic cavity?
5. What is the frontal plane?
6. Define *anterior* and *posterior*.
7. Name the three layers of the heart.
8. What is myocardial infarction?
9. What are the functions of the cerebrum?
10. What is the cochlea?

True or False: Read each statement carefully. Then write *True* or *False* by the statement number on a separate sheet of paper.

1. When cells in the lung grow out of control, they can form cancerous tumors.
2. From the cornea, images are sent to the brain through the optic nerve.
3. Type 1 diabetes occurs when the body has enough insulin but is unable to use it.
4. Alzheimer's disease is part of the normal aging process.
5. Some areas of the skin, such as the lips, have a greater number of receptors than others.

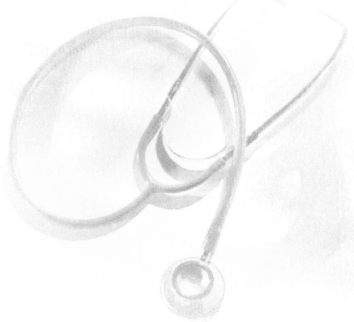

Think and Decide

Directions: Think about each of the following scenarios. Answer each question on a separate sheet of paper.

1. Clara, a resident in your care, seems depressed because her granddaughter, Josie, is coming to visit. Clara explains that Josie quickly becomes frustrated and shouts at her because she cannot hear her. This makes Clara sad and frustrated. What might you do to help?

2. A 62-year-old hospitalized patient with type 2 diabetes asks you if she will ever need to take insulin. What should you do?

3. You are a home health aide caring for an elderly male client. When you arrive this morning, he asks you to take a look at his back. He says the skin feels "rough and scratchy," but he cannot tell what is wrong with it. When you examine his back, you see a reddish rash that covers about a 5-centimeter area near the right shoulder. What should you do?

4. You are working in a long-term care facility. When you enter Rosita's room this evening, she tells you, "I had a heart attack today." You check the shift notes from the day shift and find no record of any complaint or pain. Rosita appears to be in her usual state of health. What should you do?

5. Mr. G., a resident in the long-term care facility where you work, looks troubled today. When you ask him what is wrong, he says that he has just been diagnosed with lung cancer. Mr. G. is a fairly heavy smoker and is well-known for his frequent trips outside to the smoking area. He asks you, "If I quit smoking, do you think the cancer will go away?"

6. Mrs. J. has been admitted to the convalescent center where you work while she recovers from a CVA (stroke). The CVA affected her sense of balance, so she is undergoing physical therapy. Little else seems to have been affected. However, during the last few days, you have noticed that she sometimes slurs her words and seems to lose track of what she is saying. What might this indicate? What should you do?

7. Jamie, a resident at a long-term care facility, confides to you that she does not like to go to the dining room to eat, even though she would enjoy the company of other residents at mealtime. She says the lights in the dining room are so bright that she has trouble seeing and she is afraid that, even with her walker, she may fall. What might you suggest?

CNA Certification Exam Prep

Directions: This practice test contains ten questions. Each question has four suggested answers. For each question, choose the ONE that best answers the question or completes the statement. Write your answers on a separate sheet of paper.

1. Groups of tissues that work together to perform a specific body function are called
   A. cells.
   B. organs.
   C. systems.
   D. senses.

2. The lungs are protected from the bones of the ribs by the
   A. alveoli.
   B. spine.
   C. stomach.
   D. pleural membranes.

3. Hepatitis is a disease that affects the
   A. pancreas.
   B. colon.
   C. liver.
   D. lung.

4. A coronal plane divides the body into
   A. front and back sections.
   B. left and right sections.
   C. upper and lower sections.
   D. upper right and lower left sections.

5. An injury that is inferior to the left knee is
   A. above the knee.
   B. below the knee.
   C. beside the knee.
   D. on the knee.

6. Which of the following statements correctly describes the wrist?
   A. The wrist is proximal to the hand.
   B. The wrist is proximal to the elbow.
   C. The wrist is medial to the shoulder.
   D. The wrist is distal from the thumb.

7. The two layers of the skin are the epidermis and the
   A. alveolar.
   B. endocardium.
   C. dermis.
   D. ventricular.

8. The upper chambers of the heart are the
   A. ventricles.
   B. alveoli.
   C. auricles.
   D. atria.

9. Specialized cells or nerve endings that respond to specific stimuli are
   A. islet cells.
   B. tissues.
   C. receptors.
   D. pleural membranes.

10. Which of the following statements about the lungs is correct?
    A. The right lung has three lobes, and the left lung has two lobes.
    B. The left lung has three lobes, and the right lung has two lobes.
    C. Both lungs have three lobes.
    D. Both lungs have two lobes.

CHAPTER 10

OBJECTIVES

- Explain why nursing assistants should obtain a basic understanding of anatomy and physiology.

- Describe the systems of the human body, including their basic structures and functions.

- Describe disorders and diseases related to various body systems.

Anatomy and Physiology

VOCABULARY

anatomy The basic structures of the human body.

antibodies Specialized proteins that fight disease.

artery A blood vessel that carries blood away from the heart.

capillary Small blood vessel that connects the ends of arterioles with venules.

constrict To narrow.

digestion The process of breaking down foods into usable nutrients, absorbing nutrients, and excreting waste products.

dilate To expand.

gas exchange The process of moving oxygen into the blood and removing carbon dioxide from the blood.

gland Organ that creates chemicals needed for proper body functioning.

hemoglobin An iron-containing protein in red blood cells that carries oxygen and gives blood its red color.

hemostasis The prevention of blood loss.

hormone Chemical that regulates and controls the activities of cells.

menstruation The cyclic process of the blood and tissue lining the uterus being discharged through the vagina.

peristalsis Involuntary muscular, rhythmic contraction that propels contents through an organ.

physiology The functions of systems in the human body.

plasma The liquid part of the blood that carries blood cells, nutrients, antibodies, chemicals, gases, and waste products within the body.

platelets Irregular, disc-shaped solids in the blood that play a critical role in hemostasis.

semen The fluid that transports sperm.

vein A blood vessel that carries deoxygenated blood and waste products back to the heart.

ventilation The movement of air in and out of the lungs.

Systems of the Body

Systems are groups of organs that work together to perform one or more body functions. Each body system contributes to the total functioning of the body. The systems depend on each other for proper functioning. What happens in one system affects not only other systems, but also the body as a whole. For example, when you are upset, your nervous system is stressed. If you eat while you are upset, your digestive system may have difficulty breaking down the food. In the same way, when disease or injury occurs in one system, others are affected.

As a nursing assistant, you will care for patients whose bodies are not functioning properly because of disease, illness, injury, or the aging process. Understanding **anatomy** (the basic structures) and **physiology** (functions) of the human body will help you perform your job effectively. By understanding how systems function in a healthy body, you will better understand the effects of disease and aging on the body. **See Figure 10-1.** This knowledge will help you:

- Recognize certain signs and symptoms in the people you care for.
- Understand the reasons for the procedures you are directed to perform.
- Provide patients with safe, efficient care that returns them to maximum functioning as quickly as possible, or that helps them live as comfortably as possible in a long-term care facility.

The Cardiovascular System

The cardiovascular system transports blood throughout the body. It is made up of the heart, the blood, and the blood vessels. The heart pumps the blood to all parts of the body. (Information about the structure and function of the heart is in Chapter 9.) The blood delivers important substances such as nutrients (food) and oxygen to the cells. The blood also removes waste products, such as carbon dioxide, from the cells. Blood vessels carry the blood throughout the body, to and from the heart and lungs. The cardiovascular system is also involved in regulating the body's temperature.

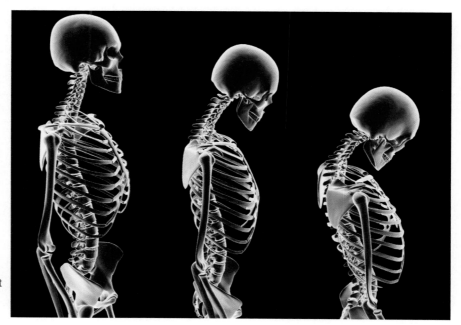

O **Figure 10-1.** Understanding body systems can help nursing assistants better understand what their patients experience as a result of disease or aging.

The Blood

The body contains 9 to 12 pints (4 to 6 liters) of blood, depending on size. Blood is connective tissue made up of plasma and blood cells. **Plasma** is the liquid part of the blood. It is about 90% water. Plasma carries blood cells, nutrients, antibodies, chemicals, gases, and waste products within the body.

Blood cells are produced in the bone marrow and lymphatic tissue. When they are no longer useful to the body, they are removed and destroyed by the spleen and liver. There are three types of blood cells: red blood cells, white blood cells, and platelets.

- Red blood cells carry oxygen to various parts of the body. **Hemoglobin** is an iron-containing protein in red blood cells that carries oxygen and gives blood its red color. As blood circulates through the lungs, hemoglobin picks up oxygen and delivers it to the cells. Oxygen-rich blood is bright red. As it delivers the oxygen to various parts of the body, the blood also picks up carbon dioxide, a waste product. Blood that is rich in carbon dioxide is dark red.
- White blood cells protect the body against infection and provide immunity to some diseases. For example, when any part of the body becomes infected, they rush to the area, multiply, and attack the infection.
- **Platelets** are irregular, disc-shaped solids in the blood that play a critical role in **hemostasis** (the prevention of blood loss). They do so by causing blood to clot and by repairing small leaks in blood vessel walls. They are produced by the bone marrow.

Blood Vessels

Throughout the body, blood vessels transport blood to cells and tissues. Blood vessels **constrict** (narrow) or **dilate** (expand) as required by the body. They vary in size. There are three types of blood vessels: arteries, veins, and capillaries. **See Figure 10-2.**

- **Arteries** are blood vessels that carry blood away from the heart, rich in oxygen and nutrients. The largest artery in the body is the aorta, which receives blood directly from the left ventricle of the heart. The aorta then branches into smaller arteries that deliver blood to all parts of the body. Arterioles are the smallest type of artery.
- **Veins** are blood vessels that transport deoxygenated blood and waste products back to the heart. As the veins approach the heart, they come together into two major veins. The inferior (lower) vena cava delivers blood to the heart from the legs and trunk. The superior (upper) vena cava carries blood to the heart from the arms and head. Venules are the smallest type of vein.
- **Capillaries** are very small blood vessels that carry blood from arterioles to venules. They pass oxygen, nutrients, and other substances to the cells and pick up waste products from the cells.

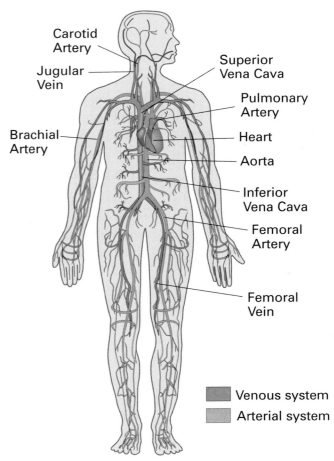

○ **Figure 10-2.** The cardiovascular system transports blood throughout the body.

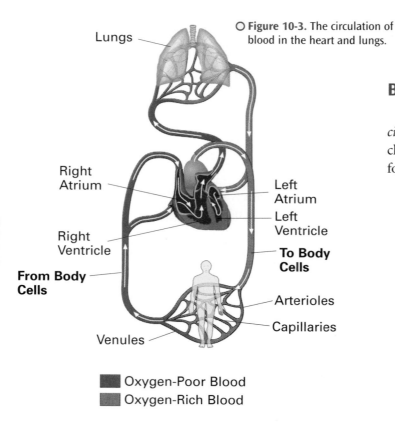

○ **Figure 10-3.** The circulation of blood in the heart and lungs.

Lungs

Right Atrium

Right Ventricle

From Body Cells

Left Atrium

Left Ventricle

To Body Cells

Arterioles

Capillaries

Venules

█ Oxygen-Poor Blood
█ Oxygen-Rich Blood

Blood Flow

The flow of blood through the body is called *circulation* because, in a way, it moves in a circle. The circulation of the blood occurs in the following sequence. **See Figure 10-3.**

1. Veins (the superior vena cava and the inferior vena cava) carry blood into the right atrium of the heart. This blood is low in oxygen and high in carbon dioxide.
2. The blood moves into the right ventricle, which pumps the blood out of the heart and into the lungs.
3. In the lungs, the blood picks up oxygen and rids itself of carbon dioxide.
4. The oxygen-rich blood returns to the left atrium of the heart through the pulmonary vein. (The pulmonary vein is the only vein in the body that carries oxygen-rich blood.)
5. This blood then passes into the left ventricle, where it is pumped out to the body through the aorta and into smaller arteries.
6. Blood is transported to the tissues by arterioles and to the cells by capillaries.
7. The capillaries provide the cells with oxygen and nutrient-rich blood in exchange for blood that is high in carbon dioxide and waste products.
8. The capillaries connect with the venules, which carry the oxygen-depleted blood back to the heart via the veins.

Diseases and Disorders

Clotting disorders include problems with blood clotting too little or too much. Blood clotting normally occurs after an injury to stop bleeding. People whose blood does not clot properly are subject to very large bruises. They could also die from losing too much blood. On the other hand, if blood clots too easily, blood clots can form in blood vessels. A blood clot can cause blockage in major blood vessels and prevent the normal circulation of blood. This blockage can be life-threatening if not treated immediately. Clots may occur in coronary arteries, pulmonary (lungs) arteries, cerebral (brain) arteries, and veins in the legs.

Coronary artery disease occurs when a coronary artery narrows. Coronary arteries supply food and oxygen to the cardiac muscle. When a coronary artery narrows, the blood supply to the parts of the heart served by that artery is reduced. A number of serious health problems can result. For example, areas of the heart muscle could die. One of the common causes of narrow arteries is atherosclerosis, a condition in which fat deposits build up on the inner walls of the artery.

SAFETY FIRST

Blood carries waste products and disease in the body. In a disease that is transmitted by contact, blood is often the vehicle of transmission. If you might have any contact with a patient's blood, follow standard precautions, the guidelines for preventing the spread of infection. Chapter 11 describes standard precautions.

Abnormally high blood pressure, or hypertension, is called the "silent killer" because it sometimes has no symptoms. People may not know they have hypertension until their blood pressure is measured. Left untreated, hypertension can cause major damage to the heart, blood vessels, liver, and kidneys. Hypertension often occurs in people who have narrow arteries. When arteries narrow, the heart has to pump with greater force to push the blood through the smaller openings in the blood vessels. This puts extra strain on the heart muscle. Over time, the heart tires and enlarges, making it more susceptible to heart failure.

The Respiratory System

Body tissues, especially the heart and brain, need a constant supply of oxygen. Oxygen provides cells with the energy they need to function effectively. The respiratory system has two functions: ventilation and gas exchange. **Ventilation** is the movement of air in and out of the lungs. (More information about the structure and function of the lungs is in Chapter 9.) When we breathe in (inhale), we bring oxygen into the lungs. When we breathe out (exhale), we eliminate the waste product carbon dioxide from the lungs. **Gas exchange** is the process of moving oxygen into the blood and removing carbon dioxide from the blood.

The respiratory system consists of two parts. The upper respiratory tract includes structures that are outside the thoracic (chest) cavity: the nasal cavities, pharynx (throat), and larynx (the voice box). The lower respiratory tract includes structures that are inside the thoracic cavity: the trachea, bronchi, lungs, bronchioles, and alveoli.

The Respiratory Process

Respiration (the combination of ventilation and gas exchange) occurs in the following sequence. **See Figure 10-4.**

1. The diaphragm, a strong muscle between the chest and abdominal cavities, contracts and moves downward, making the chest cavity expand. This causes the intake of air through the nose.
2. Air enters the nose and moves into the nasal cavities. Here, air is warmed and humidified. The mucous membrane and hair filter out dirt and germs to keep them from entering the lungs.
3. From the nasal cavities, air travels through the pharynx, a pathway for air and food.
4. Air then passes through the larynx. A small flap of cartilage, the epiglottis, covers the opening of the larynx. During breathing, the epiglottis remains open and allows air to pass through. During swallowing, the epiglottis closes over the larynx to prevent food from entering the airway.

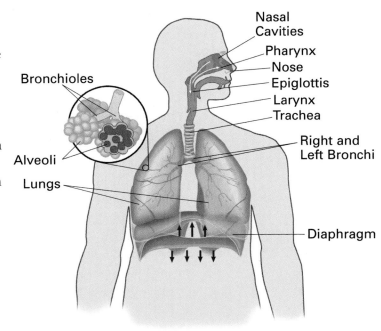

○ **Figure 10-4.** The process of respiration.

5. From the larynx, air moves down into the chest through the trachea, or windpipe.

6. The lower portion of the trachea divides into bronchi. Air from the right bronchus fills the right lung, and air from the left bronchus fills the left lung.

7. In the lungs, the bronchi divide into smaller branches called bronchioles. From the bronchioles, air moves into the alveoli. Alveoli are the millions of small, one-celled air sacs that fill with oxygen when air enters the lungs.

8. Gas exchange occurs in the alveoli. Blood in the capillaries receives oxygen from the alveoli and releases carbon dioxide.

9. When the diaphragm relaxes, the chest cavity contracts, and carbon dioxide-rich air is expelled through the lower and upper respiratory tracts.

Diseases and Disorders

Pneumonia is an inflammation of the lungs caused by a bacterial or viral infection. The alveoli fill with fluid, decreasing gas exchange. People who have pneumonia can experience painful breathing, fever, coughing, and wheezing. Many elderly people get pneumonia after having another primary infection, such as influenza.

Asthma affects the bronchi and bronchioles in the lungs. Certain triggers, such as allergies, smoke, or stress, cause these structures to constrict. Breathing then becomes very difficult. An asthma attack can be fatal.

Chronic obstructive pulmonary disease (COPD) refers to chronic conditions that affect the lungs, including emphysema and chronic bronchitis. Many people have both diseases. Chronic bronchitis is a disease of the bronchi and bronchioles. Chronic irritation of these structures (for example, from smoking) produces a thick mucus that obstructs air flow. Many people who have chronic bronchitis also get frequent infections.

Emphysema is a chronic and progressive lung disease. The alveoli become less elastic, resulting in the obstruction of air flow. A person with emphysema is unable to exhale all the air in the lungs. Carbon dioxide builds up in the lungs and further damages the alveoli. As the disease progresses, breathing becomes more difficult. The person becomes short of breath with the slightest effort. Mild emphysema often affects the elderly. Emphysema that occurs in younger adults is often a result of smoking.

The Digestive System

The digestive system (also called the gastrointestinal system) breaks down the food we eat into a form that can be used by the body's cells. It also eliminates waste from the body. The digestive system consists of the digestive tract and accessory organs.

The digestive tract includes the mouth, pharynx, esophagus, stomach, small intestine, and large intestine. Digestion occurs within the digestive tract. The accessory organs are the teeth, tongue, salivary glands, liver, gall bladder, and pancreas. These organs contribute to digestion. **Figure 10-5** shows the major organs of the digestive system.

The Digestive Process

Digestion is the process of breaking down foods into usable nutrients, absorbing nutrients, and excreting waste products. The entire process occurs in the following sequence.

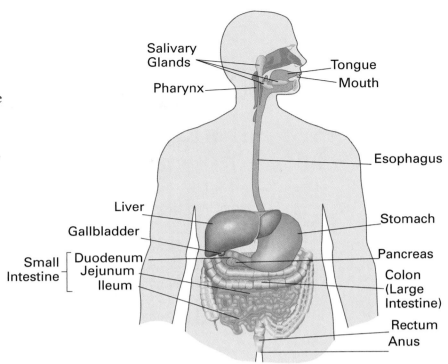

O **Figure 10-5.** The major and accessory organs of the digestive system.

1. Digestion begins in the mouth, where food is chewed and mixes with saliva. Saliva, produced by the salivary glands, contains chemicals that begin to break down the food into nutrients. Saliva also moistens food, making it easier to swallow.

2. The tongue helps push the food backward into the pharynx. When we swallow, food travels from the pharynx into the esophagus, which is a long, muscular tube.

3. From the esophagus, the food moves into the stomach. The stomach has strong muscles that churn the food to break it down even further. The stomach also secretes gastric juices, which aid in breaking down food.

4. The semiliquid mixture of partially digested food and gastric juices, called *chyme* (pronounced KIME), then leaves the stomach and travels to the small intestine. Food is moved through the intestines by **peristalsis**, the involuntary, rhythmic muscular contraction that propels contents through an organ. The small intestine is about 20 feet long and contains three main sections: the duodenum, the jejunum, and the ileum.

5. In the duodenum, the first portion of the small intestine, digestive juices from the liver, gallbladder, and pancreas work to further break down food so it can be absorbed by the body.

6. Absorption of nutrients begins in the jejunum and continues in the ileum. The walls of the small intestine are lined with thousands of tiny projections called *villi*. Villi absorb the digested food and pass the nutrients into the bloodstream via the capillaries. The capillaries then carry the nutrients to the individual cells.

7. Additional absorption takes place in the colon, or large intestine. The colon reabsorbs most of the remaining water from the chyme. The remaining waste is called *feces*. During excretion, feces pass through the colon and into the rectum. The rectum is the last 8 to 10 inches of the large intestine.

8. Feces leave the body through the anus, which is the body opening at the end of the rectum. Sphincter muscles control the opening and closing of the anus.

Diseases and Disorders

Ulcers are sores caused by tissue breakdown. They can occur anywhere in the digestive tract. Smoking, certain infections, and overuse of some pain drugs can contribute to the occurrence of ulcers. Patients with gastric (stomach) or duodenal ulcers may feel nausea or a burning sensation after eating.

The gallbladder can become diseased due to the formation of stones. These gallstones can obstruct the bile duct leading to the duodenum. Inflammation or infection can result in severe pain.

The Urinary System

The urinary system has two primary functions:
- Eliminating liquid waste from the body in the form of urine; this includes filtering blood and removing waste products and excess fluid
- Maintaining the body's homeostasis (stable internal balance)

The average adult male takes in about 3 liters of liquid per day, and the average adult female takes in about 2.2 liters. In a healthy body, approximately the same amount of fluid is output every day. Most of this fluid is eliminated through the urinary system. The remaining output is in the form of perspiration, exhalation, and tears.

The kidneys and the bladder are the major organs of the urinary system. **See Figure 10-6.** The two kidneys are bean-shaped organs located in the upper abdominal cavity, posterior to the liver and spleen. There is one on each side of the spinal column.

Formation of Urine

Each kidney contains more than a million nephrons. *Nephrons* filter the blood that passes through the kidneys. Several structures within the nephrons help to filter the blood, including specialized capillaries. Blood comes into the nephrons from the renal arteries. Filtered blood is returned to the body through the renal veins. The remaining liquid, called filtrate, accumulates in collecting small tubules. Blood vessels surrounding these tubules reabsorb water, nutrients, and other substances needed by the body. These substances are then circulated to different parts of the body via the veins. The remaining liquid and waste products make up urine.

Elimination of Urine

The primary structures responsible for the elimination of urine are the ureters, the bladder, and the urethra. Each kidney is connected to the bladder by a 10- to 12-inch tube called the *ureter*. Urine moves from the kidneys through the ureters to the bladder. The bladder is a muscular, hollow sac that stores urine. It is located in the lower part of the abdomen. The accumulation of around a half-pint (250 ml) of urine in the bladder causes an urge to urinate, or void. Urine then passes from the bladder into another tube-shaped structure, the urethra. Urine leaves the body through the meatus, which is the opening at the end of the urethra.

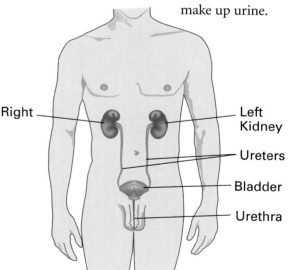

Right

Left
Kidney

Ureters

Bladder

Urethra

○ **Figure 10-6.** The urinary system eliminates liquid waste from the body.

Calculating Urinary Output

The bladder is a hollow sac that stores urine. It has an average capacity of about 1000 cc. When the bladder is about one quarter full, it sends a message to the brain that creates the urge to urinate. A person normally takes in about 3000 cc to 3500 cc of fluid each day.

Suppose you are the nursing assistant assigned to do I/O's (record intake and output) for Mr. H. He has an indwelling urinary catheter, which you empty to measure the urine. You record 850 cc of urine. You then record his intake: 450 cc from breakfast, 200 cc from lunch, and 375 cc from the water pitcher. What is Mr. H.'s intake? What is the difference between his intake and output?

Intake = 450 cc + 200 cc + 375 cc = 1025 cc

Difference = Intake − Output = 1025 cc − 850 cc = 175 cc

Practice

For another patient, you measure an output of 975 cc of urine. The patient's intake includes: 300 from breakfast, 275 from the water pitcher, 450 from lunch, and 360 from dinner. What is this patient's intake? What is the difference between intake and output?

Diseases and Disorders

Urinary tract infections can occur in the urethra, the bladder, or the kidney. Infections in the urethra and bladder may occur as a result of sexual activity. Bladder infections are more common in women because of the proximity of the meatus to the anus. Bacteria in feces can contaminate the urinary tract. A kidney infection can result if a bladder infection is not properly treated. An untreated kidney infection can cause permanent kidney damage.

Kidney stones are crystals of salts, such as calcium chloride, that can form because of decreased fluid intake or increased mineral intake. A kidney stone that forms in the kidney and enters the ureter can cause severe pain and bleeding. If a kidney stone obstructs the ureter, urine can back up in the kidney, leading to kidney damage if not treated.

The Endocrine System

Glands are organs that create chemicals needed for proper body functioning. The endocrine system is made up of glands called *endocrine glands*. **See Figure 10-7.** The endocrine glands secrete (release) hormones into the blood. **Hormones** are chemicals that regulate and control the activities of cells.

The Glands

The pituitary gland, with the hypothalamus, makes and secretes hormones that activate and control most of the other glands. It is known as the *master gland*. Located at the base of the brain, the pituitary gland is divided into two sections, or lobes. The anterior lobe secretes a number of hormones to regulate body functions.

SAFETY FIRST

A bladder infection, also called *cystitis*, can occur in patients using a urinary catheter. When caring for a patient with a catheter, standard precautions must always be followed to avoid introducing bacteria into the patient's urinary tract. Chapter 11 discusses standard precautions.

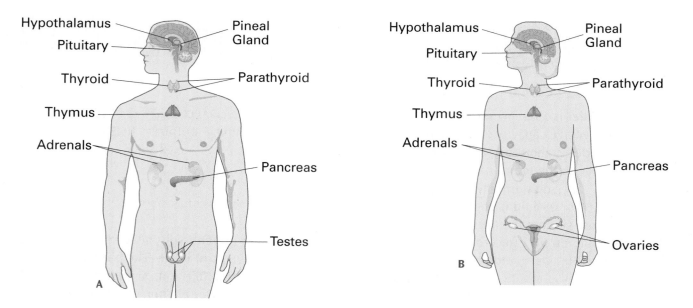

○ **Figure 10-7.** *(A). Male endocrine system. (B). Female endocrine system.* The endocrine system secretes hormones into the blood.

The pineal gland is located beneath the brain. It secretes melatonin to regulate the body's sleep cycle. The thyroid gland is located in the neck. Shaped like a butterfly, the thyroid secretes thyroxine, which regulates body metabolism. The parathyroid glands are located on either side of the thyroid. They secrete parathyroid hormone (PTH), which controls the body's use of calcium. The thymus gland impacts the body's immune system. The pancreas (which is part of the digestive system as well as the endocrine system) produces insulin.

The adrenal glands are located just above the kidneys. Each gland consists of two parts. The adrenal medulla manufactures norepinephrine and epinephrine, as well as dopamine. These are hormones that activate what is known as the "fight or flight" response, allowing you to act quickly in an emergency. The adrenal cortex produces several hormones. The reproductive glands are the ovaries in women and the testes in men. They are discussed in the section about the reproductive systems.

Diseases and Disorders

Graves' disease is caused by excessive secretion of thyroxine. This increases the body's metabolism. Patients can experience extreme hunger, weight loss, tremors of the fingers and tongue, nervousness, excessive sweating, and increased heart rate.

Cushing's disease results from excessive secretion of cortisol, caused by either a disorder of the pituitary gland or the adrenal gland. Patients develop fatty deposits in the body' trunk and face. The skin and the bones become fragile. This disease can also result from medical use of corticosteroids, which are drugs prescribed for transplant recipients and many autoimmune diseases.

The Reproductive Systems

The reproductive system is responsible for reproducing the species and producing hormones that differentiate the sexes. The male and female reproductive systems are different but work together to accomplish reproduction.

Vital Skills READING

Keeping a Vocabulary Log

This chapter introduces many new words that you will need to know as a nursing assistant. One way to remember them is to keep a log of the new words that you encounter. You can reserve a section of the learning log that you started in Chapter 7 to record new words. Don't limit yourself to just the new words in this chapter. You can include new words you come across when you study or when you begin working.

Include a short definition and the context in which you saw the word to jog your memory. For certain words, it might even be helpful to draw a picture to help you remember.

Example: If you include the word **artery** in your vocabulary log, jot down the word "away" as a reminder that **arteries** carry blood **away** from the heart.

Practice

Start a vocabulary log, either as part of your learning log or as a separate log. Pick at least three new words from each body system presented in this chapter and add them to your vocabulary log. Include a short definition, the context in which you saw the word, and perhaps a picture or reminder word to help jog your memory.

The Male Reproductive System

The major structures of the male reproductive system are illustrated in **Figure 10-8**. The primary reproductive organs in the male are the testes, or testicles. The testes (singular: *testis*) are two oval-shaped organs housed outside the body in the scrotum, a sac of skin between the thighs. The testes are responsible for producing sperm cells, the male reproductive cells. The male hormone testosterone is also produced in the testes. It is needed for the proper functioning of the reproductive organs and for the development of secondary sex characteristics in males (facial hair, deepening voice, and so on).

1. Sperm cells travel from the testes through a series of coiled tubes called the *epididymis*. This is where sperm cells are stored and mature.

2. From the epididymis, the sperm cells move through a tube called the *vas deferens*, and then into the seminal vesicles, where semen is produced. **Semen** is the fluid that transports sperm.

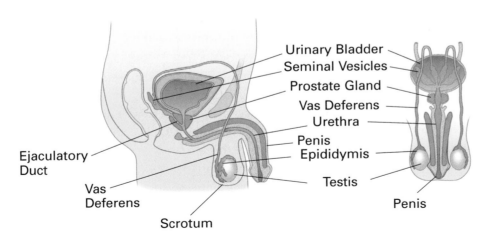

○ Figure 10-8. The male reproductive system.

3. Ducts in the seminal vesicles combine to form the ejaculatory duct. This duct passes through the prostate gland, which secretes a liquid that increases the sperm's ability to move in the semen and survive after ejaculation.

4. Semen leaves the prostate via the ejaculatory duct, where the duct joins the urethra. The urethra is located within the penis. (The urethra carries both semen and urine, but not at the same time.)

The Female Reproductive System

The major structures of the female reproductive system are shown in **Figure 10-9**. The primary reproductive organs of the female are the ovaries. These two almond-shaped organs, located on either side of the lower abdominal cavity, contain the female reproductive cells, or ova (singular: *ovum*). Ova are also called eggs. The ovaries also secrete the female hormones estrogen and progesterone. These hormones are necessary for the proper functioning of the reproductive system and for the development of secondary sex characteristics in females, such as breast enlargement and pubic hair.

All of a female's ova are present in the ovaries at birth. During the reproductive years, the ovaries release one mature ovum each month in a process called *ovulation*.

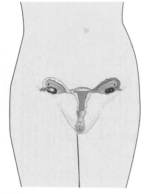

O **Figure 10-9.** The female reproductive system.

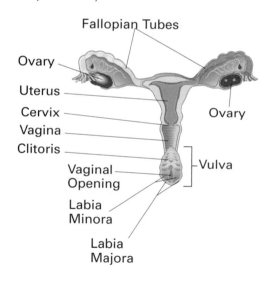

Fallopian Tubes

Ovary

Uterus

Cervix

Vagina

Clitoris

Ovary

Vaginal Opening

Vulva

Labia Minora

Labia Majora

1. When an ovary releases an ovum, it travels through one of the fallopian tubes. The two fallopian tubes connect the ovaries to the uterus, which is a hollow, pear-shaped organ located in the center of the lower abdomen, between the ovaries. When a woman is pregnant, the uterus (womb) is where the fetus grows and is nurtured throughout the pregnancy.

2. Around the time of ovulation, the endometrium (lining of the uterus) builds up in preparation for a possible pregnancy.

3. During sexual intercourse, millions of sperm cells are released into the vagina, a muscular tube connected to the uterus. Sperm cells travel up through the vagina, through the cervix (the opening of the uterus), and into the uterus.

4. The sperm cells move through the uterus and on to the fallopian tubes. This is where fertilization, or conception, takes place.

5. If a sperm cell and an ovum unite in the fallopian tube, the fertilized ovum travels back down the fallopian tube to the uterus. There, it implants in the endometrium, where it will remain and grow until birth occurs. If fertilization does not occur, blood and a layer of the endometrium are discharged through the vagina in a process called **menstruation**.

The female body has separate openings for the urinary and reproductive systems. Urine is expelled through an opening at the end of the urethra called the *urinary meatus*. The reproductive opening is the vagina.

The external genitalia and the mammary glands are also part of the female reproductive system. The primary structures of the external genitalia are the vulva and the clitoris. The vulva consists of the labia majora and labia minora, which are folds of tissue that cover and protect the other external female genitalia. The mammary glands are enclosed within the breasts. After a woman has given birth, the mammary glands secrete milk to nourish the newborn. Milk leaves the mammary glands through the nipple at the center of each breast.

Diseases and Disorders

The prostate gland tends to increase in size as men age. This condition is called *benign prostatic hyperplasia*. An enlarged prostate can press on the urethra, causing problems with urination. Some men experience difficulty urinating (delayed starting, decreased force), a sudden urge to urinate, or incontinence (loss of bladder control).

Both the male and female reproductive systems are subject to several kinds of cancer. Testicular, prostate, and penile cancer affect men. Breast, cervical, endometrial, and ovarian cancer affect women. Breast cancer is the most common type of cancer in women. Men and women should follow guidelines for testing on a regular basis for signs of these cancers.

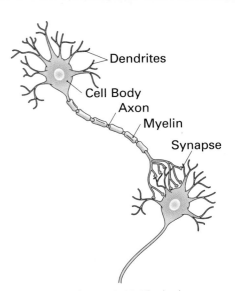

○ **Figure 10-10.** The basic structure of the neuron.

The Nervous System

The nervous system controls and coordinates the body's voluntary and involuntary functions. Some parts of the nervous system maintain day-to-day functioning. Other parts respond in stressful or emergency situations.

Neurons are the basic cells of the nervous system. **See Figure 10-10.** Dendrites are tiny fibers, or extensions, coming off the neuron that transmit nerve impulses (electrical signals) toward the neuron. The axon is a similar extension that sends impulses away from the neuron. When a neuron transmits a nerve impulse to the next neuron, the two neurons do not touch each other. The space between the axon of one neuron and the dendrites of the next neuron is called a *synapse*. Chemicals transmit the nerve impulse across the synapse.

Nerves are groups of axons and dendrites from different neurons, with blood vessels and connective tissue. Nerves are connected to the spinal cord, and the spinal cord is connected to the brain. The two major divisions of the nervous system are the central nervous system and the peripheral nervous system. **See Figure 10-11.**

The Central Nervous System

The central nervous system is made up of the brain and the spinal cord. Chapter 9 includes information about the structure and function of the brain. The spinal cord is made up of nerve tissue and extends from the brainstem down the back to just above the small of the back. It is housed within the bones of the spinal column. Messages are relayed to and from the brain via the nerves in the spinal cord.

The brain and the spinal cord are protected by three layers of tissue.
• The dura mater is the tough outside covering next to the skull.
• The arachnoid is the middle layer made up of weblike strands of connective tissue.
• The pia mater is the innermost layer of the tissue.

Cerebrospinal fluid fills the space between the pia mater and the arachnoid. It flows around the brain and spinal cord, acting as a cushion to protect these structures from injury.

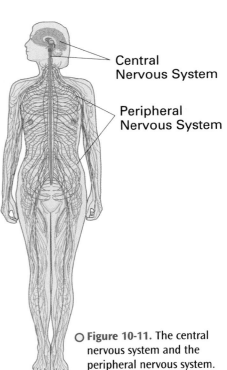

○ **Figure 10-11.** The central nervous system and the peripheral nervous system.

The Peripheral Nervous System

The peripheral nervous system is made up of 12 pairs of cranial nerves and 31 pairs of spinal nerves. Cranial nerves come from the brainstem. They carry impulses between the brain and the head, neck, chest, and abdomen for the senses and voluntary and involuntary muscle control. Spinal nerves come from the spinal cord. They carry impulses from the extremities (arms and legs), skin, and other body structures that are not served by the cranial nerves.

Diseases and Disorders

A cerebrovascular accident (CVA) is a sudden interruption in the blood supply to the brain. It is also called a *stroke*. CVAs can occur when a blood clot blocks the flow of blood in a vessel, or when a blood vessel bursts in the brain. One of the primary causes of CVAs is hypertension. A CVA can cause brain damage, leading to disabilities such as paralysis and loss of speech.

Spinal cord injuries are usually the result of an accident. If trauma causes fracture or compression of the vertebrae (bones of the spinal column), the associated nerves can be damaged. This disrupts the signals going to and from the brain. The severity and type of damage depends on where on the spinal cord the injury has occurred and how severely the nerve has been damaged. Some people with spinal cord injury recover completely. Others may have paralysis or partial paralysis.

The Sensory System

The sensory system includes the eyes and ears and those parts of other systems involved in the reactions of the five senses. As you learned in Chapter 9, sensory receptors receive information from a stimulus and transmit it to the brain. The brain then interprets the information and "instructs" the appropriate part of the body to respond.

Vital Skills — COMMUNICATION

Communicating with Patients with Speech Impairments

The effect of a CVA depends on where in the brain the blood supply is interrupted. In some cases, it can affect a person's ability to speak without necessarily changing the person's ability to hear, think, or reason. It is important not to treat these patients as though they are deaf or mentally disabled. If you are assigned to care for a CVA victim, find out what abilities the patient has and which have been affected by the CVA. Then treat the patient accordingly. For example, if speech impairment is the only effect, you may want to ask "yes or no" questions so that the person can answer you by nodding or shaking the head.

Practice

Think about how you would feel if you were perfectly able to think clearly, but could not form words or speak clearly. How would you communicate? How would you want others to treat you? Make a list of things a nursing assistant can do to communicate effectively with a person who has a speech impairment.

Muscle and Visceral Senses

The sensory organs are not the only places receptors are found. They are also found in many areas of the body, including internal organs. Receptors in the muscles provide "muscle sense." For example, we know where our legs and arms are and what they are doing without looking at them. We also know when our muscles are stretching or contracting. We do not have to think about how to move.

There is also a visceral sense that tells us when we are hungry or thirsty. It is believed that receptors for hunger and thirst are in the brain. The receptors for hunger detect changes in the level of nutrients in the blood. Hunger pangs are then felt in the stomach when it contracts. Receptors for thirst detect changes in the body's fluid level. Thirst is then felt in the mouth and throat.

Diseases and Disorders

Macular degeneration is a disorder of the eyes that can occur in elderly people. It affects the macula, which is the central part of the retina. The receptors in the macula break down, decreasing sharpness of vision and resulting in the loss of central vision. Peripheral, or side, vision is not impaired. People with macular degeneration often lose the ability to read and to drive.

Ménière's disease is a disorder of the inner ear, particularly the semicircular canals and the eighth cranial nerve. The disease affects balance and hearing. People with Ménière's disease occasionally experience the abnormal sensation of movement in space (vertigo), dizziness, loss of balance, nausea and vomiting, loss of hearing, and ringing in the ears. These symptoms are usually temporary, although permanent hearing loss can occur. During an attack, the person's balance is affected, so walking and driving can be dangerous.

The Musculoskeletal System

The musculoskeletal system consists of the bones, muscles, joints, tendons, and ligaments. The bones provide the underlying framework of the body structure. The muscles make it possible for the body to move.

The Skeletal System

The skeletal system is made up of bones and joints. The functions of the skeletal system are to:
• Support the body.
• Protect fragile internal organs, such as the heart and brain, from injury.
• Store calcium.
• Produce blood cells.

The human body contains 206 bones. **Figure 10-12** shows some of these bones. Bones vary in size and shape. **Figure 10-13** shows the four categories of bones.
• Long bones help shape and support the body. The ulna, radius, and humerus in the arm, and the femur and fibula in the leg, are examples of long bones.
• Short bones make the body flexible. They include the carpals in the wrist and the metatarsals in the foot.

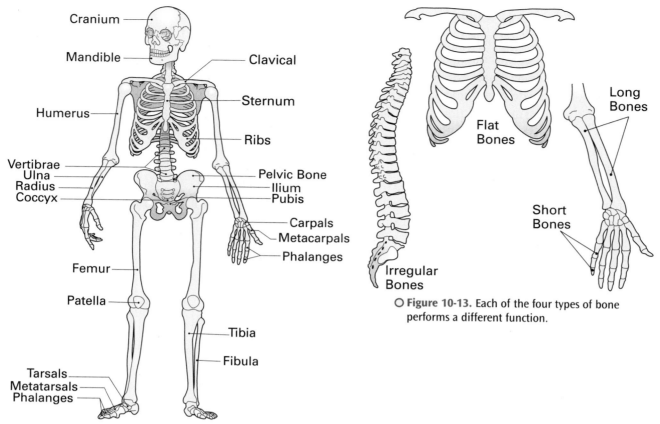

Labels on Figure 10-12 (left skeleton):
Cranium, Mandible, Humerus, Vertibrae, Ulna, Radius, Coccyx, Femur, Patella, Tarsals, Metatarsals, Phalanges, Clavical, Sternum, Ribs, Pelvic Bone, Ilium, Pubis, Carpals, Metacarpals, Phalanges, Tibia, Fibula

○ **Figure 10-12.** Some of the bones of the skeletal system.

Labels on Figure 10-13 (right):
Flat Bones, Long Bones, Short Bones, Irregular Bones

○ **Figure 10-13.** Each of the four types of bone performs a different function.

- Flat bones protect delicate body tissue and organs. The ribs and cranial bones are flat bones.
- Irregular bones allow movement and flexibility. The vertebrae and facial bones are irregular.

A joint is a place of contact for two or more bones. The knees, elbows, wrists, shoulders, ankles, and hips are joints. Joints make movement possible. There are three different types of joints: hinge joints, pivot joints, and ball-and-socket joints. **See Figure 10-14.**

Ligaments are strong bands of fibrous connective tissue that hold bones together at the joint. The tissue that connects bones to the joint, called *cartilage*, prevents the two connecting bones from rubbing against one another. Joints are also cushioned by fluid that lubricates the joint, eliminating friction and making smooth movements possible.

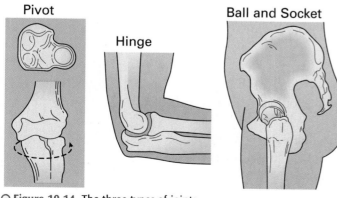

Labels: Pivot, Hinge, Ball and Socket

○ **Figure 10-14.** The three types of joints.

The Muscular System

There are more than 600 muscles in the human body. **Figure 10-15** shows some of these muscles. Muscles that we can consciously move are called *voluntary muscles*. They are the skeletal muscles, such as the muscles of the arms and the legs. Tendons are connective tissue that attaches muscles to bones. When skeletal muscles contract, or shorten, they make the bone move. The skeletal muscles are responsible for moving the body and maintaining posture.

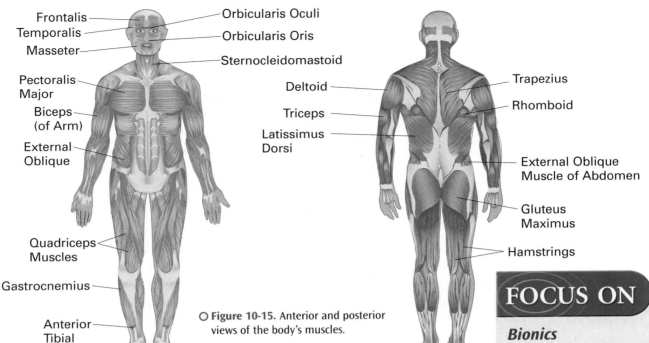

Frontalis
Temporalis
Masseter
Pectoralis Major
Biceps (of Arm)
External Oblique
Quadriceps Muscles
Gastrocnemius
Anterior Tibial

Orbicularis Oculi
Orbicularis Oris
Sternocleidomastoid

Deltoid
Triceps
Latissimus Dorsi

Trapezius
Rhomboid
External Oblique Muscle of Abdomen
Gluteus Maximus
Hamstrings

○ **Figure 10-15.** Anterior and posterior views of the body's muscles.

Muscles that we cannot consciously control are called *involuntary muscles*, or smooth muscles. These muscles are found in the blood vessels, the digestive organs, and other organs of the body. The cardiac muscle is the muscle that forms the wall of the heart.

Diseases and Disorders

Osteoarthritis is a chronic disease affecting the joints. Over time, cartilage wears away, causing bone to rub on bone. Symptoms are inflammation, pain, and stiffness at the joint. Movement of the joint becomes difficult. Many older people have osteoarthritis. It is one of the leading causes of disability.

Muscular dystrophy (MD) is a group of disorders that cause muscle weakness and loss of muscle tissue. It is a progressive disease, meaning that it gets worse over time. Some types of MD are inherited. Muscle weakness can result in frequent falls and difficulty in performing the activities of daily living. Some forms of the disorder are fatal.

The Integumentary System

The integumentary system is made up of the skin and its associated structures. **See Figure 10-16.** The skin is the body's protective covering. It is the first line of defense against infection. (See Chapter 9 for more information about the skin and its functions.)

The layer of skin beneath the epidermis is called the *dermis*. It consists of connective tissue, sweat and oil glands, nerves, blood vessels, and hair and nail follicles. The capillaries in the dermis supply the epidermis with oxygen and nutrients. The subcutaneous tissue directly under the dermis is a layer of fat. This layer connects the dermis to the muscles.

FOCUS ON

Bionics

In medicine, *bionics* involves replacing or enhancing organs or other body parts with mechanical versions. Bionic implants mimic the original part and sometimes surpass it. For example, someone who has had heart disease may get a pacemaker, an internal defibrillator, or even an artificial heart. Some people have electronic arms or legs that perform the same movements as real arms and legs.

Structures of the Skin

The structures associated with the skin include sweat glands, oil glands, hair, and nails. Sweat glands play an important role in maintaining body temperature. As sweat passes through the pores in the skin, it evaporates and cools the body. Sweating also removes waste products from the body.

Hair covers the entire body except for the soles of the feet and palms of the hands. Hair around the eyes, ears, and nose prevents dust and other objects from entering these delicate organs. The skin and the hair are kept soft by an oily substance called *sebum* that is secreted by oil glands. The nails protect the fingers and toes.

Diseases and Disorders

Pressure sores are areas of the skin that break down when the body rests in one position over a period of time. The constant pressure on the skin reduces the blood supply to the area, depriving the skin of oxygen and nutrients. The affected tissue dies. The area can develop a blister, an open sore, and then a crater that can extend to the muscle or bone. People who use wheelchairs, are bedridden, or are unable to change position are at risk for pressure sores.

Several types of cancer also affect the skin. Melanoma occurs in the cells that produce pigment. It is the most dangerous type of skin cancer, because it can spread rapidly to other parts of the body. The development of melanoma is related to sun exposure, along with other risk factors. The risk increases with age, but melanoma can also affect young people. Early symptoms usually include a change in a mole or the development of an irregular, pigmented lesion. Melanoma may be cured if treated early.

The Lymphatic System

The lymphatic system is also known as the *immune system*. Its functions include:
- Maintaining homeostasis through the removal of waste products from the circulation.
- Defending the body against disease and illness.

Structures and Function

The lymphatic system consists of lymph (a tissue fluid), lymph vessels, and lymph nodes. During blood circulation, when some tissue fluid returns to the bloodstream via capillaries, other tissue fluid is drawn off into lymphatic vessels. This fluid is called *lymph*. Lymph nodes are masses of lymphatic tissue at specific sites in the body. Lymph nodes filter the lymph as it passes through them. This filtering removes bacteria and other particles from the fluid. The filtered lymph then returns to the bloodstream.

The lymphatic system can be divided into the central organs and the peripheral organs. The central organs include the thymus and the bone marrow.

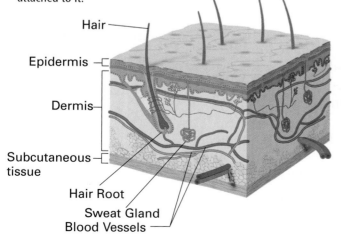

○ **Figure 10-16.** The integumentary system is made up of the skin and the structures attached to it.

Hair

Epidermis

Dermis

Subcutaneous tissue

Hair Root

Sweat Gland

Blood Vessels

The peripheral organs include the spleen, the tonsils, and the lymph nodes. **See Figure 10-17.**

A series of complex physical and chemical reactions occur within the organs of the immune system as the body responds to foreign or harmful substances. Lymphocytes are small white blood cells that arise in lymphoid organs. They are involved in immune responses and create **antibodies**, specialized proteins that fight disease. Lymphocytes that mature in bone marrow are called B cells. Lymphocytes that mature in the thymus gland are called T cells.

Diseases and Disorders

If the immune system is too weak or works too hard, the body may no longer be in balance and disease will occur. A severe allergic reaction is an example of an overactive immune response.

Acquired immunodeficiency syndrome (AIDS) is an example of a condition that results in a weakened immune system. People with human immunodeficiency virus (HIV) develop AIDS because they do not have enough T cells to assist their immune system to protect against infections and cancers.

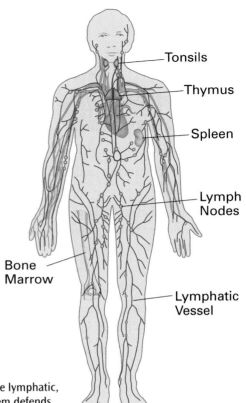

○ **Figure 10-17.** The lymphatic, or immune, system defends the body against disease.

Vital Skills — WRITING

Peer Editing

Editing and revising are essential steps in the writing process. Even the best writers need an editor to look over their work and suggest changes. In *peer editing*, classmates review each other's writing. Your classmates suggest how to improve your work, and you do the same for them.

When you edit someone else's work:

- Try to stay positive. It can sometimes be hard to hear criticism about your work. Point out what you liked about the writing. You might say something like "I really liked the way you started the paragraph."
- Make specific suggestions and avoid vague criticisms. Instead of saying, "You lost me in the first sentence," you could say, "The first sentence seemed confusing to me. Is there a way to break it up into two shorter sentences?"
- Remember: grammar, punctuation, and spelling count. Point out these errors for correction.
- Be polite! Keep in mind that you are working together to improve the writing.

Practice

Choose three of the body systems covered in this chapter. Write a paragraph about a disease state associated with each. (You can review the basics of writing a paragraph in Chapter 1.) Break into groups of three or four students and give each group member a copy of your three paragraphs. Review each other's writing and suggest improvements. Then revise your paragraphs, taking your peer editors' suggestions into consideration.

Chapter Summary

- A basic understanding of human anatomy and physiology can help nursing assistants provide safe and efficient care.

- The body's systems work together to make the body function properly. The systems are dependent on each other.

- The cardiovascular system transports blood throughout the body.

- The respiratory system brings oxygen to cells and removes carbon dioxide.

- The digestive system turns the food we eat into nutrients and removes wastes.

- The urinary system removes liquid waste from the body and helps the body maintain its stable balance.

- The endocrine system produces hormones that regulate the activities of organs and glands.

- The male and female reproductive systems are responsible for reproducing the species. They also produce hormones that differentiate the sexes.

- The nervous system controls the voluntary and involuntary functions of the body.

- The integumentary system is made up of the skin and its associated structures.

- The lymphatic system maintains homeostasis and protects the body from illness and disease.

VOCABULARY REVIEW

Directions: Match the letter of each definition in the second column with the correct vocabulary term in the first column. Write your answers on a separate sheet of paper.

Vocabulary

1. artery
2. capillary
3. constrict
4. dilate
5. gas exchange
6. hemoglobin
7. hemostasis
8. hormone
9. menstruation
10. peristalsis
11. plasma
12. semen
13. vein
14. ventilation

Definitions

A. An iron-containing protein in red blood cells that carries oxygen and gives blood its red color

B. A blood vessel that carries deoxygenated blood and waste products back to the heart

C. The prevention of blood loss

D. The cyclic process of the blood and tissue lining the uterus being discharged through the vagina

E. Chemical substance that regulates and controls the activities of cells

F. The process of moving oxygen into the blood and removing carbon dioxide from the blood

G. To narrow

H. A blood vessel that carries blood away from the heart

I. Small blood vessel that connects the ends of arterioles with venules.

J. The fluid that transports sperm

K. The movement of air in and out of the lungs

L. To expand

M. The liquid part of the blood that carries blood cells, nutrients, antibodies, chemicals, gases, and waste products within the body

N. Involuntary muscular, rhythmic contraction that propels contents through an organ

Check Your Knowledge

Review Questions: Answer each of the following questions on a separate sheet of paper.

1. Explain why it is important for a nursing assistant to have a basic understanding of anatomy and physiology.

2. Describe the function of platelets.

3. Why does the body need a constant supply of oxygen?

4. Which part of the digestive process begins in the jejunum of the small intestine?

5. Which structures are responsible for the elimination of urine?

6. What are glands?

7. Explain the purpose of the female hormones estrogen and progesterone.

8. Name the two major divisions of the nervous system.

9. What are the three functions of the skeletal muscles?

10. What body system is most affected by the human immunodeficiency virus?

True or False: Read each statement carefully. Then write *True* or *False* by the statement number on a separate sheet of paper.

1. Arteries carry blood rich in carbon dioxide from the heart to the body.

2. Blood is pumped to the lungs and then back to the heart before it is pumped out to the body.

3. Humans normally take in and eliminate about the same amount of fluid per day.

4. The knee is an example of a ball-and-socket joint.

5. One of the functions of the skin is to eliminate waste products.

Think and Decide

Directions: Think about each of the following scenarios. Answer each question on a separate sheet of paper.

1. Your three-year-old nephew falls and cuts his chin. The blood is dark red in color. Is this blood from an artery or a vein? What gives the blood the dark color?

2. Mrs. R. is a long-term care resident who was admitted to the facility yesterday and is under your care. She is scared and nervous that she has been left alone. You walk in to comfort her and check her vital signs. You note that her heart rate is 110 beats per minute. Should you notify the nurse? What might be causing the elevated heart rate?

3. Zoe, a resident in your care, is showing you her dry, flaky skin. She says it itches and asks what she should do. What layer of the skin is probably being shed? What should you do?

4. Jeremiah, a long-term resident, tells you that he cannot move his right hip. Based on your knowledge of the hip joint, what do you expect this joint to be able to do in a normal, healthy individual? Should you report this to the nurse?

5. You are walking a resident to the cafeteria. Are the muscles you and the patient are using to get to the cafeteria voluntary or involuntary? Why?

6. Carrie, a long-term resident in your care, has severe arthritis in both hands. She looks forward to a cup of coffee with her breakfast each day. On some mornings, however, she has difficulty holding her coffee cup without spilling the coffee and burning herself. What can you do to help?

7. Mr. Rio, a long-term resident in your care, has been losing weight recently, even though he is always hungry and eats more than he used to. His heart rate has increased, and he seems more nervous to you. Tonight, as he was showing you pictures of his grandson, you noticed that his fingers were trembling. What might these symptoms mean? What should you do, if anything?

8. Mrs. Chilton is a new resident at the long-term care facility where you work. She is bedridden. As you help her get settled in her new room, she mentions that she has a "sore spot" on her lower back. She asks you to take a look. You find a blister-like area that looks red and irritated. What has happened? Why? What should you do about it?

CNA Certification Exam Prep

Directions: This practice test contains ten questions. Each question has four suggested answers. For each question, choose the ONE that best answers the question or completes the statement. Write your answers on a separate sheet of paper.

1. Which of the following is the *most* accurate description of a vein?

    A. Veins carry blood to the heart.

    B. Veins carry blood away from the heart.

    C. The blood in veins is rich in oxygen.

    D. The blood in veins is low in oxygen.

2. What is the medical term for the windpipe?

    A. epiglottis

    B. esophagus

    C. trachea

    D. larynx

3. The rhythmic muscular movement that aids in food digestion is called

    A. chyme.

    B. duodenum.

    C. jejunum.

    D. peristalsis.

4. Which body system filters blood to remove waste products and excess fluid?

    A. respiratory

    B. urinary

    C. endocrine

    D. reproductive

5. What is the master gland in the endocrine system?

    A. thyroid

    B. pineal

    C. pituitary

    D. adrenal

6. The process of moving oxygen into the blood and removing carbon dioxide from the blood is

    A. gas exchange.

    B. peristalsis.

    C. hemostasis.

    D. homeostasis.

7. The chemicals that regulate and control the activities of cells are known as

    A. glands.

    B. plasma.

    C. hormones.

    D. semen.

8. The space between the axon of one neuron and the dendrites of the next neuron is called a

    A. capillary.

    B. synapse.

    C. antibody.

    D. platelet.

9. The small blood vessels in which gas exchange actually occurs are the

    A. venules.

    B. arterioles.

    C. veins.

    D. capillaries.

10. Which of the following is considered a form of chronic obstructive pulmonary disease?

    A. emphysema

    B. pneumonia

    C. Graves' disease

    D. Cushing's disease

CHAPTER 11

OBJECTIVES

- Identify four primary types of microorganisms.
- Identify the five methods of infectious disease transmission.
- Follow standard precautions and transmission-based precautions.

- Demonstrate handwashing according to standard precautions.
- Put on and remove personal protective equipment according to standard precautions.
- Care for patients in isolation using proper isolation precautions.

- Identify some infectious diseases and their methods of transmission.
- List the employer's responsibilities under OSHA's Bloodborne Pathogen Standard.
- Describe strategies for maintaining health and reducing exposure risk.

Infection Control and Standard Precautions

antisepsis Using chemicals to kill pathogens or to stop their growth.

asepsis The condition of being free of pathogens.

autoclave A pressurized steam sterilizer.

bloodborne pathogen A disease-causing organism found in blood or other body fluids.

body fluids The body's secretions: sputum, semen, mucus, vaginal excretions, urine, feces, blood, saliva, tears, vomit, sweat, cerebro-spinal fluid, amniotic fluid, breast milk, and excretions from wounds.

Centers for Disease Control and Prevention (CDC) A division of the U.S. Department of Health and Human Services (HHS) that sets standards to protect the public health.

chain of infection The series of six conditions that together produce infection.

disinfection A cleaning process that uses strong chemicals to kill most pathogens.

host A person who harbors pathogens.

immunity The body's resistance to a particular disease.

infection A disease caused by a group of pathogenic microorgan-isms that invade and multiply within the body.

infectious diseases Diseases that are transmitted from one person to another through the chain of infection.

inflammatory response The body's built-in defense mechanism.

isolation precautions Guidelines to follow to prevent the spread of infectious diseases.

medical asepsis The practice of minimizing or reducing the spread of pathogens.

microorganism A living plant or animal that is too small to be seen without magnification.

noninfectious disease A disease that cannot be transmitted from one person to another.

nonpathogen A microorganism that does not cause disease or infection.

nosocomial infection An infection that a patient acquires while in a health care facility.

pathogen A microorganism that causes disease or infection.

reservoir Any environment that allows a pathogen to live and grow.

standard precautions A set of infec-tion control guidelines designed to minimize the risk of transmitting microorganisms and disease.

sterilization The use of extremely high temperatures to kill patho-gens, nonpathogens, and spores.

surgical asepsis The practice of eliminating microorganisms.

transmission-based precautions Infection control guidelines used for patients with highly conta-gious infections.

vector A nonhuman living organism that transmits pathogens.

Microorganisms and Disease

As a nursing assistant, you will be exposed to many kinds of illnesses. Learning how to prevent the spread of disease is the best way to protect yourself and your patients. Some diseases are spread by microorganisms. **Microorganisms** are living plants or animals that are organisms that are so small that we can see them only with a microscope. Some microorganisms have a beneficial effect on our bodies, but others are harmful.

As shown in **Figure 11-1**, microorganisms are everywhere. They can be found on our skin, inside our bodies, in our mouths, in our food, and on anything we touch. Some microorganisms are necessary because they assist with normal body functions. They help break down food in the digestive tract and help the body process certain substances. These microorganisms are called **nonpathogens**, because they do not cause disease and infection.

Harmful microorganisms, called **pathogens**, do cause disease and infection. Pathogens use human tissue as their food and give off waste products called *toxins*. A toxin is a substance that is harmful to the human body.

Types of Microorganisms

There are four primary types of microorganisms. Each includes pathogens and nonpathogens.

- *Bacteria* are one-celled microorganisms that cause common diseases such as staph infections, strep throat, and infectious pneumonia.
- *Viruses* are the smallest type of microorganism. They are different from other pathogens because they need to enter a living cell to reproduce. Some of the diseases that viruses cause include influenza, the common cold, herpes, hepatitis, measles, and HIV/AIDS.
- *Fungi* (singular: *fungus)* are a group of microorganisms that live on dead organic matter. There are two types of fungi: yeast and molds. Fungi cause athlete's foot, yeast infections, and fungal toenail.
- *Protozoa* are one-celled parasitic microorganisms. A parasite is an animal or plant that lives on or in another organism and feeds from it. Protozoa can cause gastroenteritis and malaria.

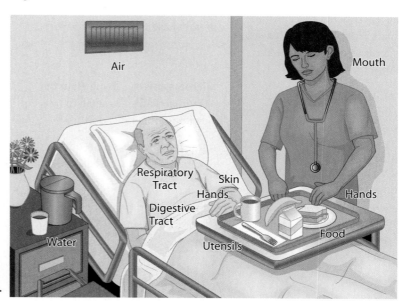

O **Figure 11-1.** Microorganisms can be found everywhere in a hospital patient's room.

How Microorganisms Grow

Microorganisms need a place to live and grow. By understanding the growth requirements of pathogens, you can help control their growth, reproduction, and transmission. The environment in which microorganisms grow is called a **reservoir**. A reservoir can be a human being, an animal, a plant, an insect, air, soil, water, food, utensils, or anything else that provides the microorganism with what it needs to live. The health care environment offers many reservoirs for microorganisms, including the patient, the environment itself, the equipment, and the health care worker.

The following conditions help microorganisms thrive:

- **Moisture.** Any damp place, such as skin folds or bathroom surfaces.
- **Warmth.** Microorganisms thrive between 50° F and 110° F (10° C and 43° C).
- **Oxygen.** Some microorganisms need oxygen to sustain life.
- **Darkness.** Microorganisms thrive in darkness. Many are destroyed by light.
- **Food.** All microorganisms need nourishment to survive. Each type requires a different food.

The Infection Process

An **infection** occurs when pathogenic microorganisms invade and multiply within the body, causing disease. However, the presence of pathogens does not always cause infection. Certain conditions must be present.

Chain of Infection

A **chain of infection** is the series of six conditions that together produce infection. These conditions occur in a cycle, beginning with the infectious agent. **See Figure 11-2.** A break in any part of the chain of infection stops the transmission of pathogens. The six conditions are:

- **Infectious agent**—a pathogen capable of producing disease.
- **Reservoir or host**—any environment that allows the pathogen to live and grow. A **host** is a person who harbors a pathogen.
- **Portal of exit**—the pathogen must have a way of exiting the reservoir. The human body provides many portals of exit, including the respiratory tract, gastrointestinal tract, urinary and reproductive tracts, blood, any break in the skin or mucous membrane, and all secretions from these portals. These secretions are called **body fluids**. They are sputum, semen, mucus, vaginal excretions, urine, feces, blood, saliva, tears, vomit, sweat, cerebrospinal fluid, amniotic fluid, breast milk, and excretions from wounds.
- **Method of transmission**—the way the infectious agent moves from the reservoir to a new, susceptible host.
- **Portal of entry into the susceptible host**—same as the portals of exit.
- **Susceptible host**—people who are ill or have weak immune systems. The elderly and the very young are also susceptible.

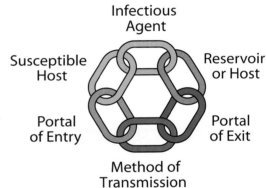

Infectious Agent

Susceptible Host

Reservoir or Host

Portal of Entry

Portal of Exit

Method of Transmission

○ **Figure 11-2.** Each link in the chain of infection must be connected and in sequential order for an infection to occur. An interruption in any one link can stop the process of infection.

Methods of Transmission

Some diseases, such as cancer or diabetes, cannot be transmitted from one person to another. These are known as **noninfectious diseases**. Diseases that are transmitted from one person to another through the chain of infection are known as **infectious diseases**. They are also called *communicable* or *contagious* diseases. One of the links in the chain of infection is the method of transmission. There are five methods of transmission.

- *Contact transmission* occurs when a person touches an infected person or the body fluids of an infected person. The nursing assistant comes into direct contact with a patient when touching, bathing, massaging, feeding, and toileting. Indirect contact occurs when a nursing assistant touches anything that has come into contact with the patient or something that is dirty, such as the floor. Clothing, linens, personal belongings, equipment, specimens, and dressings can transmit disease by indirect contact. **See Figure 11-3.**
- *Airborne transmission* occurs when microorganisms travel through the air and enter a susceptible host's respiratory tract by inhalation. Tuberculosis, measles, and chickenpox viruses are transmitted in this way.
- *Droplet transmission* occurs when large particle droplets containing microorganisms are transferred from one person to another, usually through coughing, sneezing, or talking. Influenza, strep throat, and pneumonia are transmitted by droplets.
- *Common vehicle transmission* occurs when someone eats food, drinks water, handles devices or equipment, or takes medicines contaminated by pathogens. *Salmonella* bacteria is one example. It is transmitted when a person eats food such as chicken or an egg that is contaminated. Thorough cooking destroys the

Vital Skills   READING

Comparing and Contrasting

A good way to remember what you read is to compare and contrast the concepts you encounter. When you *compare* things, you list the things they have in common. When you *contrast*, you look at the differences. One way to keep track of the similarities and differences is to organize the information into a table. For example, below is a table comparing and contrasting cats and dogs:

Characteristic	Cat	Dog
Number of legs	Four	Four
Tongue	Barbed	Smooth
Species name	Feline	Canine
Dependence on owner	Independent	Dependent

Practice

This chapter discusses infectious diseases and the agents that cause or carry them—bacteria, viruses, fungi, and protozoa. Compare and contrast these four types of agents. You may need to do some additional research using the library or the Internet. Organize the information comparing and contrasting infectious disease agents into a table like the one shown. What types of traits might you compare? As one characteristic, include the name of a disease associated with each agent.

bacteria. However, everything the raw chicken or eggs have touched must be cleaned to kill the bacteria.

- *Animal (vector-borne) transmission* occurs when an animal or insect bites a human. A **vector** is a nonhuman living organism that transmits pathogens. Some animals can maintain an infection that is harmful to humans but not to the animal. For example, mosquitoes transmit West Nile virus and deer ticks transmit Lyme disease without contracting the disease.

Risk Factors

Disease occurs in a susceptible host when pathogens enter the body, multiply, and cause damage to the body's tissues. Risk factors determine how susceptible a host is to the infection and how severe the damage will be. Risk factors include age, sex, general health, heredity, nutrition, lifestyle, stress, fatigue, and effects of medications. Indwelling medical devices, such as catheters, also increase risk.

Being in a health care facility also increases the risk of becoming infected. A **nosocomial infection** is one that a patient acquires while in a health care facility. Patients are at risk for nosocomial infection because they often have weakened immune systems and because the health care facility is an environment that harbors infections.

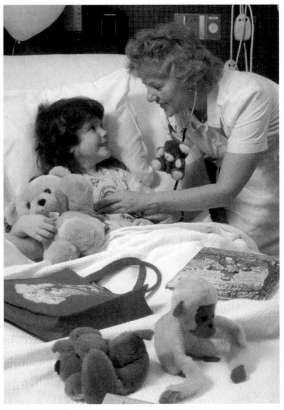

○ **Figure 11-3.** Some pathogens can be transmitted by indirect contact when handling an infected person's clothing or other personal items.

The Body's Defenses

The body has natural resources for fighting disease. Good health is the best defense. It helps maintain a strong immune system. For example:

- Healthy skin and mucous membranes protect the body from invading pathogens. If the skin is broken or cracked, bacteria can enter and cause disease.
- Saliva helps to rid the mouth of many bacteria that may enter.
- Tears defend the eyes by continually washing away harmful organisms.
- The **inflammatory response** is the body's built-in defense mechanism. It is activated when a pathogen or toxin enters the body. Changes in blood flow and a release of helpful chemicals and antibodies occur during infection to fight infectious agents and disease.
- **Immunity** is resistance the body has against a particular disease. People can build immunity to some diseases by being naturally exposed to the pathogen. For example, someone who has had measles will not get the disease a second time. *Immunization*, the process of providing protection against specific communicable diseases, also creates immunity. Children who are vaccinated against measles will not develop the disease even if exposed to it.

Signs and Symptoms of Infection

Sometimes the body is not able to fight off the invading pathogen, so infection occurs. Infections produce common signs and symptoms. If a patient shows any of these signs or symptoms, report them immediately to your supervisor. **See Figure 11-4.**

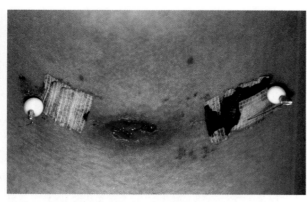

- Fever and warmth
- Pain or tenderness
- Redness and swelling
- Foul odor
- Draining fluid from open wounds
- Fatigue
- Shortness of breath
- Disorientation
- Loss of appetite
- Rash
- Nausea, vomiting, and/or diarrhea

○ **Figure 11-4.** Look for signs of infection, such as redness, swelling, and drainage.

Infection Control

Infection control involves breaking the chain of infection. It is the responsibility of all health care workers. You must be aware at all times of the need for practicing effective infection control measures.

Asepsis

Asepsis is the condition of being free of pathogens. Keeping the health care environment aseptic includes maintaining cleanliness and preventing or destroying contamination.

Any item that touches or comes near a patient with an infectious disease is considered dirty. For example, a food service tray is clean. After it is brought to the patient's room it is dirty, even if the patient does not touch it. Anything that touches the floor is considered dirty. When a dirty object comes in contact with a clean object or area, it contaminates the clean area. Health facilities have separate storage areas for clean and dirty items.

Medical asepsis, or *clean technique*, is the practice of minimizing or reducing the spread of pathogens from one area to another. Medical aseptic practices include handwashing, wearing personal protective equipment, and routine cleaning. Cleaning to achieve medical asepsis includes the following techniques.

- **Antisepsis**—using chemicals to kill pathogens or to stop their growth. For example, rubbing alcohol and antiseptic soap clean the skin and equipment surfaces.

- **Disinfection**—a cleaning process that uses stronger chemicals to kill most pathogens. Chemical disinfectants are used for cleaning equipment, a patient's room after discharge, and certain items in a client's home. They are used in everyday housekeeping to clean floors, commodes, bed frames, side rails, wheelchairs, and any equipment the patient has touched. They are *never* used to clean the skin. Wear waterproof gloves when using chemical disinfectants, because they can irritate the skin. **See Figure 11-5.**

By comparison, **surgical asepsis** is the practice of completely eliminating disease-causing organisms. It is also called *sterile technique*. Surgical asepsis is not usually within the nursing assistant's scope of practice, although some nursing assistants receive extra training in this area. It is used for surgical procedures, injections, catheters, and any other invasive procedures. (*Invasive* refers to entering the body in some way.)

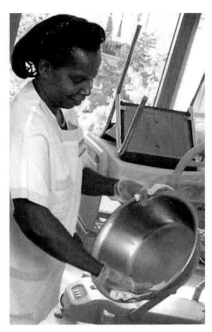

○ **Figure 11-5.** Always wear waterproof gloves to disinfect dirty equipment.

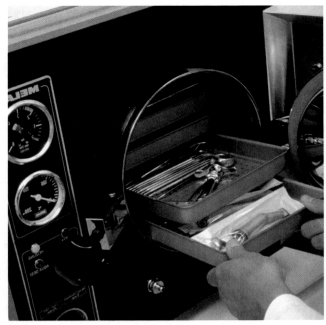

○ **Figure 11-6.** An autoclave sterilizes metal objects, glass, and surgical linens.

Sterilization uses extremely high temperatures and sometimes pressure to kill pathogens, nonpathogens, and spores. Spores are a hard outer shell that are formed by some types of bacteria. They can be killed only by extremely high temperatures. An **autoclave** is a pressurized steam sterilizer that cleans metal objects, glass, and surgical linens. **See Figure 11-6.** Plastic and rubber items are not put in an autoclave, because the high temperature will destroy them. Surgical instruments and catheters can be sterilized by autoclaving or soaking in strong chemicals. When working in a patient's home, you can sterilize small items by boiling them in a pot.

Isolation Precautions

The **Centers for Disease Control and Prevention (CDC)** is a division of the U.S. Department of Health and Human Services (HHS) that works to protect the public health. The CDC has established guidelines to help prevent the spread of disease. These guidelines are called **isolation precautions**. There are two tiers, or steps, to isolation precautions. The first tier is the set of standard precautions. **Standard precautions** are infection control guidelines that are designed to minimize the risk of transmitting microorganisms and disease. They are used with all patients. The second tier is called **transmission-based precautions**. They are used in addition to standard precautions for patients with highly contagious infections.

Standard Precautions

According to the CDC's standard precautions guidelines, health care workers must treat all patients as if they are infected with a bloodborne pathogen. A **bloodborne pathogen** is a disease-causing organism found in blood or other body fluids. Transmission occurs when blood or other body fluids from an infected person enter the bloodstream of a person who is not infected. According

Alcohol-Based Hand Rubs

Although soap and water remain the preferred method for cleaning hands, the CDC recommends alcohol-based hand rubs for *routine* hand hygiene when hands are not visibly soiled. Apply a quarter-sized drop (3–5 ml) of the product to one hand and rub all surfaces of both hands until dry. Do not apply gloves until hands are completely dry to ensure the antiseptic effect. Researchers have found that using these products for 15–25 seconds improves adherence to hand hygiene recommendations. For home care, alcohol-based products can be especially beneficial when water is not readily available.

to standard precautions, all body fluids are to be treated as if they are contaminated. **See Figure 11-7.** Standard precautions require handwashing and the use of barrier methods of prevention, such as gloves, gowns, masks, and protective eyewear to be used when in contact with:

• Blood.
• All body fluids, secretions, and excretions except sweat.
• Nonintact skin.
• Mucous membranes.

Handwashing. Handwashing is the most important procedure you have for preventing the spread of microorganisms. Handwashing:

• Is the most important control measure available to break the chain of infection.
• Prevents the spread of infection.
• Prevents cross-contamination between patients, equipment, and health care providers.
• Helps to keep the health care provider as healthy as possible.

  Procedure 11-1 shows the proper steps for washing your hands. Wash your hands before and after every procedure and any contact with a patient. Wash your hands even if you wear gloves during patient contact. Change gloves between procedures and between patients.

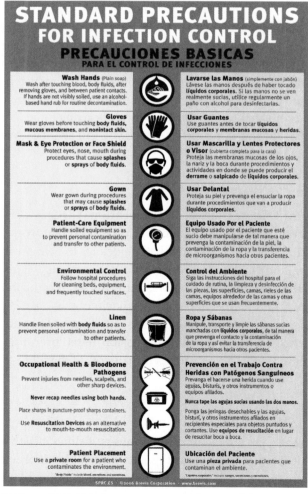

○ **Figure 11-7.** This sign may or may not be posted, but standard precautions are always followed for every patient.

Procedure 11-1

Standard Precautions: Handwashing

Equipment: soap dispenser • paper towels • waste container

Note: The sink and faucet are considered contaminated. Do not directly touch them during the handwashing procedure. Do not allow your uniform to touch the sink.

1. Push your watch up your arm or remove it. Push your sleeves at least 4 inches above the wrist.
2. Using a dry paper towel, turn on the faucet. **See Figure 11-8.** Make sure your hand does not come in direct contact with the faucet or sink. Adjust the water until it is warm. Dispose of the paper towel.

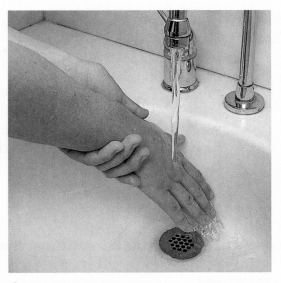

O **Figure 11-9.** Facility policy dictates whether the fingers point downward or upward. Check with your facility for instructions.

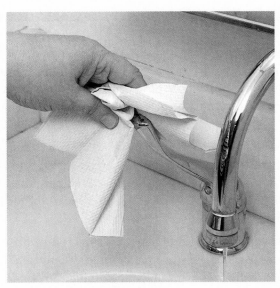

O **Figure 11-8.** Turning on the faucet.

together creates friction, which loosens microorganisms. Rub vigorously for a minimum of 15 seconds. Clean back of hands, between fingers, and each wrist. Clean under your fingernails and around each nail.

3. Wet your hands and forearms with water. Keep your fingertips pointed up or down, according to facility policy. **See Figure 11-9.**
4. Take the soap from a dispenser. Use enough soap to create lots of lather.
5. With your hands pointed downward so water does not run up your arm, rub your hands together in a circular motion. **See Figure 11-10.** The act of rubbing your skin

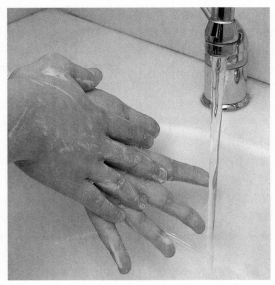

O **Figure 11-10.** Rub the hands together to create friction.

6. Rinse your hands with warm running water. Continue to hold your hands down, allowing water to flow off the fingertips. Remove all soap from your hands.
7. Dry your hands and wrists with a paper towel. Do not shake fingers or hands.
8. Discard the paper towel without touching the waste container.
9. Turn off the faucet with a clean paper towel and discard the towel immediately. **See Figure 11-11.** Make sure your uniform, hands, and wrists do not directly touch the faucet or sink.

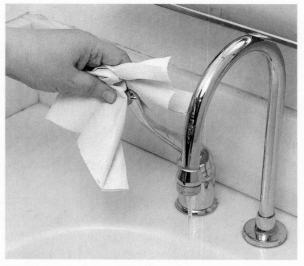

○ **Figure 11-11.** Turn off the faucet using a clean paper towel.

Personal protective equipment (PPE) provides a barrier to shield you from blood and body fluid contamination. This equipment includes gloves, gowns, masks, and protective eyewear. The purpose of wearing PPE is to protect the eyes, skin, and respiratory tract from pathogens as outlined in the standard precautions guidelines.

Gloving. Gloves help prevent the spread of disease by acting as a barrier between your hands and your patients. Do not use gloves if they are torn. Keep your fingernails short so they do not tear the gloves. Most facilities have rules about fingernail length and artificial fingernails. **Procedure 11-2** shows the proper steps for putting on and removing gloves.

Gowning. Gowns protect your clothing from a patient's microorganisms. They protect you against spills and spattering when performing patient care. They also protect a patient from microorganisms on your clothing. Gowns are made of cloth or paper. The gown's edges overlap in the back to cover your clothing completely. Note that a gown is considered unclean and needs to be changed if it becomes wet. **Procedure 11-3** shows the proper steps for putting on and removing a gown.

Masking. The face mask prevents microorganisms that you exhale from being passed to a patient. It also prevents you from inhaling the patient's microorganisms. Masks are made of paper and are disposable. The face mask fits snugly over your mouth and nose.

A mask is considered unclean if it becomes moist or wet; the inside of the mask is unclean once it touches your face. Change masks after 30 minutes of use. Remove and discard a mask when you leave a patient's room. When removing a mask, you should touch only the strings that tie at the back of your head. **Procedure 11-4** shows the proper steps for putting on and removing a mask.

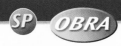

Standard Precautions: Gloving

Equipment: gloves • waste container

Putting on Gloves:

1. Remove your jewelry.
2. Wash and dry your hands.
3. Slip your hands into the gloves, one hand at a time. Be careful not to tear the gloves. If your facility requires that you use double gloves, place a second pair of gloves over the first pair. **See Figure 11-12.**
4. Do not wear torn gloves. Inspect your gloved hands before administering patient care. If holes or defects are seen, replace torn gloves immediately.

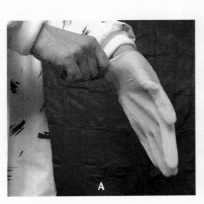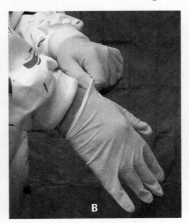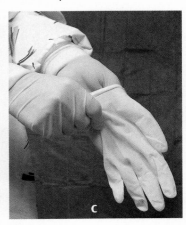

○ **Figure 11-12.** (A) Put on the first glove. (B) Put on the second glove. (C) Double-gloving.

Removing Gloves:

1. The outside of the glove is contaminated. Do not touch any part of your own skin with a gloved hand.
2. Pinch the outside of one glove at least 1 inch below the cuff. **See Figure 11-13.**
3. Pull the glove down and over your hand so that the glove is inside out. **See Figure 11-14.**

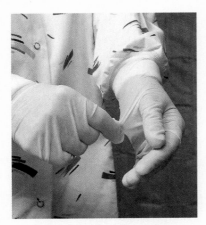

○ **Figure 11-13.** Pinch the outside surface of the glove on the palm.

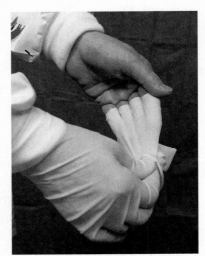

○ **Figure 11-14.** Pull the glove down, avoiding contact with the skin.

4. Hold the glove completely inside the other (gloved) hand. **See Figure 11-15.**
5. Place two fingers of the ungloved hand inside under the cuff of the glove. See **Figure 11-16.**

6. Pull the glove down and over the hand, so that the first glove is completely inside the second glove. **See Figure 11-17.**
7. Dispose of the gloves in an appropriate waste container.
8. Wash your hands.

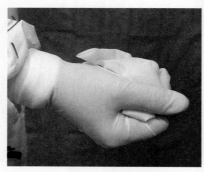

○ Figure 11-15. Hold the glove inside the other hand.

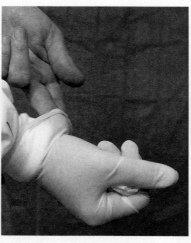

○ Figure 11-16. Put two fingers under the cuff, avoiding contact with the skin.

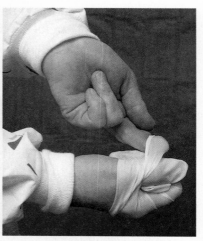

○ Figure 11-17. Pull the second glove down.

Procedure ⬤ 11-3

SP **OBRA**

Standard Precautions: Gowning

Equipment: gown • paper towels • waste container

Putting on the Gown:
1. Remove all jewelry and watches. Roll up your sleeves.
2. Wash and dry your hands.
3. Hold the clean gown in front of you so it unfolds. **See Figure 11-18.** Do not shake the gown.
4. Slip your hands and arms through the gown, making sure the gown completely covers the front of your uniform. **See Figure 11-19.**

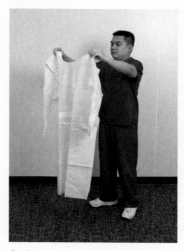

○ Figure 11-18. Hold the gown in front of you at the neck area.

5. Tie the neck strings or fasten with the adhesive strip. **See Figure 11-20.**
6. Grasp the edges of the gown at the waist and pull to the back.

7. Overlap the back of the gown. Tie the waist strings in the back. **See Figure 11-21.**
8. Make sure the back of your uniform is completely covered.

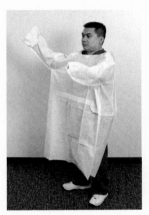

○ **Figure 11-19.** Slip your hands and arms into the gown.

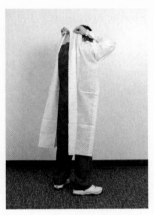

○ **Figure 11-20.** Tie the neck string. Do not touch the gown except at the neckline.

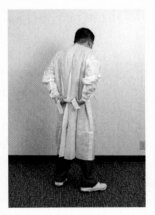

○ **Figure 11-21.** Overlap the back of the gown.

Removing the Gown:

1. Untie the waist strings.
2. Wash your hands.
3. Untie the neck strings or unfasten the adhesive strip.
4. Pull the sleeves off by grasping each shoulder of the gown at the neckline on the outside of the gown. **See Figure 11-22.**
5. Roll the gown up away from you, turning it inside out as arms are removed. **See Figure 11-23.**

6. Grasp gown by the inside of the shoulder seams and fold it inside out, bringing the shoulders together.
7. Roll the gown up with the inside out.
8. If paper, dispose of the gown in a waste container. **See Figure 11-24.** If cloth, put it in the appropriate container for washing.
9. Remove your gloves.
10. Wash your hands. Use a dry paper towel to open the door.

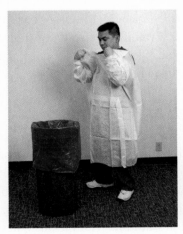

○ **Figure 11-22.** Grasp the shoulders to pull the sleeves off.

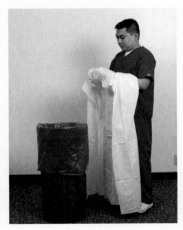

○ **Figure 11-23.** Pull the gown off, rolling it away from you as you turn it inside out.

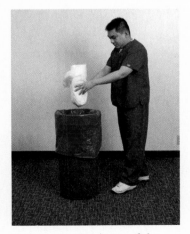

○ **Figure 11-24.** Dispose of the gown.

Standard Precautions: Masking

Equipment: mask • waste container

Putting on the Mask:
1. Wash your hands.
2. Pick up the mask by the ear loops or upper ties.
3. Place the mask over your nose and mouth, making sure that both are covered. Never walk around hallways with a dangling mask.
4. Pull the loops or upper strings over your ears. **See Figure 11-25.** Tie the strings in the back securely at the crown of your head.
5. Grasp bottom portion of mask and spread mask to cover below chin.
6. Tie the bottom strings at the back of your neck. If you wear glasses, the mask should fit snugly over your nose and under the bottom of the glasses.
7. Pinch to mold the metal strip over the bridge of your nose.
8. Wash your hands.

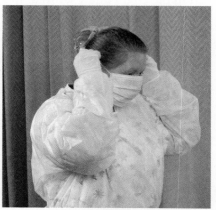

O **Figure 11-25. Put on the mask.**

Removing the Mask:
1. Wash your hands.
2. Untie the lower strings first, then the upper strings.
3. Bring the strings together in front of your face. Do not touch the inside of the mask.
4. Dispose of the mask in a waste container.
5. Wash your hands.

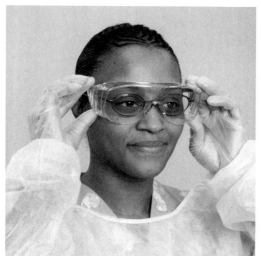

O **Figure 11-26.** Wear goggles as a barrier for splashes to the eyes when working with body fluids.

Protective Eyewear. Goggles or face shields should be worn as a protective barrier when there is a possibility of splashes or sprays of blood or body fluids to the eyes. Even if you already wear glasses, you should wear goggles over your glasses and extending around the sides of the glasses. **See Figure 11-26.**

Transmission-Based Precautions

When a patient in a health care facility is diagnosed with or is suspected to have a highly transmissible or contagious disease, standard precautions are followed. In addition, transmission-based precautions are used, depending on how the pathogen is transmitted. There are three types of transmission-based precautions: airborne, droplet, and contact precautions. The various types of precautions may be combined for diseases that have multiple routes of transmission. **See Figure 11-27.**

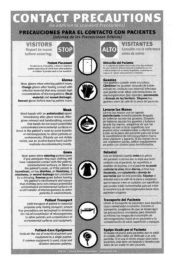
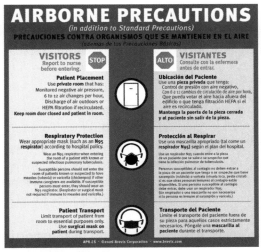
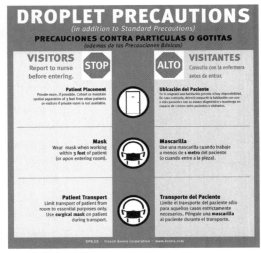

○ **Figure 11-27.** Contact, airborne, and droplet precautions.

When caring for a patient with a highly contagious disease, you must protect yourself and others from the disease. You must also protect the patient from other diseases, since the patient's resistance is low. **See Table 11-1.**

In extreme cases, the patient is placed in isolation or separated from other patients so the disease does not spread. All of the items the patient touches are also isolated. A patient touches linens, personal care supplies, medical equipment, and food service trays in the normal course of a day. All of these items are potential reservoirs for the pathogen.

Caring for the Patient in Isolation

A patient in isolation for contact, airborne, or droplet precautions is usually in a private room. If you provide care for a patient in isolation, it is important to follow the appropriate isolation procedures.

Outside the room is an isolation cart that contains supplies needed to care for the patient and to protect visitors from infection. The isolation cart usually contains PPE, linen bags and hampers for dirty linen, disposable waste bags and container, and medical supplies. Controlling the spread of tuberculosis requires additional isolation procedures, including a small, extra area where everyone

○**Table 11-1.** Isolation Precautions

Type of Precaution	Standard Precautions	Contact Precautions	Airborne Precautions	Droplet Precautions
When used	For all patient care	Used in addition to standard precautions for patients whose illnesses can be transmitted by direct or indirect contact	Used in addition to standard precautions for patients with airborne-transmitted diseases	Used in addition to standard precautions for patients with droplet-transmitted diseases
Examples of diseases requiring precautions	All	*E. coli* bacteria Impetigo Conjunctivitis Scabies Herpes	Rubella Chickenpox Tuberculosis Smallpox SARS	Diphtheria Pneumonia Scarlet Fever Mumps Influenza

entering the isolation unit puts on or removes gowns, gloves, and masks, and disposes of contaminated items. Tuberculosis is airborne, so this small area keeps contaminated air from spreading to the entire hospital.

Personal Care

When providing personal care for a patient in isolation, combine quality patient care with proper isolation techniques. For example, every time you enter the room, you must wash your hands, put on a gown, a mask, goggles, and gloves. Always wash your hands before entering and leaving the isolation room. Use a paper towel to turn faucets on and off and a separate paper towel to close the door when you leave the room. Discard the towel in the waste container inside the door before you exit.

Perform all personal care procedures in a supportive, caring manner. Observe the patient for changes in appearance or behavior, especially when performing personal hygiene care for the patient.

- **Personal Hygiene**—Skin care, oral hygiene, nail care, back rubs, bathing, and shampooing all contribute to a patient's feeling of well-being. Perform these procedures on a regular schedule. When you are with the patient, spend some extra time just talking. Remember, it is the disease that is being isolated, not the patient.

- **Personal Care Items**—Many items used in personal care, such as razors and cotton balls, are disposable. For example, plastic drinking cups are thrown out after one use. Make sure that both you and the patient wash your hands after performing a personal care procedure.

Vital Skills COMMUNICATION

Communication and Standard Precautions

Because some people in a hospital setting carry infectious diseases, you must use standard precautions for all patients. That means you must treat all patients as though they are carrying a bloodborne pathogen. Depending on the nature of a patient's illness and your institution's policies, you may be required to take additional transmission-based precautions, or to care for a patient in an isolation room. Following the proper procedures can help you protect the other patients and yourself.

How will following standard and transmission-based precautions affect your relationship and communication with your patients? It should not affect them at all. Treat each patient as an individual, with unique concerns, likes, dislikes, and needs. Explain to the patient why the precautions are necessary, but do so in a kind, matter-of-fact way that will not make the patient feel isolated or guilty for having a transmissible disease.

Practice

With a partner, practice providing a meal to patients with the following diseases: tuberculosis, pneumonia, AIDS, breast cancer, influenza (the "flu"), and conjunctivitis. One person can be the patient, and the other the nursing assistant. What should you tell the patient? How should you treat him or her? How can you help the patient feel at ease?

Food Service

The central kitchen supplies food to isolation rooms on disposable trays. Before serving a meal to a patient, wash your hands and help the patient wash his or her hands. If required, wear a gown if you need to feed the patient or assist the patient in eating. Unconsumed food and liquids are considered contaminated. Flush unconsumed liquids down the toilet. Place uneaten food, trays, and disposable containers in the contaminated waste container. (Record the amount the patient consumed before discarding.)

Contaminated Items

Everything that is removed from the isolation room is considered contaminated. Contaminated waste is disposed of according to each facility's policy. All items are bagged before they leave the room. Some facilities use color-coded waste bags to indicate contaminated waste. **See Figure 11-28.**

The CDC recommends discarding contaminated waste in a single, sturdy plastic bag if the contaminated article can be placed inside the bag without contaminating the outside of the bag. Otherwise, double bagging may be necessary. The supervisor will tell you when double bagging is needed.

Two people are needed for double bagging. The person inside the isolation room bags the contaminated items. The bag is closed and tied. The contaminated bag is placed inside the clean bag. **See Figure 11-29.** The clean bag is tied, labeled, and disposed of.

Contaminated linens should be handled as little as possible. The risk of disease transmission is small if linen is handled properly and carefully. A single linen hamper should be available in the patient's room. Linen should be bagged, removed, and laundered according to facility policy.

Specimen Collection

Patients in isolation may require certain laboratory tests that require the collection of blood, urine, feces, sputum, and other body fluids. Plan your steps prior to entering the patient's room, including applying warning labels and patient information labels to containers. Follow the recommended barriers for the specific precautions while collecting the specimen. Collect the specimen following the steps outlined in Chapter 19. Remove gloves, wash hands, and follow the policy for transporting the specimen.

Transporting Patients

Moving and transporting patients who are in isolation should be limited but is often unavoidable. Instruct the patients in ways to assist in the prevention of transmission of infectious organisms, such as wearing a mask. Then notify the personnel where the patient is to be taken of the precautions to be used. Finally, provide protective barriers (masks, gloves, gowns, eyewear) for the patient and the people assisting in the transport.

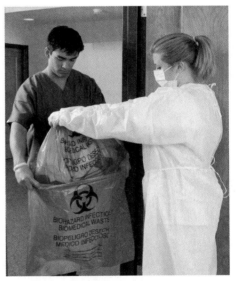

O **Figure 11-28.** Bags for contaminated waste are red.

O **Figure 11-29.** The nursing assistant in the room opens the door and places the bag inside another red contamination bag, which is then closed, tied, and removed.

Psychological Needs of the Isolation Patient

The psychological needs of the isolation patient are sometimes difficult to meet because of the strong emphasis on proper isolation procedures. Visitors may be fearful of entering the isolation room. The patient may feel depressed, unwanted, and lonely. You can help in the following ways.

- Explain the need for precautions to the patient, family, and visitors. Explain that visitors are welcome. Teach visitors how to apply PPE.
- Treat the patient with respect and dignity. Be supportive and reassuring.
- Encourage the patient to use the telephone to keep in touch with family and friends.
- Provide reading material and recreational items, such as crossword puzzles and crafts.
- Plan to do several activities in the patient's room at the same time to extend your time with the patient.

Cleaning Supplies and Equipment

Health care facilities have specific policies for disposing of contaminated material and cleaning contaminated items. Contaminated items are usually sent to a central facility for cleaning. Equipment is kept in the isolation room. It is not moved out into the general areas of the facility.

When you are cleaning the patient's room, follow these guidelines.

- Never allow linens to touch your uniform or the floor.
- Never sit on a patient's bed.
- Do not shake linens and rags, because dust particles can contain pathogens.
- Wipe dirty areas from the cleanest part toward the dirtiest part. **See Figure 11-30.** This prevents additional contamination.
- Dispose of dirty linens in special hampers for contaminated linens.
- Dispose of contaminated waste in special containers for contaminated waste.
- Disinfect and sterilize medical supplies according to the facility's policy.

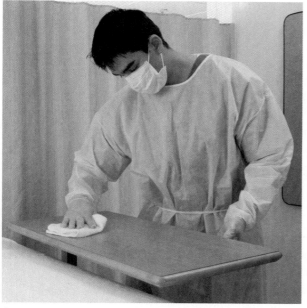

O **Figure 11-30.** When cleaning an overbed tray, always move from the clean area to the dirty area to avoid contaminating an already clean area.

Infection Control in Home Care

Breaking the chain of infection is as important in the home as it is in the health care facility. Although respect for the client's home is important, protecting yourself and your client against disease is a priority when delivering home care. Each agency providing home care will have an infection control program for you to follow. Standard precautions must be followed. You should also be alert to individual needs of clients and families in the home. The following are some guidelines for working in home care.

- **Handwashing.** Practice proper handwashing. Teach the client and family members to know when and how to wash hands. Encourage the use of antimicrobial soaps and disinfectants.
- **Personal protective equipment.** With your supervisor's instruction, encourage the client and family members to use gloves and other barriers when appropriate.

- **Food.** Encourage families to wash all raw fruits and vegetables before eating them. Refrigerate fresh and all opened and unpackaged foods. Discard expired foods.
- **Equipment.** Clean equipment with soap and water and disinfect with a chlorine bleach solution. Kitchen and bathroom areas and equipment should be disinfected using a chlorine bleach solution. Encourage the use of hot water and soap when cleaning dishes and utensils.
- **Personal items.** Discourage the use of shared personal items in the home, such as toothbrushes, washcloths, and towels.
- **Contaminated waste.** Dispose of dressings and other disposable items by placing them in a moisture-proof plastic bag and removing the bag from the home.
- **Sharps.** Needles and other sharp instruments or objects are called *sharps*. Help clients place sharps in a puncture-resistant container with a secure lid. Avoid touching sharps. Hold the container so the patient can put the sharp into it. **See Figure 11-31.**
- **Linens.** Wash soiled linens in the hottest temperature possible with an added cup of bleach if appropriate.
- **Respiratory care.** Cover nose and mouth when coughing or sneezing, and then wash your hands. Encourage the client and family members in the home to do the same.
- **Infections.** Help the client and family to identify signs and symptoms of infection and explain when to report them to the health care provider.

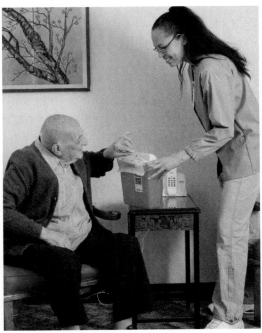

○ **Figure 11-31.** Special containers may be purchased for a home care situation, or you may use a heavy plastic detergent bottle for disposal of sharps.

Infectious Diseases

When you care for a patient with an infectious disease, you must follow standard precautions and additional precaution procedures dictated by your facility. The precautions vary with the type of disease. Ask your supervisor if you are not sure what precautions you should take.

Hepatitis B and Hepatitis C

Hepatitis B and hepatitis C are highly contagious viral infections of the liver. Hepatitis B virus (HBV) and hepatitis C virus (HCV) are caused by separate and distinct hepatitis viruses. The diseases produce mild fever, muscle and joint pain, nausea, vomiting, loss of appetite, fatigue, grayish-white stools, dark urine, and jaundiced (yellowed) skin and the whites of the eyes. HBV and HCV are usually spread through contact with infected blood and body fluids. However, both are most often transmitted by injecting illegal drugs, involving shared needles, syringes, or other equipment associated with drug use.

There is no cure for hepatitis B or hepatitis C, and the diseases can be fatal. A vaccination is available for hepatitis B and is recommended for all health care workers. Patients with active HBV and HCV are cared for in hospitals, long-term care facilities, or in their homes.

Creating Summary Notes

One way to practice your writing skill is to summarize a few pages in just a few paragraphs. A *summary* is shorter than the original source. It captures the main ideas of the source and rephrases them.

For example, read about caring for a patient in isolation on pages 265–268. The pages might be summarized into a few paragraphs as follows:

Patients with contact, airborne, or droplet precautions are usually in a private isolation room. When taking care of these patients, the proper procedures and PPE must be followed. PPE can usually be found outside the patient's room. Remember to wash your hands before entering and leaving the room.

Remember that everything that has been inside an isolation room is considered contaminated, and should be disposed of properly. Most items that a patient in isolation comes in contact with will be thrown away. If equipment is to be re-used, it must be properly cleaned and disinfected according to the facility policy.

When caring for patients in isolation, it is important to remember that the disease is being isolated, not the patient. Explain the need for the precautions to the patient, who may be fearful. Treat the patient with the same care and respect that you would extend to any patient.

Practice

Read the section in this chapter about infection control and the importance of asepsis, isolation precautions, and handwashing. Summarize this information in three to five paragraphs. (You do not need to include the procedures.)

HIV/AIDS

Acquired immunodeficiency syndrome (AIDS) is caused by the human immunodeficiency virus (HIV). AIDS attacks the immune system, which affects the body's ability to fight other diseases. The patient usually dies from infections the body cannot withstand. Such infections are called *opportunistic*. They infect only hosts with lowered resistance, where they have an opportunity to take hold. Currently, more and more patients with HIV and AIDS are living longer due to improvements in medical treatments. However, there is no known cure for AIDS, which is always fatal. Always follow standard precautions to prevent the spread of HIV/AIDS.

People who are infected with HIV are carriers for life. Some carriers never show symptoms, but they can still transmit HIV to others. HIV is transmitted when contaminated fluid enters the bloodstream. HIV is a bloodborne pathogen.

HIV/AIDS is transmitted through semen, vaginal secretions, breast milk, blood, and body fluids that contain blood. The infection can enter the body through:

- Puncture wounds from infected needles or broken glass.
- Cuts or open sores.
- Mucous membranes (nose, mouth, eyes).
- Intimate sexual contact.
- Blood transfusions with infected blood.
- Infected mothers to their unborn or newly born babies.

Emerging Infectious Diseases

Many infectious diseases have been controlled or eliminated through medical treatments and vaccinations. However, as some diseases decline, others appear. The CDC refers to these "new" diseases as *emerging diseases*. Some of these diseases have only recently been identified. Others were once confined to one part of the world but are now spreading through international travel, crowding, and lack of resources.

Examples of emerging infectious diseases include severe acute respiratory syndrome (SARS), West Nile virus, and new strains of influenza and *Escherichia coli* bacteria. Other, more dangerous versions of previously known diseases are also appearing. Examples include drug-resistant strains of tuberculosis, whooping cough (pertussis) and methicillin-resistant *Staphylococcus aureus* (MRSA).

SARS is caused by a virus that attacks the respiratory system. It is spread by droplet transmission and has been identified around the world. Symptoms include an extremely high fever, headache, and body aches. The infection develops into pneumonia. SARS has been fatal in some cases.

The West Nile virus (WNV) is spread by a common vector: the mosquito. Symptoms of fever, headache, and body aches can progress to disorientation, muscle weakness, paralysis, and death. Precautions include those that protect people from contact with the mosquito, including mosquito repellents.

Staying Healthy on the Job

It is vital for you to understand and consistently practice standard precautions and transmission-based precautions to protect yourself from infectious diseases. Unfortunately, occupational injuries involving blood and body fluids can sometimes occur.

OSHA's Bloodborne Pathogen Standard

The Occupational Safety and Health Administration (OSHA) requires every health care employer to follow the Bloodborne Pathogen Standard. This set of regulations was created to protect health care workers from being exposed to potentially infectious materials. According to OSHA, there are three modes for the transmission of infections in clinical areas. They are:
- Skin contact, when breaks or cracks in an employee's skin can come in contact with infectious microorganisms.
- Puncture wounds from accidental needle sticks or other sharp instruments.
- Mucous membrane contact such as splattering to eyes, mouth, and nose.

According to OSHA's Bloodborne Pathogen Standard, employers must:
- Develop a written exposure control program.
- Provide special training at no charge for all employees about the facility's plan and what to do if an incident occurs.
- Provide hepatitis B vaccine free to all employees who come into contact with patients' blood and body fluids. The best defense against HBV is vaccination, which is recommended for all health care workers, except pregnant or nursing women, or employees with a history of cardiopulmonary disease. Consult your doctor.

FOCUS ON

Drug-Resistant Microorganisms

Misuse of antibiotics has resulted in the resurgence of many infectious diseases that were at one time well controlled. They are now resistant to many antibiotics. The number of bacteria resistant to antibiotics increases each time bacteria are exposed to a drug but are not completely destroyed.

SAFETY FIRST

Needle-stick injuries are wounds caused by needles that accidentally puncture the skin. Needle sticks can transmit infectious disease, especially bloodborne viruses. Although the nursing assistant's scope of practice does not usually include using needles, you can be injured by needles that have not been properly disposed of in a sharps container. If you find needles left at a patient's bedside or in a regular waste container, report the incident to your supervisor at once.

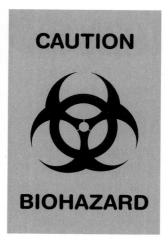

○ **Figure 11-32.** Employers in health care facilities must label all waste and containers of potentially infectious materials with the biohazard symbol.

- Use environmental and work practice controls to eliminate or reduce worker exposure to bloodborne pathogens. An example of an environmental control is a sharps container for disposal of used needles. An example of a work practice control is the facility's procedure for contaminated waste disposal.
- Provide hazard communication to warn employees of potentially hazardous material exposure. This communication includes warning labels and orange or orange-red biohazard symbols for waste and containers of potentially contaminated or infectious materials. **See Figure 11-32.**
- Develop written cleaning schedules and decontamination procedures.
- Provide handwashing facilities that are easily accessible to employees.
- Provide PPE at no charge to all employees who may come into contact with blood and other body fluids. PPE includes gloves, gowns, masks or respirators, and protective eyewear.
- Offer post-exposure evaluation and counseling and follow-up medical testing for workers who experience needle sticks or other exposures.
- Maintain confidentiality of employees who have had an exposure incident.

Your Responsibilities

All health care providers are responsible for preventing the spread of disease to patients and for keeping themselves healthy and free of disease. Follow these basic procedures to decrease the risk of transmitting disease.

- Wash your hands whenever they are visibly soiled, before and after direct contact with all people, after contact with anything that might be contaminated with blood or body fluids, before and after performing any procedure, before and after handling food, before and after using the bathroom, before gloving, and immediately after putting on or removing gloves.
- Wear a gown and gloves during procedures when you will be exposed to blood, any body fluids (other than sweat), broken skin, or mucous membranes.
- Wear a mask and protective eyewear if blood or body fluids are likely to splatter.
- Have mouth-to-mouth resuscitation barrier devices readily available.
- Immediately clean blood and other body fluid spills with a disinfectant solution. Your facility will instruct you on how to clean spills. Discard cleaning implements in a plastic bag and dispose of the bag according to facility procedure. In a home care situation, use a chlorine bleach solution to clean up any spills of body fluid.

General Exposure Guidelines

Refer to your employer's exposure control plan regarding exposure to bloodborne pathogens. However, follow these general guidelines if an exposure incident occurs in the workplace.

- **Treatment.** First aid or other emergency care is always a priority. Know where to seek immediate treatment.
- **Reporting procedures.** Find out who to contact and what forms to fill out.
- **Evaluation.** Identify the source of the exposure as well as any necessary testing (with consent) to determine if further treatment is needed.
- **Follow-up.** Further testing of an employee may be required for a prolonged period of time. Medical and psychological counseling may be necessary, depending on the circumstances of the exposure.

- **Always remember:** Use standard precautions at all times. Patients can be carriers of disease even if they show no symptoms.

Maintaining Your Health

Staying healthy is the best defense against disease. Maintain good health by getting plenty of rest, proper nutrition, and exercise. Stress management techniques are also helpful to maintain a healthy frame of mind.

- Before reporting to work, cover any cuts or open sores with a clean, waterproof bandage.
- Notify your supervisor if you have flu symptoms, if you are running a fever, or if you are coughing or sneezing.
- Keep your fingernails clean and short. CDC recommends that artificial nails not be worn for direct patient care.
- Carefully handle razors and other sharps. Dispose of all sharps in special sharps containers.
- Always maintain a barrier, such as gloves, masks, and gowns, between yourself and an infection.
- Receive appropriate vaccinations as required by your employer or state.

Vital Skills MATH

Calculating Vaccination Schedules

The federal government requires all health care facilities to provide the hepatitis B vaccine to employees who come in contact with potential exposure. The vaccine is given in a series of three injections and a booster. The second injection is given 30 days after the first injection. The third injection is given 6 months after the first shot. The booster is given in 10-year intervals.

Example: If you started the series on January 20, 2007, when would you complete the initial series of injections? When would you receive the first booster?

Let's think it through. There are 12 months in a year, and January is the first month. You would receive the third injection 6 months after the first injection, and 1 + 6 = 7. You would receive your third injection in the seventh month, or July. Your first booster would be 10 years from 2007. 2007 + 10 = 2017, so you would receive your first booster in the year 2017.

Practice

1. If you received your first hepatitis B vaccination injection on May 5, 2004, when would you have completed the initial series of injections? When will your first booster be due?
2. If you received your first hepatitis B vaccination injection on March 15, 2006, when would you have completed the initial series of injections? When will your first booster be due?

Chapter Summary

- Nursing assistants work with people with a variety of illnesses in a variety of environments, so knowing how to prevent disease transmission is vital.

- There are four primary types of microorganisms responsible for infection and transmitting disease.

- Six conditions must be present for the chain of infection to occur.

- Infectious disease is transmitted in five basic ways.

- Nursing assistants must be able to recognize the signs and symptoms of infection and report them to a supervisor.

- Medical asepsis and surgical asepsis are practices for reducing and eliminating microorganisms.

- Precautions control the spread of infection and are divided into two categories: standard precautions and transmission-based precautions.

- Caring for patients in isolation requires using standard precautions and the appropriate transmission-based precautions.

- Nursing assistants must be aware of how highly contagious diseases are transmitted so they can follow appropriate infection control precautions when caring for patients.

- OSHA's Bloodborne Pathogen Standard requires employers to protect health care workers from being exposed to potentially infectious materials.

VOCABULARY REVIEW

Directions: Match the letter of each definition in the second column with the correct vocabulary term in the first column. Write your answers on a separate sheet of paper.

Vocabulary

1. asepsis
2. bloodborne pathogen
3. chain of infection
4. disinfection
5. infection
6. infectious disease
7. medical asepsis
8. microorganism
9. noninfectious disease
10. nonpathogen
11. nosocomial infection
12. pathogen
13. reservoir
14. surgical asepsis
15. vector

Definitions

A. A disease caused by a group of pathogenic microorganisms that invade and multiply within the body

B. A microscopic living plant or animal

C. The practice of minimizing or reducing the spread of pathogens

D. The condition of being free of pathogens

E. An infection that a patient acquires while in a health care setting

F. A microorganism that does not cause disease or infection

G. The practice of completely eliminating microorganisms

H. A disease-causing organism found in blood or other body fluids

I. A cleaning process that uses strong chemicals to kill most pathogens

J. A microorganism that causes disease or infection

K. A disease that cannot be transmitted from one person to another

L. The series of six conditions that together produce infection

M. A nonhuman living organism that transmits pathogens

N. A disease transmitted from one person to another through the chain of infection

O. Any environment that allows a pathogen to live and grow

Check Your Knowledge

Review Questions: Answer each of the following questions on a separate sheet of paper.

1. What are the four primary types of microorganisms?
2. Name the five methods by which a microorganism can be transmitted.
3. What is a susceptible host?
4. What are the signs and symptoms of infection?
5. Describe the standard precautions a nursing assistant takes to prevent the spread of infection. Which is the single most important precaution?
6. Name the three types of transmission-based precautions.
7. What steps should you take when transporting a patient with a highly contagious disease?
8. List two bloodborne pathogens and describe how you would protect yourself from infection.
9. What is OSHA's Bloodborne Pathogen Standard?
10. List ways that you can maintain your personal health to protect yourself and your patients.

True or False: Read each statement carefully. Then write *True* or *False* by the statement number on a separate sheet of paper.

1. Microorganisms need a warm, moist, dark environment to thrive.
2. The elderly and young are more susceptible hosts than healthy, middle-aged people.
3. A nosocomial infection can always be successfully cured with antibiotics.
4. All health care workers must follow standard precautions.
5. A patient in isolation may feel unclean and unwanted.

Think and Decide

Directions: Think about each of the following scenarios. Answer each question on a separate sheet of paper.

1. Harvey is a long-term care resident in your care. He has pneumonia, and the nurse tells you to take him to the X-Ray Department for a chest x-ray. Should you take him? Explain.

2. You are getting ready to change the diaper of Willi, a 3-month-old child in the Pediatric Department. She has been hospitalized for diarrhea. Upon applying your gloves, you notice a hole in the thumb of one of the gloves. What should you do?

3. You are assisting with the care of Brian, a home health patient who has AIDS. Brian has sores around his mouth and genital areas. How should you protect yourself while helping with his personal hygiene needs?

4. You arrive at the home of the Carrera family to care for Mr. Carrera (the father), who has cancer. When you go to the sink to wash your hands, you realize that the home has no running water. What should you do?

5. Mr. U., a long-term care resident, is in isolation because he has methicillin-resistant *Staphylococcus aureus* (MRSA). What PPE should you wear when entering this patient's room?

6. After working for three years in a long-term care facility, you have decided to accept a job as a home health aide. Your first assignment is at the home of Roxanne, a woman who has viral pneumonia. Compare and contrast infection control measures you will need to use in the home care environment with those used in the long-term care facility.

7. You have been working in an isolation room and are washing your hands prior to leaving the room. You perform all of the handwashing steps properly. However, when you go to dry your hands on a clean paper towel, you notice that this paper towel is the last one in the towel dispenser. There will not be a paper towel with which to turn off the faucet. What should you do?

8. You are following airborne precautions as you help Ms. P., who has severe acute respiratory syndrome (SARS), with her personal hygiene. Suddenly, she sneezes violently, and droplets fall on your mask. What should you do?

CNA Certification Exam Prep

Directions: This practice test contains ten questions. Each question has four suggested answers. For each question, choose the ONE that best answers the question or completes the statement. Write your answers on a separate sheet of paper.

1. What is the difference between pathogens and nonpathogens?

   A. Pathogens do not cause disease or infection.

   B. Nonpathogens do not cause disease or infection.

   C. Nonpathogens cause disease or infection.

   D. Pathogens do not give off toxins.

2. What factors contribute to the growth of microorganisms?

   A. moisture, warmth, light

   B. darkness, oxygen, dryness

   C. moisture, food, darkness

   D. cool temperature, darkness, moisture

3. Which type of microorganism causes common diseases such as strep throat?

   A. fungus

   B. virus

   C. protozoa

   D. bacteria

4. One way a disease can be transmitted is by

   A. direct contact.

   B. wearing gloves.

   C. following standard precautions.

   D. following isolation precautions.

5. Airborne transmission can occur when

   A. microorganisms are inhaled by the host.

   B. one person touches another person.

   C. an infected person is kept in isolation.

   D. autoclaves are used.

6. A disease is transmitted by a mosquito bite. This type of transmission is

   A. airborne transmission.

   B. indirect contact.

   C. direct contact.

   D. vector-borne transmission.

7. For which of the following diseases is a vaccine available?

   A. arthritis

   B. hepatitis B

   C. AIDS

   D. Alzheimer's disease

8. The most important method for preventing the spread of infection is to

   A. wash your hands.

   B. avoid touching patients.

   C. take a daily shower.

   D. bathe the patient every day.

9. This organization's primary purpose is the prevention or spread of highly infectious diseases.

   A. FDA

   B. OSHA

   C. CDC

   D. NIH

10. Which of the following is an example of a direct mode of contact transmission?

    A. using contaminated utensils

    B. sharing drinks

    C. massaging

    D. coughing

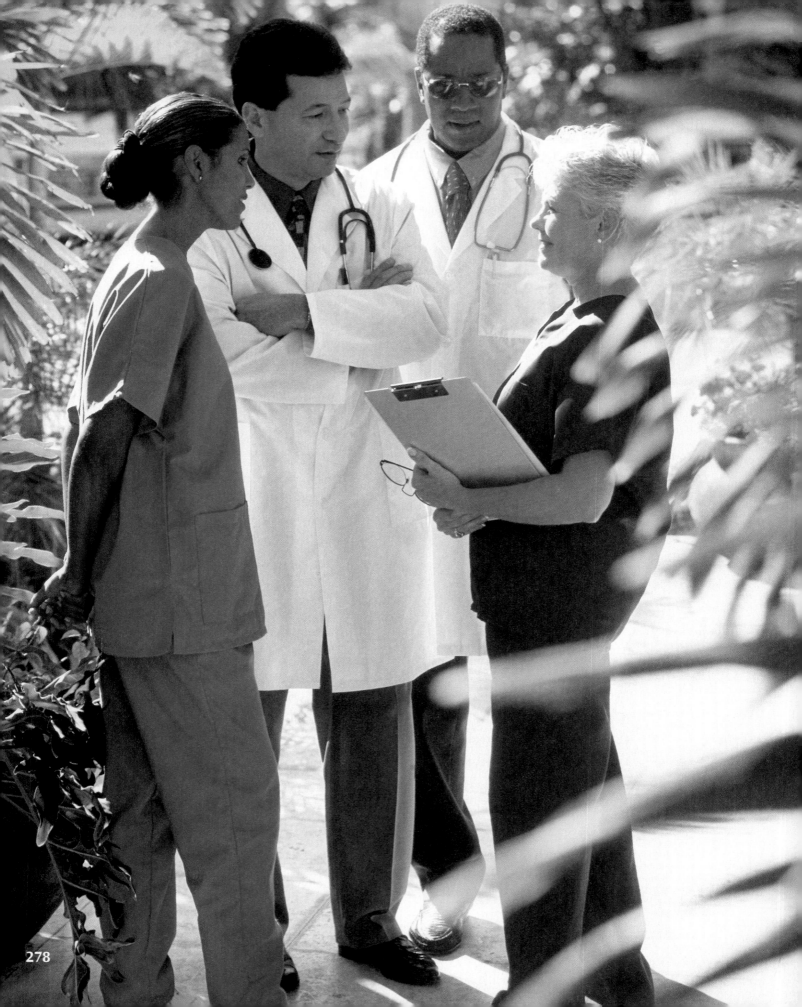

UNIT 3

Medical Communication

Chapter 12	Medical Technology
Chapter 13	Observing, Charting, and Reporting

Unit 3 presents the language that health care workers use to report and record their observations and actions on the job. Chapter 12 explains how medical terms are made up, listing common medical root words, prefixes, and suffixes. It also describes the abbreviations and symbols used in health care. Chapter 13 describes how nursing assistants observe and report on patient conditions and maintain records.

OBJECTIVES

- Name the four basic word parts used in medical terminology.
- Break medical terms into their word parts.
- Recognize and use common medical terminology.
- Identify abbreviations and symbols commonly used in health care.
- Recognize abbreviations that should not be used according to JCAHO guidelines.

Medical Terminology

abbreviation A shortened form of a word or phrase.

acronym An abbreviation made up of the first letters of each word in a phrase.

combining form A word part plus a vowel to make the word easier to pronounce.

medical terminology The specialized language used by the health care professions.

prefix A word part that comes before a root word or a combining form and modifies its meaning.

root word The basic part of a word that gives the word meaning.

suffix A word part that comes after a root word or a combining form and modifies its meaning.

symbol A written or printed sign that has meaning.

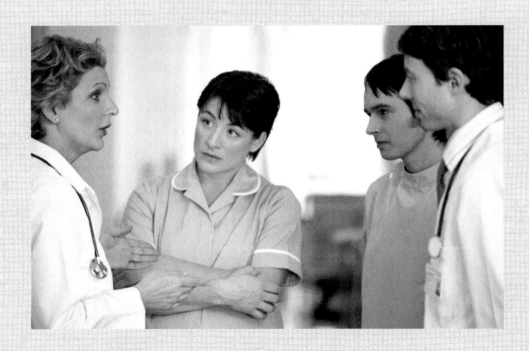

The Language of Health Care

Professionals of all kinds need to communicate with one another about their work. They use specialized or technical language that describes the work they do. It also describes the objects and equipment they use.

The specialized language used by the health care professions is called **medical terminology**. Medical knowledge has increased over many years, and so has the need for new terms to describe this knowledge. New medical terms are continually created as new illnesses, therapies, and medicines are identified and discovered.

People use some medical terms every day, such as *doctor, nurse, pharmacy, virus, pneumonia,* and *strep throat*. However, nursing assistants must learn more specific medical terminology. You will read charts, write observations, and discuss patients' concerns with other members of the health care team. You will need to recognize and use the words and abbreviations that are the special language of health care.

Word Building

Some medical terms are *compound* words, or words made up of two or more distinct words. You already know many compound words. For example, *heartbeat* is a compound of *heart* and *beat*. It means "one complete pulsation of the heart." Some compound words are hyphenated (*well-being*). Some are made of two or more separate words (*adrenal gland*).

Many medical terms, however, are more complex. Most come from early Latin and Greek words. Over time, these ancient words have been combined to make the medical terms used today. They are generally made up of several combined words and word parts. Each part has meaning by itself.

The four basic word parts used in medical terminology are root words (stems), combining forms, prefixes, and suffixes. Some word parts can be used as either a combining form, a prefix, or a suffix.

Root Words and Combining Forms

A **root word**, or stem, is the basic part of a word that gives the word meaning. For example, *cephal* comes from a Greek word that means "head." A **combining form** is a word part plus a vowel to make the word easier to pronounce. *Cephal(o)-* is a combining form also meaning "head." A *cephalometer* is an instrument for measuring the head. **Table 12-1** lists many root words and combining forms with their meanings and examples of their use in medical terminology. **Figure 12-1** shows the human body with some of the combining forms used in medical terminology.

Vital Skills   READING

Using Context Clues

As you read the charts of your future patients, you may encounter some words or abbreviations with which you are not familiar. You can try to figure out the meaning of the word or abbreviation using context clues. *Context clues* are clues to the meaning of a word. They can help you make a logical guess about the meaning of a word.

Example: Mr. Smith was hospitalized for a <u>hepatectomy</u>. He was concerned about how much of his liver function he would have after his operation.

From the sentence, can you guess what a *hepatectomy* is?

Answer: hepa (liver) + ectomy (surgical removal of): hepatectomy is surgical removal of all or part of the liver.

Practice

In the sentences below, see if you can **figure out** the meaning of the underlined words using context clues.

1. When cleaning a room between patients, it is important to use a <u>bactericide</u> to help minimize the risk of spreading an infectious disease.
2. Mrs. Garcia had a <u>circumoral</u> rash that made it difficult for her to bite and chew her food.
3. The swelling from the injection she received was <u>unilateral</u>, so she could still use her left hand.

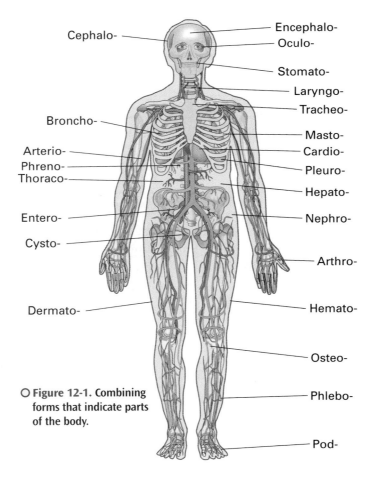

Cephalo-
Encephalo-
Oculo-
Stomato-
Laryngo-
Tracheo-
Broncho-
Masto-
Arterio-
Cardio-
Phreno-
Pleuro-
Thoraco-
Hepato-
Entero-
Nephro-
Cysto-
Arthro-
Dermato-
Hemato-
Osteo-
Phlebo-
Pod-

○ **Figure 12-1.** Combining forms that indicate parts of the body.

○ **Table 12-1.** Root Words/Combining Forms

Root Words/Combining Forms	Meaning	Example Medical Term
arteri(o)	artery	arteriosclerosis—hardening of the arteries
arthr(o)	joint	arthritis—a disease marked by inflammation of the joints
bacteri(o)	bacteria	bactericide—something that kills bacteria
bronchi(o)	bronchus	bronchitis—inflammation of the bronchial tubes
carcin(o)	cancer	carcinogen—an agent that contributes to or causes cancer
cardi(o)	heart	cardiomegaly—enlargement of the heart
cephal(o)	head	cephalomegaly—enlargement of the head
cyst(o), cysti	bladder, cyst	cystitis—inflammation of the urinary bladder
cyt(o)	cell	cytotoxic—poisonous to cells
dent(o)	tooth or teeth	dentifrice—a preparation for cleaning the teeth, such as toothpaste
derm(o), derma, dermat(o)	skin	dermatitis—inflammation of the skin
dextr(o)	right	dextromanual—right-handed
dors(o), dorsi	back	dorsiflex—to bend backward
echo	reflected sound	echocardiogram—test that measures the reflected sound of the heart
electr(o)	electricity	electrocardiogram—record of the electrical activity of the heart
encephal(o)	brain	encephalomyelitis—inflammation of the brain and spinal cord
enter(o)	intestines	enteritis—inflammation of the intestines
erythr(o)	red	erythrocyte—red blood cell
fibr(o)	fibers	fibroma—a tumor made of fibrous tissue
gluc(o)	sweetness, glucose	glucometer—instrument for measuring glucose
gyn(o), gyne, gynec(o)	woman, female	gynecology—specialty dealing with the care of the female reproductive system
hem(o), hema, hemat(o)	blood	hematoma—a mass of clotted blood
hepat(o), hepatic(o)	liver	hepatitis—inflammation of the liver
hydr(o)	water	hydrated—sufficient water in the body
juxta	near or adjoining	juxtacardiac—near or beside the heart
kerat(o)	cornea	keratotomy—incision through the cornea
laryng(o)	larynx	laryngitis—inflammation of the larynx
leuk(o)	white	leukocyte—white blood cell
lip(o)	fat	lipoprotein—compound containing both fats and proteins
mast(o)	breast	mastitis—inflammation of the breast
megal(o)	large	megalocephaly—abnormal enlargement of the head

Root Words/Combining Forms	Meaning	Example Medical Term
men(o)	pertaining to the menstrual cycle	menopause—end of the menstrual cycle
necr(o)	death	necropathy—a condition with death of certain tissues
nephr(o)	kidney	nephritis—inflammation of the kidney
neur(o)	nerves or nervous system	neuritis—inflammation of the nerves
ocul(o)	eye	oculofacial—of the eyes and face
odont(o)	tooth or teeth	odontalgia—toothache
orth(o)	straight, normal, correct	orthopedics—surgery dealing with restoring the function of the skeletal system
oste(o)	bone	osteomyelitis—inflammation of the bone and bone marrow
path(o)	disease	pathogen—an agent that causes disease
ped(o), pedi	foot	pedopathy—any disease of the foot
pedi(o)	child	pediatrics—medical specialty that deals with children
phleb(o)	vein or veins	phlebitis—inflammation of a vein
phot(o)	light	photosensitive—sensitive to light
phren(o)	diaphragm	phrenalgia—pain in the diaphragm
physi(o)	physical or nature	physiotherapist—a physical therapist
pleur(o), pleura	the membrane surrounding the lungs	pleurisy—inflammation of the pleura
pneum(o), pneuma, pneumat(o)	air, lungs, gas, respiration	pneumonia—inflammation of the lungs
pod(o)	foot	podiatry—specialty concerned with diagnosis and treatment of the foot
pyel(o)	pelvis	pyelogram—x-ray of the renal pelvis
py(o)	pus	pyonephritis—inflammation of the kidney with pus
radi(o)	x-ray, radiation	radiotoxemia—radiation sickness
rect(o)	the rectum	rectoabdominal—relating to the rectum and abdomen, as in an examination
retr(o)	behind, backward	retroversion—a turning backward, especially of the uterus
rhin(o)	nose	rhinoplasty—plastic surgery of the nose
sarc(o)	fleshlike	sarcoma—a malignant mass
scler(o)	hardness	scleroderma—hardening and thickening of the skin
scoli(o)	twisted or crooked	scoliosis—crooked spine
sinistr(o)	left, left side	sinistrotorsion—twisting toward the left
somat(o)	body	psychosomatic—having physical symptoms of emotional or mental origin

Root Words/Combining Forms	Meaning	Example Medical Term
sten(o)	contracted or narrow	stenosis—narrowing of a duct, canal, or valve
stoma, stomat(o), stom(o)	mouth, opening	stomatitis—inflammation inside the mouth
therm(o)	heat	thermometer—a device for measuring temperature
thorac(o)	chest	thoracoscope—a scope for examining the pleural cavity
thromb(o)	clot, thrombus	thrombosis—stationary blood clot within a blood vessel
tox(o), toxi, toxic(o)	poison	toxicology—the study and science of poisons
trache(o)	trachea, windpipe	tracheoplasty—surgical repair of the trachea
ventr(o), ventri	the belly or the front of the body	ventricumbent—lying on the belly

Prefixes

A **prefix** is a word part that comes before a root word or a combining form and modifies its meaning. Prefixes are written like this: *auto-*. *Auto-* means "against." *Autoimmune* means "against one's own tissue." An autoimmune disease is one in which the body produces immune responses against itself. **Table 12-2** lists common prefixes used in medical terms. **Figure 12-2** shows prefixes that indicate location and direction of sections of the body.

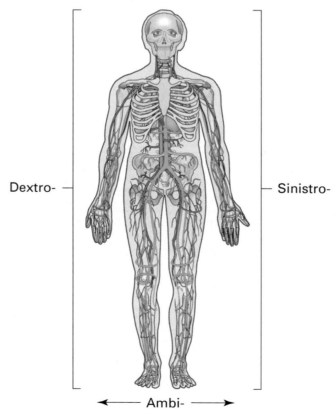

○ Figure 12-2. Prefixes that refer to the location and direction of sections of the body.

○ Table 12-2. Prefixes

Prefix	Meaning	Example Medical Term
a-	without	asepsis—without living organisms (sterile)
ab-, abs-	away from	abduct—to draw away from a position
ad-	toward, to	adduct—to draw toward (as a limb)
ambi-	both, around	ambidextrous—having dexterity on both sides
an-	without	anencephalic—without a brain
ante-	before, in front of	antemortem—before death
anti-	against	anti-inflammatory—reducing inflammation
aut(o)-	self	autoimmune—against one's own tissue
bi-	two, double, twice	bisection—division into two parts
brady-	slow	bradycardia—abnormally slow heartbeat
circum-	around	circumoral—around the mouth
co-, col-, com-, con-, cor-	together	codependent—dependent on each other (usually extremely or abnormally so)
contra-	against, opposed	contraindicated—not recommended
de-, di-, dif-, dir-, dis-	not, separated	dehydrated—not hydrated
dys-	abnormal, difficult, painful	dysfunction—abnormal functioning
ect(o)-	outside	ectopic—occurring outside of the normal place (an ectopic pregnancy)
end(o)-	within	endocarditis—inflammation of the innermost part of the heart
epi-	over	epicystitis—inflammation of the tissue around the bladder
eu-	well, normal	euglycemia—normal blood glucose
ex-	out of, away from	exhale—to breathe out
exo-	external, on the outside	exopthalmus—protusion (sticking out) of the eyeball
extra-	outside of, beyond	extrahepatic—outside the liver
hemi-	half	hemiplegia—paralysis on one side of the body
hyper-	above, beyond, above normal	hyperactive—abnormally restless and inattentive
hypo-	beneath, under, below normal	hypothyroidism—decrease in thyroid activity
infra-	under, beneath, below	infracostal—below the rib
inter-	between	interrenal—between the two kidneys
intra-	within	intramuscular—within the substance of the muscles
iso-	equal, same	isometric—of equal dimensions
meg(a)-	large	megacolon—abnormally large colon
met(a)-	change, transformation; after	metatarsus—the part of the foot between the instep and toes
micr(o)-	unusually small	microdont—having abnormally small teeth
mon(o)-	single	monomania—obsession with a single thought or idea

○ **Table 12-2.** Prefixes continued

Prefix	Meaning	Example Medical Term
non-	not	nonspecific—not due to any known cause (such as a disease)
pan-	all	pandemic—widespread epidemic
para-	near, beside, abnormal, or two similar parts	paraplegia—paralysis of the lower extremities
peri-	near, around	perienteric—near or around the intestine
poly-	many	polyarthritis—inflammation of several joints at once
post-	after, following, behind	postmortem—after death
pre-	before	prenatal—before birth
pro-	before, forward	proglossis—the tip of the tongue
quadra-, quadri-	four	quadriplegia—paralysis of all four limbs
re-	again, backward	retraction—the act of drawing back
semi-	half, partial	semicomatose—drowsy and inactive but not in a full coma
sub-	less than, under, inferior	subcutaneous—beneath the skin
super-	more than, above, superior	superinfection—an infection in addition to one already present
supra-	above, over	suprarenal—above the kidney
tachy-	fast	tachycardia—rapid heartbeat
trans-	across, through	transfusion—transfer of blood from one person to another
ultra-	excess, beyond	ultrasonic—concerning sounds inaudible to humans
un-	not	unconscious—insensible, not conscious
uni-	one	unilateral—on one side only

Vital Skills COMMUNICATION

Pronunciation of Medical Terms

Many of the medical terms you encountered in this chapter are probably new to you. The best way to familiarize yourself with them is to practice using them. That means saying them out loud! Include a pronunciation guide for the word to help you remember how to say it. (You can find out how to say a word by looking in the dictionary. See the Vital Skills: Writing section in this chapter.)

Practice

In groups of four, practice using the words listed in Tables 12-1 through 12-4. One person should pick twenty words from Table 12-1; a second person should pick twenty words from Table 12-2, etc. Say the word out loud, and then define it. You might need to ask your instructor to say the words for you first.

Suffixes

A **suffix** is a word part that comes after a root word or a combining form and modifies its meaning. Suffixes are written like this: -*oma*. This suffix means "tumor." A melanoma is a skin tumor. **Table 12-3** shows common suffixes used in medical terminology.

○ **Table 12-3. Suffixes**

Suffix	Meaning	Example Medical Term
-ad	to, toward	cephalad—toward the head
-algia	pain	neuralgia—nerve pain
-ase	enzyme	protease—an enzyme that combines with a protein
-ate	salt (in chemistry)	carbonate—a salt of carbonic acid
-blast	immature, forming	neuroblast—an embryonic cell that develops into a nerve cell
-cidal, -cide	killing	germicide—agent that kills pathogens
-crit	separate	hematocrit—volume of whole blood separated from plasma
-cyte	cell	lymphocyte—lymph cell
-derma, -dermic	skin	hypodermic—applied beneath the skin
-ectomy	removal of	appendectomy—removal of the appendix
-emia	blood	hypoglycemia—low blood sugar
-form	having the shape of	uniform—having the same shape throughout
-gen	producing	carcinogen—an agent that produces cancer
-gram	a recording	encephalogram—recording of brain activity
-graph	an instrument for recording	encephalograph—an instrument for measuring brain activity
-ia	a condition	hysteria—extreme emotional excitability
-iasis	a condition	psoriasis—a chronic skin disease
-ic(s)	pertaining to	orthopedic—pertaining to skeletal disorders
-ism	condition, disease	autism—in psychiatry, a condition in which interest is focused only on the self
-itis	inflammation	nephritis—inflammation of the kidneys
-(o)logy	study or practice of	histology—study of tissue
-lysis	destruction of	electrolysis—removal of unwanted hair using electrical current
-mania	obsession	kleptomania—obsession with stealing
-megaly	large	acromegaly—a condition including enlargement of the hands, face, and feet
-meter	a measuring device	audiometer—an electronic device for measuring hearing
-metry	measurement	optometry—the professional practice of examining and measuring eye health and function

○ **Table 12-3. Suffixes** continued

Suffix	Meaning	Example Medical Term
-oma	tumor	sarcoma—a tumor of the connective tissue
-osis	condition or process, usually denoting an increase	necrosis—the death of cells, tissues, or an organ
-ostomy, -stomy	opening	colostomy—a surgical opening in the colon
-otomy, -tomy	incision, act of cutting	gastrotomy—incision into the stomach
-pathy	disease	osteopathy—any disease of the bone
-penia	deficiency	leukopenia—a condition with a deficient number of white blood cells
-phobia	extreme fear	acrophobia—irrational fear of heights
-plasty	surgical repair	rhinoplasty—plastic surgery of the nose
-plegia	paralysis	quadriplegia—paralysis of all four limbs
-rrhage, -rrhagia	abnormal flow or discharge	hemorrhage—abnormally heavy bleeding
-rrhea	rapid and abnormal flow	diarrhea—abnormally frequent and loose bowel movements
-scope	an instrument for examining or viewing	laparoscope—an instrument for viewing the abdominal cavity
-stasis	stopping, constant	homeostasis—a state of equilibrium in the body
-stat	something that stops	bacteriostat—an agent that inhibits bacterial growth
-stomy (see -ostomy)		
-tomy	a cutting, incision	laparotomy—incision in the abdominal wall
-uria	of the urine	pyuria—pus in the urine

Vital Skills (WRITING)

Using a Dictionary

This chapter is full of new words that you will need to learn in order to work in the health care setting. You will often need to use them when you write patient care notes. A good way to find out the meaning of unfamiliar words is to look them up in the dictionary. Some of these words may not be found in a regular dictionary. You may need to look in a medical dictionary. Your library should have a medical dictionary in its reference collection. Some dictionaries are also available online.

Different dictionaries might use slightly different formats, but usually you will see the word broken into syllables, followed by a symbol indicating what part of speech it is, a pronunciation guide, and the meaning or meanings of the word. The most commonly used meaning is listed first. If you have trouble understanding the pronunciation, look at the guide to common pronunciation symbols at the beginning of the dictionary.

For example, here is a typical entry for the noun *physician*:

phy·si·cian *n.* (fə-ˊzi-shən) **1** someone licensed to practice medicine **2** someone who heals or exerts a healing influence

> **Practice**
>
> Pick ten words from each table (Tables 12-1 through 12-4). Look the word up in a dictionary and note its meaning, pronunciation, and spelling. Then write a new sentence using the word.

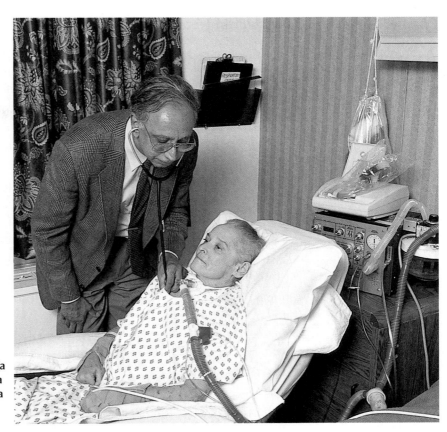

○ **Figure 12-3.** A specialist is a physician who concentrates on treating one body organ or system. Here, a pulmonologist (a lung specialist) examines a patient with a lung disorder in a subacute care unit of a nursing home.

Interpreting Medical Terms

Many of the medical words you will see and hear are very long. It may seem hard to understand them at first. However, you can learn to interpret words you do not recognize by following these steps.

1. First, break down the long words into a series of short word parts. If you see a word part that you do not recognize, look it up in a medical dictionary. For example, the word *cardiomyopathy* is made of these word parts:

    cardi(o) + *my(o)* + *-pathy*
    (meaning "heart") (meaning "muscle") (meaning "disease")

2. Then put the meanings of the word parts together to learn the meaning of the whole word.

Cardiomyopathy refers to a general diagnosis of heart muscle disease. The word parts were put together to make one word when this condition was first identified. The word *cardiologist* uses the same combining form, *cardi(o)*. A cardiologist is a doctor who specializes in treating heart disease. A pulmonologist specializes in treating lung disease. *Pulm(o)* and *pulmon(o)* mean "lung." **See Figure 12-3. Table 12-4** lists medical terms, their word parts, and their meanings.

○Table 12-4. Interpreting Medical Terms

Medical Term	Word Parts	Meaning
arteriosclerosis	arteri(o) + scler(o) + -osis (arteries) (hard) (condition)	a condition in which the arteries become hardened
bronchitis	bronch(o) + -itis (bronchus) (inflammation)	inflammation of the bronchial tubes
cystalgia	cyst + -algia (urinary bladder) (pain)	pain in the urinary bladder
dysmenorrhea	dys- + men(o) + rrhea (painful)(menstrual)(abnormal flow)	painful menstruation
erythrophobia	erythr(o) + -phobia (red) (fear of)	irrational fear of the color red (and sometimes of blood); morbid flushing
gastroenterology	gastr(o) + enter(o) + -logy (stomach) (intestines) (study of)	study of/treatment of the stomach and intestinal disorders
hepatectomy	hepat + -ectomy (liver) (removal of)	surgical removal of all or part of the liver
hydrocephalic	hydr(o) + cephal + -ic (water) (head) (pertaining to)	accumulation of water (fluid) in the skull
interpleural	inter- + pleural (between) (membrane surrounding the lungs)	between two layers of the pleura
mastectomy	mast- + -ectomy (breast) (removal of)	surgical removal of a breast
nephromegaly	nephr(o) + -megaly (kidney) (large)	enlargement of the kidney
orthodontics	orth(o) + odont(o) + -ics (correct) (teeth) (pertaining to)	the branch of dentistry concerned with correcting tooth irregularities and malocclusion
pathology	path(o) + -logy (disease) (study of)	study of the effects of disease on tissue and body fluids
rhinitis	rhin + -itis (nose) (inflammation of)	inflammation of the mucous membranes of the nose
thrombosis	thromb + -osis (clot) (condition)	formation or presence of a stationary blood clot within a blood vessel

Abbreviations and Symbols

Health care workers must communicate a great deal of information about patients. They read and write reports and notes in patient charts to keep everyone on the health care team informed. They often use abbreviations and symbols to save time and space.

Abbreviations

A shortened form of a word or phrase is called an **abbreviation**. An abbreviation may be just one letter, such as *C* for *Celsius*. It can be just a few letters, such as *in.*, which is short for *inch*. An **acronym** is an abbreviation made up of the first letters of each word in a phrase. For example, *ICU* is an acronym for *intensive care unit*. Some abbreviations have periods in them and others do not.

Some abbreviations seem to be completely unrelated to the original phrase. For example, *b.i.d.* means "twice a day." It is an abbreviation of the Latin phrase, *bis in die*, which means "twice a day."

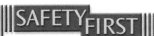

SAFETY FIRST

You may see some of the abbreviations on JCAHO's lists (p. 294) still in use in some health care facilities. Do not use those abbreviations! Doing so could cause confusion and affect the health and safety of your patients.

Vital Skills MATH

Determining Medication Times

In most states, nursing assistants do not give medications to patients. However, especially if you work in home health care, you should be familiar with the terminology used. You should be able to calculate when a medication should be taken based on the number of times per day it has been prescribed.

Example: Recall that b.i.d. means "twice a day." If the client takes the first daily dose at 0800, when should the second dose be taken?

Answer: There are 24 hours in a day, so divide 24 by 2 to get the number of hours between doses: $24 \div 2 = 12$. Then add 12 to the hour the first dose was taken to find out when the second dose should be taken: 12 + 0800 = 2000 hours, or 8:00 PM.

Practice

1. The abbreviation t.i.d. means "three times a day." If a medication is ordered t.i.d., and the patient takes the first dose at 0700 hours, when should the other doses be taken?
2. The abbreviation q.i.d. means "four times a day." If a medication is ordered q.i.d., and the patient takes the first dose at 0530 hours, when should the other doses be taken?

Abbreviations can be confusing. Some can be mistaken for other abbreviations. For example, *IU* (meaning "international unit") might look like *IV* (meaning "intravenous"). If chart notes or medication orders are written too quickly, abbreviations can be misinterpreted. Errors in prescribing a medication could be made that would endanger a patient. To prevent confusion, the Joint Commission for Accreditation of Healthcare Organizations (JCAHO) has created a "Do Not Use" list and an "Undesirable" list of abbreviations. They have also listed preferred terms. **See Figure 12-4.**

The abbreviations listed in **Table 12-5** are common ones you will probably encounter as a nursing assistant. They are the abbreviations most likely to appear on a patient's chart or in a doctor's note.

"Do Not Use" List		
Abbreviation	**Meaning**	**Preferred Term**
U	unit	unit
IU	international unit	international unit
Q.D.	daily	daily
Q.O.D.	every other day	every other day
MS	morphine sulfate	morphine sulfate
MSO4 or MgSO4	magnesium sulfate	magnesium sulfate

"Undesirable" List		
Abbreviation	**Meaning**	**Preferred Term**
μg	microgram	mcg
H.S.	half-strength or Latin abbreviation for bedtime	half-strength **OR** at bedtime
T.I.W.	three times a week	3 times weekly **OR** three times weekly
S.C. or S.Q.	subcutaneous	sub-Q **OR** subQ **OR** subcutaneously
D/C	discharge	discharge
c.c.	cubic centimeter	mL (for milliliters)
A.S., A.D., A.U.	Latin abbreviation for left, right, or both ears	left ear **OR** right ear **OR** both ears

○ **Figure 12-4.** JCAHO has created lists of abbreviations that should not be used because they cause confusion. You will use the preferred terms instead.

Table 12-5. Commonly Used Medical Abbreviations

Abbreviation	Meaning
$\overline{a}$	without
abd	abdomen
ABR	absolute bed rest
ac, a.c. (source: Latin, *ante cibum*)	before meals
ADLs	activities of daily living
adm, ADM, AD	admitting, admission
amb	ambulatory, able to walk
amt	amount
ARDS	adult respiratory distress syndrome
AZT	azidothymidine (an AIDS medication)
BaE, BE	barium enema
BB	bed bath
B&B	bladder and bowel retraining
b.i.d., bid, BID (source: Latin, *bis in die*)	twice a day
BM	bowel movement
BP	blood pressure *or* boiling point
br, BR, b.r., B.R.	bed rest
BRP	bathroom privileges
BSC	bedside commode
$\overline{c}$	with
C	Celsius
Ca	calcium
CA	cancer
cath	catheter
CBC	complete blood count
CBR	complete bed rest
c/o	complains of
CO_2	carbon dioxide
COLD	chronic obstructive lung disease
COPD	chronic obstructive pulmonary disease
CPR	cardiopulmonary resuscitation
CRD	chronic renal disease
C-section, CS	cesarean section
CVA	cerebrovascular accident, stroke
DNR	do not resuscitate
DOB	date of birth
drsg	dressing

○ **Table 12-5. Commonly Used Medical Abbreviations continued**

Abbreviation	Meaning
DX, Dx	diagnosis
EEG	electroencephalogram
ER	emergency room
F	Fahrenheit *or* female
FBS	fasting blood sugar
Fe	iron
fld	fluid
Fx, fx	fracture
g	gram
GI, G.I.	gastrointestinal
gt, gtt (source: Latin, *gutta*)	a drop (of a liquid)
GU	genitourinary
gyn	gynecology
h, hr, hr.	hour
HAV	hepatitis A virus
HBV	hepatitis B virus
HDL	high-density lipoprotein
HOB	head of bed
HS	at night (hour of sleep)
ht, ht.	height
Hx	history
I&O, I/O	intake and output
IM	intramuscular
irr	irregular
isol	isolation
IV	intravenous
L	liter *or* left
lb. (source: Latin, *libra*)	pound
LLQ	left lower quadrant
lt, L	left
LUQ	left upper quadrant
M	male
med, meds	medicine, medications
min	minute
mL	milliliter
mn, Mn	midnight
MRI	magnetic resonance imaging

○ Table 12-5. Commonly Used Medical Abbreviations continued

Abbreviation	Meaning
NG	nasogastric
NPO (source: Latin, *nil per os*)	nothing by mouth
O$_2$	oxygen
OB, O.B.	obstetrics
OD (source: Latin, *oculus dexter*)	right eye
OOB	out of bed
OR	operating room
OS (source: Latin, *oculus sinister*)	left eye
OT	occupational therapy/occupational therapist
OTC	over-the-counter (medication)
OU (source: Latin, *oculus uterque*, each eye)	both eyes
pc (source: Latin, *post cibum*)	after a meal
p.o. (source: Latin, *per os*)	by mouth
pos	positive
PPBS	postprandial (after meal) blood sugar
preop	preoperative
prep	preparation
prn, PRN, p.r.n. (source: Latin, *pro re nata*)	as necessary
pt	pint
Pt	patient
PT, P.T.	physical therapy/physical therapist
Px	physical exam
q (source: Latin, *quaque*)	every
qam (source: Latin, *quaque matin*)	every morning
qh (source: Latin, *quaque hora*)	every hour
q2h, q3h, etc.	every two hours, every three hours, etc.
q.i.d. (source: Latin, *quater in die*)	four times a day
qt, qt.	quart
R	rectal *or* right
RBC	red blood cell
RLQ	right lower quadrant
rt, R	right
RT	respiratory therapy/respiratory therapist
RUQ	right upper quadrant
Rx (source: Latin, *recipe*)	prescription
s̄ (source: Latin, *sine*)	without

○ **Table 12-5. Commonly Used Medical Abbreviations** continued

Abbreviation	Meaning
SOB	shortness of breath
spec	specimen
SSE	soap suds enema
stat (source: Latin, *statim*)	immediately
STD	sexually transmitted disease
Surg	surgery
T, temp	temperature
tbsp	tablespoon
tid, TID, t.i.d. (source: Latin, *ter in die*)	three times a day
TPR	temperature, pulse, and respiration
tsp	teaspoon
TWE	tap water enema
Tx	treatment
U/A, u/a	urinalysis
VS, v.s.	vital signs
WBC, W.B.C.	white blood count
w/c, W/C	wheelchair
wt.	weight

FOCUS ON

Patient Care

You must understand medical terms, abbreviations, and symbols in order to give proper care. For example, if a patient is to receive a certain kind of enema and is given another, the patient may be harmed. If a patient exercises more or less than ordered, the patient may suffer. Always check and recheck written orders and ask questions when in doubt. **See Figure 12-5.**

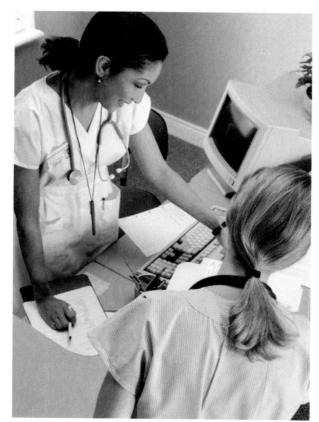

○ **Figure 12-5.** If you cannot understand the written order, ask your supervisor.

Symbols

A **symbol** is a written or printed sign that has meaning. **See Figure 12-6.** Some symbols have universal meaning and are used around the world. Even if people do not speak each other's languages, they usually understand the meaning of certain international symbols, such as @ for *at*. **Table 12-6** shows some symbols that are commonly used in health care.

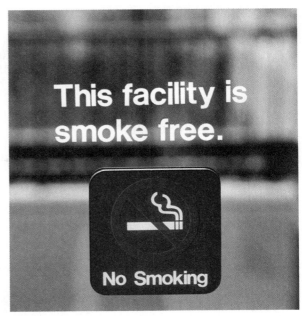

○ **Figure 12-6.** The "no-smoking" symbol, found on almost all medical facilities, is universally understood.

○ **Table 12-6. Commonly Used Medical Symbols**

Symbol	Meaning
@	at
°	degrees
+	plus, positive
−	minus, negative
+/−	plus or minus
×	times
*	important
Ø	zero, nothing
Δ	change to
>	greater than
≥	greater than or equal to
<	less than
≤	less than or equal to
↑	up, increase
↓	down, decrease
☠	poisonous
🚭	no smoking

Chapter Summary

- Medical terminology is the special language used in health care.

- Most medical terms are made up of several word parts, including root words, combining forms, prefixes, and suffixes.

- Most medical terms can be interpreted by breaking them into their word parts.

- Abbreviations and symbols are shortened forms of words or phrases that are widely used in medical terminology.

VOCABULARY REVIEW

Directions: Match the letter of each definition in the second column with the correct vocabulary term, word part, or abbreviation in the first column. Write your answers on a separate sheet of paper.

Vocabulary

1. abbreviation
2. ac
3. acronym
4. BM
5. brady-
6. combining form
7. enter(o)
8. HOB
9. HS
10. -oma
11. prefix
12. root word
13. suffix
14. symbol
15. u/a

Definitions

A. A word part plus a vowel to make the word easier to pronounce
B. Intestines
C. Urinalysis
D. A word part that comes after a root word or a combining form and modifies its meaning
E. At night
F. The basic part of a word that gives the word meaning
G. A shortened form of a word or phrase
H. Slow
I. Before meals
J. Bowel movement
K. A written or printed sign that has meaning
L. An abbreviation made up of the first letters of each word in a phrase
M. Head of the bed
N. Tumor
O. A word part that comes before a root word or a combining form and modifies its meaning

Check Your Knowledge

Review Questions: Answer each of the following questions on a separate sheet of paper.

1. What is a compound word? Give an example.

2. Name the four basic word parts used in medical terminology.

3. What is the combining form meaning "liver"?

4. Define the suffix *-logy*. Give an example of a word ending in *-logy*.

5. Define the word parts that make up the word *tracheotomy*.

6. What is a tracheoscopy?

7. What is a gynecologist?

8. What are JCAHO's "Do Not Use" and "Undesirable" lists?

9. Translate the following abbreviations: Pt c/o UGI pain.

10. What does the symbol @ mean?

True or False: Read each statement carefully. Then write *True* or *False* by the statement number on a separate sheet of paper.

1. *Neur(o)* is an example of a suffix.

2. The suffix *-scopy* means the use of a viewing instrument.

3. A medical term ending in *-osis* usually means that the patient has a tumor.

4. A gastroenterologist is a doctor who treats diseases of the stomach and intestines.

5. The symbol Δ means "change."

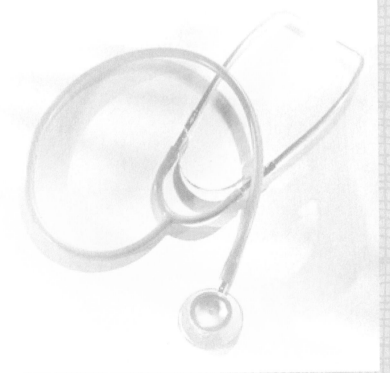

Think and Decide

Directions: Think about each of the following scenarios. Answer each question on a separate sheet of paper.

1. The charge nurse writes instructions for you prior to leaving the unit for a lunch break. She writes, "Assist Mr. B. with his ADLs and check V.S. a.c." What does this mean to you?

2. If a patient is allowed to get OOB, is he on B.R.? Explain.

3. You are reading your daily assignment. Mrs. S. cannot have a blood pressure check done in one of her arms. The abbreviation is unclear. You cannot tell whether the assignment says, "take the patient's BP only on the R" or "take the patient's BP only on the L." What should you do?

4. Mrs. J. was diagnosed last week with severe salpingitis and has been admitted to the hospital today for a salpingectomy. What is wrong with Mrs. J.? What type of operation will she have?

5. Mr. P., an 84-year-old resident in your care, is telling you about a recent visit from his physician. Mr. P. thinks the physician said that his hearing is failing, and he wants Mr. P. to see a specialist called an *andensologist*. Mr. P. misunderstood his physician (or didn't hear him correctly). What specialist is Mr. P. most likely to need to check his hearing?

6. Mrs. W. is a 72-year-old resident in your care. She has had trouble with urinary tract infections off and on for the last year. Today, her doctor diagnosed pyelonephritis. What does this mean? Look up the term in the dictionary. Given her history of urinary infections, does the diagnosis of pyelonephritis surprise you? Explain.

7. R. Pickens, one of your patients in ICU, is recovering from her surgery yesterday to remove a colorectal carcinoma. Specifically, what was wrong with Ms. Pickens? What did the surgeon remove?

8. Mr. H., a long-term care patient, tells you that his doctor told the nurse to "Get the phlebotomy tech in here to draw some samples." Mr. H. is nervous. He doesn't know what phlebotomy means, but he thinks it sounds like a major operation. Based on your knowledge of medical terminology, what can you tell Mr. H.?

9. Mrs. V., a long-term care resident who has throat cancer, can no longer take oral medications. Her doctor has prescribed medications that can be absorbed transdermally. How will she receive her medications?

CNA Certification Exam Prep

Directions: This practice test contains ten questions. Each question has four suggested answers. For each question, choose the ONE that best answers the question or completes the statement. Write your answers on a separate sheet of paper.

1. What does the medical term *dermatitis* mean?
   A. cell inflammation
   B. skin inflammation
   C. bladder inflammation
   D. eye inflammation

2. The medical term *cephalomegaly* means
   A. enlarged heart.
   B. enlarged head.
   C. smaller-than-normal heart.
   D. smaller-than-normal head.

3. A patient has a hematoma, which is a(n)
   A. liver tumor.
   B. mass of blood.
   C. mass of tissues.
   D. abnormal tumor.

4. It is important to use correct spelling of medical terms so that
   A. patients will understand what you mean.
   B. you can prevent misunderstandings that might harm a patient.
   C. family members become familiar with important terms.
   D. you can demonstrate how smart you are.

5. A word part that is placed before a root word to change its meaning is a
   A. suffix.
   B. adjective.
   C. pronoun.
   D. prefix.

6. Which of the following is the abbreviation for "every hour"?
   A. qh
   B. q.i.d.
   C. hs
   D. ht

7. The basic parts of words used in medical terminology are
   A. medials, lateral words, root words, and suffixes.
   B. distals, compound words, suffixes, and root words.
   C. prefixes, suffixes, root words, and combining forms.
   D. root words, combining forms, saggital forms, and suffixes.

8. A patient diagnosed with "Fx R tibia" has
   A. fluid buildup in the right eardrum.
   B. a fractured right tibia.
   C. a fractured rear tympanic membrane.
   D. iron deficiency.

9. The abbreviation for "intake and output" is
   A. I/O
   B. IAO
   C. IPT
   D. IOT

10. Your supervisor asks you to perform a procedure stat. You should perform it
    A. this afternoon.
    B. tomorrow.
    C. at 3:00 PM.
    D. immediately.

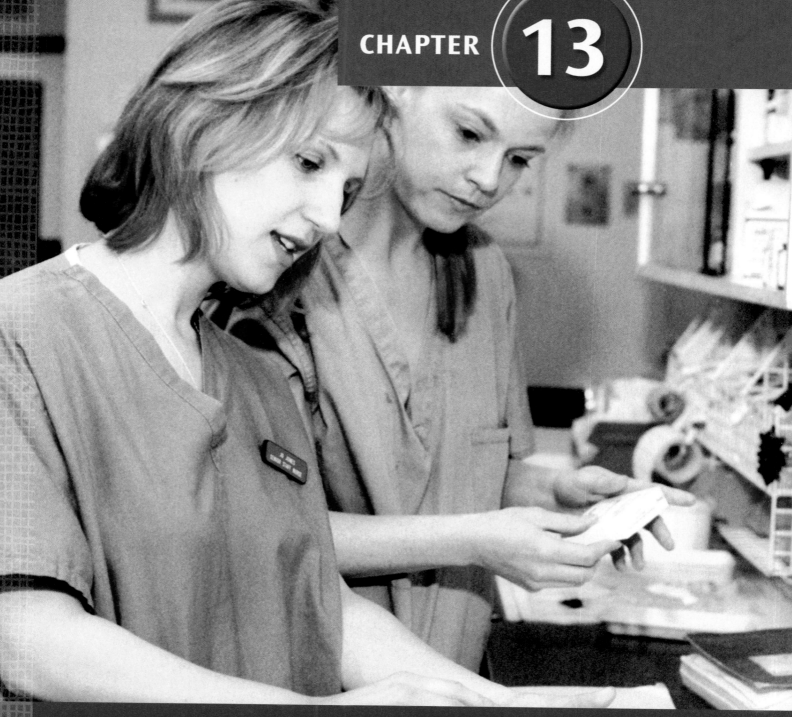

CHAPTER 13

OBJECTIVES

- Describe the sender-receiver communication model.
- Explain the difference between verbal and nonverbal communication.
- List guidelines for effective communication.
- Identify common barriers to effective communication.

- Identify ways to communicate effectively with patients.
- Identify the purposes of communication with members of the health care team.
- Describe the technologies used for communication in the health care setting.

- Explain how a nursing assistant observes patients.
- Explain how a nursing assistant reports observations.
- Identify methods of recording information about patients.

Observing, Reporting, and Recording

VOCABULARY

active listening A listening technique that consists of restatement, reflection, and clarification.

body language All of the mannerisms and gestures used in communication.

call signal A one-way communication device that must be kept within the patient's easy reach. The signal goes off at a main terminal.

charting The process of writing down the observations you make and the treatments and procedures you perform.

communication The exchange of information.

data Information entered and stored in a computer.

feedback The response to a communication message.

flow sheet A chart in the medical record used to record different types of data.

graphic chart A chart in the medical record used to record observations and measurements.

intercom A two-way device in a patient's room that permits patients to talk and to listen to a health care worker at a main terminal.

log-in The unique ID a person uses to access a secure computer system.

medical record A written or computerized record documenting a patient's care, condition, treatment, and response to treatment.

medium The way or means in which information is sent or received.

message The information a sender wants to convey.

nonverbal communication All forms of communication except words.

nurses' notes Nurses' written documentation about a patient's condition.

nursing care plan A document that details the care required for a patient. Nursing care plans are developed by the health care team and coordinated by a nurse.

objective information Information you collect about a patient using your senses.

observation Something that you can see, hear, smell, or touch that provides information about a patient, such as a physical change or a change in behavior.

password A secret code made up of letters, numbers, and/or symbols, used to access a secure computer system.

receiver The person who receives a communication message.

recording The process of writing down the observations you make and the treatments and procedures you perform.

reporting The process of describing observations and care given.

sender The person who sends a communication message.

sign Something about a patient that you can see, hear, feel, or smell.

subjective information Information the patient tells you.

symptom Something the patient tells you that he or she feels.

verbal communication Communication through the use of words.

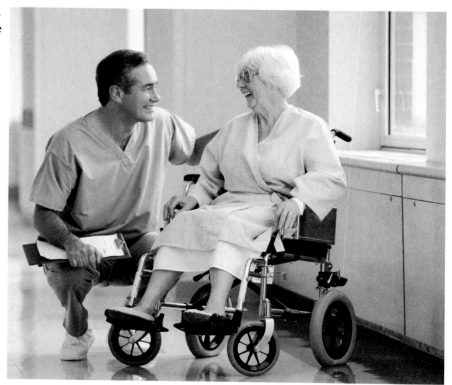

○ **Figure 13-1.** As a nursing assistant, you want to communicate information to your patient.

Communication

In the health care setting, communication is important. To provide the best care for patients, the health care team must be able to communicate effectively with each other and with patients and their family members.

Communication is the exchange of information. The process works like this.

1. A **sender** creates a **message**, which is the information the sender wants to convey.
2. The sender sends the message (by talking or writing, for example).
3. A **receiver** receives the message (by listening or reading, for example).
4. The receiver interprets, or understands, the message.
5. The receiver responds to the message. This response is called **feedback**. It lets the sender know that the message was received and understood. In some cases, feedback lets the sender know that the message was not understood. Then the sender can try again.

The **medium** is the way the information is sent or received. In **Figure 13-1**, speaking is the medium used by the sender. Listening is the medium used by the receiver.

There are two types of communication: verbal and nonverbal. **Verbal communication** is communication through the use of words. The words can be spoken or written. When the sender speaks the words, the receiver listens. When the sender writes the words, the receiver reads them. **See Figure 13-2.**

Nonverbal communication includes all forms of communication except words. Sounds, such as laughing, crying, sighing, and moaning, are examples of nonverbal communication. **Body language**—mannerisms and gestures—is also a form of nonverbal communication. It includes appearance, facial expressions, eye contact, posture, movement, and touch.

Guidelines for Effective Communication

Just speaking does not guarantee communication. If your listener does not understand your meaning, there is no communication. If you do not pay attention when someone else is speaking, there is no communication. If your verbal communication does not send the same meaning as your nonverbal communication, the receiver will not understand you.

Your communication on the job should always be straightforward, understandable, accurate, and timely. The following guidelines will help make sure that you communicate successfully.

Speaking. Follow these guidelines to develop effective speaking skills.

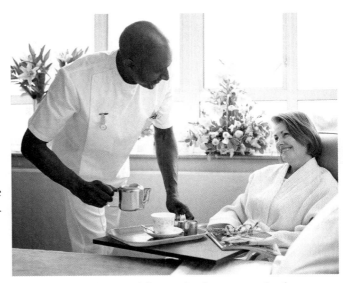

○ **Figure 13-2.** Enjoying a joke together is one example of verbal communication.

- Be courteous and respectful. Never use slang or vulgar words.
- Speak clearly.
- Control your voice volume. Do not speak too loudly, but make sure your listener can hear you.
- Maintain eye contact with your listener.
- Ask open-ended questions to encourage feedback from your listener and to make sure you understand—or have been understood—correctly. These questions cannot be answered by a simple yes or no. Closed-ended questions can be answered by a yes or no, and may not show that your listener understands. Imagine this situation: You have told your home health care client that there will be a change in the next day's routine. You want to make sure the client understands you.

  Closed-ended question: "Do you know what you are going to do tomorrow?" The client can say yes or no, even if he does not understand the plan for the next day.

  Open-ended question: "What are you going to do tomorrow?" The client must explain the new routine. Then you will know if he understands.

Listening. There is a difference between hearing and listening. Listening means understanding what you hear and then giving feedback. **See Figure 13-3.** Whether you are listening to patients or to instructions, requests, or other information, use the following listening techniques.

- Give full attention to the speaker.
- Listen carefully to what is being said.
- Do not interrupt while someone is speaking. Let the speaker finish before you respond.

Active listening is a listening technique that consists of restatement, reflection, and clarification.

- *Restatement* is repeating what the speaker said using different words.
- *Reflection* is thinking about what the speaker has said and then expressing your thoughts about the message. When you reflect, you consider the speaker's words and feelings.

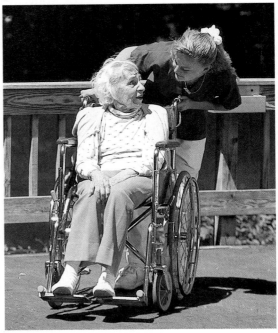

○ **Figure 13-3.** Listening is an important part of communication.

- *Clarification* is asking questions to make sure you understand what was said. Clarifying allows you to summarize the speaker's message.

Being Consistent. The sender's verbal and nonverbal messages should always communicate the same information. Otherwise, the receiver might be confused. For example, when you ask a patient how he is feeling, make eye contact and direct all your attention toward him. In this way, your nonverbal message expresses interest and attentiveness.

If you ask the patient how he is feeling and then tap your foot and look away from him, you are giving a mixed message. Your words express interest, but your body language does not. You are indicating nonverbally that you are impatient and have no interest in the patient.

Writing. Sometimes you will need to communicate in writing to patients. For example, a home care worker might need to write instructions for a client who has trouble remembering. Before you use written communication, however, be sure that the person receiving the message can read it. Some people cannot read, cannot understand English, or may have a vision impairment. Talk with the client or family members first to find out about these potential challenges.

Communicating with Patients

Many people who enter a health care facility are anxious and frightened. They are away from home in an unfamiliar place. They are worried about their health, especially if they are facing a serious illness or major surgery. They may be worried about how they are going to pay their medical bills or about how their family will manage without them. You can help ease patients' concerns, show sensitivity, and establish trust by using these communication techniques.

- Introduce yourself. In the health care setting, patients meet many people who take care of them. It is common courtesy to tell the patient your name and title each time you enter the room.
- Use words the patient understands. If you must use medical terms, clearly explain what they mean if the patient does not understand them.
- Use active listening techniques. Patients who are nervous or worried often feel better when they have someone to talk to. You can be that person. Listen attentively to a patient to show your interest and concern. Be sure to maintain eye contact and express empathy when appropriate.
- "Listen" also to the patient's nonverbal messages. If a patient says she feels fine but constantly rubs her shoulder, the verbal and nonverbal messages do not match. Ask a question for clarification: "I notice you keep rubbing your shoulder. Is anything bothering you?"
- Ask the patient for feedback by using open-ended questions. Remember to listen and focus on the patient's feedback. If your message has not been understood, you may have to say it in a different way.
- Touch the patient's arm gently when speaking or listening. A caring touch is a form of nonverbal communication. **See Figure 13-4.** Note that touch can be a culturally sensitive area. Touch should be discussed with the person, family, and coworkers.
- Let your patients know you care just by being there. Sometimes patients do not want you to respond. They want you to just listen.

- At times you may provide care for a person who has a condition that causes strong, disagreeable odors. To avoid making that person feel rejected, keep your face calm and your expression even.

Avoiding Barriers to Effective Communication

Some commonly used phrases are actually barriers to communication. They can make communication unsuccessful. Try to avoid the following when you care for patients.

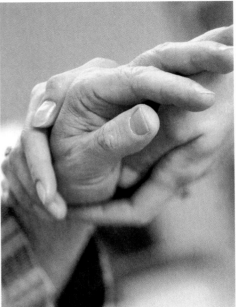

○ **Figure 13-4.** A concerned look and a touch of the hand communicate caring without words. This is an example of nonverbal communication.

- **Asking "why" questions.** When you ask *why*, a patient may feel put on the spot or threatened. It appears to be a type of open-ended question, but it can be hard to answer—we do not always know why. For example, if a patient is not eating, do not ask, "Why don't you eat the food I brought you?" Instead, you might say, "You usually enjoy your meals. Perhaps you aren't hungry today?" This would encourage the patient to think about and explain the reasons for not eating.
- **Using pat answers or clichés.** Pat answers and clichés are expressions that are overused and have become almost meaningless. People repeat them without thought. Responding to patients in this way may make them feel that you are not really paying attention to them. For example, suppose your patient expresses fear about a procedure. If you say, "Don't worry, everybody goes through this," your patient might feel that you are not focusing on him or her as an individual. Instead of relying on these phrases, you can encourage the patient to express feelings by saying, "Tell me what concerns you."
- **Being judgmental, expressing opinions, or giving advice.** Do not make judgments or express your opinions about the patient or patient's situation. If you do, the patient might feel reluctant to talk to you about problems or feelings. If the patient asks for advice, refer the questions to the supervisor or nurse.
- **Avoiding topics patients want to discuss.** When you change a topic to avoid listening to something a patient wants to discuss, the patient cannot express concerns or fears. Part of your job is to talk with and listen to those in your care, even though you may feel uncomfortable. Let the patient bring up or change subjects, rather than leading the conversation yourself.
- **Gossiping about patients or coworkers.** When you communicate with others, patients need to be certain that the information exchanged is kept confidential. Otherwise, they will be reluctant to confide in you.

Adapting Communication to Fit Patient Needs

You will care for patients who have visual, hearing, or speech impairment, or who cannot speak English. Very young children in your care may not be able to tell you how they feel in words. Patients and family members with different cultural backgrounds may use different words to express themselves. Some may use different body language than you are used to. Try to understand these special situations and think of other ways to communicate. In many cases, the patient's care or treatment plan will include specific guidelines for communicating with the patient.

Patients with Visual Deficiency. Patients may have visual impairment caused by a disease such as diabetes. Elderly people may have blurred vision because of cataracts, a condition that causes gradual loss of vision as the eye lens becomes clouded over. These people may be totally or partially blind.

- Do not alarm the patient by entering or leaving the room quickly. Instead, knock on the door and say hello, introducing yourself right away. Say good-bye when you leave.
- Speak in a normal tone of voice.
- Tell the patient what you are going to do. If you are helping a patient at mealtime, for example, you could say, "We are going to the dining room now. Let's start down the hall."
- Explain what is happening. For example, if a visitor arrives, you can help by saying, "Mrs. Lowery, your friend Mrs. Chan is here to visit." On a walk outdoors, describe the flowers you see and perhaps allow the patient to smell them. **See Figure 13-5.**

Patients with Hearing Deficiency. Hearing loss may be complete or partial. Some patients may use a hearing aid. Some may have hearing in one ear only.

- Approach from the front, so you do not surprise the patient.
- Face the patient when speaking.
- Use body language and facial expressions to make your meaning clear.
- Reduce or eliminate background noise.
- Speak slowly and clearly, without shouting, and use short sentences.
- Some people are able to lip-read, so do not cover your mouth when you speak.
- If necessary, write a message or draw a picture.

Patients with Speech Deficiency. The ability to speak or understand speech can be impaired by a stroke or brain damage.

- Face the patient when speaking.
- Speak slowly and clearly. Use short sentences.
- If the patient has trouble speaking, you may provide writing equipment or electronic speaking aids to help communicate.

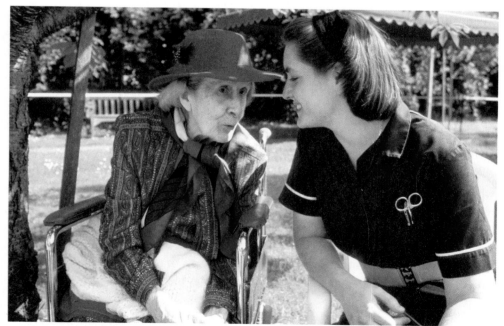

○ **Figure 13-5.** On an outing with a patient with visual impairment, describe the view.

Non-English Speakers. If a patient does not speak English, you may need to adapt your method of communicating.

- Sometimes, a family member or friend can interpret for you.
- Some health care facilities employ interpreters.
- If an interpreter is not available, you may use gestures and other body language, as well as pictures. For example, you might point to an object so the patient can understand what you are saying.

Children. Very young children may not be able to communicate in words, so try to understand their nonverbal messages. If they are crying, try to figure out why. They may need a diaper change or they may be hungry. If they do not need physical care, comfort them by gently touching or hugging them. They may be unhappy and frightened in the health care setting. Call the child by name or nickname. It may be appropriate to encourage family members to help care for the child.

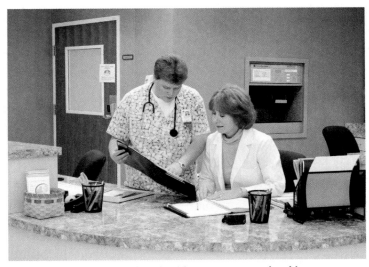

○ **Figure 13-6.** Members of the health care team must be able to communicate patient information clearly and accurately.

Communicating with Members of the Health Care Team

To provide the best care, members of the health care team share the following information about patients. **See Figure 13-6.**

- The patient's current condition and treatment
- What has been done for the patient as part of the plan of care
- What needs to be done for the patient
- The patient's response to treatment

When communicating with other team members about a patient's condition, use precise language. Avoid words that have more than one meaning. For example, do not say, "Mr. Kelly has a small sore on his back." "Small" could mean 1 inch to one person and ¼ inch to someone else.

Using Technology to Communicate

In addition to talking directly with health care team members and with people in your care, you will communicate using intercoms and call signals, telephones, fax machines, and e-mail. You will use computers to communicate and store information about patients. When used properly, these technologies enhance the efficiency of the health care facility.

Intercoms and Call Signals. An **intercom** is a two-way device in a patient's room that permits patients to talk and to listen to a health care worker at a main terminal. Patients often use intercoms to ask for assistance.

Patients who must remain in bed or a chair use a **call signal**. This is a one-way communication device that must be kept within the patient's easy reach. **See Figure 13-7.** When a patient presses or pulls

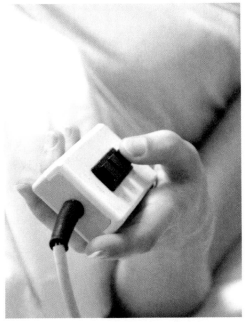

○ **Figure 13-7.** The call signal should be within easy reach, so the patient can communicate with staff when necessary.

the call signal, a bell sounds or a light flashes at the main terminal. To respond, go to the patient's room and ask how you can help. Answer the call bell as soon as possible, but make sure it is answered within 3 to 5 minutes. Then press the "cancel" button on the unit to turn off the call signal. This lets the health care team know that the patient is being looked after.

Respond to patient's requests at once. Regularly check on children and adults who are confined to bed—at least every 2 hours—since they may not be able to use the call signal or intercom.

Telephones. You may have to answer the phone in a patient's or resident's room, a client's home, or at the nurses' station. Always be professional and courteous when using the telephone. **See Figure 13-8.** Follow facility procedure for answering the telephone. Here are some general rules.
- Answer the call on the first ring if possible, and always by the fourth ring.
- Answer the phone in a calm manner, and speak slowly enough to be understood.
- Use a pleasant tone of voice.
- Give a courteous greeting. Give your name, title, and department.
- When taking a message, record the following:
  - The caller's name and telephone number
  - Date and time
  - Message and whether the person should call back
- Repeat the message and phone number to verify.
- If you must put the person on hold, ask the caller for permission. Before putting the caller on hold, get the name and telephone number. Place the person on hold. Check back if the person has remained on hold for 30 seconds. Never put a person on hold if it is an emergency call.
- Never lay the phone down or cover the receiver with your hand while you are talking. The caller could overhear confidential information.
- In all cases, observe patients' rights for confidential handling of information about them and their care. Avoid repeating what you know or think about patients on the phone.
- End the conversation politely, thank the person for calling, and say good-bye.
- Give all messages to the person intended.

Fax Machines. Health care facilities use fax machines to send print documents for doctors' signatures, to verify information, or to send orders between departments. Pharmacies also fax information to nursing facilities. Most documents that are faxed contain confidential information. Be very careful when entering the fax number, so you do not send the fax to a wrong number. Here is the usual procedure for sending a fax.
1. Place the document in the fax machine.
2. Enter the fax number on the keypad. Fax machines use telephone lines, and fax numbers are like telephone numbers.
3. Push the "start" button. The paper then feeds through the machine.

Computers. Most health care facilities use computers for several purposes:
- To record and store information about patients. This information, or **data**, can be quickly and easily retrieved as needed.
- To send messages and reports to the nursing unit and other departments. Sharing patient information in this way saves time and ensures accuracy. This increases the quality and safety of care.

- To monitor measurements such as blood pressure, temperature, heart rate, and heart function. If an abnormal reading occurs, an alarm alerts the nursing staff. This type of computer is used in the specialty units of a hospital, such as ICU.

You may use e-mail to communicate with other members of the health care team. Follow these etiquette tips when using e-mail:
- Be professional and courteous, just as when you are talking on the phone. Do not write anything in an e-mail that you wouldn't want someone else, such as your supervisor, to read.
- Fill in the subject line to let the receiver know what the e-mail is about.
- Be concise and to the point.
- Do not open another person's e-mail or message.

The computers in the workplace are to be used for work only. Your employer has the right to monitor computer use within the workplace. Do not send personal e-mail or messages. Remember that any communication can be read by someone other than the intended receiver. Even deleted messages can be retrieved by authorized personnel.

Observing

As a nursing assistant, you will spend more time with patients than other members of the health care team. An important part of your job will be making observations about your patients' condition. An **observation** is something that you notice about a patient, such as a physical change or a change in behavior. Observations are made up of objective and subjective information.

Objective information is the information you collect about a patient using your senses. This includes signs. A **sign** is something about a patient that you can see, hear, feel, or smell. For example, when a patient wheezes, you use your sense of hearing to observe the wheezing. The wheeze is a sign that gives you objective information. Objective information can also be measured. When you measure vital signs, such as blood pressure and heart rate, you are collecting objective information.

Vital Skills (READING)

Objective vs. Subjective Information

When you are caring for a patient, you will need to share information about that patient with other members of the health care team. The information you share may be objective or subjective.

Practice

The paragraphs below describe a nursing assistant's interaction with a patient. Read the paragraphs and determine what information is important. What information should Anna include in her report? Which items are objective? Which are subjective?

Anna, the nursing assistant, entered Mr. Johnson's room at 8:35 AM on Wednesday. Mr. Johnson was in bed. He was awake and said "hello" to Anna when she entered the room. Anna drained the urine from the collection bag on his Foley catheter into a cylinder so she could measure it. She measured 190 milliliters of clear, yellow urine.

Mr. Johnson said he was in pain and that he "didn't sleep all night." He rates his pain as 7 out of 10. He asked Anna to lower the blinds. Anna observed that he seemed to be in a bad mood. She noticed that his breakfast was still on his tray—he hadn't eaten any of it. She checked his vital signs: temperature 98.8°F; blood pressure 168/110; respirations 17; pulse 68. Anna told Mr. Johnson's nurse about his pain and the nurse gave him his PRN pain medication.

Anna changed his sheets and helped him with a bed bath. She noticed that the incision from his recent abdominal surgery looked red and was oozing a yellowish-white pus.

Subjective information is the information the patient tells you. You cannot observe it yourself. This includes symptoms. A **symptom** is something the patient tells you that he or she feels. When a patient says "I have a pain in my right leg," you are getting subjective information. You cannot see, hear, feel, or smell the pain. You are relying on information given to you by someone else. Subjective information cannot be measured.

To recognize unusual signs and symptoms, you must first be able to recognize normal body appearance and functioning. (The structure and functions of a healthy body are discussed in Chapters 9 and 10.) To do your job effectively, you also need to know about diseases and injuries. For example, if a patient has diabetes, it is important to recognize the signs and symptoms of hyperglycemia, hypoglycemia, and insulin shock. If a patient has a wound, it is important to know the signs of infection. **Figure 13-9** lists some basic questions you can ask yourself to get started observing patients. Your observations should be as complete as possible. For example, when observing whether a patient is mobile, record your observation in detail: Can the patient stand without assistance? Can the patient walk with or without a walker?

When observing your patients, pay close attention to anything that seems unusual. For example, you might see that a patient's skin looks yellowish. You might hear a change in the sound of a patient's cough. You might smell a strange odor. You might notice that an area of skin feels hot.

Guidelines for Observing Patients

Senses

How well can the patient see objects close by? At a distance?
Is the patient able to hear when you speak in a normal tone of voice?
Can the patient smell strong odor?
Can the patient sense temperature accurately?
Does the patient complain of food or beverages not tasting right?

Responses

Is the patient awake and alert?
Is the patient calm or restless?
Is the patient aware of people, place, and time?
Can the patient speak clearly?
Can the patient follow instructions?
What is the patient's emotional state? (Does the patient appear happy, worried, withdrawn?)

Activities of Daily Living

How much personal care can the patient perform without help?
Can the patient eat without assistance?
Can the patient use the toilet, bedpan, urinal, or commode?
With what level of assistance?

Appetite

How is the patient's appetite?
How much of the food served does the patient eat (at all three meals)?
Does the patient eat between meals?
How often does the patient drink fluids?
How much fluid does the patient drink?
Does the patient complain of nausea?
Is the patient gaining or losing weight?

Respiration (Assess the patient's breathing by watching the chest go up and down, listening to the sounds.)

What is the breathing rate?
Does the patient have difficulty breathing?
Are there any noises when the patient inhales or exhales?
If the patient has a cough, is it dry or does it produce mucus?
What is the quantity and color of the sputum?

Pain or Discomfort (Remember that pain is individualized—it does not mean the same thing to all people.)

Where is the pain or discomfort?
How long has the patient been experiencing pain or discomfort?
How long does the pain or discomfort last?
Ask the patient to describe the pain (sharp or dull, throbbing or stabbing, etc.).
How does the patient rate the pain on a scale from 1 to 10, with 10 being the greatest pain?
What medication, if any, has been given to relieve the pain or discomfort?
Has the medication helped?
Is the pain or discomfort interfering with sleep?

Elimination

Does the patient have difficulty urinating?
Does the patient complain of burning or soreness when urinating?
How much urine is passed?
What color is the urine?
How often does the patient urinate?
Does the patient complain of gas?
How often does the patient have bowel movements?
Is there any bleeding with bowel movements?

Skin (Assess the skin by looking and a gentle touch. Bath time is a good time to assess the skin.)

What color does the skin appear to be (pale, yellowish, gray, flushed, etc.)?
Is the skin dry or moist?
Is the skin hot, cold, or warm?
Are there any abnormalities on the skin (rashes, sores, bruises, etc.)?

Movement

How well does the patient walk? With or without assistance?
Is the patient able to move all parts of the body?
Is the patient able to get out of bed without assistance? Sit up in bed?

○ **Figure 13-9.** Ask yourself these questions as you observe your patients while providing daily care.

Listen carefully to what your patients tell you about how they feel. Observe changes you see in their behavior or body language. For instance, a patient who usually sits up when you knock and enter the room may not do so one morning. This may be a sign to you that the patient is tired, not feeling well, or depressed. **See Figure 13-10.** In this case, you can ask the patient to describe how he or she is feeling to get more information. You will then have objective and subjective information.

All observations, objective and subjective, should be recorded and communicated to other members of the health care team. Many nursing assistants carry a notebook or pad of paper to jot down observations as they make them. **See Figure 13-11.** Later, when reporting to other members of the health care team, they can refer to these notes to refresh their memories.

A **nursing care plan** is a document written and developed by the health care team and coordinated by a nurse. It details the care required for a patient. Each patient has a unique care plan. The nurse usually gets input from other members of the health care team. The care plan includes goals for the patient to meet. It also includes physical needs, specific medical treatments (such as dressing changes) and the frequency of such treatments, and long-term discharge plans, if applicable. The plan is used to communicate the patient's needs and goals to the health care team. Care plans are continually updated as the patient's condition changes. Care plan formats vary from facility to facility. Some are written as short essays. Others are completed forms.

Nurses use care plans to assign patient care tasks to members of the health care team. As a nursing assistant, you must read and be thoroughly familiar with the care plans for each of your patients. Your role in implementing the care plan may include:

• Observing the patient.
• Providing specific care as outlined in the care plan.
• Reporting on the patient's progress and response to treatment.

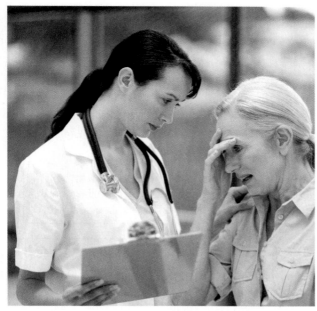

O **Figure 13-10.** The nursing assistant observes the way the resident is turning away and not looking at her. This is a type of body language communication.

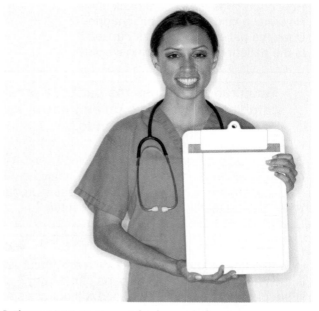

O **Figure 13-11.** Carry a notebook or pad of paper so you can write down what care you provide for each resident.

Reporting

Reporting is the process of describing your observations and the care you give. You report your observations so that nurses and other health care team members can stay up-to-date on the care and condition of the patient. Reports must always be accurate and thorough.

The frequency of observation and reporting varies from facility to facility. At a minimum, reports are given at shift change, when they are requested by the nurses, and when a change in a patient's condition is observed. In a hospital setting, reports are given at the end of one shift to the team beginning the next shift. The *end-of-shift report* ensures that the incoming team is up-to-date on the patient's condition. **See Figure 13-12.** The report also includes information about treatment, procedures, and reportable events that have taken place during the shift that is ending. A *reportable event* is anything that happens during the shift that is out of the ordinary and may affect patient care. Most states have specific guidelines for events that are considered reportable. In long-term care facilities, such as nursing homes, reporting may be done on a weekly or monthly basis, depending on the resident's condition.

Some nursing assistants tape-record their reports. When reports are given by one health care team member to another orally, there is less patient coverage. One person is delivering the report, and at least one other person is listening to the report. With tape-recorded reports, two people do not need to be present to exchange information. This ensures that someone is providing patient coverage during the reporting period. However, it can be more difficult to find a specific fact in a taped report. You must sometimes listen to the entire report to find the information you need.

When taping your report, limit it to vital information, abnormal findings, and patient responses. If you have any questions after listening to another person's report, ask the person who taped the summary for clarification.

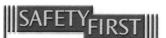

SAFETY FIRST

Communication is more accurate with the 24-hour clock. If someone forgets to write "AM" or "PM" when using conventional clock time, a serious error could result. The time noted could be misinterpreted. The patient could be harmed.

		STATS				7-3	3-11	11-7
		Admission	Medical Leave of Absence Return	Discharge	Critical			
	7-3				Serious			
	3-11				Oxygen			
Date: _____ Unit: _____	11-7				Catheter			
					Reportable Event			

Resident's Name	New Order/Change of Condition	7-3	3-11	11-7

Open Areas				
Bowel/Bladder Management				
		❑ Doctor's orders checked	❑ Doctor's orders checked	❑ Doctor's orders checked
		❑ Chargeable items accounted for	❑ Chargeable items accounted for	❑ Chargeable items accounted for
		❑ Narcotics count correct	❑ Narcotics count correct	❑ Narcotics count correct

Signature _____

○ **Figure 13-12.** An end-of-shift report ensures a smooth transition in the care given to patients or residents after a shift change.

Vital Skills (COMMUNICATION)

End-of-Shift Report

The end-of-shift report is a way to make sure that the incoming team is up-to-date. The report includes information about treatments and procedures that have taken place during the shift that is ending. The report may also alert the arriving shift to upcoming tests or procedures for which they might need to prepare the patient.

Practice

Read the patient care scenario below and decide what information you would include in your end-of-shift report. Use a tape recorder to record the report you would give.

Tammy is the night nursing assistant for Mrs. Templeton. Mrs. Templeton did not sleep very well last night. She got up to void at 1:00 AM and couldn't fall back to sleep. Tammy noticed Mrs. Templeton's light on and went to her room to ask if she was OK. Mrs. Templeton said she was afraid of her upcoming surgery and whether she would be able to walk properly afterwards. Tammy sat with Mrs. Templeton for about ten minutes from 1:30 AM to 1:40 AM. She listened while Mrs. Templeton talked about her fears. Mrs. Templeton asked if the nurse could come in the morning and go over the schedule for the day of surgery again. After they talked Mrs. Templeton said she was feeling tired and would try to get some sleep. Tammy helped her get comfortable in bed and put her call light within reach. When Tammy checked on Mrs. Templeton at 2:40 AM she appeared to be sleeping.

Follow these guidelines when reporting:

- Be specific and use precise language to describe your observations.
- Report only the facts, not your personal opinion.
- Include the patient's name, room number, bed number, and the time of your observation.
- Report abnormal observations to the nurse immediately. Do not wait until the end-of-shift report if there appears to be a problem.
- Report events in the order in which they happen. For example, if you were working the 7–3 shift and Mrs. Jones seemed upset in the morning but was calm by lunch, make sure to say this so that the incoming staff doesn't think she was upset all day.
- If there were external forces that upset the resident (such as a family member who had a disagreement with the resident), report the event and what you did to calm the resident.
- Report any part of your assignment that you did not complete.

Recording

Recording is the process of writing down the observations you make and the treatments and procedures you perform. Recording is also called **charting**. Information needs to be accurate, concise, and legible. **See Figure 13-13.** This information goes into the patient's medical record.

The Medical Record

Health care facilities are legally required to keep written records for every patient. The **medical record** is written documentation about a patient's care, condition, treatment, and response to treatment. This record is also called a *patient record* or *chart*. The main purpose of the medical record is to communicate information about the patient to members of the health care team.

Each patient has a medical record. It is usually a folder that is clearly labeled and dated. The record contains the patient's name, doctor's name, room number, location, and hospital or facility number. It is made up of forms that contain information written by members of the health care team about the patient's condition and care. Some sections of the record are maintained by the doctor or nurse. Other sections may be the responsibility of the nursing assistant. During your orientation to the facility, you will be trained in recording procedures. Some facilities do not allow nursing assistants to write directly in the medical record. Instead, the nursing assistants keep logs and notes, which they submit to the supervisor.

Medical records are an important part of a patient's total care. They are saved and stored for many years after the patient has been discharged. These records are also legal documents that may be used as evidence in a court of law.

In most facilities, all team members have access to medical records and contribute information to the record. However, medical records are confidential. If you have permission to read medical records, you may not discuss them with anyone outside your team. That would be a violation of the patient's right to privacy.

The parts of the medical record that are most important to nursing assistants are the graphic chart, nurses' notes, and the activities of daily living flow sheet.

Graphic Chart. The **graphic chart** is a document used to record observations and measurements, such as blood pressure, temperature, pulse, and respiration rate. **See Figure 13-14.** Abbreviations are used on the graphic chart: BP for blood pressure, T for temperature, P for Pulse, and R for respiration. A quick glance at this information gives any member of the team an overview of the patient's condition. In a hospital environment, observations and measurements on the graphic chart are recorded several times a day. In a long-term care facility, vital signs are taken once a month unless the resident's condition requires more frequent monitoring.

Nurses' Notes. The documentation written by the nurse on duty containing information about treatments provided and the patient's response to treatment are the **nurses' notes**. Nursing assistants read nurses' notes to learn how the patient is responding. **See Figure 13-15.**

Flow Sheets. The **flow sheet** is a chart used to record many different types of data, depending on the type of facility and the particular needs of the patient. In a hospital, a nursing assistant might use a flow sheet to record a patient's fluid intake and output. In a nursing home, flow sheets are also used to chart residents' activities of daily living. The patient's medical record will likely contain several different flow sheets. **See Figure 13-16.**

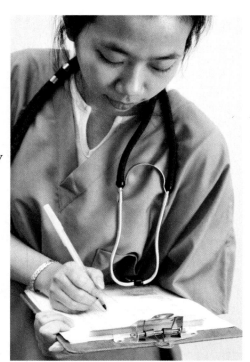

O Figure 13-13. The nursing assistant fills out forms required by the facility to keep a record of all care given.

FOCUS ON

Legal Issues

A medical record is a confidential document. The health care staff may read the chart, but no unauthorized person may see it. For instance, the record may contain information that the patient does not wish a particular family member to have. Never discuss what is in a patient's medical record with anyone outside the health care team.

| YEAR: _____ |
| RESIDENT'S NAME: _____ PHYSICIAN: _____ |
| MEDICAL RECORD # _____ ROOM # _____ ADMISSION DATE: _____ |

DATE	TIME AM/PM	T	P	R	BP	DATE	TIME AM/PM	T	P	R	BP

○ **Figure 13-14.** The graphic chart is used to record observations and measurements.

Guidelines for Recording

Each agency has policies about medical records and who can see them. Policies address:

- Who records
- When to record
- Approved abbreviations (See Chapter 12 for lists of approved and "Do Not Use" abbreviations.)
- How to correct errors
- Ink color
- Signing entries

Recording is an important job responsibility for nursing assistants. Follow these general guidelines when recording.

- Record entries in the required ink color with a ballpoint pen.
- Sign each entry with the date, your first initial, last name, and title.
- Make entries in chronological order (the order in which they occurred).
- Make entries objective and factual. Do not offer your opinion.

NURSES' NOTES
(Side One)

DATE	TIME	
8/15	0300	*Tagamet 300 mg PO*
		Aspirin enteric 325 mg
		Nitrospray 0.4 mg subl.
	0700	*Apply SS (Medid) shampoo*

Resident's Name: _____ Doctor: _____

○ **Figure 13-15.** Nurses' notes are written by nurses and contain information about treatments provided and the responses to treatments.

NAME		DOCTOR			ROOM #		MEDICAL RECORD #	

DATE:		SUN.	MON.	TUES.	WED.	THUR.	FRI.	SAT.
1. PERSONAL CARE	N							
Oral Hygiene	D							
	E							
AM Care								
PM Care								
HS								
2. BATH								
Tub-Bed-Shower								
Shampoo								
Dressing	N							
	D							
	E							
3. DIET								
Method	B							
Appetite (E-G-F-P)	L							
	S							
4. ELIMINATION								
BLADDER	N							
Foley–BR–BP–COMM–UR	D							
Inc. c peri-care	E							
BOWEL	N							
"See Kardex for BR-BP/BM's."	D							
Inc. c peri-care	E							
5. MOBILITY								
Nacs (AM & PM)								
OOB (Code & Hrs.)								
W/C G/C* Ch								
Ca-Walker-Assist (1 or 2)								
Must record # Ft.								
6. RECREATION								
Lounge/DR Activity								
Rec. Room								
Relig. Service								
Visitors								
7. SLEEP PATTERN (Code Hrs.)								
Observed (How freq.)								
Side Rails (Up/down)								
8. RESTRAINTS: VEST–WAIST–GERI–CHAIR								
CHECK:								
q 1/2 hr. Released q 2 hrs.								
for: ROM & Skin Check								

INITIALS:	N	D	E	N	D	E	N	D	E	N	D	E	N	D	E	N	D	E	N	D	E

CODE: A = Assist, T = Total, I = Independent, S = Supervised, *R = Refused (* Requires Narrative Note)

APPETITE, ROM – P = 0-25%   F = 26-50%   G = 51-75%   E = 76-100%

P = Poor   F = Fair   G = Good   E = Excellent

○ **Figure 13-16.** A resident's ADLs are recorded on a flow sheet.

- Make entries brief, exact, and complete.
- Do not erase or use correction fluid on the chart. If you make a mistake, mark a single line across the word or sentence and write your initials next to the line.
- Do not leave any open spaces. Draw a line through the unused lines. (This prevents someone else from reporting when you were caring for the person.)
- Make entries in a timely manner.
- Do not use ditto marks. Use appropriate abbreviations.
- If the chart is more than one page, make sure the patient's name is on every sheet.

Vital Skills (WRITING)

Sequencing Ideas

As discussed in this chapter, health care facilities keep written records of their patients. You might be required to contribute to that record by recording your observations and the care you give. You may be asked to write this in a log or other form, or directly in the medical record.

Before you write anything, organize your thoughts. You will need to report events in the order they happened. What information do you want to include? See the example of a nursing assistant's log notes in **Figure A**.

Practice

Below is a description of a nursing assistant's interaction with a patient during morning care. Read the account and then prepare an entry for the medical record.

Robert, the nursing assistant, arrived at Mrs. Rodriguez's room at 7:15 AM. Mrs. Rodriguez asked Robert if her morning paper had arrived. She said she liked to read the Sunday comics. Robert helped her out of bed and into the bathroom. She was able to walk with her cane and Robert's assistance. She voided 250 mL of clear, yellow urine. Robert ran the water for her, and helped her wash, brush her teeth, and comb her hair. He then helped her back into bed. Then her breakfast arrived. Robert set up the tray for her and asked if she needed anything. She said she did not and that she was comfortable. He made sure her call bell was in reach and left the room.

○ Figure A

NOTES			Rodriguez, Rita PT ID# 791338
Date	Time	Notes	
5/4/07	1320	Foley bag emptied of 800 mL clear, yellow urine. Assisted Pt in repositioning herself. Call bell within reach. ———— J. Dillon, CNA	
5/4/07	1330	Brought lunch tray to Pt. She stated she is "not hungry." Asked to have lunch tray removed from room. ———— J. Dillon, CNA	

- When you record subjective information, or symptoms, put quotation marks around statements made by the patient. This reduces the chance that patients' subjective statements will be misinterpreted. For example, "Pt says, 'I have been extremely thirsty all day.'"
- Enter the time a procedure was performed, according to facility policy.
- Record only what you observed and did yourself. Never record for a coworker.

- Record safety measures such as placing the call light within reach or reminding someone not to get out of bed. This demonstrates that you have followed correct procedures.

Recording on Computers

You may be asked to record patient observations on a computer instead of on a form or chart. **See Figure 13-17.** In some facilities, computers are used at the bedside for recording. In others, there is a central computer located near the nurses' station for entering vitals, ADLs, and other data.

Some computer recording is done in a series of windows that have lists of normal procedures and ADLs. In this case, you simply enter check marks on the list to show what

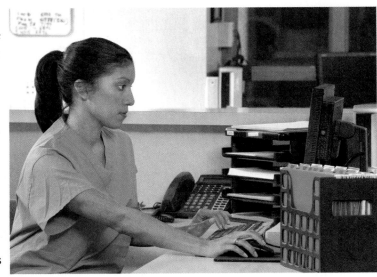

O **Figure 13-17.** In some facilities, nursing assistants record patient information directly on a computer.

you have done for the patient. Sometimes you will record only abnormal events or measurements. This is called *charting by exception*.

The patient's right to privacy must be protected, so the computers in health care facilities are secure. *E-records* (electronic records) containing medical information or patient-specific observations are considered legal documents.

When you use the computer, you will need to enter a **log-in**, which is usually your first and last name. Then you will enter a **password**, a secret code made up of letters, numbers, and symbols. You will choose the password. Do not tell your password to anyone. Your log-in and password verify that you are the person who completed the care on a certain patient at a certain time. Other health care team members and other departments also access the patient's record. Everyone uses their own log-in and password.

Vital Skills (MATH)

Working Out a Schedule

Your shift begins at 1400. Susan, the RN, informs you that you will work on the rehab wing (300 hall) this afternoon. You check your assignment list. You will care for eight residents, in rooms 301, 302, 303, 304, 305, 307, 308, and 310. All of these residents must walk before supper. Supper is served at 1730. You will need to figure out a schedule for walking the residents.

Practice

1. If you begin walking the first resident at 1500, how much time do you have to walk all of the residents on your assignment sheet?
2. How much time do you have to walk with each resident?

Chapter Summary

- When a sender sends a message to a receiver, and the receiver responds with feedback, communication has taken place.
- Nursing assistants use both verbal and nonverbal communication with patients and coworkers.
- Guidelines for effective communication include speaking and writing clearly, listening actively, and being consistent.

- Many technologies are used to make communication in the health care setting efficient.
- Nursing assistants observe patients for signs and symptoms of illness.
- Nursing assistants report their observations to supervisors, coworkers, and other shifts.
- The patient's medical record includes information from all members of the health care team.

VOCABULARY REVIEW

Directions: Match the letter of each definition in the second column with the correct vocabulary term in the first column. Write your answers on a separate sheet of paper.

Vocabulary

1. body language
2. communication
3. feedback
4. medium
5. message
6. nonverbal communication
7. objective information
8. observation
9. receiver
10. sender
11. subjective information
12. verbal communication

Definitions

A. The response to a communication message
B. Information you collect about a patient using your senses
C. Something that you notice about a patient, such as a physical change or a change in behavior
D. The person who receives a communication message
E. Communication through the use of words
F. All of the mannerisms and gestures used in communication
G. The person who sends a communication message
H. The way or means in which information is sent or received
I. All forms of communication except words
J. The information a sender wants to convey
K. The exchange of information
L. Information a patient tells you

Check Your Knowledge

Review Questions: Answer each of the following questions on a separate sheet of paper.

1. What is the difference between open-ended and closed-ended questions?

2. List three active listening techniques.

3. List two ways you can communicate with patients with visual impairment.

4. What is the difference between an intercom and a call signal?

5. Is a sore on a patient's back a sign or a symptom?

6. What is another word for *recording*?

7. What information is recorded on a graphic chart?

8. What kind of information might be recorded on a flow sheet?

9. What kind of information is found in nurses' notes?

10. What is a log-in?

True or False: Read each statement carefully. Then write *True* or *False* by the statement number on a separate sheet of paper.

1. Subjective information is information obtained by using your senses.

2. Nursing care plans communicate information about the patient's condition to all members of the health care team.

3. Statements the patient makes about how he or she is feeling do not belong in your report.

4. Medical records are legal documents.

5. Medical records are destroyed when the patient is discharged from the facility.

Think and Decide

Directions: Think about each of the following scenarios. Answer each question on a separate sheet of paper.

1. Mr. Phillips has trouble seeing. He is used to his room and knows where to find everything easily. When his family members visited today, they rearranged the furniture. They explained to him that it will be friendlier to visitors this way. What happens to Mr. Phillips' security? What should you say, and to whom?

2. Mrs. Y. puts on her call light. You knock and enter her room to see what she needs. She tells you she has a "terrible headache." What action or actions should you take?

3. You are just ending a very busy shift. You are getting ready to tape-record your end-of-shift report for the oncoming shift. What important points should you communicate to the next shift?

4. You are charting Mr. Spencer's 10:00 AM vitals on the graphic chart. You know that this will become part of the patient's medical record and that it is a legal document. You accidentally write 30 instead of 20 in the Respirations column. What should you do?

5. You are a home health aide working in Mrs. A.'s home. The phone rings, and she asks you to answer it. You answer pleasantly, only to have Mrs. A.'s adult son yell at you over the phone because he is not happy with his mother's health, and he blames you. How should you handle this situation?

6. You answer the call light in Mrs. Olsen's room. She has aphasia (difficulty forming speech), and has trouble communicating her needs. You observe that she is getting frustrated, but you find it hard to understand what she wants. What should you do to meet her needs?

7. Mr. L. is a new resident at the long-term care facility where you work. You have come to his room to welcome him and to explain where things are, the daily routines, and the activities provided for the residents. As you are talking, Mr. L. is gazing out the window and nodding absently. Is communication taking place? Explain. What should you do?

8. Mrs. G. has been diagnosed with colon cancer and was admitted to the hospital today for surgery tomorrow. She is fearful about the surgery and the cancer and wants to talk about it. Due to a recent experience with colon cancer in your own family, this is a painful subject for you to discuss. How should you react to Mrs. G.'s conversation?

9. Vicki is a new nursing assistant at the facility where you work. She has just finished school and is excited about the job. However, she confesses to you that she is very timid about using a tape recorder to record end-of-shift reports. She is afraid she'll say something wrong or sound silly. What tips might you give her?

CNA Certification Exam Prep

Directions: This practice test contains ten questions. Each question has four suggested answers. For each question, choose the ONE that best answers the question or completes the statement. Write your answers on a separate sheet of paper.

1. The sender-receiver model of communication involves a sender, a receiver, a message, and a
   A. sign.
   B. symptom.
   C. medium.
   D. report.

2. Sounds such as laughing or sighing are
   A. verbal communication.
   B. unsuccessful communication.
   C. abstract communication.
   D. nonverbal communication.

3. Active listening consists of restatement, reflection, and
   A. feedback.
   B. clarification.
   C. resubmission.
   D. response.

4. One technique for communicating with a patient who has a hearing deficiency is to
   A. shout so that she can hear you.
   B. face her while speaking.
   C. whisper softly.
   D. ignore her.

5. A nursing assistant records that a patient with diabetes complains of numbness in his right leg. This is an example of a(n)
   A. subjective observation.
   B. singular observation.
   C. regular observation.
   D. objective observation.

6. The purpose of the graphic chart is to record
   A. a patient's intake and output.
   B. the medications a patient receives.
   C. nurse's notes about the patient.
   D. the patient's vital signs.

7. When answering the phone on the job, you should always answer by the
   A. second ring.
   B. third ring.
   C. fourth ring.
   D. fifth ring.

8. Something about a patient that you can see, hear, feel, or smell is known as a
   A. symptom.
   B. fever.
   C. message.
   D. sign.

9. A document that is written and developed by a nurse and describes the care required for a patient is a
   A. graphic chart.
   B. I/O report.
   C. nursing care plan.
   D. activity log.

10. The written documentation that health care facilities are required to keep for every patient is the
    A. end-of-shift report.
    B. medical record.
    C. graphic chart.
    D. flow sheet.

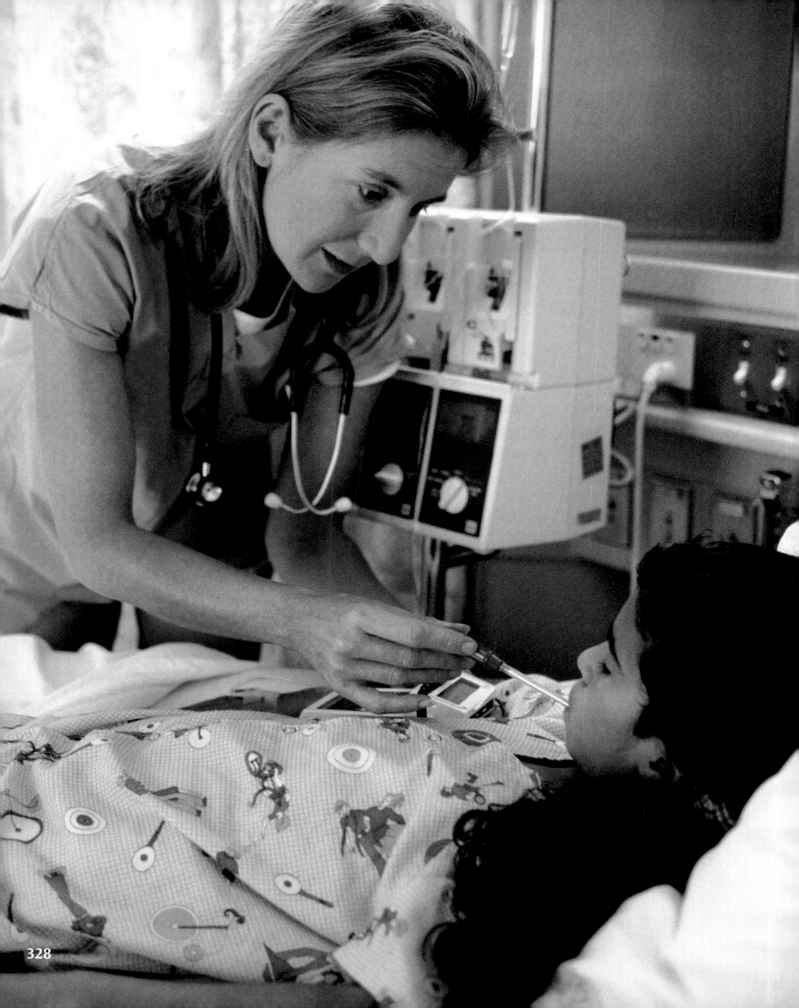

UNIT 4

Patient Care

Chapter 14 Care of the Patient's Room

Chapter 15 Admission, Transfer, and Discharge

Chapter 16 Body Mechanics

Chapter 17 Emergency Care

Chapter 18 Examinations and Therapies

Chapter 19 Elimination and Sample Collection

Chapter 20 Caring for the Surgical Patient

Chapter 21 Patient Rehabilitation

Unit 4 presents specific information about tasks nursing assistants perform in providing patient care. Each chapter focuses on a specific type of care or task. Procedures for carrying out specific tasks are described in detail.

CHAPTER 14

OBJECTIVES

- Identify environmental conditions in the patient's room that affect comfort and safety.
- List the minimum furniture and equipment provided in the patient's room.

- Identify personal belongings that patients and residents might have in their rooms to promote their well-being.
- Explain why clean, dry bed linens and proper bedmaking are important to the patient's safety and well-being.

- List guidelines for handling and changing bed linens to ensure good health, comfort, infection control, and safety.
- Demonstrate proper bedmaking procedures.

Care of the Patient's Room

bath blanket A lightweight blanket used to provide warmth and privacy when changing the bed while the patient is in it and when the patient is bathing or using the bedpan.

bed pad An absorbent pad placed between the bottom sheet and the patient to protect the linen from becoming wet or soiled.

closed bed A bed in a health care facility that is not currently in use.

draw sheet A small sheet placed over the middle of the bottom sheet to help lift and move a person up in bed.

fanfold Turn back (bed linens) in an accordion fashion.

mitered corner A corner of bed linens that is angled and tucked to lie flat against the mattress.

occupied bed A bed that is made while the patient or resident is in it.

open bed A bed that is used by a resident who gets up during the day.

surgical bed A closed bed that has been opened to the side to allow safe, easy transfer of a patient who is being moved from a stretcher to a bed.

toe pleat A pleat made at the bottom of the bed linens to allow room for the toes and feet to move freely.

unoccupied bed A bed that is empty.

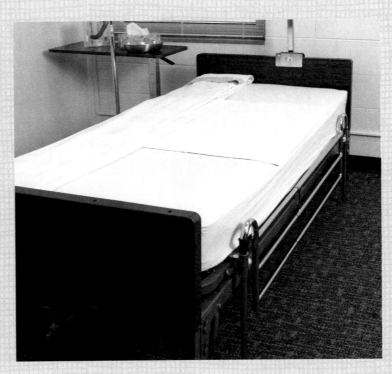

A Safe, Pleasant Environment

It is important that the health care environment be pleasant, comfortable, and safe for patients. Health care facilities regulate environmental conditions that affect patients. In addition, federal and state legislation regulates the following conditions in long-term care facilities.

- **Space.** The size of rooms is regulated to provide patients with enough space for comfort and safety. This ensures that the room will not be so crowded that the patient risks falling.

- **Lighting.** Dimly lit rooms can cause eyestrain, headache, and falls. Rooms generally have overhead lighting in addition to sunlight. A wall-mounted light over the bed, a bedside lamp, or a floor lamp may be provided for reading, writing, or doing other close work. This directed lighting also helps health care workers see properly when they provide care. **See Figure 14-1.**

- **Temperature.** The facility must maintain the temperature at a safe, comfortable level. Most people are comfortable at temperatures between 68° F (20° C) and 74° F (23° C). Elderly or sick people, however, may feel cold at these temperatures. It is not possible to keep room temperatures at a setting that pleases all residents, but an effort should be made to accommodate individual requests.

- **Air quality.** Unpleasant odors interfere with comfort and safety. People who are sick can be more sensitive to odors and more susceptible to nausea. Prompt emptying of bedpans, cleaning up spills, and changing soiled bed linens are crucial for good hygiene and for preventing odors. Good ventilation systems also help minimize unpleasant odors. These systems can cause drafts, however, so make sure the patient does not sit or sleep in a draft.

- **Noise control.** Many people and constant activity can make the health care environment very noisy. It is important to control the noise level as much as possible. Carpeting, curtains, and ceiling tiles in patient rooms help absorb noise. In addition, caregivers can keep their voices down and report equipment that is too noisy.

- **Storage.** There must be adequate, secure storage space in the room for patients' personal belongings.

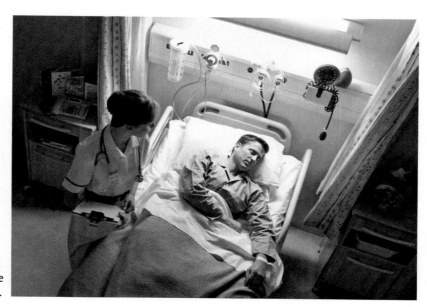

○ **Figure 14-1. Directed lighting helps the nursing assistant see to provide care to the patient.**

Vital Skills READING

Skimming and Scanning

When you read new material, the reading technique you choose depends on your purpose for reading and the material to be read. For example, if you are going to the beach, you might take a novel to read for pleasure. You would read each sentence. But when you come back home and read your mail and newspaper, you might choose a different reading technique, such as skimming or scanning.

When you *skim* reading material, you read through it quickly to grasp the main idea. For example, when you read a magazine, you might skim the articles to see which ones appeal to you, and then take your time with those. There are different techniques for skimming. You might read just the first and last sentence of each paragraph, or just the first and last paragraphs. When skimming a research paper, you might read just the titles and subtitles, and look at any illustrations.

When you *scan* reading material, your eyes move quickly over the text, looking for key words or ideas. For example, if you had to write a research paper on infection control, you might select a nursing textbook and scan the table of contents for the word *infection*.

Practice

1. Skim the text in the chapter describing patient rooms. What are the main points you should remember? Write a few sentences summarizing those points.
2. Scan the text for points related to patient safety. What key words did you look for? List some patient safety concerns you found in the text.

Furniture and Equipment

Whether in a hospital or long-term care facility, patient rooms contain, at a minimum, certain furniture and equipment needed for comfort.

- **Bed.** The beds in health care facilities are generally called *hospital beds*. The head and foot of these beds can be raised and lowered for the patient's comfort. Most hospitals use electronic beds. They allow bed positions to be changed by pushing buttons that control the movement of the bed frame. Some nursing homes use electronic beds. Others use manual hospital beds, which have a hand crank that is turned to change bed positions. **See Figure 14-2.**
- **Chairs.** Most rooms have two chairs—a straight-backed chair without arms and an upholstered chair with arms for use by the patient and visitors.
- **Bedside stand.** A bedside stand is a cabinet positioned next to the head of the bed. It is used to store the patient's personal belongings and personal hygiene items, such as soap, deodorant, a wash basin, and a washcloth and towel. A telephone and personal belongings may be kept on top of the bedside stand.
- **Overbed table.** This table swings over the bed and is used for items the patient needs often, such as a water pitcher and cup, and for meal trays. It is on casters and can be pushed out of the way when necessary. **See Figure 14-3.**

In long-term care facilities, the room also may include a dresser for clothing and other personal items. Rooms also have a closet for hanging clothes.

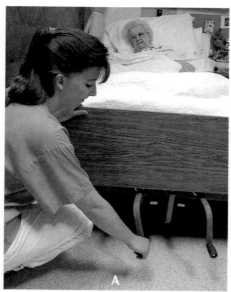

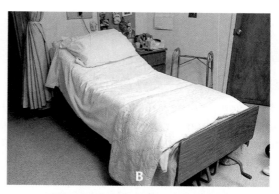

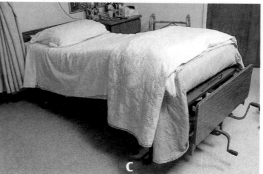

○ Figure 14-2. (A) The manual bed is raised or lowered in sections or as a whole, using cranks at the bend of the bed. (B) The head of the bed raised. (C) The foot of the bed raised.

Equipment in rooms usually includes a wastebasket, a call system (intercom or call signal), privacy curtains or screens, and medical equipment. Some patients may have a walker, wheelchair, or other assistive device in the room.

Personal Belongings

Upon admission to a health care facility, a list of the person's belongings, including clothing, is completed. This list becomes part of the medical record. Facilities vary in what belongings they will allow patients to keep in their rooms.

In a hospital, patient belongings typically include personal hygiene items, such as a hairbrush and comb, toothbrush, deodorant, and so on. Patients also receive get-well cards and flowers from friends and family. Hospital patients may have their cash, checkbook, credit cards, and jewelry locked up by security personnel.

Long-term care facility residents usually have more personal belongings, such as clothing and a television. Personal belongings such as photos, craft items, and plants provide enjoyment, remind residents of their past, and help them feel close to family and friends. Patients might bring books, pictures, and other familiar items from home. These items help them stay connected to the activities and people important to them and help reduce stress. See Figure 14-4. Respect each resident's personal needs and honor individual wishes as much as possible.

When a resident moves into a nursing home, personal belongings are marked with his or her name. Most are kept in the resident's room. Valuable items, such as jewelry, may be kept in a safe in the facility. When the resident requests the item, a staff member removes it from the safe and delivers it to the resident.

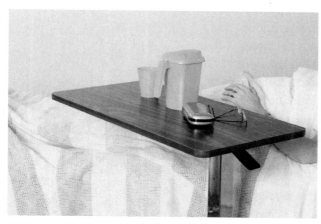

○ Figure 14-3. The overbed table provides easy access to items the patient uses often.

Bed Linens and Bedmaking

Providing clean, dry bed linens and proper bedmaking are essential for the patient's well-being. Following guidelines and procedures in this area will:

- Ensure the patient's comfort
- Avoid wrinkles that can cause pressure sores
- Promote infection control
- Provide for patient safety

Bed Linens

The following bed linens are used when making a hospital bed:

- Mattress pad
- Bottom sheet. This can be a flat or contour (fitted) sheet.
- Bed linen protector, such as a draw sheet or a bed pad
- Blanket
- Top sheet
- Bedspread
- Pillows
- Bath blanket. A **bath blanket** is a lightweight blanket used to provide warmth and privacy when changing the bed while the patient is in it.

Keeping Bed Linens Clean and Dry. Linens and the mattress can become wet or soiled when

- Food or drink is spilled in bed.
- Wounds drain onto the bed linen.
- The linen becomes wet with perspiration.
- Patients have *incontinence*, which is the inability to control elimination.

To help keep the linens and mattress clean and dry, a cotton draw sheet may be used. A **draw sheet** is a small sheet that is placed over the middle of the bottom sheet to lift and move a person up in bed. It lies beneath the patient from the shoulders to the buttocks. Some facilities use a plastic draw sheet. When plastic is used, a cotton draw sheet must be used over it. The plastic should never come in contact with the patient's skin.

Some facilities use **bed pads**, which are absorbent pads placed over the bottom sheet to protect the linen from becoming wet or soiled. The pad is changed when it becomes soiled or damp. They are more comfortable for the patient because a full bed change is not required.

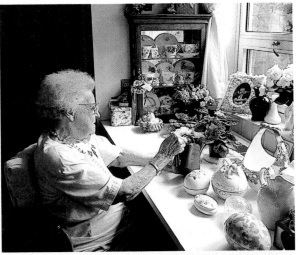

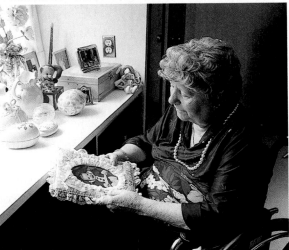

○ **Figure 14-4.** Gardening was the hobby of the resident in the top photo for many years, and she continues to nurture African violets in her room. Her roommate has chosen a photo of her great-grandson to personalize her surroundings.

FOCUS ON

Handling Residents' Clothing

At times, you may handle residents' personal clothing. As with bed linens, wear gloves to handle dirty clothing. Place the clothing in the hamper or handle according to facility policy. Then wash your hands. You might also help residents put clean clothing away in the closet or dresser. Do not allow either clean or dirty clothing to touch your clothing.

Pads may be washable or disposable. Using disposable pads provides these advantages:

- Cuts down on the amount of laundry that must be done
- Provides increased infection control because soiled pads are simply disposed of

Guidelines for Handling Bed Linens. For the patient's health and safety, special guidelines must be followed when handling bed linens. This includes the following infection control practices.

- Place clean bed linens on a clean surface until they are used in bedmaking.
- Do not shake clean or dirty linens in the air. Doing so could spread germs.
- Place dirty linens in the hamper or in the laundry bag, never on the floor.
- If body fluids or other substances leak or spill on the mattress or bed frame, wipe it down with cleaning solution, according to facility policy.

O **Figure 14-5. When carrying clean or dirty linens, never allow them to come into contact with your uniform.**

Schedule for Changing Bed Linens. Policies for when and how often to change bed linens vary. Bed linens are always changed when someone is discharged and when linens are wet, soiled, or extremely wrinkled. There is usually a regular schedule for complete bed linen changes. You will receive this information in your daily assignment. Some facilities follow the shower or bath schedule to completely change bed linens. In some facilities, not all linens are changed every time the bed is made. Some linens are reused for the same bed if they are not wet or soiled. For example, the bedspread and blanket are reused in some facilities.

Bedmaking

Bedmaking is an important part of a nursing assistant's job. Making the bed properly includes making sure the linens fit tightly and that there are no wrinkles. They create friction or pressure against the patient's skin, causing irritation.

Beds are either unoccupied or occupied. An **unoccupied bed** is one that is empty. There are several ways to make an unoccupied bed: closed, open, and surgical. If the patient is in the bed while it is made, it is an **occupied bed**.

Closed Bed. A **closed bed** is a bed not currently in use. Top linens are not turned back. **See Figure 14-6.** In a hospital, the room is cleaned and the bed linens changed when a patient is discharged. The bed is made closed and remains closed until a new patient is assigned to that bed number. In a long-term care facility, beds are made closed for residents who are not confined to bed during the day.

Open Bed. An **open bed** is a bed that is used by a resident who can get in and out of bed during the day. It is also one that is made ready for a newly admitted patient or resident. The top linens in an open bed are **fanfolded**, or turned back in an accordion fashion. The patient can easily get into the bed when ready. **See**

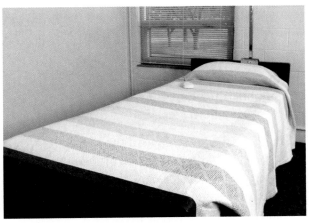

○ Figure 14-6. A closed bed is a bed that is not currently in use. Top linens are not turned back.

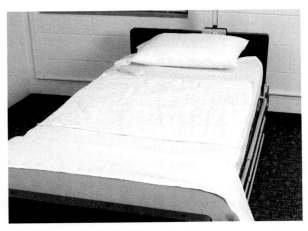

○ Figure 14-7. An open bed has the top sheet and blanket fanfolded to the bottom of the bed. The bedspread has been removed for sleeping.

Figure 14-7. Open beds are usually made while the patient or resident is out of the room for some reason, such as bathing, eating, or having medical tests.

Surgical Bed. A **surgical bed** is a closed bed that has been opened to the side to allow safe, easy transfer of a patient who is being moved from a stretcher to a bed. It is also called a post-operative bed. The patient might be returning to the room from surgery (post-operative), returning by stretcher from a treatment, or arriving by ambulance.

Occupied Bed. An **occupied bed** is a bed that is made while the patient or resident is in it. The patient turns and faces away from you as you make each side of the bed. Be sure to provide privacy and explain what you are doing to reassure the patient.

Vital Skills (COMMUNICATION)

Giving and Following Directions

A patient who is unable to get out of bed may have a Foley catheter (a device that drains urine from the bladder). The patient may also have other medical equipment, such as IVs, oxygen tubing, cardiac monitor leads, or chest tubes. You will need to be very careful not to dislodge this medical equipment.

Before you move a patient to make an occupied bed, note the equipment in use. If it is the first time you are moving the patient, ask the nurse if there is anything specific you should be aware of. Ask a coworker for help lifting the patient.

Practice

Review the steps in this chapter for making an occupied bed. With a partner, practice making an occupied bed. One of you can be the patient while the other makes the bed. Then switch. What instructions can you give to the patient to make the process easier? How might you change your techniques for someone who is unresponsive and cannot move on his or her own? For someone who had recent shoulder surgery or a hip replacement?

Procedure 14-1

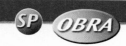

Making a Closed Bed and Making an Open Bed

Equipment: bedspread • blanket • plastic draw sheet (optional) • cotton draw sheet or pad • mattress pad • bottom sheet (flat or contour) • top sheet• two pillowcases

1. Wash your hands.
2. Gather the clean bed linens you will need and place them on a clean surface such as the overbed table or a chair. If you have questions about the cleanliness of the surface, put them on a clean towel. Place the pillow at the head of the bed.
3. Arrange the linens in the order you will put them on the bed. The items needed first should be on top, and items needed last on the bottom.
4. Raise or lower the bed so it is at a comfortable working height.
5. Slide the mattress forward toward the head of the bed until it reaches the headboard.
6. If facility policy is to use a mattress pad, place the pad on the mattress, even with the top of the mattress.
7. Place the bottom sheet, sewn side down, on the mattress and unfold it lengthwise. (If using a contour sheet, starting at the top, hook the corner of the sheet under the corner of the mattress. Then repeat at the bottom.)
   a. Align the center crease in the sheet with the center of the mattress. **See Figure 14-8.**

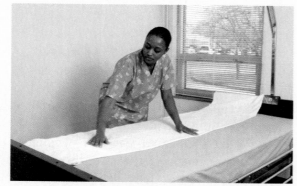

O Figure 14-8. Align the center crease in the sheet with the center of the mattress.

   b. Place the lower edge of the sheet so it lines up with the bottom of the mattress.
8. Open the bottom sheet. Make sure that about the same length of sheet hangs over each side.
9. Check to make sure that about 12 to 18 inches of sheet is available to tuck under each side.
10. At the head of the bed, lift the mattress slightly and tuck the top of the sheet under the mattress.
11. Make a mitered corner at the head of the bed. A **mitered corner** is a corner of the bed linens that is angled and tucked to lie flat against the mattress. Mitered corners help the bed linens stay in place. **See Figure 14-9.** Tuck the sheet underneath the mattress along the sides of the bed. Work on one side of the bed until it is complete before working on the other side.
12. Place a pad, a plastic draw sheet, or other moisture-resistant product on the mattress about 14 inches from the head of the bed. **See Figure 14-10.** (Some patients do not need a pad. Follow your supervisor's instructions.)
13. Open the plastic draw sheet (optional) and tuck it under the mattress.
14. Place the cotton draw sheet over the pad or plastic draw sheet to completely cover the plastic sheet. **See Figure 14-11.**
15. Open the cotton draw sheet and tuck it under the mattress, making sure it is tight and wrinkle free.
16. Place the top sheet on the mattress and unfold it lengthwise.
   a. Check to be sure the stitching on the hem is facing upward, away from the patient's skin.

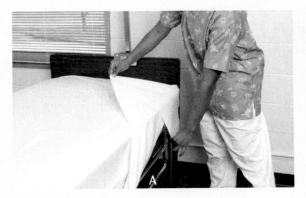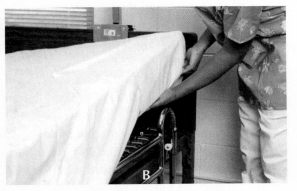
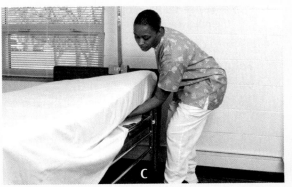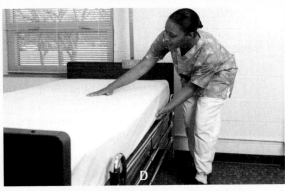

○ **Figure 14-9.** (A) Make an angle with the corner of the sheet at the head of the bed. (B) Tuck the angle tightly under the mattress. (C) Tuck the excess draping of the sheet tightly under the mattress along the side of the bed. (D) Smooth the sheet and make sure it fits tightly.

  b. Align the top of the sheet with the head of the mattress.
  c. Align the center crease in the sheet with the center of the mattress.
17. Place the blanket on the bed and unfold it.
  a. Align the center crease in the blanket with the center of the mattress.
  b. Place the top hem of the blanket about 6 to 8 inches from the head of the mattress.
18. Place the bedspread on the bed and unfold it.
  a. Align the center crease in the bedspread with the center of the mattress.
  b. Align the top of the bedspread with the head of the mattress.
  c. Check that the side of the bedspread facing the door is even and covers all the bed linens.
19. Tuck the top linens in together at the foot of the bed. Make a mitered corner on both sides. Check that the bed linens are smooth and tight.

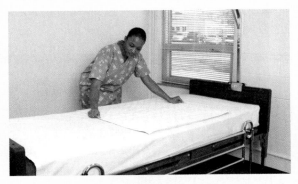

○ **Figure 14-10.** Place the bed pad so that the bottom of the pad is about 14 inches below the head of the bed.

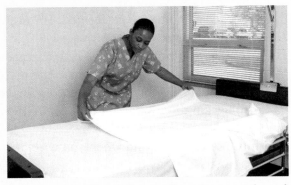

○ **Figure 14-11.** Place the cotton draw sheet over the pad.

20. Turn the top of the bedspread down over the blanket about 6 inches to make a cuff.
21. Turn the top sheet down over the bedspread.
22. Lay the pillows on the bed.
23. Open each pillowcase and lay it flat on the bed.
24. Place the pillow inside the pillowcase. **See Figure 14-12.** Fold the corners of the seam end of the pillow inward to make a "V." Open the pillowcase, slide the "V" end of the pillow into the pillowcase, and then flatten out the corners.
25. Place the pillow at the head of the bed, with the open end facing away from the door. Fold the extra pillowcase material under the pillow.

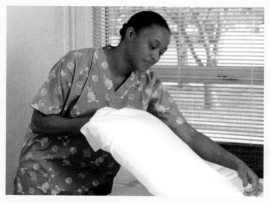

O Figure 14-12. Place the end of the pillow into the pillowcase.

Follow these steps to finish making a closed bed.

26. Pull the bedspread up over the pillows.
27. Lower the bed to its lowest position.
28. Place the signal light near the head of the bed.
29. Check to make sure the bed and room look neat and clean.
30. Wash your hands.

Follow these steps to finish making an open bed.

26. Grasp the top cuff of the bedding in both hands.
27. Fanfold the bed linens to the foot of the bed.
28. Lower the bed to its lowest position.
29. Place the signal light near the head of the bed.
30. Check to make sure the bed and room look neat and clean.
31. Wash your hands.

Vital Skills (WRITING)

Process Analysis List

One way to remember the steps of a procedure is to write a process analysis list. List each step in the order it should be performed. For example, you could write a process analysis list for how to light a campfire. The list would explain the process in a step-by-step format. The reader should be able to complete the task, and have a burning campfire, based on the instructions in the essay.

Things to keep in mind when you write a process analysis essay include:

• What is the intended audience for the list?
• What items or tools are needed to carry out the procedure?
• Can someone else perform this task adequately by following the steps in your list?

Practice

Choose one of the bedmaking procedures described in this chapter and write a process analysis list instructing the reader on how to make that particular type of bed.

Procedure 14-2

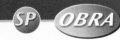

Making a Surgical Bed

Equipment: bedspread • blanket • plastic draw sheet (optional) • cotton draw sheet or pad • mattress pad • bottom sheet (flat or contour) • top sheet • two pillowcases • emesis basin • tissues • other equipment requested by the nursing team

1. Wash your hands.
2. Gather clean bed linens. Arrange the linens on a clean surface in the order you will put them on the bed. The items needed first should be on top, and items needed last on the bottom.
3. Raise or lower the bed so it is at a comfortable working height.
4. Remove the signal light from the bed.
5. Slide the mattress forward toward the head of the bed until it reaches the headboard.
6. If facility policy is to use a mattress pad, place the pad on the mattress, even with the top of the mattress.
7. Place the bottom sheet, sewn side down, on the mattress and unfold it lengthwise. (If using a contour sheet, starting at the top, hook the corner of the sheet under the corner of the mattress. Then repeat at the bottom.)
   a. Align the center crease in the sheet with the center of the mattress.
   b. Place the lower edge of the sheet so it lines up with the bottom of the mattress.
8. Open the bottom sheet. Make sure that about the same length of sheet hangs over each side.
9. Check to make sure that about 12 to 18 inches of sheet is available to tuck under each side.
10. At the head of the bed, lift the mattress slightly and tuck the top of the sheet under the mattress.
11. Make a mitered corner at the head of the bed. Tuck the sheet underneath the mattress along the sides of the bed. Work on one side of the bed until it is complete before working on the other side.

12. Place a pad, a plastic draw sheet, or other moisture-resistant product on the mattress about 14 inches from the head of the bed. (Some patients do not need a pad. Follow your supervisor's instructions.)
13. Open the plastic draw sheet (optional, rarely used) and tuck it under the mattress.
14. Place the cotton draw sheet over the pad or plastic draw sheet to completely cover the plastic sheet.
15. Open the cotton draw sheet and tuck it under the mattress, making sure it is tight and wrinkle free.
16. Place the top sheet on the mattress and unfold it lengthwise.
    a. Check to be sure the stitching on the hem is facing upward, away from the patient's skin.
    b. Align the top of the sheet with the head of the mattress.
    c. Align the center crease in the sheet with the center of the mattress.
17. Place the blanket on the bed and unfold it.
    a. Align the center crease in the blanket with the center of the mattress.
    b. Place the top hem of the blanket about 6 to 8 inches from the head of the mattress.
18. Place the bedspread on the bed and unfold it.
    a. Align the center crease in the bedspread with the center of the mattress.
    b. Align the top of the bedspread with the head of the mattress.
    c. Check that the side of the bedspread facing the door is even and covers all the bed linens.

19. Do not tuck the top bed linens under the mattress. Fold the bottom of the top bed linens back up onto the bed. The fold at the foot of the bed should be even with the edge of the mattress.
20. Fanfold the bedspread, blanket, and top sheet to the far side of the bed. **See Figure 14-13.**
21. Place a clean pillowcase on the pillow. Don't tuck the pillow under your chin to hold it while changing the pillowcase.
22. Place the pillow upright against the head-board, with the open end facing away from the door.
23. Raise the bed to stretcher height.
24. Be sure that all side rails are down.
25. Put a box of tissues and an emesis basin on top of the bedside stand.
26. Move furniture that would be in the way of the stretcher.
27. Wash your hands.

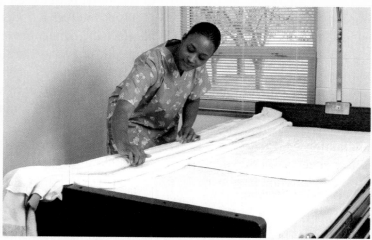

○ **Figure 14-13.** When making a surgical bed, fanfold the bedspread, blanket, and top sheet to the far side of the bed.

Procedure 14-3

SP OBRA

Making an Occupied Bed

Equipment: disposable gloves • bath blanket • bedspread • blanket • plastic draw sheet (optional) • cotton draw sheet or bed pad • mattress pad • bottom sheet (flat or contour) • top sheet • two pillowcases

1. Wash your hands.
2. Gather the clean linens you will need, arranging them in the order you will place them on the bed. The items needed first should be on top, and items needed last on the bottom.
3. Provide privacy.
4. Remove the signal light from the bed.
5. Raise the bed to a comfortable working position.
6. Lower the head of the bed as flat as possible for patient comfort and safety.
7. Lower the side rail on the side of the bed that is closest to you. The other side rail should be in the upright position and locked.

8. Put on gloves and a protective barrier (apron or gown) if bed linens are soiled.
9. Loosen the top bed linens at the foot of the bed.
10. Take off the bedspread. Fold it neatly if it will be reused.
11. Take off the blanket. Fold it neatly if it will be reused.
12. Place a bath blanket over the top sheet, if it is still covering the patient.
13. Ask the patient to hold the top edge of the bath blanket. If he or she cannot, tuck the blanket under both shoulders. **See Figure 14-14.**
14. Gently reach under the bath blanket and pull the top sheet down toward the foot of the bed. When it reaches the foot of the bed, remove the sheet from the bed and place in the hamper or laundry bag.
15. Slide the mattress to the head of the bed.
16. Ask the patient to turn onto his or her side, facing away from you. **See Figure 14-15.** If needed, help the patient turn in bed. One or two health care workers should help position the patient on the far side of the bed in proper body alignment. (Chapter 16 discusses proper body alignment.)
17. Move the pillow to the far side of the bed and place it under the patient's head. Adjust it for the patient's comfort.

18. Loosen the bottom bed linens, starting at the head of the bed and working towards the foot.
19. Fanfold or roll the bottom bed linens toward the patient, one at a time.
20. If the mattress pad will be replaced, fanfold it also. If it will be reused, straighten it, making sure there are no wrinkles.
21. If appropriate, place a clean mattress pad on the bed.
    a. Unfold it lengthwise.
    b. Make sure the center crease in the pad aligns with the center of the mattress.
    c. Fanfold or roll half of the pad toward the patient.
22. Place a clean bottom sheet on top of the pad.
    a. Unfold it lengthwise.
    b. Make sure the center crease in the sheet aligns with the center of the mattress.
    c. Make sure the stitching on the hem is facing away from the patient.
    d. Check to see that the hem is even with the bottom of the mattress.
    e. Fanfold the sheet toward the patient.
    f. If using a contour bottom sheet, tuck the top and bottom over mattress, making sure they are wrinkle free.
23. Make a mitered corner at the head of the bed.
24. Tuck the sheet underneath the mattress along the side of the bed closest to you.

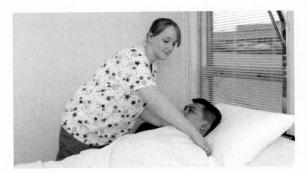

○ **Figure 14-14.** If the patient cannot hold the top edge of the bath blanket, tuck it under both shoulders.

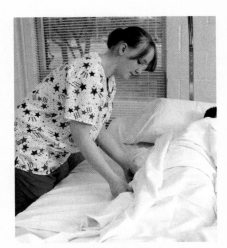

○ **Figure 14-15.** Each side of the occupied bed is made while the patient turns and faces away from the nursing assistant.

25. Place the plastic draw sheet (optional, rarely used) about 14 inches from the head of the bed.
26. Place the bed pad, or place the cotton draw sheet so that it covers the entire plastic draw sheet if one is used. If a draw sheet is used instead of a pad, do the following:
    a. Fanfold half of the cotton draw sheet toward the patient.
    b. Tuck in the excess under the mattress.
27. Raise the side rail on the side of the bed closest to you. Lock it in the upright position.
28. Walk to the other side of the bed and lower the side rail.
29. Ask the patient to turn onto his or her other side. If necessary, help the patient turn in the bed. The patient should be positioned on the side of the bed away from you, in proper body alignment. Explain to the patient there will be a "bump" to roll over.
30. Remove the soiled pillowcase and place a clean one over the pillow.
31. Raise the patient's head and adjust the pillow to a comfortable position.
32. Remove the soiled bottom bed linens from the bed and place in the hamper or laundry bag.
33. Straighten out the mattress pad.
34. Grasp the clean bottom sheet and pull it toward you.
    a. Make a mitered corner at the head of the bed.
    b. Tuck the sheet in along the side.
    c. If using a contour sheet, pull over and hook under mattress at the top and bottom, making sure they are wrinkle free.
35. Bring the plastic draw sheet (if used) and bed pad or cotton draw sheets toward you. Tuck both draw sheets under the mattress.

36. Ask the patient to lie on his or her back in the middle of the mattress. Assist the patient if necessary. Arrange the pillow in a comfortable position for the patient.
37. Place the clean top sheet on the bed.
    a. Unfold it lengthwise.
    b. Make sure the center crease in the sheet aligns with the center of the mattress.
    c. Make sure the stitching on the hem is facing away from the patient.
    d. Check to see that the hem is even with the head of the mattress.
38. Ask the patient to hold the top sheet. If he or she cannot, tuck it under both shoulders.
39. Gently remove the bath blanket and place in the hamper or laundry bag.
40. Place the blanket on the bed.
    a. Unfold it lengthwise.
    b. Make sure the center crease in the blanket aligns with the center of the mattress.
    c. Make sure the upper hem of the blanket is 6 to 8 inches from the head of the bed.
41. Place the bedspread on the bed.
    a. Unfold it lengthwise.
    b. Make sure the center crease in the bedspread aligns with the center of the mattress.
    c. Make sure the upper hem of the bedspread lines up with the top of the mattress.
42. Turn the top 6 inches of the bedspread down over the blanket to form a cuff.
43. Turn the top sheet down over the bedspread to make a cuff.
44. Go to the foot of the bed and tuck in the top bed linens, making mitered corners.

45. Then make a **toe pleat**, a pleat made at the bottom of the bed linens to allow room for the toes and feet to move freely. Grasp each corner of the bed linens and pull up 3 to 4 inches. Then pull down, making a pleat. **See Figure 14-16.**

46. Raise the side rail on the side of the bed where you just finished working. Lock it in the upright position.

47. Place the signal light in a position the patient can easily reach.

48. Raise the head of the bed to a position that is comfortable for the patient.

49. Lower the bed to its lowest position.

50. Open the curtain.

51. Remove soiled linens and place in the hamper or laundry bag.

52. Wash your hands.

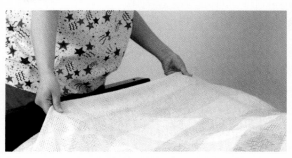

○ **Figure 14-16.** A toe pleat allows toes and feet to move freely. Grasp each corner of the bed linens and pull up 3 to 4 inches. Then pull down, making a pleat.

Vital Skills   (MATH)

Converting Fractions to Percentages

People often talk casually in terms of fractions. For example, you may be told that half of the beds you will make today will be closed beds. What percentage of the beds will be closed?

Percentages are based on the number 100. For example, 15% really means "15 per 100."

So, to convert a fraction, such as ½, to a percentage, you divide the upper part of the fraction (numerator) by the bottom part of the fraction (denominator) and then multiply by 100:

$$1 \div 2 = .50$$
$$.50 \times 100 = 50\%$$

Practice

You have been assigned to make the beds in Hall 100. One half (½) of the beds will be closed beds, ¼ of the beds will be complete linen changes, and ⅓ of the beds will be occupied beds. Change each of these fractions to percentages.

Chapter Summary

- Environmental conditions in the patient's room affect comfort and safety.

- Health care facilities generally provide certain types of furniture and equipment in the patient's room.

- Most health care facilities allow patients and residents to have personal belongings in their rooms to promote their well-being.

- Clean, dry bed linens and proper bedmaking are important to the patient's safety and well-being.

- Follow guidelines for handling and changing bed linens to ensure good health, comfort, and infection control.

VOCABULARY REVIEW

Directions: Match the letter of each definition in the second column with the correct vocabulary term in the first column. Write your answers on a separate sheet of paper.

Vocabulary

1. bath blanket
2. bed pad
3. closed bed
4. draw sheet
5. fanfold
6. mitered corner
7. occupied bed
8. open bed
9. surgical bed
10. toe pleat
11. unoccupied bed

Definitions

A. A small sheet placed over the middle of the bottom sheet

B. A corner of bed linens that is angled and tucked to lie flat against the mattress

C. Turn back (bed linens) in an accordion fashion

D. A bed that is used by a resident who gets up during the day

E. A lightweight blanket used to provide warmth and privacy when changing the bed while the patient is in it

F. A bed that is made while the patient or resident is in it

G. A pleat made at the bottom of the bed linens to allow room for the toes and feet

H. A bed in a health care facility that is not currently in use

I. A bed that is empty

J. An absorbent pad placed over the bottom sheet to protect the linen from becoming wet or soiled

K. A closed bed that has been opened to allow safe, easy transfer of a patient who is being moved from a stretcher to a bed

Check Your Knowledge

Review Questions: Answer each of the following questions on a separate sheet of paper.

1. List the six environmental conditions in a patient's room that affect comfort and safety.

2. Name the types of furniture usually found in a patient's room.

3. What is an overbed tray used for?

4. List three reasons why bed linen and bedmaking guidelines and procedures should be followed.

5. Why might a health care facility use disposable bed pads instead of washable ones?

6. How can you save steps when bedmaking?

7. What are the three types of unoccupied bed?

8. Why are mitered corners used in bedmaking?

9. Why are the top linens fanfolded in an open bed?

10. How do you make a toe pleat?

True or False: Read each statement carefully. Then write *True* or *False* by the statement number on a separate sheet of paper.

1. Soiled linens should be shaken thoroughly before placing them in the hamper.

2. Soiled linens should be placed on the floor until you are finished making the bed.

3. Some bed linens can be reused when making an occupied bed.

4. Bed linens must be changed whenever they are wet or soiled.

5. A closed bed is an example of an occupied bed.

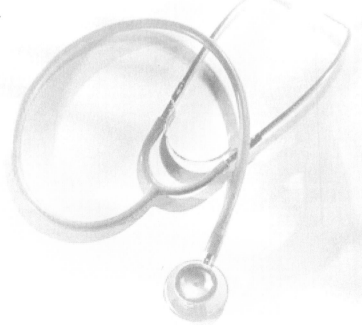

Think and Decide

Directions: Think about each of the following scenarios. Answer each question on a separate sheet of paper.

1. Mrs. A., a new resident, appears to be sad and refuses to participate in any activities. You notice that she does not have any personal items in her room. She does have family in the area. In fact, her son visits frequently. What might you say or do for Mrs. A. to make her feel better?

2. You are working the second shift on a medical floor in a busy hospital. You have just been notified by your charge nurse that a new patient will be coming from the Emergency Department. The patient will be coming to your floor via stretcher and is very ill. Your charge nurse asks you to prepare the room. What will you do?

3. You are making rounds and see you have to do a complete linen change in room 612. What does this mean? What special precautions will be needed?

4. Mr. P. was transferred from the hospital to the long-term care facility two weeks ago. On the first day, he requested an extra blanket on a permanent basis. Today he tells you that he is still cold, even with two blankets, and he has been cold ever since he arrived at the facility. What measures should you take?

5. Mrs. L., a long-term care resident, has complained constantly since a new resident, Mrs. E., was placed in the room next to hers. Mrs. L. explains that Mrs. E. has a very loud speaking voice and stays on the phone all day long. Mrs. L. is accustomed to taking naps in the morning and afternoon, but she cannot sleep because of the noise. How should you handle this situation?

6. Mrs. G. is a long-term care resident whose forgetfulness has been increasingly evident in the last 6 months. She often complains that "someone has taken" her toothbrush. When you look, you find her toothbrush with the rest of her personal hygiene items, inside a little case her daughter brought for her to store the toothbrush. What should you do to relieve Mrs. G.'s mind?

7. Mr. D. is a new long-term care resident. Your facility's policy is to do a complete linen change every other day, unless the bedding is soiled, wet, or extremely wrinkled. The bedding was completely changed yesterday. Today, Mr. D. wants to know why all of the bedding wasn't changed again today. He says he feels "uncomfortable" lying in yesterday's linens. What should you do?

CNA Certification Exam Prep

Directions: This practice test contains ten questions. Each question has four suggested answers. For each question, choose the ONE that best answers the question or completes the statement. Write your answers on a separate sheet of paper.

1. Which of the following helps make the patient's room a pleasant environment?
    A. good lighting
    B. high noise level
    C. visitors allowed 24 hours
    D. slick floors

2. When handling linens,
    A. place dirty linens on the floor.
    B. hold linens away from your uniform.
    C. shake them to remove crumbs.
    D. put wet linens in the utility room.

3. A complete linen change is done when
    A. the bottom linens are wet and soiled.
    B. the bed is made for a new resident.
    C. it is Monday.
    D. there are crumbs in the bed.

4. Most patients are comfortable at temperatures between
    A. 60° and 65° Fahrenheit.
    B. 65° and 70° Fahrenheit.
    C. 68° and 74° Fahrenheit.
    D. 76° and 83° Fahrenheit.

5. What is the difference between a closed bed and an occupied bed?
    A. A closed bed is made while the patient is in it.
    B. An occupied bed is a bed that is not currently in use.
    C. An occupied bed is one being prepared for a new patient.
    D. A closed bed is a bed that is not currently in use.

6. One purpose of a draw sheet is to
    A. lift and move a patient up in bed safely.
    B. remind the patient not to soil the linens.
    C. take the place of a top sheet.
    D. take the place of a bottom sheet.

7. Fanfolded linens are linens that have been
    A. arranged decoratively over the patient.
    B. turned back in accordion fashion.
    C. shaken out to reduce wrinkles.
    D. folded into 12-inch squares.

8. A closed bed that has been opened to allow safe transfer of a patient who is moving from a stretcher to the bed is called a(n)
    A. surgical bed.
    B. occupied bed.
    C. unoccupied bed.
    D. temporary bed.

9. The item that provides warmth and privacy for a patient in bed while the bed is being changed is a
    A. bed pad.
    B. draw sheet.
    C. bath blanket.
    D. top sheet.

10. A table that swings over a patient's bed and holds items the patient needs often is a
    A. bedside stand.
    B. standing table.
    C. overbed table.
    D. end table.

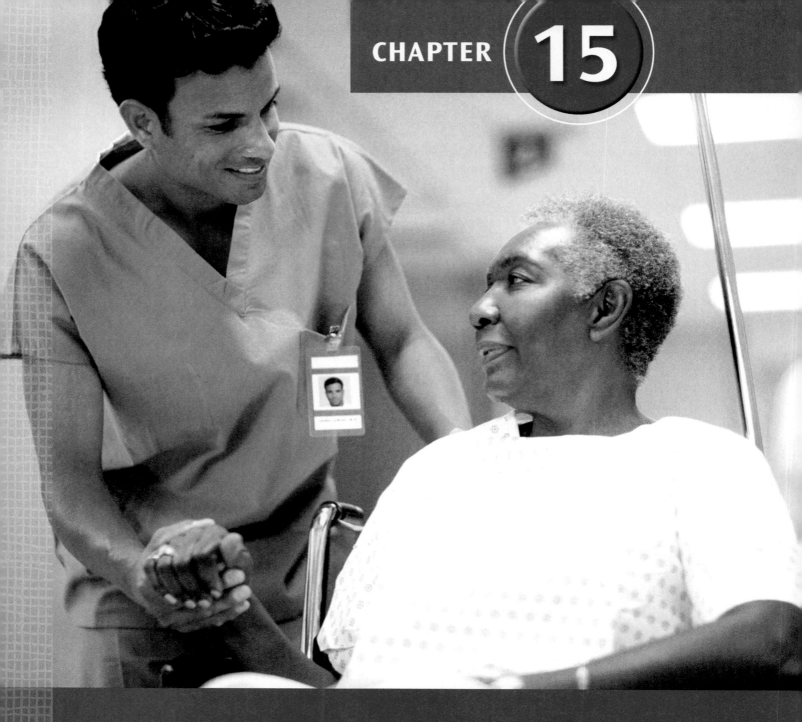

CHAPTER 15

OBJECTIVES

- Describe the nursing assistant's role in the admission process.
- Demonstrate how to prepare a room for a new admission.
- Explain how to take an inventory of the patient's belongings during admission.

- Explain how the nursing assistant helps the new patient get settled in the room.
- Demonstrate the steps in safely admitting a new patient.
- Identify the reasons for transferring a patient or resident.

- Describe the nursing assistant's role in transferring a patient or resident.
- Demonstrate the steps in safely transferring a patient.
- Describe the nursing assistant's role in the discharge process.
- Demonstrate the steps in safely discharging a patient.

Admission, Transfer, and Discharge

VOCABULARY

admission The official entry of a person into a health care facility.

admissions checklist A standard form a health care facility uses for initial impressions and a baseline assessment of a new patient.

discharge A patient's authorized release from a health care facility.

discharge instructions Written documents that outline the information the patient needs about ongoing care.

discharge interview A meeting of the patient, family members, caregivers, and other interested parties with the nurse to learn how to continue the healing process and provide patient care.

discharge plan A plan that outlines ongoing patient care following discharge.

transfer Moving a patient from one unit or room in a facility to another unit or room in the same facility or to a different facility.

transfer form A document that authorizes a patient's transfer and ensures that the patient's care plan is understood by the new staff.

unit A specialized area within a health care facility.

Admission

A person's official entry into a health care facility is called **admission**. The person may arrive from home, from an accident site, or from another health care facility. In the case of an emergency admission to a hospital, the patient arrives directly from the emergency room. Other admissions to long-term care facilities are arranged in advance.

This time is stressful for the patient and family members. Patients are entering an unknown environment. They may be overwhelmed, confused, and frightened. People entering a long-term care facility may also regret leaving home. A nursing assistant's job is to make patients comfortable, both physically and emotionally. You can help by understanding that admission is an important life event to the patient. You can assist the patient by listening and being reassuring.

The patient's first impressions of the health care facility are important. **See Figure 15-1.** A nursing assistant does everything possible to make the admissions process as pleasant as possible for the patient and the family. Your professional, courteous, and caring manner will give the patient confidence about the facility.

The Admissions Process

The admissions process covers the period from the time the patient enters the facility until he or she is settled in the room. The process described here is what happens in most health care facilities. Some facilities have other rules for admitting patients, but the general process and your role in it will be similar. When you start a new job, you will learn the specific rules for that facility.

In a hospital, an admitting clerk in the admitting office or emergency room obtains information about the patient and completes the admissions record. A patient entering a hospital receives an ID bracelet that will be used to identify the patient for all future procedures and medication therapy.

Residents entering long-term care facilities may or may not receive an ID bracelet, depending on the facility's policy. During the admissions process, a picture of the resident is taken and kept in his or her medical record.

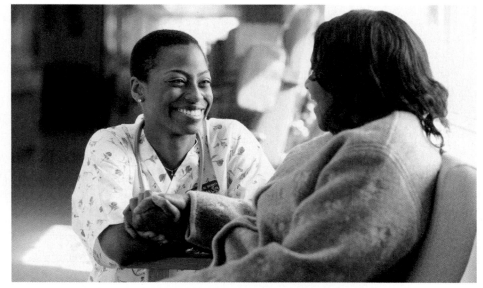

○ Figure 15-1. A new patient entering a facility is likely to be apprehensive at first. A warm greeting from a nursing assistant helps the patient begin to feel more at ease.

After check-in, a nurse or volunteer brings the patient to the nursing unit. In a small long-term care facility, you may meet the patient at the front entrance of the building, along with your supervisor. In a larger facility, you meet the patient in the nursing unit. From this point, a nurse is responsible for the admissions process. Nursing assistants usually help with the following tasks under the supervision of the nurse:

- Preparing the room
- Completing some or all of the questions and procedures on the admissions checklist
- Settling the patient in the room
- Orienting the patient to the new environment

Preparing the Room

A room is prepared for a new resident or patient as soon as the nursing unit is notified that someone is expected. The room should look welcoming so the patient knows that he or she is expected. **See Figure 15-2.** It is the nursing assistant's responsibility to prepare the room. You will need to:

- Find out how the patient will arrive—ambulatory (walking), in a wheelchair, or on a stretcher.
- Lower the bed if the patient is ambulatory or in a wheelchair, or raise the bed if the patient will arrive by stretcher.

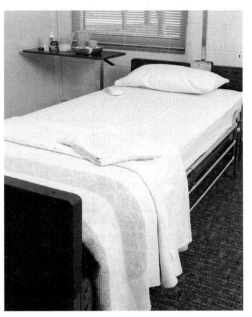
○ **Figure 15-2. This hospital room is ready for a new patient.**

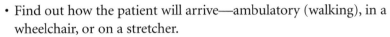
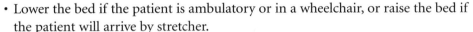

WRITING

Creative Writing—Keeping a Journal

Being a patient in the hospital can be difficult. Some people may be angry at being hospitalized; others may be afraid and wonder if they will be OK. Sometimes people have difficulty expressing their feelings, and it may seem like they are "taking it out" on the hospital staff.

One way for you to understand how a patient might feel is to put yourself in his or her place. For example, maybe you or a loved one has spent some time in the hospital. Do you remember how it felt to be in that strange environment? Were there people on the hospital staff who were particularly helpful (or unhelpful)?

Practice

Imagine that you have just been admitted to the hospital. (You can choose the reason for your admission.) You have been keeping a journal at home, so you decide to continue writing in your journal while you are hospitalized. Write a journal entry of two to three paragraphs for each of three days that you are in the hospital. What kinds of things bothered you? Were you bored, anxious, scared? Was it hard to sleep at night because of all the activity in the hospital? What would it feel like if you had to ask for help every time you needed to go to the bathroom? Include these feelings in your journal.

Procedure 15-1

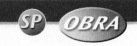

Preparing a Room for a New Admission

Equipment: gown or pajamas (for hospital admission) • admissions checklist • clothing or inventory list • valuables envelope • patient pack (including washbasin, water pitcher, cup, personal care items, emesis basin, tissues, bedpan, or urinal) • urine specimen container, sphygmomanometer, stethoscope, thermometer (for hospital admission)

1. Wash your hands.
2. Open the bed. Fanfold the linens to the bottom of the bed.
3. Neatly fold the gown or pajamas and place them at the foot of the bed.
4. Unpack the patient pack and place the contents in the bedside stand.
5. Arrange the admissions checklist, clothing list, and valuables envelope on the overbed table. For hospital admissions, also collect

a sphygmomanometer, stethoscope, thermometer, and specimen container.
6. Lower the bed if the patient is ambulatory or arriving by wheelchair. Raise the bed if the patient is arriving by stretcher.
7. Clip the signal cord to the linens at the top of the bed within easy reach of the patient.
8. Wash your hands.
9. Report to the supervisor that the room is ready for the patient.

• Open the bed if you work in a hospital. In long-term care, the bed is usually not turned down unless the resident is bedridden.
• Lay out clean hospital clothes if you work in a hospital.
• Prepare initial paperwork and supplies for the patient.
• Find out what specimens are needed and gather the appropriate containers (a necessary step for a hospital admission, but not for a long-term care facility, unless specifically instructed by the nurse).

The Admissions Checklist

In most facilities, the admissions process includes completion of an **admissions checklist**. This is a standard form the facility uses for initial impressions. It also provides a baseline assessment of the new patient. The nurse is responsible for thoroughly completing the checklist. You may be asked to assist in completing some or all of the admissions checklist procedures. **See Figure 15-3.** Observe the patient carefully when you first meet. Listen carefully to what the patient tells you. This information is part of the initial assessment.

The checklist generally includes four areas of information:
• Basic information: name, sex, languages spoken or understood, and mode of transportation for admission
• Condition on admission: mental status, emotional state, scars, disabilities, and any complaints of pain
• Baseline information: vital signs, known allergies, and a list of medications the patient takes. For instance, patients are screened for latex allergy, because many of the tubes, drains, equipment, and gloves used in caregiving are made of latex.

- Orientation to the environment: list of what the patient needs to learn, such as how to operate the television and bed, how to summon help from the nursing staff, and hospital policies about visiting hours and mealtimes

Settling the Patient in the Room

Part of the admissions process is making the patient comfortable in the room. The room may be a permanent home for a resident in a long-term care facility. You can help the person feel physically and emotionally secure in the new surroundings by doing the following:

- Smile. Introduce yourself and give your title. Explain what you do in the facility and how you will be available to help the patient.
- Introduce the patient and family members to a roommate.
- Make the patient comfortable in the chair or bed. Provide seating for family members.
- Put away or help put away the patient's belongings in the closet and drawers. If the room is shared, show the patient which closet and dresser to use.
- Show the patient how to call for help using the call signal.
- Explain how to operate equipment, such as the bed, television, and telephone.
- Briefly explain policies such as visiting hours and how to purchase newspapers.
- Orient the patient to the different areas in the facility by going on a short tour.
- Explain when meals are served and how to complete menus to order meals.
- Answer questions about the facility's services.
- Explain a typical daily routine.
- Answer questions and concerns from the patient, family members, and others.

Rockview Nursing Home ADMISSION FACT SHEET					PATIENT NUMBER
FAMILY NAME	FIRST NAME	MIDDLE NAME	SEX M F	MARITAL STATUS M S W D SEP.	AGE
HOME ADDRESS	CITY	STATE ZIP	HOME PHONE		ALIEN REGISTRATION NO.
SOCIAL SEC. NO.	BIRTH MO. DAY YR. DATE	PLACE OF BIRTH	VETERAN OF WHICH WAR	PREVIOUS OCCUPATION	
NAME OF HUSBAND OR MAIDEN NAME OF WIFE		ADDRESS			BIRTHPLACE
NAME OF FATHER		BIRTHPLACE	MAIDEN NAME OF MOTHER		BIRTHPLACE
NOTIFY IN CASE OF EMERGENCY		RELATIONSHIP	ADDRESS		PHONE
GUARDIAN OR NEAREST RELATIVE		RELATIONSHIP	ADDRESS		PHONE
RELIGION	NAME OF CLERGY		ADDRESS		PHONE
ADMITTED FROM (NAME OF HOSPITAL, INSTITUTION, OR HOME)					
ADMISSION ARRANGED BY:		ADDRESS			PHONE
ATTENDING PHYSICIAN		ADDRESS			PHONE
ADMISSION DATE	A.M. P.M.	MODE OF TRANSPORTATION			

○ Figure 15-3. A standard admissions checklist used in a long-term care facility.

Vital Skills [COMMUNICATION]

Teaching a Patient About the Call Signal

When you first begin working at a facility, familiarize yourself with the call signal. (Different institutions might use different types of call signals.) In some institutions, the call signal is combined with the television remote control. Take a few minutes and practice using the call signal in an empty room.

As a nursing assistant you may be required to teach a patient how to operate a call signal. Explain to patients that they should use the call signal if they need help, particularly when getting out of bed. Call signals are especially important for patients at risk for falling. After you have shown a patient how to use the call light, have him or her demonstrate its use back to you to be sure the patient understands.

Practice

With a partner, pretend that one of you has just been admitted to a hospital room. As the nursing assistant, what would you tell a patient about the call signal? When is it OK for the patient to use the call signal?

The Patient's Personal Belongings

Help the patient unpack all clothing and change into a hospital gown or pajamas in a hospital, or into comfortable clothing in a long-term care facility. List the patient's personal clothing on the clothing sheet or inventory slip according to the facility's policy. Explain that you are going to list each item of clothing on the clothing list. (Items other than clothing can be listed in a section called "Other Belongings," usually at the bottom or on the back of the sheet.) Remember to include the clothes the person wore into the facility. Describe each item but do not assign a dollar value to any item. Both you and the resident (and/or a family member) should sign the clothing list, indicating that you both agree with the inventory. **See Figure 15-4.** Place the clothing neatly in the drawers and closet.

It's best to send items of value, such as jewelry or money, home with the family. However, if the resident prefers to keep valuable items, place them either in a valuables envelope for the facility's safe or in a locked drawer in the resident's room, depending on the facility's policy. In both cases, list each valuable item individually on the valuables envelope. Describe each piece of jewelry by color (yellow if gold, white if silver), without assigning a dollar value to it. Place the items in the envelope. Count the resident's money, place it in the envelope, and seal the envelope. Both you and the resident should sign the envelope. Then take the envelope to the nurse's station. A resident may choose to keep a small amount of money in the bedside stand to purchase newspapers and items from the sundries cart.

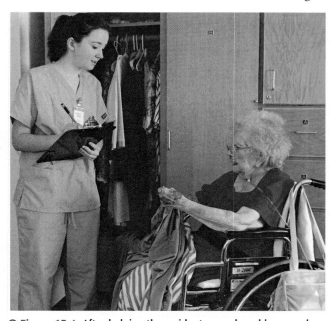

O **Figure 15-4.** After helping the resident unpack and hang up her clothes, the nursing assistant makes a list of the clothes. Both the nursing assistant and the resident sign the list.

Procedure 15-2

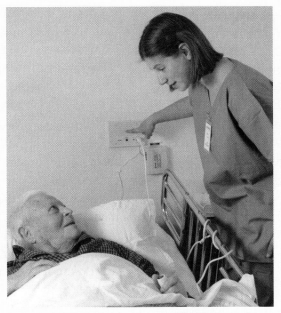

SP · OBRA

Admitting a New Patient

Equipment: none

1. Wash your hands.
2. Greet the patient by name. Check the ID band. Introduce yourself by name and title to the patient and family members. Be friendly and courteous.
3. Introduce the patient to the roommate.
4. Assist the patient to the bed or chair.
5. Provide for patient privacy if the patient feels more comfortable getting settled without family members in the room. Ask the family members to step out of the room. Tell them how long you will be with the patient and direct them to a comfortable waiting area.
6. For a hospital admission, help the patient undress and put on the gown or pajamas. Help the long-term care facility resident into comfortable clothing.
7. Make the patient comfortable in bed or a chair.
8. Put away the patient's street clothes. Complete the clothing list or inventory slip. Put the clothes in the closet or pack them for the family to take home.
9. Place the patient's valuables in the valuables envelope. Complete the form according to policy.
10. Place personal items in the bedside stand.
11. Collect medications the patient has brought from home.
12. Complete the procedures needed on the admissions checklist according to facility policy. These may include measuring the patient's vital signs. Ask about current medications and any medication allergies.
13. If a urine sample is required, describe the procedure for collecting urine. Assist the patient to the bathroom or provide a urinal or bedpan. If you assist the patient to the bathroom, point out the call signal and other safety measures. Practice standard precautions when in contact with urine and other body fluids. Label the specimen according to facility policy.

14. Assist the patient back to the bed or chair.
15. If the patient is allowed to have water, fill the water pitcher and place it within the patient's reach. Some patients entering a hospital have NPO orders, which means they may have no food or fluids by mouth.
16. Orient the patient to the new environment by explaining:
    • A typical daily routine.
    • How to operate the call signal. **See Figure 15-5.**
    • How to operate the bed.
    • The contents of the bedside stand and how each item is used.
    • How to operate the lights.
    • How to operate the telephone and television.

○ **Figure 15-5.** It is important to show the patient how to use the call signal and explain that you will respond and turn off the signal when you come to the room.

- When meals are served and how to fill out a menu. Ask about special dietary preferences (kosher, low-salt, etc.).
- Visiting hours.
- Smoking rules and locations.
- Names of the nursing team members.
- Location of the chapel, library, dining room, and other places of interest.

17. Ask the patient if he or she has any questions.
18. Complete the admissions checklist.
19. Open the curtains or remove the screen if the patient had requested privacy.
20. Deliver the urine specimen, medications, clothing list, valuables envelope, and admissions checklist to the nurse's station.
21. Wash your hands.
22. Invite family members and visitors back in the room if they were asked to leave earlier. Explain visiting hours and policies.
23. Ask the patient if anything else is needed.
24. Before leaving the room, make sure the room is neat, the call signal is within reach of the patient, and the patient is comfortable.
25. Report your observations to the nurse.

FOCUS ON

Transferring a Resident to the Hospital

One of the most difficult transfers is moving from a nursing home to a hospital. The resident has to cope with changing environments and fears about the severity of the medical condition. Residents often express their anxieties to a familiar caregiver. You can respond by being a good listener.

Transfer

A **transfer** occurs when a patient or resident is moved from one unit or room to another in the same facility or to a different facility. A **unit** is a specialized area within a health care facility. For example, hospitals have intensive care units, where patients with acute conditions are cared for. Many long-term care facilities have an Alzheimer's unit, where residents with Alzheimer's disease can get the special care they need. *Note:* The word *transfer* is also used to mean moving a person from a bed to a wheelchair or a stretcher. That type of transfer is covered in Chapter 16.

There are several reasons for transferring a patient:
- A patient may request a transfer if the type of room requested at the time of admission becomes available. For example, a patient in a semiprivate room may move to a private room.
- The family may request a transfer to a facility closer to home.
- A member of the health care team may request a transfer because of a change in the patient's medical condition.

The transfer procedure is carried out according to the policy of the health care facility. The policy ensures that there is no interruption in care. A **transfer form** is a document that provides a doctor's authorization of the transfer and ensures that the patient's care plan is understood by the new staff. This document includes much of the same information about the patient that is found in the medical record.

If the transfer has been ordered by a doctor, the patient may be confused or alarmed. The doctor or nurse will explain the reasons to the patient and family. You can reassure the patient by being supportive and optimistic about the change.

Vital Skills (MATH)

Counting Money

You are admitting Mr. Garcia to your facility. Part of your responsibility is to unpack and put away Mr. Garcia's belongings. You and Mr. Garcia do this together. You then ask Mr. Garcia if he has any belongings he wants to have locked up. He says he has money in his wallet, but adds that he wants to keep three dollars for ready spending and lock up the rest.

You and Mr. Garcia count his money. He has 2 ten-dollar bills, 3 five-dollar bills, and 6 one-dollar bills. How much money does Mr. Garcia have?

$10 + $10 + $5 + $5 + $5 + $1 + $1 + $1 + $1 + $1 + $1 = $41

How much will you lock up?
$41 − $3 = $38

Practice

1. You are helping Mrs. Bailey count her money prior to having it locked up for security. You find that she has 1 twenty-dollar bill, 2 five-dollar bills, and 4 one-dollar bills. How much money does Mrs. Bailey have?
2. Mrs. Bailey wants to keep five dollars in her room. How much do you lock up?

Procedure 15-3

SP OBRA

Transferring a Patient

Equipment: transport equipment according to the patient's needs: wheelchair or stretcher • patient bed cart to transport personal belongings • transfer bag or luggage

1. Before moving the patient, check that the room is ready and that the nurse in the new area is ready to receive the patient. This is usually done via telephone.
2. Find out how the patient will be moved and bring the transport device and cart to the patient's room.
3. Identify the patient. Match the patient's ID bracelet with the ID on the transfer form.
4. Wash your hands.
5. Explain to the patient that you are going to transfer him or her to a new room or unit.
6. Collect the patient's personal belongings. Place them in the patient's luggage or in the transfer bag. **See Figure 15-6.** Place the luggage or bag on the bed, cart, or patient's lap to ensure items are not lost. Use the admissions clothing list to make sure you have all belongings. Have a coworker or family member push the patient cart if necessary.

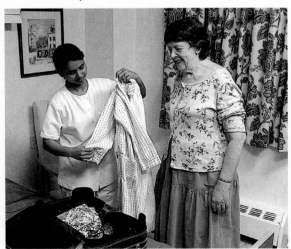

O **Figure 15-6.** The nursing assistant helps the resident pack for a transfer.

7. Physically transfer the patient. (Chapter 16 explains how to do this in greater detail.)
   • By wheelchair: Place the wheelchair near the patient and lock the wheels. Assist the patient into the wheelchair and unlock the wheels. Wheel the patient to the new location.
   • By stretcher: Place the stretcher next to the bed at the proper height. Lock the wheels. Get a coworker to help you move the patient onto the stretcher. Raise the side rails of the stretcher and fasten the safety straps for transport. Unlock the wheels. Push the stretcher to the new location.

SAFETY FIRST

When transferring a patient, wash your hands before gathering belongings, chart, and other items for transfer. Wash them again after you return from transferring the patient. If necessary, follow other standard precautions. Remember, handwashing is the first line of defense protecting you and others from the transmission of pathogens.

8. Introduce the patient to the nursing staff. **See Figure 15-7.** Deliver the patient's chart to the charge nurse (done by the nurse in some facilities).
9. Introduce the patient to the roommate.
10. If the patient prefers privacy while getting settled, provide for privacy.
11. Make the patient comfortable in the bed or chair.
12. Bring the belongings to the new room. Place the clothes in the closet and personal items in the bedside stand.
13. Open the curtains or remove the screen if the patient had requested privacy.

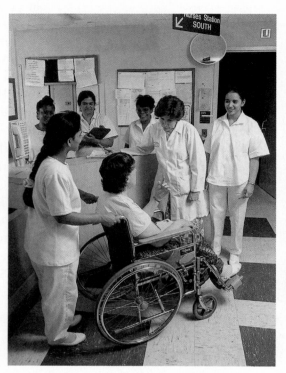

○ **Figure 15-7. It is usually the nursing assistant's responsibility to introduce a new resident to the nursing staff.**

14. Ask the patient if he or she needs anything else.
15. Wash your hands.
16. Hand the medical records to the nurse in the new unit. Do not leave medical records unattended. Point out any medication allergies specifically. Report how the patient tolerated the transfer and relate any observations you made during the transfer.
17. Return to your unit. Report to the nurse that the patient has been transferred and provide the time of the transfer, how the patient tolerated it, and any observations you made during the transfer.
18. Follow your facility's procedure for cleaning the room the patient has vacated.
19. Wash your hands.

Discharge

A patient's authorized release from a health care facility is called a **discharge**. A doctor's order is required for a patient to be discharged from a hospital. In most states, it is also required for a discharge from a long-term care facility. Patients may be discharged home, or they may be discharged to another health care facility.

The discharge process can make patients anxious. Patients may be unsure of their ability to take care of themselves and may wonder who will help them. A patient who is being moved to another health care facility may be nervous about new routines and meeting new people. You can help the patient with this transition by showing empathy, respect, and courtesy during the transfer process.

Occasionally, a patient might decide to leave the health care facility without a doctor's permission. Immediately notify the nurse if a patient tells you he or she is planning to leave or if you see preparation to leave. In other cases, a family member may decide to take a resident out of a facility without a doctor's permission. This also should be reported immediately to the nurse.

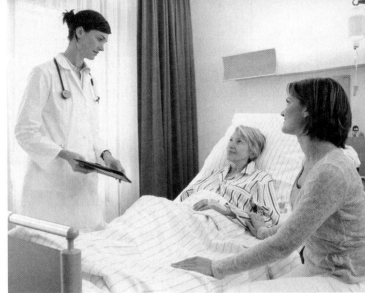

O **Figure 15-8.** During the discharge interview, the nurse instructs the patient and family members about ongoing care.

Discharge Plan

The health care team develops a patient **discharge plan**, a plan that outlines ongoing patient care following discharge. The plan may include instructions and arrangements for home health care, physical therapy, special meals, and other services. A nurse is responsible for the actual discharge process. You may be asked to assist under the supervision of the nurse.

Before leaving a facility, the patient, family members, caregivers, and other interested parties meet with the nurse to learn how to continue the healing process and provide patient care. This meeting is called the **discharge interview. See Figure 15-8.** The nurse provides detailed instructions from the discharge plan to help the patient understand the following concepts.

Discharge Instructions. A patient who leaves a health care facility receives **discharge instructions**, written documents that outline the information the patient needs about ongoing care. **See Figure 15-9.** Most facilities have preprinted discharge forms that the nurse completes with specific information for the patient. The form summarizes the discharge plan. The patient has time to review the instructions before leaving the facility. In some facilities, both patient and nurse are required to sign the instructions in duplicate to verify that they have been explained and that the patient understands them. One copy of the instructions remains in the patient's medical chart.

Disease, Disability, or Illness. Patients have a legal right and a personal need to know about their disease, disability, or illness. The more patients know, the better equipped they are to assist with treatment. The nurse will explain the disease, disability, or illness to the patient, along with any body changes caused by it. The nurse will also describe usual and unusual symptoms and complications that require calling the doctor.

Discharge Instructions After Heart Surgery

Prior to your discharge, you should have received information on the following:

Medications

Upon discharge your nurse and doctor will give you an explanation of all your medications. These instructions will include the medication names, dosage, schedule, and possible side effects.

Diet

You should follow a low-cholesterol diet. Instructions regarding this diet will be given by the dietitian prior to your discharge.

Risk Factors

Your risk factors for the development of arteriosclerosis have been discussed. You should be aware of these risk factors and make plans to modify your lifestyle to reduce these risk factors.

Common Activities

Bathing. Showers are usually allowed within 24 hours after you are allowed out of bed. Wash normally, with any kind of soap and water but do not apply unusual pressure at the site of the catheter insertion. Pat dry instead of rubbing the skin dry around the site. No baths for three days because the bath water may be a medium for infection into the bloodstream.

Site Care. A band-aid may or may not be applied. If it is, it can be removed. Bruising will gradually fade within one to two weeks. A hematoma (collection of blood in the tissue) may be painful to touch but should also reduce in size and tenderness within one to two weeks. If increased bruising, swelling, or infection is noted, your doctor should be notified immediately. Also, watch for any signs of infection such as drainage, warmth, redness, or increased temperature from the site.

Activity. Most patients who have had angioplasty, atherectomy, or stent can return to their daily routine within three days to one week unless they have heart damage (heart attacks). Patients with heart damage may be told to resume activity more slowly. Check with your doctor. All patients should avoid lifting anything greater than 5–10 pounds during the first few days home.

Driving. Driving can be resumed within a few days to one week unless you have been told you had heart damage (heart attack). Patients with heart damage should check with their cardiologist before driving. All patients should arrange to have someone drive them home from the hospital.

Working. Ask your doctor when you will be able to return to work. The nature of your occupation plus your progress will determine this. Patients may return within several days to several weeks.

Sex. If you are able to climb a flight of stairs comfortably, you can resume sexual activity.

Exercise. The day after you go home, begin walking 2–3 times per day. Start out walking about the same amount you did in the hospital. Increase the distance based on tolerance. Extreme shortness of breath, dizziness, extreme fatigue, or chest discomfort are all signs that you are doing more than your heart is ready for. If these occur, stop and rest. Next time you walk, slow down and/or cut back on the distance. If these symptoms persist after resting, notify your physician.

Office Visit

Follow up with your physician in 1–2 weeks after discharge from the hospital. A follow-up treadmill test will be performed to determine the success of the procedure and the current status of your physical and cardiac condition. Then you will be required to enter a Cardiac Rehab Phase II program located closest to your home as part of your recovery program.

For more information, call the Cardiac Unit at University Hospital at 800-555-0000.

○ **Figure 15-9.** Sample discharge instructions used in a hospital cardiac unit.

Ongoing Treatments. Treatments that have been provided in a health care setting often must be continued at home. The nurse explains and demonstrates these procedures to the patient and makes sure the patient or a family member can perform the procedures correctly.

Physical Activity. Before resuming normal activity, the patient needs to heal. The activities of daily living he or she can engage in are increased as the patient gains strength. The nurse will explain the expected progression to normal activity. He or she will also describe restrictions or limitations in physical activity and demonstrate special exercises to help the healing process.

Nutrition and Diet. A healthy diet is important to strengthen the body and help the healing process. A doctor may order a special diet. Most facilities have a *dietitian*, a health care professional who plans nutritious meals based on special needs. A dietitian will develop a special diet for the patient to follow outside the facility. The nurse or dietitian will teach the patient the purpose of the special diet, what foods are allowed, and the amounts of foods to be eaten.

Medications. Patients often need to continue taking medications after they leave a health care facility. The nurse will teach the patient the name and purpose of each medication, when to take it, how much to take, and expected side effects. The nurse will also describe side effects that the patient should report to a doctor.

Future Appointments. Continuing care is usually needed to track the patient's condition. The nurse will tell the patient the name of the doctor providing care and the dates and times of future appointments.

Referral Agencies. Many communities have agencies that provide services to patients and their families. These agencies can provide emotional support, medical and financial assistance, and special services, such as hot meals and home health care. Referrals are often made before discharge to maintain continuity of care. The patient is given the names and phone numbers of local agencies, and the types of services each agency provides.

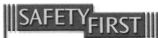

SAFETY FIRST

When transporting patients by wheelchair or stretcher, make sure to lock the wheels before you assist the patient onto the device. If the wheels are not locked, the device could move and the patient could fall and be injured.

Procedure 15-4

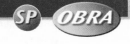

Discharging a Patient

Equipment: transport equipment according to the patient's needs: wheelchair or stretcher • patient bed cart to transport personal belongings

1. Check that the doctor has ordered the discharge. Make sure that all written orders and other paperwork are complete before you begin the patient discharge procedure.
2. Ask the nurse if any equipment or supplies are going home with the patient. Make sure they are clean.
3. Wash your hands.
4. Identify the patient. Check the patient's ID bracelet against the ID on the discharge order.
5. Provide privacy for the patient.
6. Explain that you are preparing the patient to be discharged.

7. Help the patient dress.
8. Help the patient collect all personal belongings. Check the clothes against the clothing list that was completed when the patient was admitted. Have the patient sign the list to indicate that all clothing has been returned.
9. Pack the patient's personal belongings. Check drawers, closet, bedside stand, and bathroom for belongings.
10. Return valuables according to facility policy. Check the valuables against the inventory made at the time of admission. Have the patient sign the list to indicate that all valuables have been returned.
11. Tell the nurse that the patient is ready for the discharge interview. The nurse will give the patient discharge instructions and prescriptions for medications.
12. After the interview, physically transfer the patient.
    - By wheelchair: Place the wheelchair near the patient and lock the wheels. Assist the patient into the wheelchair and unlock the wheels.
    - By stretcher: Place the stretcher next to the bed at the proper height. Lock the wheels. Get a coworker to help you move the patient onto the stretcher. Raise the side rails of the stretcher and fasten the safety straps for transport. Unlock the wheels.
13. Place the patient's belongings on the cart.
14. Carry out the discharge procedure according to the facility. Patients may be required to visit the business office or discharge desk before leaving. Make sure the charge nurse or the business office removes the ID bracelet if one was given at admission. Give the discharge paperwork to the patient or family member according to facility policy.
15. Take the patient to the front entrance. Have someone follow with the patient's belongings. Remember, the patient is the facility's responsibility until he or she leaves the facility. The patient must be safely escorted

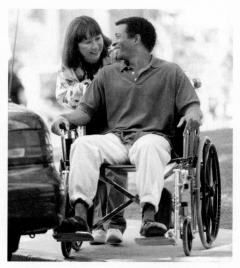

○ **Figure 15-10.** In many facilities, the nursing assistant escorts the patient to a waiting car at the facility's entrance after the discharge process.

out of the building to the waiting transport vehicle (car or ambulance). **See Figure 15-10.** Send off the patient and family members pleasantly.
16. Lock the wheelchair or stretcher wheels. Assist the patient from the wheelchair or stretcher and into the waiting vehicle.
17. Place the patient's luggage in the transport vehicle.
18. Say good-bye to the patient and close the vehicle door.
19. Return the wheelchair or stretcher to the unit. Clean and return the equipment.
20. Wash your hands.
21. Return to the patient's room. Strip the bed and place the linen in the dirty linen hamper according to the facility's policies and procedures, using standard precautions.
22. Notify the housekeeping department that the room is ready to be cleaned.
23. Wash your hands.
24. Take the paperwork to the nurse according to facility policy. Report the time of the patient's discharge, the transport device used (wheelchair, etc.), who accompanied the patient (parent, child, etc.), how the patient tolerated the procedure, and observations of anything unusual.

Concept Map or Web

One way to remember what you read is to organize the information into a *concept map*, also called a *concept web*. Concept maps are a good way to organize information visually and to help you see how ideas are connected. A concept map has one central idea or point. Related points are arranged around the center like spokes around a wheel.

To construct a map, read the assigned text and write down the central point in the middle of a sheet of paper. Place secondary, or related, ideas around the map, radiating out from the central point. Add secondary information to the map quickly by jotting down ideas as they pop into your head. Don't edit or think too much about what you should add; just let your ideas flow.

When secondary ideas are related to each other, they can be connected with a line. You may also have ideas branching from the secondary ideas. Concept maps can also have lists or notes explaining an idea. Arrows can point from one idea to a related one. You can be as creative as you'd like. The point is to organize the information in a way that makes sense to you and will help you remember it. **Figure A** is a concept map for a patient being admitted to the hospital.

Practice

After reading the section in this chapter about patient discharge, draw a concept map similar to the one in Figure A. Include at least five secondary ideas.

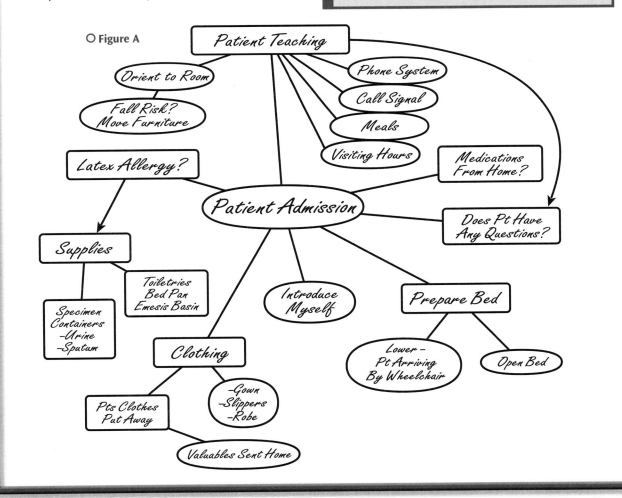

○ **Figure A**

Patient Teaching
- *Orient to Room*
- *Fall Risk? Move Furniture*
- *Phone System*
- *Call Signal*
- *Meals*
- *Visiting Hours*
- *Medications From Home?*
- *Does Pt Have Any Questions?*

Latex Allergy?

Patient Admission
- *Supplies*
  - *Toiletries Bed Pan Emesis Basin*
  - *Specimen Containers –Urine –Sputum*
- *Introduce Myself*
- *Prepare Bed*
  - *Lower – Pt Arriving By Wheelchair*
  - *Open Bed*
- *Clothing*
  - *Pts Clothes Put Away*
  - *–Gown –Slippers –Robe*
  - *Valuables Sent Home*

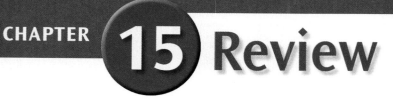
Chapter Summary

- The nursing assistant assists the nurse in the admission process by preparing the room for the new patient, completing part of the admissions checklist, taking an inventory of the patient's personal belongings, and helping the patient get settled and oriented.

- Patients can be transferred to a new room, unit, or facility at their request, at their family's request, or by doctor's orders.

- The nursing assistant helps in the transfer process by making sure the new location is ready, helping the patient get ready, collecting the patient's belongings, safely transferring the patient, and introducing the patient to new staff and other patients.

- The nursing assistant helps the nurse in the discharge process by helping the patient gather belongings, retrieving valuables from the safe, making sure the patient has a discharge interview and receives discharge instructions, and safely assisting the patient to a waiting transport vehicle.

- During the discharge interview, the nurse teaches the patient about all aspects of ongoing care, treatment, and healing.

VOCABULARY REVIEW

Directions: Match the letter of each definition in the second column with the correct vocabulary term in the first column. Write your answers on a separate sheet of paper.

Vocabulary

1. admission
2. admissions checklist
3. discharge
4. discharge instructions
5. discharge interview
6. discharge plan
7. transfer
8. transfer form

Definitions

A. A document that authorizes a patient's transfer and ensures that the patient's care plan is understood by the new staff

B. Written documents that outline the information the patient needs about ongoing care

C. A plan that outlines ongoing patient care following discharge

D. A standard form a health care facility uses for initial impressions and a baseline assessment of a new patient

E. Moving a patient from one unit or room in a facility to another unit or room in the same facility or to a different facility

F. The official entry of a person into a health care facility

G. A patient's authorized release from a health care facility

H. A meeting of the patient, family members, caregivers, and other interested parties with the nurse to learn how to continue the healing process and provide patient care

Check Your Knowledge

Review Questions: Answer each of the following questions on a separate sheet of paper.

1. Who is responsible for the admissions process?

2. List four tasks the nursing assistant may help with during the admissions process.

3. What kinds of baseline information is included on the admissions checklist?

4. Who needs to sign the clothing list?

5. Why might a patient be transferred from a long-term care facility to a hospital?

6. Who physically transfers the patient from one room to another room?

7. What is required for a patient to be discharged from a hospital?

8. What should you do if a resident tells you that he or she is planning to leave the nursing home?

9. During the discharge interview, who teaches the patient about ongoing treatments and medications?

10. What does the dietitian teach the patient about nutrition and a special diet before discharge?

True or False: Read each statement carefully. Then write *True* or *False* by the statement number on a separate sheet of paper.

1. The patient's room is prepared after the patient arrives in the nursing unit.

2. A patient's valuables should be hidden in the bedside stand or closet.

3. When transferring a patient, first take the patient's belongings to the new unit, and then come back for the patient.

4. A patient must have a written doctor's order to be discharged.

5. Patients need to understand their disease or illness so they can assist in their ongoing care.

Think and Decide

Directions: Think about each of the following scenarios. Answer each question on a separate sheet of paper.

1. John Taylor just entered a long-term care facility. How might the admissions process be stressful to John and his family?

2. Mrs. F. is recovering from a broken hip. She has been in the hospital for four days. Her care plan now says that she is ready for transfer to the skilled nursing unit for rehabilitation. How will you prepare Mrs. F. for transfer?

3. Emma Johnson can no longer take care of herself at home. Her family feels she needs constant care. Emma will be arriving at the long-term care facility by car. The Admissions Coordinator tells you that Emma will be arriving at 1400. What will you do for Emma when she arrives?

4. Mrs. T. is a first-time resident who has been living at home with her son and his wife. As you are settling her into her new room and making the admission clothing list, Mrs. T. confides to you that she has brought her jewelry with her "for safekeeping." Upon further examination, you find that she has a case containing a diamond ring and several other expensive pieces of jewelry. You suggest that Mrs. T. allow you to have the jewelry locked up for safety, but she insists that she "must" keep it with her. She becomes very agitated during the discussion. What should you do?

5. Mr. D. wants to leave the long-term care facility where he has lived for the last 13 months. He asks you to take him out to the side entrance of the facility. He states that his son will pick him up. What should you do in this situation?

6. E. H. is a new resident who is just being admitted to the long-term care facility where you work. He seems to be very nervous and afraid, and he replies hesitantly, "I don't know" whenever anyone asks him a question. What can you do to ease E. H.'s stress?

7. Mr. Y. is finally ready to go home after being hospitalized for several days for major surgery. During the discharge interview, Mrs. Y. seems not to be paying much attention to the nurse's instructions, and Mr. Y. looks confused. How can you be sure the discharge instructions are carried out?

8. Mrs. W., P.C.'s roommate at the long-term care facility, was transferred to the hospital yesterday for surgery. Every time you enter P.C.'s room, she asks you again, "How is Mrs. W. doing? How did the surgery go?" What should you tell P.C.?

CNA Certification Exam Prep

Directions: This practice test contains ten questions. Each question has four suggested answers. For each question, choose the ONE that best answers the question or completes the statement. Write your answers on a separate sheet of paper.

1. Who is responsible for the admissions process?

    A. the nursing assistant

    B. the nurse

    C. the physician

    D. the dietitian

2. The patient's valuables are handled according to facility policy. In most facilities, they are placed

    A. in the patient's suitcase.

    B. in the bedside table.

    C. in the facility safe.

    D. in the closet.

3. The patient's discharge order is written by

    A. the patient's family.

    B. a member of the clergy.

    C. the nurse.

    D. the patient's doctor.

4. What do you do if a patient tells you she is leaving the health care facility without a doctor's orders?

    A. help her pack

    B. notify the nurse immediately

    C. try to talk her out of it

    D. lock her door

5. Which of the following is considered the patient's personal property?

    A. dentures

    B. bedpan

    C. bed linens

    D. visitor's chair

6. When discharging a patient, transport the patient

    A. to the front door of the building.

    B. out of the building to a waiting vehicle.

    C. to the elevator.

    D. to the patient's home.

7. A patient's authorized release from a health care facility is a(n)

    A. admission.

    B. transfer.

    C. discharge.

    D. exchange.

8. When a patient is ready to leave a facility, who needs to meet to discuss the patient's discharge instructions?

    A. patient, doctor, and nursing assistant

    B. doctor, nurse, and nursing assistant

    C. patient, family/caregivers, and nurse

    D. patient, doctor, and nurse

9. The list of a resident's clothing and personal belongings that is made and signed when the resident first arrives is a(n)

    A. admission clothing list.

    B. admissions checklist.

    C. discharge checklist.

    D. discharge interview.

10. The written instructions given to a patient being discharged from a facility are the

    A. discharge instructions.

    B. discharge interview.

    C. transfer form.

    D. discharge form.

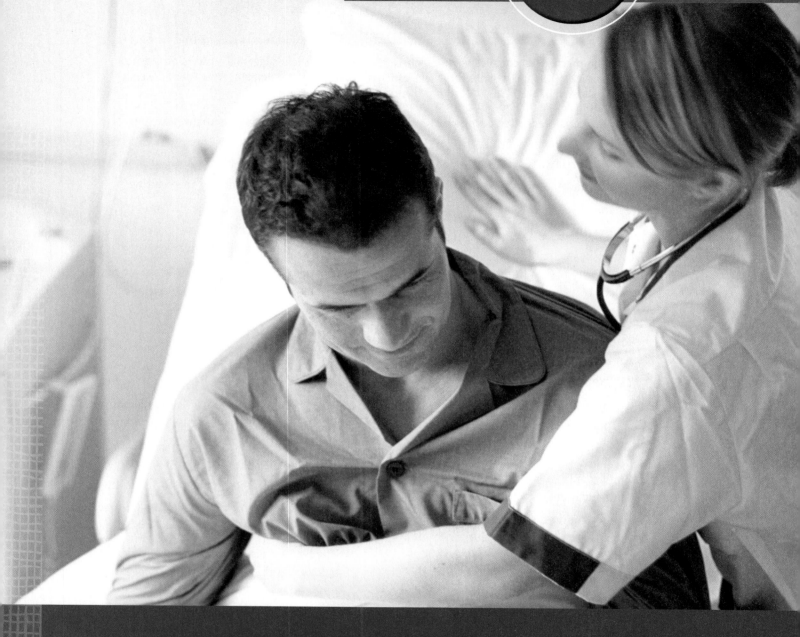

OBJECTIVES

- Explain the importance of proper body mechanics, posture, and body alignment.
- Identify principles of using proper body mechanics.
- Identify various positioning and draping techniques.

- Explain ways to reduce friction and shearing force when moving patients.
- Demonstrate safe and effective methods for moving patients in bed.
- Identify assistive devices for moving and transferring patients safely.

- Demonstrate safe and effective methods of transferring patients.
- Describe safe and effective methods of transporting patients.

Body Mechanics

bedridden Confined to bed.

body alignment The proper positioning of the head, back, and limbs in a straight line.

body mechanics The positions and movements that help the body maintain proper posture and prevent injury.

body support A brace that supports the back when worn properly to perform lifting, moving, or transferring tasks.

dangle To sit up and allow the legs to hang loosely over the side of the bed for a short while.

dorsal recumbent position The patient is positioned lying flat on the back with the legs close together, the knees flexed, and the soles of the feet flat on the mattress.

draping Covering part or all of a patient's body with a sheet, blanket, or other material.

Fowler's position A semi-sitting position with the head of the bed raised between a 45° and 60° angle and the knees slightly flexed.

friction A force caused by the rubbing of one surface against another.

horizontal recumbent position The patient is positioned lying flat on the back with the legs close together.

knee-chest position The patient lies face down with knees flexed at a 90° angle and the chest touching the bed or table.

lateral position The patient is lying on his or her side.

logrolling A method for turning the patient onto the side in one movement to keep the spine aligned.

mechanical lift A lifting device that assists in raising, lowering, and transferring patients.

orthostatic hypotension A drop in blood pressure when a change in position occurs.

pressure sore An area on the skin that is broken down.

prone position The patient lies on the abdomen.

reverse-Trendelenburg's position A position in which the entire bed is tilted so that the patient's head is slightly higher than the feet.

semi-Fowler's position A semi-sitting position with the head raised to a 45° angle and the portion of the bed under the knee raised 15°, if possible.

shearing force A combination of friction and pressure.

Sims' position The patient lies in a semi-prone position on the left side with the right knee flexed up toward the abdomen. The left knee is also flexed, but not as much as the right knee.

slide board A device used to assist in patient transfers at even levels.

stretcher A cart with wheels for transporting patients from one place to another while they are lying down.

supine position The patient is positioned lying flat on the back.

transfer To move a patient from one item of furniture or equipment to another.

transfer belt A belt that buckles around a patient's waist and provides a handle for the nursing assistant to hold onto when transferring a patient.

transport To move a patient from place to place using a transport device, such as a wheelchair or stretcher.

Trendelenburg's position A position in which the entire bed is tilted so that the patient's feet are slightly higher than the head.

turning sheet A sheet used by two nursing assistants to move or turn a patient in bed; another term for *draw sheet*.

Using Proper Body Mechanics

Your tasks as a nursing assistant involve almost constant movement. You will make beds, assist patients to use the commode, move medical equipment, and generally be on the go. You will move patients into different positions in bed and transfer patients from beds to wheelchairs and stretchers. You will also push the wheelchairs and stretchers from place to place. To avoid injury and keep patients safe, nursing assistants (and all other health care employees) use proper body mechanics to bend, lift, push, and pull.

Body mechanics are the positions and movements that help the body maintain correct posture and prevent injury to muscles and bones. Maintaining correct posture puts muscles and other body parts into alignment. **Body alignment** is the proper positioning of the head, back, and limbs in a straight line. **See Figure 16-1.** The body performs more efficiently when it is properly aligned. Correct posture and body alignment promote proper blood flow, prevent injuries and deformities, and enhance comfort.

Some facilities require nursing assistants to wear a brace called a **body support** to support the back. **See Figure 16-2.** Body supports come in a variety of sizes. If you wear a body support, make sure it fits snugly when you are performing a task that requires strength.

Some states have a "no lift" policy that prevents health care workers from lifting patients at all. If your state allows health care workers to lift patients, follow these principles of good body mechanics to prevent injury and fatigue.

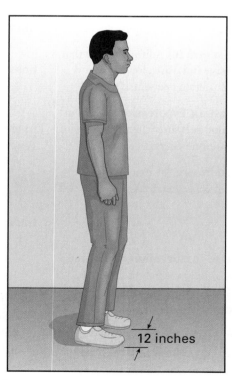

O **Figure 16-1.** Correct standing posture. Feet are flat on the floor, 12 inches apart. Back is straight, knees are slightly flexed, and arms hang at the sides.

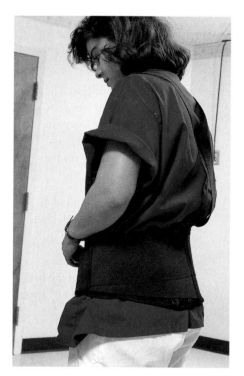

O **Figure 16-2.** Body supports, also called back braces, surround the waist and hip area and provide extra support.

- The muscles in your back are not as large and powerful as the muscles in your shoulders, arms, hips, and legs. When lifting or moving patients or heavy objects, use the stronger, larger muscles or groups of muscles. Bend your knees and lift using the muscles of your legs, not your back. **See Figure 16-3.**
- When moving a heavy object, use the weight of your body to push, roll, or pull it instead of lifting it.
- When lifting a heavy object, keep it close to your body. Keep your back straight and place your feet 12 inches apart. This provides a wide base of support.
- If an object feels too heavy to lift, get help. Do not even attempt to lift an object that appears heavy or unwieldy.
- Do not lift heavy items higher than chest level.
- Always lift in a smooth motion to prevent injury. If you are working with another person to lift or move a patient, count "one, two, three" before starting, so your movements will be smooth and coordinated.
- Maintain good body posture and alignment. Keep your back straight and distribute your weight evenly on both feet with a broad base of support.
- Avoid twisting your body. Turn your whole body to face the object you will be moving or lifting. Pivot your feet in the direction you move.

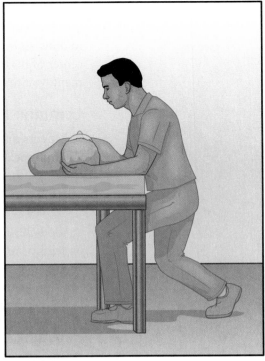

○ **Figure 16-3.** Proper body mechanics for lifting include bent knees and a wide base of support.

Positioning and Draping Patients

One of the nursing assistant's responsibilities is to position and drape patients. Some patients are able to move themselves into new positions. Other patients, such as those who are paralyzed or recovering from surgery, will need your assistance. Always check the rules for your facility before positioning a patient.

Vital Skills READING

Asking Questions

Asking yourself questions about what you read is an excellent reading technique. Good readers are constantly asking questions as they read. You can ask questions about the writer and the material, or even question yourself as you read.

For example, as you read the section on proper body mechanics, you might ask yourself, "How is this information useful in my own life?" Where lifting techniques are described,

you might wonder, "Do I always use proper posture and lift using my legs instead of my back?"

Practice

As you read this chapter, compile a list of at least five questions related to the material. They can be questions about the author or the material. They can also be questions that you ask yourself. Share your questions with the class.

Positioning the patient includes making sure that the body is in proper alignment. When you stand at the foot of the bed or exam table, you should be able to draw an imaginary straight line from the top of the patient's head through the center of his or her body to a spot between the feet. To keep the body in alignment, you may need to use support devices, such as pillows or rolled-up towels.

Common Positions

Patients may need to be moved into different positions for several reasons:
- For physical comfort, as well as for general well-being
- For examinations and medical procedures
- To improve circulation to extremities and prevent medical complications such as pressure sores, especially for patients who are bedridden

You will need to know the most common positions so that you can help patients or residents when these positions are required. Refer to **Figure 16-4** as you read about the various positions.
- **Supine**—patient lies on the back. There are two types of supine positions:
  - **Horizontal recumbent**—patient lies flat on the back with the legs close together.
  - **Dorsal recumbent**—patient lies flat on the back, with legs separated, knees flexed and supported, and the soles of the feet flat on the mattress.

Vital Skills   MATH

Estimating Angles

Some of the common patient positions specify the angles to which the patient's head and knees are raised. Unfortunately, hospital beds are not marked with angles, so you may need to estimate the angle at which you position a patient's head and knees. In **Figure A**, a *protractor* (instrument for measuring angles) is used to show the three angles most often used in positioning patients. Study these angles and try to visualize patients positioned with their heads and knees in the appropriate positions for Fowler's and semi-Fowler's positions.

Practice

Remember that in Fowler's position, the head of the bed may be raised anywhere from 45° to 60°. Use the protractor in Figure A as a guide to create the following sketches.

1. Sketch a patient in Fowler's position with the head of the bed raised to 50°.
2. Sketch a patient in Fowler's position with the head of the bed raised to 55°.

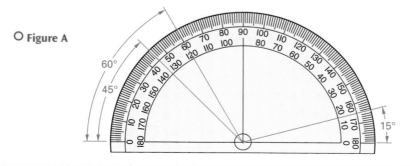

O **Figure A**

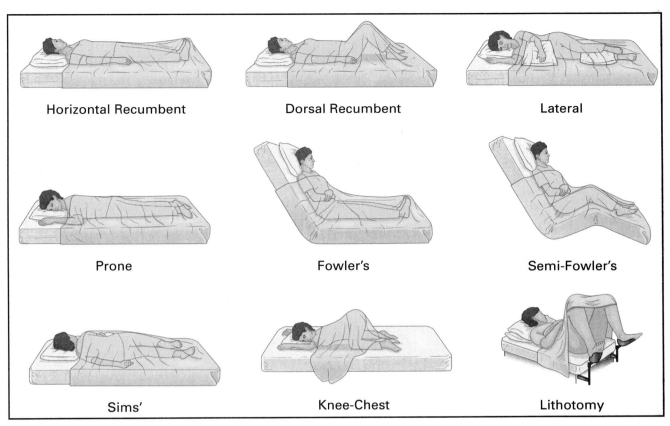

Horizontal Recumbent	Dorsal Recumbent	Lateral
Prone	Fowler's	Semi-Fowler's
Sims'	Knee-Chest	Lithotomy

○ **Figure 16-4.** Common patient positions. Notice the draping for each position.

- **Lateral**—patient lies on his or her side. The hips are closer to one side of the bed than to the other. The knees are flexed, the top leg more than the other and supported with a pillow. This position may be used to prevent skin breakdown around the coccyx (tailbone).
- **Prone**—patient lies on the abdomen. The arms are either straight alongside the body or flexed at the elbows. The patient's head is turned to one side.
- **Fowler's**—a semi-sitting position with the head of the bed raised to between a 45° and 60° angle and the knees slightly flexed. Fowler's position is commonly used for people with breathing difficulties or with heart disease, such as congestive heart failure.
- **Semi-Fowler's**—a semi-sitting position with the head raised to a 45° angle. The portion of the bed under the knee, or the knee hinge of the bed, is generally raised 15°. This position is used for patients with head injuries to minimize swelling in the head. Raising the knees may interfere with circulation, so check with your supervisor before putting a patient into this position. Check the patient's circulation periodically.
- **Sims'**—the patient lies in a semi-prone position on the left side with the right knee flexed up toward the abdomen. The left knee is also flexed, but not as much as the right knee. The left arm lies straight down behind the body. The right arm is supported by a pillow and lies in front of the body in a comfortable position. This position is used when measuring a rectal temperature, cleaning the perineum, or giving an enema.
- **Knee-chest**—patient lies face down with knees flexed at a 90° angle and the chest touching the bed or table. The head is turned to one side. The arms extend forward beyond the head and are flexed slightly. This position is used mostly for examinations.

- **Lithotomy**—the patient lies on the back, with the thighs flexed on the stomach and the lower legs on the thighs. This position is often used for women's surgical procedures or exams that involve the perineum and the bladder.
- **Trendelenburg**—the entire bed is tilted so that the feet are slightly higher than the head. The patient is supine. Trendelenburg's position used to be thought to increase blood pressure for patients in shock. However, research has shown that elevating the legs is just as effective and does not promote swelling in the brain. Trendelenburg's also creates breathing problems by constricting heart and lung functions. This position is rarely used.
- **Reverse Trendelenburg**—the entire bed is tilted so that the head is slightly higher than the feet. The patient is supine. The position is used for visualization and examination of the head and neck, but only rarely.

Draping Patients

Draping is covering part or all of a patient's body with a sheet, blanket, or other material. This maintains privacy and dignity. Draping is usually done after positioning a patient. Patients are often covered in preparation for surgery or during an examination. Notice the position of the drapes in **Figure 16-4**.

Safely Moving Patients in Bed

Some patients are **bedridden**, or confined to bed, for long periods of time. Even if these patients are in proper body alignment, serious injury to skin, blood vessels, muscles, and bones can occur if they are left in one position for too long.

Moving and positioning patients who cannot move themselves is an important part of a nursing assistant's work. To maintain your safety and the patient's safety, comfort, and dignity when moving or lifting patients:
- Know when to get assistance.
- Use proper body mechanics. Never twist your body when lifting.
- Plan your movements to avoid putting yourself or the patient at risk for injury.
- Take your time and move slowly and carefully.
- Speak normally and explain what you are doing. Even an unconscious patient may be able to hear.
- Maintain the patient's privacy.
- Make sure the patient's body is in alignment.

Getting Assistance

You may be able to move children and lightweight adults by yourself. However, two or more helpers may be necessary, depending on the weight of the patient and the patient's ability to assist. For example, a patient who has had back surgery or a spinal injury must be moved very carefully by several people using a technique called **logrolling**. This is a method for turning the patient onto the side in one movement to keep the spine aligned, preventing further injury.

Avoiding Pressure Sores

The integumentary system is at risk in patients who are bedridden. The skin may rub against the bed linens, creating **friction**. This is a force caused by the rubbing of one surface against another. **Shearing force** is a combination of fric-

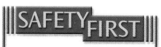

SAFETY FIRST

Always use proper body mechanics when moving patients, especially patients who cannot assist. It is wise to have a helper whenever possible.

Read Your Writing Out Loud

A good way to improve your writing is to read it out loud. When you hear yourself speak what you have written, you might catch mistakes that may otherwise slip through. You can also pick out sentences that don't sound quite right, are too "wordy," or are repetitive. After you read your writing out loud, you can go back and edit your work.

For example, below are two notes describing the same event. Read each note out loud. Does one sound better than the other?

1. Mary went down the hall to Mrs. Tyler's room because she saw that Mrs. Tyler had rung the call signal and she wanted to go see what she wanted. When Mary got to Mrs. Tyler's room, Mrs. Tyler was crying and said to Mary that she was upset that she couldn't get up out of the bed on her own because she felt like she wasn't strong enough to do it and she won-

dered if Mary could help. So Mary helped her out of bed and into a chair that was next to the bed.

2. Mrs. Tyler rang her call signal and Mary went to see what she needed. Mary arrived at Mrs. Tyler's room to find her crying. Mrs. Tyler said she was upset because she did not feel strong enough to get out of bed. She asked Mary for help. Mary helped her out of bed and into a chair.

Did the second paragraph sound better to you? It is more concise and easier to read.

Practice

Read the section describing different ways patients can be positioned in bed. Write a paragraph describing at least two of the positions. Read the paragraph aloud and make changes if you catch any errors or find a way to improve it.

---

tion and pressure. It can occur when a patient is moved by sliding or dragging instead of lifting. Shearing force can cause serious injury to delicate skin and the tissues under the skin. The skin may then develop **pressure sores**, areas that are broken down because of constant pressure or friction. (See Chapter 22 for more information about pressure sores.)

To minimize friction and shearing force, do not slide or drag the patient in bed. Instead, roll or lift the patient using a turning sheet. A **turning sheet** is a sheet used by two nursing assistants to move or turn a patient in bed.

Preventing Orthostatic Hypotension

Patients who are bedridden are also at risk for **orthostatic hypotension**, which is a drop in blood pressure when a change in position occurs. Bed rest is not the only cause of orthostatic hypotension, so you should always be cautious when a patient changes position from lying to sitting or from sitting to standing.

To prevent symptoms of orthostatic hypotension, assist the patient slowly to a sitting or standing position to allow time for the cardiovascular and nervous systems to adjust. If the patient experiences lightheadedness or dizziness, help the patient lie down. Check blood pressure, pulse, and respirations, and report the patient's condition to the nurse.

In some cases, such as recovering from surgery, you will be ordered to assist a patient to **dangle**, or to sit up and allow the legs to hang loosely over the side of the bed for a short time.

Procedure 16-1

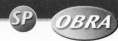

Helping a Patient Sit and Dangle

Equipment: none

1. Identify the patient, check the patient's ID band, and call the patient by name.
2. Introduce yourself and explain the procedure to the patient.
3. Wash your hands.
4. Provide privacy.
5. Decide which side of the bed the patient will sit on.
6. Check to make sure the wheels of the bed are locked.
7. Raise the bed to a working height that is appropriate for good body mechanics.
8. If the patient is not positioned properly in bed, help the patient move up in bed.
9. Fanfold the top linens down to the foot of the bed.
10. If the patient can move in bed, ask the patient to move to the side of the bed. Provide assistance as necessary.
11. Raise the head of the bed until the patient is sitting up.
12. Lower the side rail.
13. Place one arm under the patient's neck and shoulders. Place your other arm under the patient's knees. **See Figure 16-5.**
14. Gently turn the patient so the legs hang over the edge of the bed. This is dangling. **See Figure 16-6.**

15. Observe the patient's condition. Check the pulse and respirations. Help the patient lie down immediately if he or she does not feel well, has difficulty breathing, becomes dizzy or lightheaded, or is uncomfortable sitting up. Report to the nurse.
16. Stay with the patient while he or she is sitting up.
17. Assist the patient in putting on a robe and slippers, if appropriate. The robe should be nearby. Never leave the patient alone.
18. When the patient is ready to lie down, reverse the steps you followed to move the patient into a sitting position.
19. Once the patient is back in the center of the bed, lower the head of the bed to an appropriate position.
20. Check to make sure the patient is comfortable and that the body is aligned properly.
21. Cover the patient with the top linens that were fanfolded to the foot of the bed.
22. Make sure the call signal is within the patient's reach.
23. Raise the side rail on the side of the bed where the patient had been sitting.
24. Lower the bed and open the screen or curtain.
25. Wash your hands.

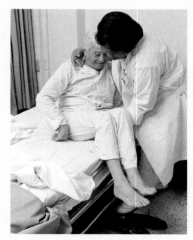

○ **Figure 16-5.** Moving a patient to a sitting position.

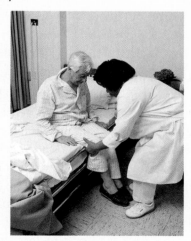

○ **Figure 16-6.** Positioning the patient for dangling.

Procedure 16-2

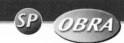

Moving a Patient Who Can Assist You Up in Bed

Equipment: none

1. Identify the patient, check the patient's ID band, and call the patient by name.
2. Introduce yourself and explain the procedure to the patient.
3. Wash your hands.
4. Provide privacy.
5. Check to make sure the wheels of the bed are locked.
6. If the bed is a hospital bed, raise it to a working height that is appropriate for good body mechanics.
7. Lower the head of the bed. If appropriate for the patient, the bed should be totally flat.
8. If the patient can be without it, move the pillow up against the headboard to protect the patient's head during the move.
9. Make sure the rail on the far side of the bed is in a raised and locked position. Lower the side rail near you.
10. Ask the patient to bend his or her knees and put the feet flat on the bed. The patient may also put the hand away from you flat on the bed and use it to help push off.
11. Ask the patient to place the arm closest to you under your arm and behind your shoulder. The patient's hand should rest on your shoulder. To prevent injury, be sure the patient does not put pressure on the back of your neck.
12. Place your arm under the patient's arm that is closest to you. Your hand is on the patient's shoulder.
13. Place your other arm gently under the neck and shoulders. **See Figure 16-7.**
14. On the count of three, pull the patient up in bed or to a sitting or semi-sitting position, if appropriate. If not, the patient can be pulled to a supine position.

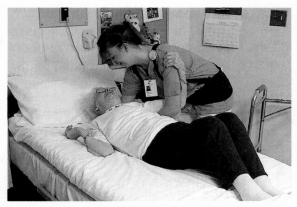

○ **Figure 16-7.** When helping a patient move, the nursing assistant puts her arm under the patient's shoulder. This patient is able to help by pushing off with her feet.

15. Use your free arm to tie the patient's gown, readjust the pillow, and so on.
16. Help the patient lie back down. With your locked arm, provide support to the patient. Use your other arm to support the neck and shoulders.
17. Place the pillow under the patient's head. Place a small pad under the knees, as needed for comfort, without causing the knees to bend.
18. Check to make sure the patient is comfortable and that the body is aligned properly.
19. Straighten the bed linens, and make sure the call signal is within the patient's reach.
20. Raise and lock the side rail on your side of the bed, if specified for the patient.
21. Lower the bed and open the screen or curtain.
22. Wash your hands.

Procedure 16-3

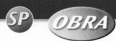

Moving a Helpless Patient in Bed

Equipment: none

1. Ask a team member to help you.
2. Identify the patient, check the patient's ID band, and call the patient by name.
3. Introduce yourself and your helper and explain the procedure to the patient.
4. Wash your hands.
5. Provide privacy.
6. Check that the bed's wheels are locked.
7. Raise the bed to a working height that is appropriate for good body mechanics.
8. Lower the head of the bed. If appropriate for the patient, the bed should be totally flat. Apply padding if ordered.
9. If the patient can be without it, move the pillow up against the headboard to protect the patient's head during the move.
10. Ask your helper to stand on one side of the bed. Stand on the opposite side.
11. If appropriate, lower the side rails.
12. Ask for the patient's cooperation.
13. Place your feet about 12 inches apart. Have one foot pointed toward the head of the bed and the other foot pointed toward the side of the bed. Bend your knees, and keep your back straight.
14. Place your arm under the patient's shoulder closest to you. Place your other arm under the patient's hips. Ask your helper to do the same on the other side. **See Figure 16-8.**
15. If the patient does not have a back injury or pressure sores, hold your helper's forearm and have the helper hold yours.
16. On the count of three, move the patient up in the bed. **See Figure 16-9.**
17. If the patient has not moved as far as necessary, repeat Steps 13 through 16.
18. Place the pillow under the patient's head.
19. Check to make sure the patient is comfortable and that the body is aligned properly.
20. Straighten the bed linens and make sure the call signal is within the patient's reach.
21. Raise and lock the side rails, if specified for the patient.
22. Lower the bed and open the screen.
23. Wash your hands.

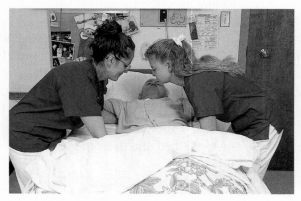

○ **Figure 16-8.** Both nursing assistants place their arms under the patient's shoulders and hips.

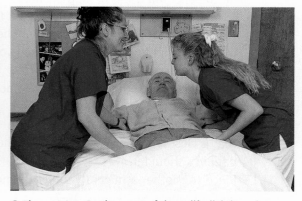

○ **Figure 16-9.** On the count of three, lift slightly and move the patient toward the head of the bed.

Procedure 16-4

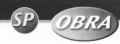

Moving a Helpless Patient Using a Turning Sheet

Equipment: turning sheet

1. Ask a team member to help you.
2. Identify the patient, check the patient's ID band, and call the patient by name.
3. Introduce yourself and your helper and explain the procedure to the patient.
4. Wash your hands.
5. Provide privacy.
6. Check to make sure the wheels of the bed are locked.
7. Raise the bed to a working height that is appropriate for good body mechanics.
8. Lower the head of the bed. If appropriate for the patient, the bed should be flat.
9. If the patient can be without it, move the pillow up against the headboard to protect the patient's head during the move.
10. Ask your helper to stand on one side of the bed. Stand on the opposite side.
11. Make sure the rails are down.
12. Ask for the patient's cooperation.
13. Roll both sides of the turning sheet up against the patient. **See Figure 16-10.**
14. With one hand, firmly grasp the turning sheet near the patient's buttocks. Use the other hand to do the same near the patient's shoulders. **See Figure 16-11.**
15. Place your feet about 12 inches apart, bend your knees, and keep your back straight.
16. On the count of three, move the patient up in the bed.
17. Unroll the turning sheet and place the pillow under the patient's head.
18. Check to make sure the patient is comfortable and that the body is aligned properly.
19. Straighten the bed linens, raise the head of the bed to a comfortable position, and make sure the call signal is within the patient's reach.
20. Raise and lock the side rails, if specified.
21. Lower the bed and open the screen.
22. Wash your hands.

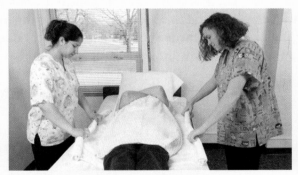

O **Figure 16-10.** Two nursing assistants roll both sides of the turning sheet in close to the body.

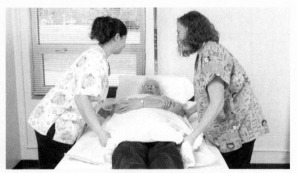

O **Figure 16-11.** The nursing assistants move the patient by grasping the turning sheet and moving toward the head of the bed.

Procedure 16-5

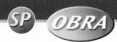

Turning or Rolling a Patient to Position onto Side

Equipment: two pillows • one small pillow

1. Identify the patient, check the patient's ID band, and call the patient by name.
2. Introduce yourself and explain the procedure to the patient.
3. Wash your hands.
4. Provide privacy.
5. Check to make sure the wheels of the bed are locked.
6. Raise the bed to a working height that is appropriate for good body mechanics.
7. Lower the head of the bed. The bed should be as flat as possible.
8. Make sure the side rail on the opposite side of the bed is raised and in a locked position. Lower the side rail near you. Apply padding if ordered.
9. Position your feet about 12 inches apart and flex your knees.
10. Ask for the patient's cooperation. Explain that the move will not take place all at once, but in several steps.
11. Cross the patient's arms over his or her chest.
12. Position one arm under the patient's neck and shoulders and your other arm under the middle of the patient's back. **See Figure 16-12.**

13. Grasp the patient's far shoulder with your hand and move the patient's upper body toward you. As you do, shift your weight to your back leg.
14. Put one of your arms under the patient's thigh and the other under the patient's waist. **See Figure 16-13.**
15. Move the patient's lower body toward you. As you do, shift your weight onto your back leg.
16. Put one of your arms under the patient's calf and the other under the patient's feet.
17. Move the patient's lower legs and feet toward you. As you do, shift your weight onto your back leg.
18. If the patient needs to be turned onto his or her side also, complete Steps 19 and 20. If the patient does not need to be turned, go to Step 21.
19. Place your hand on the patient's shoulder and hip on the far side of the bed.
20. Gently roll the patient toward you.
21. Check to make sure the patient is comfortable and that the body is aligned properly. Adjust the lower shoulder to prevent direct body pressure upon it.

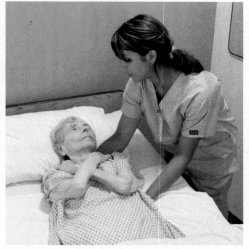

○ **Figure 16-12.** The nursing assistant first positions her arms for turning the patient.

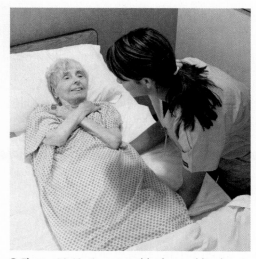

○ **Figure 16-13.** Correct positioning enables the nursing assistant to turn the patient.

22. Position pillows for the patient's comfort and support. **See Figure 16-14.**
    a. Place a pillow under the patient's head and shoulders.
    b. Place a pillow against the patient's back.
    c. Place a pillow between the patient's legs. Gently flex the knee of the top leg.
    d. Place a small pillow under the patient's upper hand and arm. Position the lower arm with appropriate elbow flexed and palm up or with elbow straight and arm alongside of body to promote comfort.
23. Straighten the bed linens and make sure the call signal is within the patient's reach.
24. Raise and lock the side rail on your side of the bed, if specified for the patient.
25. Lower the bed and open the screen.
26. Wash your hands.

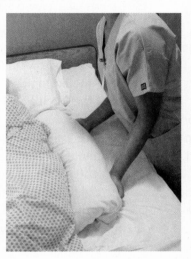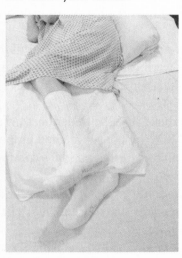

○ **Figure 16-14.** Position pillows after the patient is turned onto the side.

Procedure 16-6

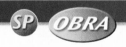

Logrolling a Patient and Positioning onto Side

Equipment: turning sheet • two or three pillows • one small pillow

1. Ask team members to help you move the patient.
2. Identify the patient, check the patient's ID band, and call the patient by name.
3. Introduce yourself and your helpers and explain the procedure to the patient.
4. Wash hands.
5. Provide privacy.
6. Check to make sure the wheels of the bed are locked.
7. Raise the bed to a working height that is appropriate for good body mechanics.
8. Lower the head of the bed. The bed should be as flat as possible.
9. Make sure the rail is up on the side of the bed toward which the patient will be turned. Lower the side rail near you.
10. Ask for the patient's cooperation.
11. Using the turning sheet and with your helpers' assistance, move the patient to the side of the bed near you.
12. Place a pillow or two between the patient's legs.
13. Position the patient's arms crossed on the chest.

14. Raise the rail on the side of the bed where you are working. Go to the other side of the bed and lower the side rail.
15. Stand near the patient's upper body. Ask your helpers to stand by the patient's waist and thighs, on the same side of the bed.
16. Position your feet about 12 inches apart. Place one foot in front of the other.
17. If the patient can assist, ask him or her to keep the body as rigid as possible during the rolling.
18. In cooperation with your helpers, roll the patient toward you. You may also use a turning sheet for this procedure. **See Figure 16-15.**
19. Check to make sure the patient is comfortable and that the body is aligned properly.
20. Position pillows for the patient's comfort and support.
    a. If appropriate for the patient's condition, place a pillow under the patient's head and shoulders.
    b. Place a pillow against the patient's back.

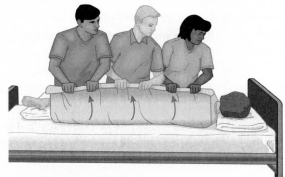

○ **Figure 16-15.** Logrolling a patient.

   c. Place a pillow on the bed over the knee of the bottom leg. Gently flex the knee of the top leg and place the leg on the pillow.
   d. Place a small pillow under the patient's hand and arm.
21. Straighten the bed linens and make sure the call signal is within the patient's reach.
22. Raise the side rail on your side of the bed.
23. Lower the bed and open the screen.
24. Wash your hands.

Vital Skills COMMUNICATION

Pressure Sores: Explaining Planned Movement

Preventing pressure ulcers is a vital part of nursing care. As a nursing assistant, you help reposition clients who cannot move themselves to help ensure that pressure sores don't develop or to promote the healing of existing pressure sores.

Likely pressure sore locations include the lower back (sacrum), the heels, the skin over the hips, ears, back of the head, and shoulder blades. In patients who use a wheelchair, pressure sores can form on the ankles, shoulder blades, sacrum, elbows, spine, and the back of the head.

Before you reposition a client, always explain what you are about to do. Assume that even unresponsive clients can hear you. Understanding what is being done will help

calm any fears the client has. The client may also be able to help you. Encourage the client to make even small shifts of weight.

Practice

In teams of three, practice moving clients in bed to prevent pressure sores. One student can be the client, and the other two are nursing assistants.

1. Practice moving a client who is partially mobile. Explain what you are doing and how the client might help you.
2. Practice moving a client who is completely immobile. Explain what you are doing in a normal speaking voice. Even an apparently unconscious patient may be able to hear you.

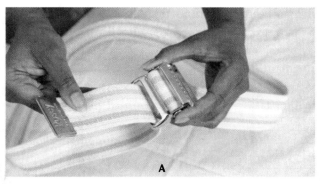
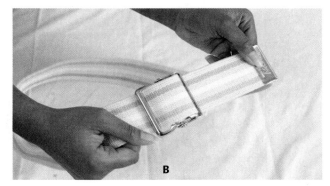

○ **Figure 16-16.** Transfer belts have Velcro or buckles. (A) Pull the strap through the buckle. (B) Tighten the belt by pulling the belt over the buckle and through the other side of the buckle.

Transferring Patients

To **transfer** a patient is to move the patient from one item of furniture or equipment to another. Patients may need to be transferred from a bed to a stretcher or wheelchair and later back into bed. Some patients are capable of moving themselves in and out of bed, but others need some assistance or are totally helpless. These patients require a nursing assistant plus one or two helpers to accomplish the transfer safely. When you transfer a patient, follow the guidelines for good body mechanics to prevent injury and strain to yourself and the patient.

A **transfer belt** is a belt that buckles around a patient's waist and provides a handle for the nursing assistant to hold onto. It is used for safety when transferring the patient. **See Figure 16-16.** It is called a *gait belt* in some facilities.

Procedure 16-7

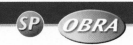

Applying a Transfer Belt

Equipment: transfer belt

1. Identify the patient, check the patient's ID band, and call the patient by name.
2. Introduce yourself and explain the procedure to the patient.
3. Wash your hands.
4. Provide privacy.
5. Help the patient move to a sitting position.
6. Place the transfer belt around the patient's waist, over the patient's clothes. **See Figure 16-17.**
7. Position the buckle off center in the front or to the side, but never at the back.
8. Tighten the belt snugly around the patient's waist. Do not make the belt too tight. It should not interfere with breathing or comfort. Two of your fingers should fit comfortably under the belt.
9. Wash your hands.

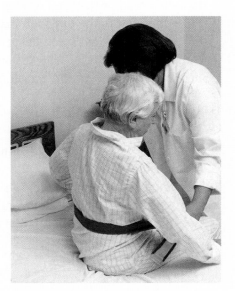

○ **Figure 16-17.** Always put the transfer belt over pajamas or clothes, never immediately next to the skin.

Using a Slide Board

A **slide board** is a device used to assist in patient transfers at even levels. A slide board may also be called a *transfer board*. Slide boards are used to transfer a patient from bed to chair or wheelchair, wheelchair to commode, or bed to stretcher.

Procedure 16-8

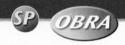

Transferring a Patient Using a Slide Board

Equipment: chair • slide board • transfer belt • robe • nonskid slippers or shoes • bath blanket

1. Identify the patient, check the patient's ID band, and call the patient by name.
2. Introduce yourself and explain the procedure to the patient.
3. Wash your hands.
4. Provide privacy.
5. Decide which side of the bed you will use. If necessary, move furniture to clear enough room to work. Always put the chair on the patient's strong side, if the patient has an impairment on one side.
6. Position the chair alongside the head of the bed on the side where you will be working. Place the chair in the direction that best enhances the patient's well-being.
7. If the patient needs it, put a cushion, bed pad, bath blanket, or other covering on the seat of the chair.
8. Move the bed to its lowest position and make sure the wheels are locked.
9. Fanfold the top bed linens down to the foot of the bed.
10. Help the patient move to the edge of the bed, assist to a sitting position, and dangle the feet. Be sure the patient's feet touch the floor.
11. Put shoes or nonskid slippers on the patient's feet and help the patient put on a robe.
12. Apply the transfer belt.
13. Place one end of the slide board under the patient's buttocks and the other over the seat of the chair.
14. Position yourself in front of the patient.
15. Have the patient push up with the arms and legs to assist.
16. Grasp both sides of the transfer belt, maintaining proper body mechanics at all times.
17. Continue to help the patient slowly slide sideways and push on the slide board all the way over to the chair.

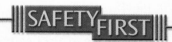

When you are transferring a patient, make sure that IV and catheter tubes and drains are also moved carefully to avoid pulling them and injuring the patient.

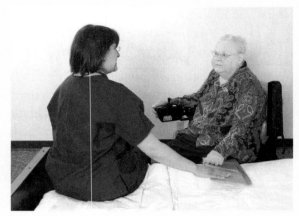

O **Figure 16-18.** The patient is now ready to get back in bed.

18. Position the patient comfortably and in good body alignment. The patient's buttocks should be positioned far back on the seat.
19. Place a bath blanket over the patient's lap and legs if necessary.
20. Remove the transfer belt.
21. Arrange the call signal so the patient can easily reach it.
22. Wash your hands.
23. When the patient is ready to return to bed, reverse the procedure. **See Figure 16-18.**

Using a Mechanical Lift

Use a mechanical lift when transferring patients who are helpless or obese. A **mechanical lift** is a lifting device that assists in raising, lowering, and transferring patients. In some facilities, use of a mechanical lift requires at least two people. Check your facility's policy before transferring a patient in this way.

Procedure 16-9

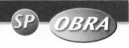

Using a Mechanical Lift

Equipment: mechanical lift • wheelchair or armchair • slippers • bath blanket

1. Ask for a helper to assist you.
2. Identify the patient, check the patient's ID band, and call the patient by name.
3. Introduce yourself and your helper and explain the procedure to the patient.
4. Wash your hands.
5. Provide privacy.
6. Center the sling of the mechanical lift under the patient. To get the sling under the patient, move him or her as you would if you were making an occupied bed. Position the lower edge of the sling underneath the patient's knees. **See Figure 16-19.**
7. Position the wheelchair (with locked wheels) or armchair alongside the head of the bed on the side where you will be working. Fold a bath blanket and place it in the chair. A cushion may also be used.

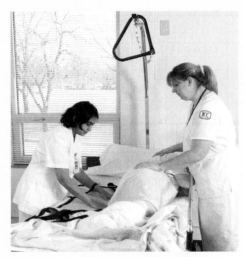

O **Figure 16-19.** You will need a partner to position the sling correctly under the patient.

8. Lower the bed to its lowest position. Make sure the wheels are locked.

9. Raise the head of the bed to bring the patient into a sitting position.
10. Move the release valve on the lift to the closed position.
11. Raise the lift so it can be positioned over the patient.
12. Spread the legs of the lift to provide a solid base of support. The legs *must* be locked in this position, or the lift may topple over with the patient in it and hurt both the patient and the nursing assistants.
13. Move the lift into position over the patient. **See Figure 16-20.**
14. Fasten the sling to the straps or chains. Turn the hooks away from the patient. **See Figure 16-21.**
15. Attach the sling to the swivel bar. The short side should be attached to the top of the sling. The long side should be attached to the bottom of the sling.
16. Cross the patient's arms across the chest. The patient may hold on to the straps. Do not let the patient hold on to the swivel bar.
17. Raise the lift until the patient and the sling are clear of the bed.
18. Have your helper support the patient's legs as you move the lift from the bed to the chair. **See Figure 16-22.** Make sure the patient's head is supported.

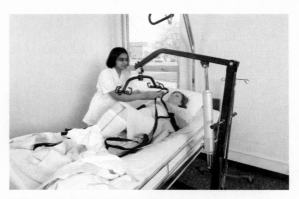

○ **Figure 16-20.** Position the lift over the patient.

19. Turn the patient so he or she is facing the support pole and is centered over the base.
20. Position the lift so the patient's back is facing toward the chair.
21. Move the lift so the patient is over the seat of the chair.
22. Slowly open the release valve on the lift. Gently lower the patient into the chair. **See Figure 16-23.**
23. Lower the bar so that you can unhook the sling. Leave the sling under the patient.
24. Place slippers on the patient's feet. If using a wheelchair, position the patient's feet on the footrests.

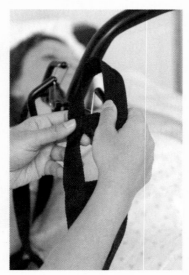

○ **Figure 16-21.** Fasten the straps so the knobs face outward.

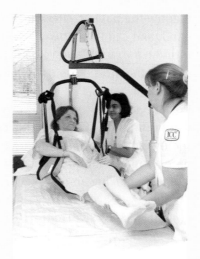

○ **Figure 16-22.** Support the patient's legs as the lift is moved over the chair.

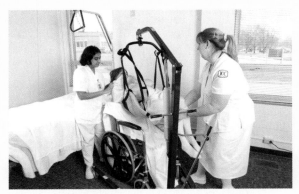

O **Figure 16-23.** Gently lower the patient into the chair.

25. Place a covering over the patient's lap and legs if necessary.
26. Arrange the call signal so that the patient can easily reach it.
27. Wash your hands.
28. Report your observations to the nurse, including how the patient tolerated the activity and any complaints of dizziness, difficulty breathing, weakness, and so on.
29. When the patient is ready to return to bed, reverse the procedure.

Transferring to a Wheelchair

Patients use wheelchairs for a number of reasons. Some are not able to walk or cannot walk very far. Some patients use wheelchairs at the time of their discharge from a facility. In long-term care facilities, residents may use a wheelchair to go to meals and activities.

Once you have transferred a patient into a wheelchair, make sure the patient is covered. If the patient does not have a robe, use a blanket or sheet. Make sure the patient's feet are covered with slippers, shoes, or a blanket. Unsteady patients may fall, so exercise extreme care when guiding a patient into a wheelchair. Be sure that the wheels are locked until the patient is seated.

Procedure 16-10

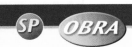

Transferring a Patient to a Wheelchair

Equipment: wheelchair • robe • nonskid slippers or shoes • bath blanket

1. Identify the patient, check the patient's ID band, and call the patient by name.
2. Introduce yourself and explain the procedure to the patient.
3. Wash your hands.
4. Provide privacy.
5. Decide which side of the bed you will use. If necessary, move furniture to clear enough room to work. Always put the wheelchair on the patient's strong side, if the patient has an impairment on one side.
6. Position the wheelchair alongside the head of the bed on the side where you will be

working. The front of the chair should face the head of the bed, with one side of the chair firmly against the side of the bed.
7. Put a cushion, bed pad, bath blanket, or other covering on the seat of the chair. Most patients should not sit directly on the plastic seat for extended periods.
8. Make sure the wheels are locked and the footrests are in the raised position and out of the way or removed.
9. Move the bed to its lowest position and make sure the wheels are locked.

10. Fanfold the top bed linens down to the foot of the bed.
11. Help the patient move to the edge of the bed and dangle his or her feet. Be sure the patient's feet touch the floor.
12. Put shoes or nonskid slippers on the patient's feet and help him or her put on a robe.
13. If you will be using a transfer belt, apply it now.
14. Help the patient move to a standing position. *Note:* This procedure should only be used for patients who can bear weight on at least one leg.

When using a transfer belt, follow steps (a) through (e):
   a. Position yourself in front of the patient.
   b. Have the patient put his or her hands on your shoulders, not around your neck.
   c. Grasp both sides of the transfer belt.
   d. Brace the patient by blocking the patient's knees with your knee and the patient's feet with your foot. **See Figure 16-24.**
   e. As you straighten your knees, raise the patient into a standing position. **See Figure 16-25.**

When not using a transfer belt, follow steps (f) through (j):
   f. Position yourself in front of the patient.
   g. Put your hands under the patient's arms so your hands are around the patient's shoulder blades.
   h. Brace the patient by blocking the patient's knees and the patient's feet with your feet.

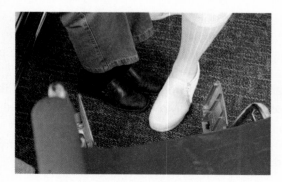

○ **Figure 16-24.** Brace the patient's feet against your foot.

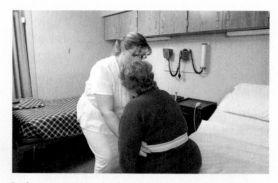

○ **Figure 16-25.** Help the patient to a standing position.

   i. Ask the patient to assist you by making fists with both hands. On the count of three, ask the patient to push both fists into the mattress and lean forward.
   j. On the count of three, straighten your knees and raise the patient to a standing position.
15. While the patient is standing, either hold the transfer belt or continue to brace the patient's knees and feet.
16. Turn the patient so that he or she can reach the arm on the far side of the wheelchair.
17. Continue to turn the patient slowly so he or she can reach and hold the other arm of the wheelchair.
18. Ask the patient to flex the knees and elbows and lean forward. Have the patient touch the front of the wheelchair seat with the back of the knees before sitting. Gently lower the patient into the wheelchair. **See Figure 16-26.** As you do, be sure to flex your knees and hips.
19. Position the patient comfortably and in good body alignment. The patient's buttocks should be positioned far back on the seat.
20. Replace and position the footrests and arrange the patient's feet on them.
21. Place a bath blanket over the patient's lap and legs if necessary. Make sure the blanket is not hanging on the floor or over the wheels of the wheelchair. Make sure the patient is secured in the wheelchair according to facility policy.

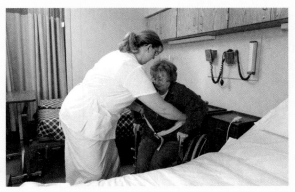

O **Figure 16-26.** Lower the patient into the wheelchair.

22. If you used a transfer belt, remove it.
23. Arrange the call signal so the patient can easily reach it.
24. Wash your hands.
25. Report your observations to the nurse, including how the patient tolerated the activity, the pulse rate (if measured), and any complaints of dizziness, difficulty breathing, weakness, and so on.
26. When the patient is ready to return to bed, reverse the procedure.

Transferring to a Stretcher

You will sometimes need to transfer a patient to a stretcher. **Stretchers** are carts with wheels for moving patients from one place to another while they are lying down. When you transfer a patient from bed to a stretcher, you will need one or more assistants.

Procedure 16-11

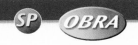

Transferring a Conscious Patient to a Stretcher

Equipment: stretcher • bath blanket

1. Ask two helpers to assist you.
2. Identify the patient, check the patient's ID band, and call the patient by name.
3. Introduce yourself and your helpers and explain the procedure to the patient.
4. Wash your hands.
5. Provide privacy.
6. Decide which side of the bed you will use.
7. If necessary, move furniture to clear enough room to work.
8. Raise the bed to a height even with the stretcher and lock the bed wheels.
9. Place a bath blanket over the patient's body up to the shoulders.
10. Fanfold the top linens down to the foot of the bed.
11. Lower the side rail on the side of the bed where the stretcher will be positioned.
12. Position the stretcher parallel to the bed, up against the bed. **See Figure 16-27.**

13. Lock the wheels of the stretcher.
14. Ask one of your helpers to go to the opposite side of the bed and lower the side rail. Ask the other helper to stand on the far side of the stretcher to prevent it from moving.
15. Go behind the headboard of the bed and place your hands gently under the patient's pillow.

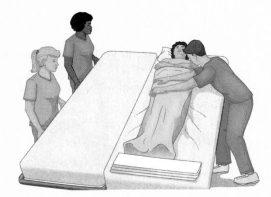

O **Figure 16-27.** Line the stretcher up against the bed.

16. Have the patient cross the arms across the chest.

17. Ask your helper alongside the bed to gently place his or her hands under the patient's back and lower legs. The helper on the far side of the stretcher should place his or her hands under the patient's back and legs also. **See Figure 16-28.** *Note*: If the patient's bed has a turning sheet, grasp it. See Procedure 16-4.

18. Turn or move the patient closer to the stretcher in one move. Then, on the count of three, move the patient onto the stretcher.

19. Fasten the stretcher straps and raise both side rails on the stretcher.

20. Wash your hands.

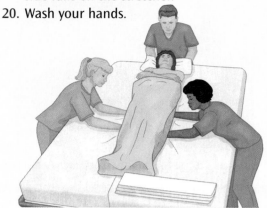

○ **Figure 16-28.** At least two people work together to move the patient onto the stretcher.

Procedure 16-12

SP OBRA

Transferring an Unconscious Patient to a Stretcher

Equipment: stretcher • bath blanket • turning sheet

1. Ask three helpers to assist you.
2. Identify the patient, check the patient's ID band, and call the patient by name.
3. Introduce yourself and your helpers and explain the procedure to the patient.
4. Wash your hands.
5. Provide privacy.
6. Decide which side of the bed you will use. If necessary, move furniture to clear enough room to work.
7. Raise the bed to a height even with the stretcher.
8. Place a bath blanket over the patient's body up to the shoulders.
9. Fanfold the top linens down to the foot of the bed.
10. Position yourself and your helpers as follows:
    a. One helper on the far side of the bed.
    b. One against the far side of the stretcher.
    c. One at the head of the stretcher facing toward the foot of the stretcher.
    d. The nursing assistant at the foot of the bed, facing the head of the bed.
11. Lower the side rails on both sides of the bed.
12. Position the stretcher parallel to the bed, up against the bed.
13. Lock the wheels of the stretcher. Make sure the wheels of the bed are locked also.
14. Roll in both sides of the turning sheet close to the patient's body.
15. The person at the patient's head orchestrates the move by counting to three. On the count of three, all helpers lift and guide the transfer of the patient, carrying out the following procedures at the same time:
    a. The nursing assistant at the foot of the bed raises the patient's lower legs and feet.
    b. The helper against the far side of the bed grasps and raises the turning sheet.
    c. The helper on the far side of the stretcher grasps the turning sheet with both hands, raises the sheet, and guides the patient toward the stretcher.

d. The helper at the head of the stretcher positions both arms together under the patient's shoulders to support the patient's head and neck. **See Figure 16-29.**

16. Position the patient in the center of the stretcher and fasten the stretcher restraints.
17. Raise and lock the side rails on the stretcher.
18. Wash your hands.

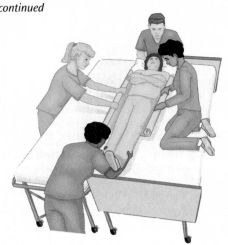

○ **Figure 16-29.** The nursing assistant and helpers transferring an unconscious patient to a stretcher.

Transporting Patients

Once a patient is seated or lying comfortably, you may transport the patient. To **transport** is to move a patient from place to place using a transport device, such as a wheelchair or stretcher.

Transporting Patients in Wheelchairs

To transport a patient in a wheelchair, first make sure the wheels are unlocked. Be sure to cover the patient before going out into the hall. Stand behind the chair and push the chair forward slowly. Go slowly around corners.

When moving a wheelchair on and off an elevator, pull the wheelchair toward you. Angle the wheelchair so that only one wheel crosses the opening between the elevator floor and the hallway floor at the same time. **See Figure 16-30.** This technique will prevent the wheelchair from getting caught if the opening is wide. When you are ready to move the patient into the elevator, turn the wheelchair around and pull it backwards into the elevator. This allows the patient to face the front along with everyone else. When leaving an elevator, turn the chair around and pull it backwards out of the elevator at a slight angle.

When transporting a patient in a wheelchair down a ramp, move the chair down the ramp backwards. This method places you between the patient and any possible fall from the wheelchair.

Transporting Patients on Stretchers

When transporting a patient on a stretcher, unlock the wheels. Make sure the straps and belts are in place and the side rails are in the up position and locked. Stand behind the stretcher and push it forward. You stand at the head of the stretcher, so the end of the stretcher holding the patient's feet is moving first.

When moving the stretcher into an elevator, pull the stretcher in backwards, so the end of the stretcher holding the patient's head enters the elevator first. When exiting an elevator, push the stretcher out, with the end of the stretcher holding the feet exiting first.

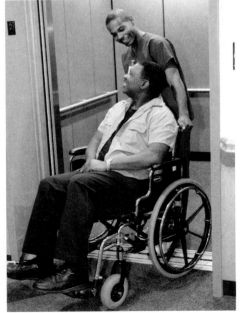

○ **Figure 16-30.** Angling a wheelchair onto the elevator.

CHAPTER 16 Review

Chapter Summary

- Proper body mechanics, posture, and body alignment are essential for the nursing assistant to prevent injury to self and patients.

- Patients must sometimes be placed in special positions for physical examinations, treatments, or to improve their well-being.

- Moving and positioning patients should be done properly to prevent friction or shearing force.

- Patients must be safely and effectively moved to different positions in bed.

- Patients must be safely and effectively transferred from bed to a chair, wheelchair, or stretcher.

- Assistive devices, including the transfer belt and the mechanical lift, are used to help move patients who cannot move themselves.

- Patients must be safely and effectively transported in wheelchairs and on stretchers.

VOCABULARY REVIEW

Directions: Match the letter of each definition in the second column with the correct vocabulary term in the first column. Write your answers on a separate sheet of paper.

Vocabulary

1. body alignment
2. body mechanics
3. dangle
4. dorsal recumbent position
5. draping
6. Fowler's position
7. friction
8. lateral position
9. logrolling
10. orthostatic hypotension
11. prone position
12. semi-Fowler's position
13. shearing force
14. Sims' position

Definitions

A. A combination of friction and pressure
B. A method for turning the patient onto the side in one movement to keep the spine aligned
C. A drop in blood pressure when a change in position occurs
D. The positions and movements that help the body maintain proper posture and prevent injury
E. A semi-sitting position with the head raised to a 45° angle and the portion of the bed under the knee raised 15°, if possible
F. The patient lies on the abdomen
G. The patient lies in a semi-prone position on the left side with the right knee flexed up toward the abdomen
H. The patient is positioned lying flat on the back with the legs close together, the knees flexed, and the soles of the feet flat on the mattress
I. Covering part or all of a patient's body with a sheet, blanket, or other material
J. The patient is lying on his or her side
K. A semi-sitting position with the head of the bed raised between a 45° and 60° angle and the knees slightly flexed
L. To sit up and allow the legs to hang loosely over the side of the bed for a short while
M. The proper positioning of the head, back, and limbs in a straight line
N. A force caused by the rubbing of one surface against another

Check Your Knowledge

Review Questions: Answer each of the following questions on a separate sheet of paper.

1. Why is it important to maintain correct posture and body alignment for both you and your patients?

2. List four rules to follow when carrying a heavy object.

3. The nurse instructs you to keep a resident with breathing difficulties in a semi-Fowler's position. At what level should the head of the bed be placed?

4. What can you do as a nursing assistant to minimize friction when moving patients?

5. What do you do when you assist a patient to dangle?

6. When turning a patient onto the side, what step can you take to prevent the patient from rolling on top of the arm?

7. Give one medical reason for logrolling a patient.

8. What is a slide board?

9. How should you exit an elevator when transporting a patient in a wheelchair?

10. When you transport a patient on a stretcher, where should you stand?

True or False: Read each statement carefully. Then write *True* or *False* by the statement number on a separate sheet of paper.

1. The rules of good body mechanics apply to transferring patients as well as moving patients in bed.

2. The muscles in the back are larger and more powerful than the muscles in the legs.

3. A patient in Sims' position should be draped up to the shoulders.

4. Transferring an unconscious patient from a bed to a stretcher requires at least two assistants.

5. A transfer belt is a lifting device that requires at least two people to operate.

Think and Decide

Directions: Think about each of the following scenarios. Answer each question on a separate sheet of paper.

1. Mr. K. is a 72-year-old man who recently suffered a stroke. He has been on bed rest for three days. The nurse asks you to assist Mr. K. to the side of the bed and dangle his legs for 15 minutes. As soon as you sit Mr. K. up to dangle, he becomes dizzy and tells you he might pass out. What should you do?

2. The facility where you are working uses mechanical lifts and requires two people to transfer patients into a wheelchair if the patient is unable to stand. You are working with Mrs. M. You and a helper have assisted her many times into the wheelchair to take her to the dining room to eat. All of your coworkers are busy and Mrs. M. is very hungry. Should you attempt to move her using the lift by yourself? Why or why not?

3. You are assisting a coworker to move Mr. T. up in bed. Mr. T. cannot help you because he is a quadriplegic. Your coworker grabs the turning sheet and asks you to do the same. The bed is in the low position. What should you do?

4. One of the residents in the long-term care facility where you work has chronic obstructive pulmonary disease. She is so tired and short of breath that she is unable to pull herself up in bed today and asks for your help. Should you lower the head of the bed to make it easier to pull the resident up in bed? Why or why not?

5. You have been asked to transfer a resident downstairs to the second floor. To transfer the patient properly into and out of the elevator, in what direction should you point the wheelchair?

6. Mr. V., a long-term care resident, walked to the dining room for lunch today as usual. He walks well with the help of his walker, so he is allowed to walk unaided by a staff member. Today, as he was turning a corner, he almost collided with someone. Startled, he fell, and although he is not hurt, he is not strong enough to get up by himself. How can you get him up and assist him to bed without causing injury to Mr. V. or to yourself?

7. Mrs. I. is returning to the long-term care facility after having been transported to the hospital for back surgery. You have been asked to accompany the stretcher to her room and transfer her from the stretcher to the bed. What procedure should you use? How many people should you ask to help?

8. Mrs. B. is a new resident at the long-term care facility. She is obese, partly due to a medical condition, and she is very sensitive about her weight. You have been asked to help her move from her bed to the armchair. When you bring in the mechanical lift and a helper, she asks what "all that" is for. What will you tell Mrs. B.?

CNA Certification Exam Prep

Directions: This practice test contains ten questions. Each question has four suggested answers. For each question, choose the ONE that best answers the question or completes the statement. Write your answers on a separate sheet of paper.

1. What device can a nursing assistant wear to support the back while lifting?
   A. body support
   B. neck brace
   C. gait belt
   D. transfer belt

2. Which of the following positions may be ordered when a patient needs to lie on his back?
   A. knee-chest
   B. prone
   C. lateral
   D. supine

3. In which of the following positions is a patient placed on her abdomen?
   A. knee-chest
   B. prone
   C. lateral
   D. supine

4. Covering part or all of a patient's body with a sheet or blanket is called
   A. dressing.
   B. draping.
   C. damping.
   D. dangling.

5. In Fowler's position, the head of the bed is raised
   A. 15° to 30°.
   B. 30° to 40°.
   C. 45° to 60°.
   D. 90°.

6. A force caused by one surface rubbing against another is known as
   A. shearing force.
   B. pressure.
   C. lifting force.
   D. friction.

7. A flat, board-like device that is used to help patients move from a bed to a chair at even levels is a
   A. slide board.
   B. transfer belt.
   C. gait belt.
   D. walker.

8. The proper positioning of the head, back, and limbs in a straight line is body
   A. mechanics.
   B. support.
   C. alignment.
   D. transport.

9. To avoid injury, do not lift heavy objects higher than
   A. knee level.
   B. waist level.
   C. chest level.
   D. head level.

10. Logrolling is used to move people who have had a
    A. knee injury.
    B. back injury.
    C. foot injury.
    D. arm injury.

CHAPTER 17

OBJECTIVES

- Describe the importance of being certified in first aid and basic life support procedures.
- Explain how to assess the scene after an emergency has occurred.

- Explain how to get help, including activating the emergency medical services system.
- Identify the signs and symptoms of respiratory arrest and cardiac arrest.
- Review the basic life support procedures to be used for adults, children, and infants.

- Explain the importance of the automated external defibrillator and review the steps for its use.
- Describe signs, symptoms, and emergency care for patients with common types of injuries or conditions.

Emergency Care

VOCABULARY

automated external defibrillator (AED) An automatic, portable device that is used to deliver an electric shock to someone in cardiac arrest.

basic life support The series of actions taken to maintain life in an emergency.

cardiac arrest The condition that occurs when the heart and breathing suddenly stop.

cardiopulmonary resuscitation (CPR) A form of basic life support that includes activation of EMS and procedures that support both breathing and circulation.

defibrillation The delivery of an electric shock to a patient's chest to re-establish the heart rhythm.

emergency An event that calls for immediate action.

emergency medical services (EMS) system A community network of equipment, facilities, and specially trained personnel set up to provide treatment and care during emergencies.

epilepsy A disease in which a person has recurrent seizures.

external bleeding Loss of blood on the outer surface of the body.

first aid The first care given to an injured or ill person in an emergency before medical help arrives.

foreign body airway obstruction (FBAO) The prevention of air from entering the lungs caused by a foreign object caught in the throat.

generalized seizure Convulsions that involve all or part of the body and are characterized by a loss of consciousness.

heat exhaustion A condition caused by prolonged exposure to heat over hours to days that results in a slightly elevated body temperature and signs of dehydration.

heat stroke A severe and possibly fatal condition caused by exposure to extreme heat and characterized by confusion and high fever.

Heimlich maneuver A first-aid procedure for dislodging an item that is causing a person to choke.

hemorrhage The sudden and extreme loss of blood.

hyperthermia A dangerous condition in which body temperature is elevated above the normal range.

hypothermia A condition in which the core body temperature drops below 95° F (35° C) caused by prolonged exposure to the cold.

internal bleeding Loss of blood inside the body or under the skin from an organ, blood vessels, or other internal tissues.

partial seizure A seizure in which the patient remains conscious and appears to stare blankly.

poison Any substance that is toxic to humans and can change the function of body organs and adversely affect the patient's health.

rescue breathing A step in basic life support, in which the rescuer forces oxygen into the patient's lungs to support or restore breathing.

respiratory arrest The condition that occurs when breathing stops but the heart continues to work for several minutes.

seizure An electrical disturbance in the brain that results in uncontrollable spasms or jerking of the muscles of the body.

shock A condition that occurs when an inadequate blood supply is delivered to the body's tissues.

stroke A condition that occurs when there is damage to a blood vessel in the brain.

universal distress signal A sign used to indicate that one is choking by clutching the neck with one or both hands.

Responding to an Emergency

An **emergency** is an event that calls for immediate action. Emergencies can happen to anyone at any time. Some emergency situations include:

- Accidents in the home, outside the home, and in the workplace
- Heart attack and cardiac arrest
- Respiratory arrest
- Airway obstruction
- Shock
- Stroke
- Severe bleeding
- Seizures
- Fires, smoke, and burns
- Poisoning
- Weather emergencies

First aid is the first care given to an injured or ill person in an emergency before medical help arrives. The goals of first aid are to keep the patient alive and to prevent further injury.

As a nursing assistant, you may encounter any of the above emergencies. Consider these possible events: A resident in a long-term care facility has a stroke while you are providing care. A three-year-old hospital patient chokes on food lodged in her throat. Your home client seems to be experiencing cardiac arrest. By learning how to respond to these emergencies, you could save lives.

The best way to prepare for emergencies is to learn how to give basic first aid and basic lifesaving care. The American Heart Association, the American Red Cross, adult education programs, and community colleges offer CPR certification courses. Some offer first aid courses as well. Perhaps your own school offers these courses. Whether or not your state requires this training for nursing assistants, consider taking a course. You will increase your skills and may possibly save someone's life. In this textbook, the 2005 American Heart Association guidelines are followed.

Assessing the Scene

When you approach an emergency situation, you must quickly assess the scene by using your senses. To assess the emergency scene:

- Check for further danger to the victims or yourself.
- Determine how many victims are affected.
- Determine whether the victims are breathing, bleeding, choking, or in acute pain.
- Listen to what witnesses and the victims tell you.
- Look at the obvious injuries.
- Look for signs and symptoms of other injuries or conditions that may not be as easily observed. For example, a patient could be in shock or have internal injuries.

Getting Help

When an emergency occurs, follow facility emergency procedures. Most hospitals have emergency staff on call to handle emergencies. In other situations, such as nursing homes or home health care, take immediate measures as directed by

Writing Concisely

As a nursing assistant, you may be required to write a description of events that occurred in an emergency. Your writing should be factual and concise. When you write, avoid adding words that do not contribute to sentence meaning. Eliminating unnecessary words or phrases and "filler" words makes your writing easier to understand and more enjoyable to read. Here are some tips for being concise:

• **Eliminate unnecessary modifiers.**
Example: Mrs. Watson was kind of upset that she had to wait for such a long time when she got to the emergency room.

Better: Mrs. Watson was upset that she had to wait in the emergency room.

• **Change phrases into single words.**
Example: Michael Conners, our head of maintenance for the hospital, said the air conditioning equipment in the waiting area should be in working order sometime before the end of the day.

Better: Maintenance head Michael Conners said the air conditioner in the waiting area would be fixed today.

• **Use active rather than passive verbs.**
Example: The emergency room coat closet was checked by Rachel.

Better: Rachel checked the emergency room coat closet.

Practice
Rewrite the following sentences for conciseness.
1. The medications which have been ordered for Mrs. Gottleib were checked by the doctor.
2. Mr. Albert was sort of confused when I asked him some questions about where he lives.
3. All of the nursing assistants who are listed on the schedule are to report to Mrs. Quarry's office sometime before Monday.
4. Mr. Reale, who is the patient in room 324, said he wants to have his bath in a little while.

your facility and dial 9-1-1. This activates the **emergency medical services (EMS) system**, a community network of equipment, facilities, and specially trained personnel set up to provide treatment and care during emergencies. **See Figure 17-1.**

Dialing 9-1-1 connects you to an emergency dispatcher who has access to emergency medical personnel, police, firefighters, a poison control center, and doctors. Give the operator the following information:
• Your location and telephone number
• A brief description of the scene

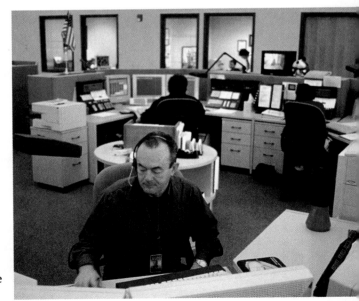

O **Figure 17-1.** Activating the EMS system will connect you with an emergency dispatcher who will send the appropriate emergency personnel to help.

- The number of people injured
- The types of injuries
- The type of aid needed

Do not hang up the phone until the operator hangs up. The operator is trained to walk you through basic lifesaving steps.

Providing Initial Care. Once help has been called, check for these life-threatening signs:
- Inadequate breathing
- Faint pulse or no pulse
- Lack of circulation (bluish skin)
- Signs of bleeding
- Signs of shock
- Additional injuries

If you see any of these signs, provide first aid and basic life support according to facility protocol or the instructions in this chapter.

Providing Supportive Care. While waiting for emergency medical services to arrive, stay with the patient. Follow these guidelines:
- Do not move the patient any more than is necessary to sustain life. If there is further danger at the scene, such as a fire or potential explosion, move the patient if possible. Do not move a patient if you will endanger your own life.
- Do not allow the patient to get up or walk. This could cause further injury.
- Keep the patient warm and safe. Cover the patient with blankets, coats, or whatever is available. For example, you can use newspaper if there is no fire danger. Do not remove the patient's clothing unless absolutely necessary.
- Do not give the patient food or fluids.
- Explain to a conscious patient that help has been called. Reassure the patient.

Emergency situations can be frightening and complex. Knowing how to perform will help you respond quickly and confidently. It is important to remain calm. When you function calmly, your patients will feel safe and secure.

Advance Directives

Advance directives should also be considered when delivering emergency care. You must respect the patient's wishes given in an advance directive. When you are working in long-term care, your supervisor is responsible for obtaining advance directives and notifying caregivers what each resident's wishes are. During an emergency, however, if you do not know if the patient has advance directives, begin basic life support immediately (if you are certified). See Chapter 4 for more information about advance directives.

Basic Life Support

The series of actions taken to maintain life in an emergency is called **basic life support**. There are two levels of basic life support. In **rescue breathing**, the rescuer forces oxygen into the patient's lungs to support or restore breathing. Rescue breathing is used on a person who is in **respiratory arrest**—one who is not breathing but still has a pulse. **See Figure 17-2.**

Vital Skills ⟨ READING ⟩

Analyzing Advance Directives

Laws regarding advance directives vary from state to state. When you begin working, you should familiarize yourself with the laws in your state. All hospitals in the United States are required to inform patients about advance directives upon admission.

However, not all patients have advance directives. If a patient has an advance directive, it will be in his or her chart. When you receive a new patient, you should read the chart to find out whether that person has an advance directive. Then read it so you will know what to do in the event of an emergency.

Practice

Read the following scenarios and discuss your feelings about advance directives with your classmates.

1. A woman with metastatic (spreading) lung cancer is admitted to the hospital for pneumonia. She does not have an advance directive. Two days later, she stops breathing and you cannot feel a pulse. What should you do?
2. A 98-year-old woman arrives from a nearby nursing home. She is unconscious. She is diagnosed with a urinary tract infection which has possibly spread to her blood. She has a living will that specifies that she does not want to be kept alive by means of artificial feeding. If her heart stops, will health care workers initiate CPR? Why or why not?

The second level of basic life support is **cardiopulmonary resuscitation (CPR)**. CPR is performed when a person is in **cardiac arrest**—when the heart and breathing suddenly stop. CPR includes both rescue breathing and chest compressions. The chest compressions cause blood to move through the heart and circulatory system.

The signs of cardiac arrest include:
- Loss of consciousness
- Absence of breathing
- Absence of pulse
- Cool, pale skin

One of the many things that can cause cardiac arrest is myocardial infarction. In myocardial infarction (heart attack), the flow of blood to an area of the heart decreases or stops completely. The signs of myocardial infarction include:
- Sudden severe chest pain not relieved by rest or nitroglycerine tablets
- Chest pain that radiates to the neck and jaw or down the arm
- Indigestion

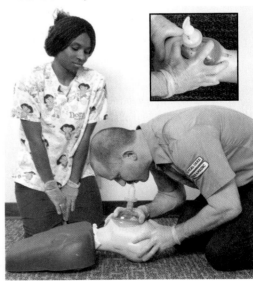

O **Figure 17-2.** Rescue breathing using a face mask with a one-way valve.

FOCUS ON

Rapid Response

In a health care facility, a nursing assistant facing an emergency should always call for help from the staff. The speed with which help is delivered can make the difference between life and death or between minimal and extensive brain damage.

• Dizziness
• Confusion
• Seizure
• Feelings of doom

Always use standard precautions when administering basic life support. Use a special face shield, barrier, or mask with a one-way valve between your mouth and the patient's mouth.

Learning the ABCs

The initial assessment in an emergency includes the ABCs of basic life support. The purpose of the ABC assessment is to locate and correct life-threatening conditions.

> **A = Airway:** Assess and open the patient's airway.
> **B = Breathing:** Assess for breathing and begin rescue breathing if indicated.
> **C = Circulation:** Check for a pulse and begin chest compressions if the patient has no pulse.

Airway: Is the Airway Open? The patient's airway must be open for breathing to occur. If the patient is breathing or conscious, the airway is open. In an unconscious patient, the tongue may fall toward the back of the throat and block the airway. This prevents air from entering the lungs and causes respiratory arrest.

The head-tilt/chin-lift procedure is used to open the airway. If you are certified in basic life support procedures, follow these steps to open the airway:
• Place one hand on the patient's forehead.
• Apply pressure with the palm of your hand to tilt the head back.
• Place the fingers of the other hand under the bony part of the chin and lift the chin forward. The head of an adult is hyperextended (if no neck injury is suspected). **See Figure 17-3.** The head of a child or infant is tilted to a normal position.

Breathing: Is the Patient Breathing? Conscious victims are usually breathing adequately. If the patient is unconscious, keep the airway open. Look at the chest to see if it is rising and falling. Listen for breathing and feel to see if air is coming out of the nose and mouth. **See Figure 17-4.** If the patient is not breathing, or is breathing inadequately, perform rescue breathing.

Circulation: Is the Patient's Heart Beating? If the patient has a pulse, the heart is beating. Feel for the pulse on the carotid artery, located on the side of the neck. **See Figure 17-5.** If you cannot feel a pulse, perform CPR. The chest compressions performed in CPR provide artificial circulation.

Basic Life Support Procedures

Learning the following basic life support procedures will *not* qualify you to perform them. It will simply provide you with a basic understanding. You must take a course to be certified to perform basic life support. Basic life support certification courses teach the following steps for performing CPR on adults. First, check the patient's ABCs and respond according to Procedure 17-1 for adults or Procedure 17-2 for infants and children.

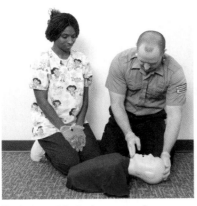

○ **Figure 17-3.** An instructor shows a nursing assistant how the correct head-tilt/chin-lift procedure is used to open the airway.

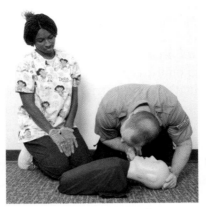

○ **Figure 17-4.** An instructor demonstrates listening for breathing.

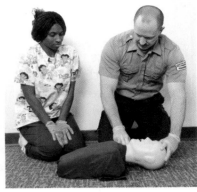

○ **Figure 17-5.** Feeling for a pulse on the carotid artery.

Procedure 17-1

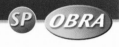

Basic Life Support for Adults

Equipment: face shield, barrier, or mask

1. Check the patient's responsiveness. Tap the patient gently on the shoulder and shout near the patient's ear, "Are you OK?"
2. If no response, call for help. Activate the EMS system.
3. Roll the patient on his or her back. Roll the entire body as a single unit.
4. Open the airway using the head-tilt/chin-lift method. **If you suspect a spinal cord injury, do not move the patient's neck. Lift the patient's chin, but do not tilt the head back.**
5. Check for adequate breathing. Place your ear over the patient's mouth and nose for 5 to 10 seconds while keeping the airway open. Look at the patient's chest to see if it is rising and falling.
6. If adequate breathing is not present, apply a mouth shield, barrier, or mask. Keep the head tilted back to keep the airway open. Pinch the nose shut. Give 2 breaths, each lasting 1 second. Take a breath between

each breath you give to the patient. Watch the patient's chest rise with each breath. Wait for the chest to deflate before giving another breath.

7. Check for a pulse. Maintain head-tilt with hand nearest the patient's head on the forehead. With the other hand, slide your fingers into the groove of the neck and feel for the carotid pulse for 5 to 10 seconds. It is important not to take more than 10 seconds for the pulse check.
8. Based on your assessment, perform the following rescue procedures.

When there is a pulse but no breathing:

9. Give 1 rescue breath every 5 to 6 seconds. Stop and check once every minute to make sure there is still a pulse.
10. Continue until the patient starts to breathe independently, until emergency medical help or another rescuer arrives and takes over, or until you are completely exhausted.

When there is no breathing and no pulse:

9. Place the heel of your hand on the center of the chest between the patient's nipples, and place your other hand on top of your first hand. **See Figure 17-6.**

10. Compress the patient's chest at a rate of 100 per minute. **See Figure 17-7.**
    - Place your shoulders directly over your hands on the patient's chest.
    - Keep your arms straight and elbows locked.
    - Push the patient's sternum (breastbone) down 1½ to 2 inches.

11. After every 30 compressions, give 2 rescue breaths.

12. Continue for a total of 5 cycles of 30 compressions to 2 breaths.

13. Recheck breathing and pulse every few minutes. If the patient still is not breathing and has no pulse, restart CPR with chest compressions.

14. If two rescuers are available, one rescuer should administer rescue breaths and the other should perform chest compressions. The rescuers should switch positions every 2 minutes.

15. Continue CPR until the victim revives, until emergency medical help arrives or another rescuer takes over, or until you are completely exhausted.

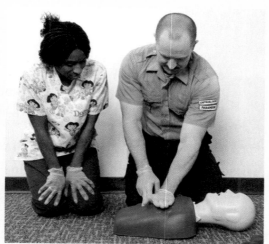

○ Figure 17-6. The instructor demonstrates the correct position for giving chest compressions to an adult.

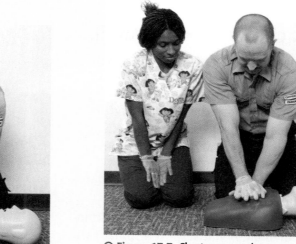

○ Figure 17-7. Chest compressions are performed by first placing your shoulders directly over your hands on the patient's chest, keeping your arms straight and elbows locked, and pushing.

Procedure 17-2

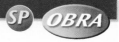

Basic Life Support for Infants and Children

Equipment: face shield, barrier, or mask

1. For infants, check responsiveness by tapping gently on the shoulder or foot. For children, tap gently on the shoulder and shout near the ear, "Are you OK?"

2. Send a second rescuer, if available, to activate the EMS system.

If alone and no second rescuer is available, perform 5 cycles of CPR before activating EMS by doing the following:

3. Roll the infant or child on the back by rolling the entire body as a single unit. **See Figure 17-8.** Avoid twisting the body.

4. Unless neck injury is suspected, open the airway using the head-tilt/chin-lift method. To lift the chin, place your finger under the bony part of the jaw and lift. **See Figure 17-9.**

5. Check for the presence or absence of adequate breathing. This should take 5 to 10 seconds. Place your ear over the mouth and nose while keeping the airway open, and then look at the chest to see if it is rising and falling.

6. If breathing is absent, give 2 *gentle* rescue breaths each lasting 1 second, using a face shield, barrier, or mask. An infant's lungs cannot tolerate the same amount of air as an adult's. **See Figure 17-10.**

   • Watch the chest rise with each breath. Wait for the chest to deflate before giving another breath.

   • If the chest did not rise with the first attempt, reposition the airway and try a second breath. If this is unsuccessful, you can suspect some kind of airway obstruction.

7. Check for a pulse. **See Figure 17-11.** Maintain head-tilt with the hand nearest the head on the forehead. Feel for a pulse on the inside of the upper arm in an infant by

gently pressing two fingers inside the arm closest to you. Check a carotid pulse in a child. This should take 5 to 10 seconds.

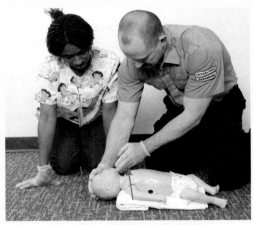

○ **Figure 17-9.** Open the infant's airway using the head-tilt/chin-lift method (unless spinal injury is suspected).

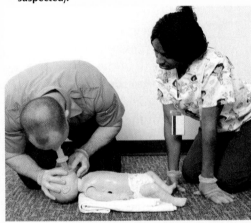

○ **Figure 17-10.** Cover the infant's nose and mouth with a barrier to deliver breaths.

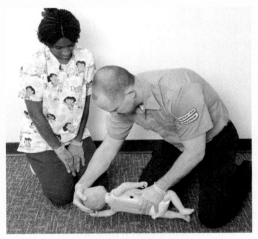

○ **Figure 17-8.** Gently roll the infant's head, body, and legs over at the same time.

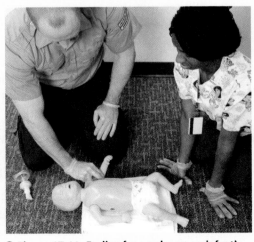

○ **Figure 17-11.** Feeling for a pulse on an infant's brachial artery.

8. Based on your assessment, perform the following rescue procedures.

When there is a pulse or signs of circulation but no breathing, do the following:

9. Give one rescue breath every 3 to 5 seconds. Stop once every minute to make sure there is still a pulse.

10. Continue until the patient starts to breathe independently, until emergency medical help arrives and takes over or another rescuer arrives, or until you are completely exhausted.

When there is no breathing and no pulse, do the following:

9. Find the finger position for an infant or the hand position for chest compressions for a child.

    Chest compression landmarks for an infant: Maintain the infant's head tilt. Place 2 fingers just below the nipple line. **See Figure 17-12.** Depress the chest approximately ⅓ to ½ the depth of the chest.

    Chest compression landmarks for a child: Maintain the child's head tilt. Depending on the size of the child, use two hands with the heel of one hand on the center of the child's chest and the other hand on top, or use the heel of only one hand across the center of the child's chest. **See Figure 17-13.** Depress the chest approximately ⅓ to ½ the depth of the chest.

10. Perform compressions at a rate of at least 100 per minute.

11. Continue cycles of 30 compressions to 2 breaths for 5 cycles (2 minutes).

12. *If two rescuers are available*, the ratio of chest compressions to rescue breathing is 15:2 for 20 cycles. The rescuers should switch positions every 2 minutes.

13. If CPR is unsuccessful after 5 cycles, activate the EMS system. Continue CPR until the infant (or child) revives, until emergency medical help arrives and takes over or another rescuer arrives, or until you are completely exhausted.

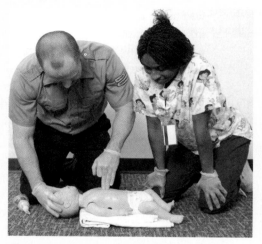

○ **Figure 17-12.** The correct finger position for chest compressions on an infant. Place two fingers just below the nipple line.

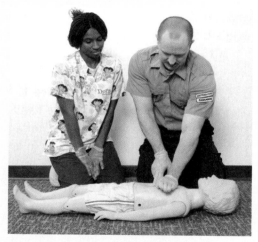

○ **Figure 17-13.** Use the heel of only one hand across the center of a small child's chest.

Automated External Defibrillator

Sudden cardiac arrest is a major complication of cardiovascular disease. It is most often related to an irregular, uncoordinated, and ineffective heart rhythm known as *ventricular fibrillation*. The most effective treatment for ventricular fibrillation is the delivery of an electric shock to a patient's chest, known as **defibrillation**. This shock can re-establish the heart's rhythm.

An **automated external defibrillator (AED)** is an automatic, portable device that is used to deliver an electric shock to someone in cardiac arrest. **See Figure 17-14.** It is easy to use and can be used by almost anyone who receives the proper training. The AED is applied to the outside of the body with two large electrode pads. It automatically analyzes a person's heart rhythm. It then directs the rescuer to deliver a shock, if needed, to restore a normal heart beat.

AEDs can be found in airports, shopping malls, hotels, and other public places. Because cardiac arrest is fatal if not treated within a few minutes, the AED has become an important lifesaving device.

An AED should be used only when a patient has the following clinical signs:
- Unresponsiveness
- Absence of breathing
- Absence of pulse

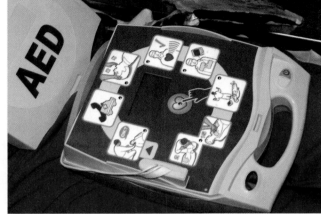

○ **Figure 17-14.** The automated external defibrillator (AED).

Procedure 17-3

Using the Automated External Defibrillator

Equipment: automated external defibrillator trainer • disposable gloves • face shield or mask

The following are general steps for the use of an AED. Be aware that each manufacturer may have slightly different steps to operate the device.

1. Establish unresponsiveness, absence of breathing, and absence of pulse.
2. Activate EMS. Request the AED.
3. Begin CPR while AED is being assembled.
4. When the AED arrives, open the carrying case or the top of the AED and push the power-on button.
5. Choose the correct pad (adult or child). **Do not use an AED on children under 1 year of age.**
6. Peel the backing away from the electrode pad.
7. Stop CPR.
8. Attach the adhesive electrode pads to the patient's bare chest. **See Figure 17-15.**
9. Attach the AED connecting cables to the AED device if not already connected.

10. Shout "Clear" and have everyone step away from the person. Press the "analyze" button on the AED. (This step is automatic on some devices.)
11. If shock is indicated by the device, make sure that no one is touching the person. Press the "shock" button to deliver the shock.
12. After the initial shock is delivered, the AED may tell you to resume CPR for 5 cycles of chest compressions (2 minutes); then repeat from Step 10.

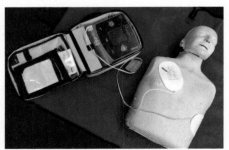

○ **Figure 17-15.** The electrode pads of the AED are applied to the patient's chest.

Airway Obstructions

A **foreign body airway obstruction (FBAO)** occurs when a foreign object is caught in the throat, preventing air from entering the lungs. A person can choke on food, vomit, the tongue, or a small object inserted in the mouth.

FBAO in adults most often occurs when a piece of food becomes lodged in the airway. People who are not able to chew properly are at great risk of choking on food. Children are also at risk of choking on food, since they do not always chew properly. FBAO can also occur when a child swallows a small object, such as a toy.

The **universal distress signal** is a sign used to indicate one is choking by clutching the neck with one or both hands. When you ask the person if he or she is choking, the person will usually attempt to nod the head up and down.

Signs and Symptoms

A choking patient is unable to communicate verbally the need for help and is usually panicking. Look for the following signs and symptoms of FBAO:
- The person cannot speak, breathe, or cough.
- High-pitched sounds may come from the throat.
- The person gives the universal distress signal.
- The skin turns blue.
- The person has lost consciousness.

If a patient can speak or is coughing vigorously, do not interfere. Stay near the patient and encourage coughing. This is the body's most effective way to dislodge a foreign object.

Heimlich Maneuver and Emergency Care

The **Heimlich maneuver** is a first-aid procedure for dislodging an item that is causing a person to choke. The Heimlich maneuver uses abdominal thrusts to dislodge a foreign body and force it upward, out of the throat. This procedure must be attempted immediately after you ask whether a person is choking and he or she nods yes. Every second is important, since the person is at risk for respiratory and cardiac arrest.

The technique for clearing an obstructed airway differs depending on whether the patient is conscious or unconscious. The Heimlich maneuver is not effective on obese people or pregnant women. You must perform chest thrusts.

Procedure 17-4

Helping a Conscious Patient with an Obstructed Airway

Equipment: none

When a patient is conscious and cannot speak, breathe, or cough, ask, "Are you choking?" If the patient nods, continue the procedure.
1. Stand behind the patient. Spread your feet apart to get a broad base of support.

2. Wrap your arms around the patient's waist.
3. Make a fist with one hand and place the thumb side just above the patient's navel and well below the tip of the sternum. **See Figure 17-16.**

4. Grasp your fist with your other hand.
5. Press the fist into the patient's abdomen with a quick upward thrust.
6. Give 5 thrusts. Each thrust should be a separate and distinct effort to dislodge the object.
7. After every 5 abdominal thrusts, check the patient and your technique.
8. Repeat cycles of 5 thrusts until one of the following occurs:
   • The patient coughs up the object.
   • The patient becomes unconscious (see Procedure 17-5, Helping an Unconscious Patient with an Obstructed Airway).
   • You are relieved by emergency medical personnel or another trained person.

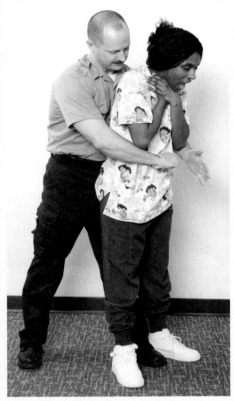

○ **Figure 17-16.** The rescuer makes a fist with one hand and places the thumb side just above the navel and well below the tip of the sternum.

Procedure (17-5)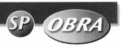

Helping an Unconscious Person with an Obstructed Airway

Equipment: face shield, barrier, or mask • disposable gloves

1. Call for help. Activate the EMS system.
2. Assist the victim to the floor or a hard surface if necessary. **See Figure 17-17.**
3. Open the airway and check breathing.
4. Put on a face shield, barrier, or mask and attempt rescue breathing as described in Procedure 17-1.
5. If the chest does not rise with the rescue breathing attempt, reposition the head and attempt rescue breathing again.
6. If rescue breathing is still unsuccessful, begin chest compressions.
7. Compress the patient's chest at a rate of 100 per minute.
   • Place your shoulders directly over your hands on the patient's chest.
   • Keep your arms straight and elbows locked.
   • Push the patient's sternum (breastbone) down 1½ to 2 inches.

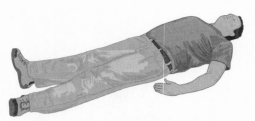

○ **Figure 17-17.** Position for helping an unconscious victim with an obstructed airway.

8. After 30 compressions, check the mouth visually for a FBAO. Remove the obstruction if you can see it. **See Figure 17-18.**
9. Repeat Steps 6 and 7 until you have an open airway or until emergency medical help arrives.
10. If you achieve an open airway, check for a pulse and continue CPR if needed until emergency medical help arrives.

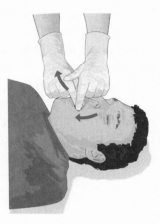

○ **Figure 17-18.** Check the mouth for a foreign object. If an object comes within reach, grab and remove it.

Shock

Shock is a condition that occurs when an inadequate blood supply is delivered to the body's tissues. This is a dangerous medical emergency. The decreased blood supply causes less blood to be pumped from the heart to the lungs. The blood picks up less oxygen, depriving the body of nourishment.

Shock can be caused by severe injury, cardiac arrest, hemorrhage, severe pain, excessive loss of body fluids, or allergic reaction. A patient in shock has some or all of the following signs and symptoms:

- Pale or bluish skin, lips, or nails
- Cool, clammy skin
- Heavy sweating
- Rapid breathing and heart rate
- Difficulty breathing
- Staring eyes
- Decreased blood pressure
- Extreme thirst
- Nausea and vomiting
- Loss of consciousness, mental confusion, or disorientation

Shock victims need immediate medical attention to save their lives. Check the person's ABCs and provide basic life support if necessary. Make the patient warm and comfortable. Reassure and calm the patient.

Procedure 17-6

Helping a Patient in Shock

Equipment: face shield, barrier, or mask, if necessary

1. Call for help.
2. Check ABCs. Administer basic life support if necessary.
3. Place the patient on his or her back if no spinal cord injury is suspected. Position the patient to lie flat on the back. **See Figure 17-19.**
4. Keep the patient warm. Cover with a coat, blanket, or whatever is available.
5. Control bleeding if necessary.
6. Turn the patient's head to the side if he or she is vomiting.
7. Try to keep the environment as quiet as possible.

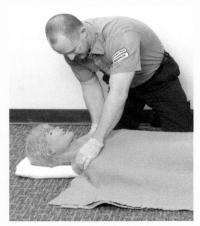

O **Figure 17-19.** A shock victim in the correct body position. For many years, guidelines required elevating the feet. However, current guidelines require that the patient lie flat.

Stroke

A **stroke** is a condition that occurs when there is damage to a blood vessel in the brain. It is also called a *cerebrovascular accident (CVA)*. A stroke can be caused by a blockage in a blood vessel, a blood clot in the brain, a blood clot carried to the brain, bleeding in the brain, or an embolism. Stroke is the third greatest cause of death in the United States and is also a major cause of disability.

Signs and symptoms of stroke depend on which area of the brain is involved. A stroke patient exhibits some of the following signs and symptoms:

• Unexplained dizziness, unsteadiness, or a sudden fall
• Sudden, severe headache
• Change or loss of consciousness
• Difficulty breathing
• Sudden numbness or weakness in the face, arm, or leg, on one side of the body
• Drooping eyelid or mouth
• Drooling from one side of the mouth
• Loss of speech or trouble talking and understanding speech
• Dimness or loss of vision, often in only one eye
• Loss of bladder or bowel control

About 10 percent of stroke victims experience little strokes, called *transient ischemic attacks (TIAs)*, before experiencing a full-fledged stroke. TIAs are an important warning sign of a larger stroke and should not be ignored. They may occur hours, days, weeks, or even months before major stroke occurs. They generally last for only a few minutes, and their symptoms are similar to those of a stroke. The patient needs immediate medical attention.

Emergency care for stroke includes calling EMS as soon as the patient begins to experience signs and symptoms. Keep the patient warm and comfortable until medical help arrives or until he or she can be transported to an emergency room.

Procedure 17-7

Helping a Patient Who Seems to Be Having a Stroke

Equipment: none

1. Call for help.
2. Check ABCs. Administer basic life support if necessary.
3. Place the patient in the semi-Fowler's position and monitor the airway.
4. Loosen tight clothing.
5. Keep the patient warm.
6. Keep the patient as calm as possible.
7. Stay with the patient until medical help arrives.

Hemorrhage

The human body needs an adequate blood supply to function properly. **Hemorrhage** is the sudden and extreme loss of blood. **External bleeding** is loss of blood on the outer surface of the body. **Internal bleeding** is loss of blood inside the body or under the skin from an organ, blood vessels, or other internal tissues. Both external and internal bleeding can result in death.

The most obvious sign of external bleeding is blood coming from a wound. The blood may not be immediately visible, however, if it is under layers of clothing. Bleeding injuries may involve arteries, veins, or capillaries.

• Bright red blood spurting from a wound indicates a damaged artery.
• Dark red blood flowing steadily from a wound indicates a damaged vein.
• A slow oozing of blood indicates damaged capillaries.

Internal bleeding cannot be seen, so it is more difficult to detect. Internal bleeding is a true medical emergency. If left untreated, the patient can go into shock, and death will soon result. Signs and symptoms include:

• Blood from the mouth or rectum, or blood in the urine
• Nonmenstrual vaginal bleeding
• Bruises or contusions
• Cold, clammy skin
• Rapid and/or weak pulse
• Dilated pupils
• Excessive thirst
• Coughing or vomiting blood
• Swollen, painful, tender, or bruised abdomen, chest, or back near the kidney area

The most important care you can first give to a patient who is hemorrhaging is to maintain an airway and restore breathing. The second thing to do is to stop the bleeding.

Always practice standard precautions when administering care to a bleeding patient. Wear disposable gloves when handling blood or body fluids. Wash your hands thoroughly as soon as your role in the patient's care is complete.

The most effective way to stop bleeding is to apply direct pressure on the wound, elevate the area (whenever possible, to a level above the heart), and apply pressure to the nearest pulse site.

Procedure 17-8

SP

Helping Stop a Hemorrhage

Equipment: disposable gloves

1. Identify the location of the bleeding.
2. Put on disposable gloves, if available. In a home situation, you can use a plastic bag or other nonabsorbent material if gloves are not available.
3. Apply direct pressure over the wound. Use a sterile dressing or the cleanest cloth available. **See Figure 17-20.**
4. Elevate the wound above the patient's heart. **See Figure 17-21.**
5. Call for help.
6. If blood seeps through the dressing, apply additional dressing on top of it. Never lift or remove a dressing once it is on the wound.
7. If bleeding has not stopped, locate a pulse site or artery above the site of the wound and apply pressure. **See Figure 17-22.** For example, if the wound is on the thigh, place pressure on the femoral artery in the groin area.
8. If bleeding has not stopped, and the bleeding is from the arm or leg, activate EMS.
9. Lay the patient down and keep warm until trained medical personnel arrive to assist.

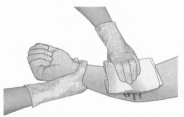

○ **Figure 17-20.** Place a sterile dressing over a wound and apply pressure.

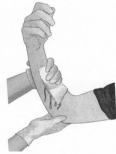

○ **Figure 17-21.** Elevate the wounded limb above the heart.

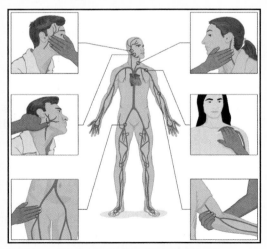

○ **Figure 17-22.** Some of the body's pulse sites.

Vital Skills COMMUNICATION

Nonverbal Messages

Emergencies can be stressful for everyone involved. When you communicate with a patient in an emergency situation, it is important to project a calm attitude so that the patient's stress level does not increase. We communicate with more than just words; our body language and other nonverbal cues can send messages about how we are feeling. It is important to be aware of the nonverbal messages you might be sending to a patient in an emergency. Some nonverbal communication tips to keep in mind:

- Touching a patient can be reassuring. If appropriate, you can hold a patient's hand while waiting for help to arrive.
- Be aware of your facial expressions. The scene of a traumatic accident, or the injury itself, can be bloody and a little scary. Be aware that the patient might be looking at your face. Try not to show signs of fear or disgust as you help the victim.
- Make eye contact with the victim or patient. Avoiding eye contact can convey fear or uncertainty.

Practice

With two of your classmates, role-play the following emergency situation: One person has been in a car accident and is admitted to the emergency room. A family member has come after receiving a call from the police. As a nursing assistant, how can you help keep the family member calm? What nonverbal cues might you be unknowingly sending to the family? Rotate roles so that everyone can practice being the nursing assistant. Discuss ways to handle the situation.

Seizures

A **seizure**, sometimes called a *convulsion*, is an electrical disturbance in the brain that results in uncontrollable spasms or jerking of the muscles of the body. Seizures can happen to anyone. They may be caused by:

- Tumors
- Head injury
- Drug overdose
- Chemical imbalance
- Fever
- Hypoglycemic reactions (See Chapter 23 for more about hypoglycemia.)
- Stroke
- Fumes in a confined space
- Seizure disorder, such as epilepsy
- Failure to take prescribed antiseizure medication

The two primary types of seizures are generalized and partial. **Generalized seizures** are convulsions that involve all or part of the body and are characterized by a loss of consciousness. They are also called *tonic-clonic* or *grand mal seizures*. The seizure may last up to several minutes. The person's body may become rigid or display uncontrolled convulsions. Other signs include:

- Falling down
- Frothing at the mouth

- Clenching of the teeth
- Yelling out or moaning
- Skin turning blue
- Jerking movements of an arm or leg
- Loss of bladder and bowel function

Partial seizures are seizures in which the patient remains conscious and appears to stare blankly. They are also known as *petit mal* or *absence seizures*. The patient may experience some mild shaking or lip smacking. These seizures last only a few seconds and may occur frequently.

People with **epilepsy**, a disease in which a person has recurrent seizures, may experience generalized or partial seizures. Epileptic seizures can be controlled or at least partially controlled with medication. An uncomplicated epileptic seizure is not a medical emergency, even though it looks like one. Look for a bracelet or other identifying information on a person who is having a seizure.

Depending on the type and underlying cause of the seizure, the seizure should gradually lessen and the patient will recover. After a generalized seizure, the patient may be confused, disoriented, combative, or exhausted. Most people fall into a deep sleep, called a *postictal state*. The patient usually does not remember the seizure.

The most important way to help patients who are having a seizure is to protect them from injury. Move anything that could cause injury away from the patient. Never restrain the patient during the seizure and never place anything in the mouth. Allow the seizure to run its course naturally. Remain with the patient throughout the seizure. Protect the head from injury.

Procedure 17-9

Helping a Patient Who Is Having a Seizure

Equipment: pillow or blanket

1. Call for help. Do not leave the patient.
2. Lower the patient to the floor unless already in bed.
3. Do not restrain movements.
4. Do whatever is possible to protect the patient from injury. Place a pillow or blanket under the patient's head, or cradle the head in your lap.
5. Turn the patient to the side to prevent choking.
6. Loosen tight clothing. **See Figure 17-23.**
7. Move furniture and equipment out of the way so the patient does not strike it.
8. After the seizure stops, help the patient to bed and raise the side rails.
9. Make the patient comfortable and allow him or her to rest.
10. Get medical attention for the patient.
11. Report and record seizure activity, including length of seizure in minutes and seconds, body parts involved, and patient reaction.

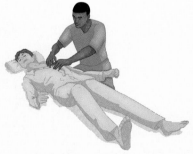

○ Figure 17-23. Loosen the clothing of someone who is having a seizure if you can do so without being injured.

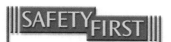
Burns

Burns are caused when body tissue is in contact with extreme heat, corrosive chemicals, radiation, or high voltage. Skin damage occurs when skin touches anything over 111° F (44° C).

Burns occur quickly and can be devastating. Any burn that affects the skin beyond the top layer requires immediate medical attention. The burn victim is at severe risk for infection, shock, pain, loss of body heat and fluids, swelling of breathing passages, and death.

Burns are categorized by the extent of tissue damage and the percentage of the body affected. The categories include minor, moderate, and major burns.

Minor Burns. A minor burn affects only the skin's outer layer. **See Figure 17-24.** The skin will be red and tender, with mild swelling and moderate pain.

Moderate Burns. A moderate burn affects the entire outer skin layer and into the inner skin layer. **See Figure 17-25.** A minor burn that covers more than 15 percent of an adult's body surface or more than 5 percent of a child's or elderly person's body surface is also considered a moderate burn. Signs of a moderate burn include blister formation, swelling, oozing of fluids from the skin, and severe pain.

Major Burns. A major burn affects all the skin layers and possibly underlying fat, muscle, and bone. **See Figure 17-26.** A moderate burn that covers more than 25 percent of an adult's body surface or more than 20 percent of a child's or elderly person's body surface is also considered a major burn. All burns of the hands, face, eyes, feet, and perineum, as well as burns resulting from inhalation injury, electrical injury, and major trauma, are categorized as major burns. Signs of a major burn include skin discoloration, leathery skin, and no pain (because the nerve endings are destroyed).

First aid for burns is intended to prevent further injury and to minimize complications in the healing process. The most important action is to remove the patient from the source of the burn. If the patient has an electrical burn, do not make contact with the electrical current.

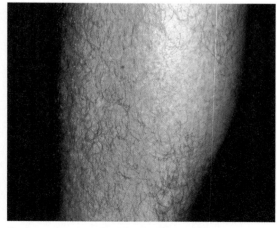

○ Figure 17-24. Redness and mild swelling are signs of a minor burn.

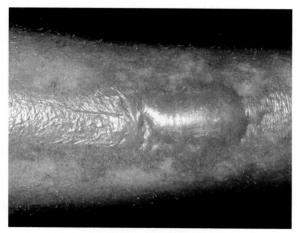

○ Figure 17-25. Blistering, swelling, and oozing or "weeping" are signs of a moderate burn.

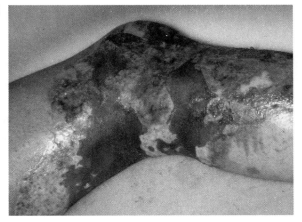

O **Figure 17-26.** Discolored and leathery skin are signs of a major burn.

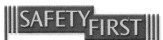

When a patient has a chemical burn, remove clothing containing the chemical and flush the burn thoroughly with a large amount of water. Be sure to direct the water flow away from areas not already exposed to the chemical. If the chemical is a dry powder, carefully brush off as much as possible before flushing the area with water. The chemical burning process can continue for a long time after initial contact. Check the patient's ABCs and provide basic life support if necessary.

Treat burns according to their severity. Moderate and major burns require immediate medical treatment. Many regions have burn centers that specialize in the treatment of burns.

Procedure 17-10

Helping a Patient with Burns

Equipment: face shield, barrier, or mask, if necessary • sterile dressing • sterile cloth • disposable gloves

1. Call for help.
2. Remove the patient from the source of the burn (fire, smoke, flames, chemical, sun).
3. Check ABCs. Administer basic life support if necessary.
4. When a patient has a minor burn, immerse the body part in cold water and then cover the area with a dry, sterile dressing.
5. When a patient has a moderate burn, cool the body part with cold water and then:
   • Blot the part dry with a sterile cloth.
   • Treat for shock.
   • Get medical attention.

6. When a patient has a major burn:
   • Remove clothing from the burn site to expose it. Do not remove clothing that is stuck to the burn.
   • Cover the burn site with a sterile cloth or a sheet to protect it from infection.
   • Treat for shock.
   • Watch for breathing difficulty.
   • Get immediate medical attention.
7. When a patient has a chemical burn:
   • Remove surrounding clothing.
   • Flush the burn site with large quantities of water.
   • Get medical attention.
8. Keep the patient comfortable until help arrives.

Poisoning

A **poison** is any substance that is toxic to humans and can change the function of body organs and adversely affect the patient's health. Poisons can be inhaled, swallowed (ingested), absorbed through touch, or injected. Many of the products we use in daily living can be poisonous if inhaled or ingested, such as household cleaners, insecticides, rat poisons, lye, and disinfectants. A patient can also be poisoned by a drug overdose or by food.

The signs and symptoms of possible poisoning include:
- Abdominal pain and cramping
- Nausea, vomiting, or diarrhea
- Burns, odor, and stains in and around the mouth
- Drowsiness or unconsciousness

In addition to assessing the patient for signs and symptoms, assess the scene for any clues of the poison, such as poison containers, needles, medications, or poisonous plants.

Procedure 17-11

Helping a Conscious Patient Who Has Been Poisoned

Equipment: none

1. Check the patient's ABCs. Maintain a clear airway.
2. Call for help.
3. Observe the patient.
4. Check the mouth for burns and odor.
5. Question the patient and other people present to determine the poison, the quantity, the time it was taken, and the age of the patient.
6. Look for a poison container and other clues.
7. Call the Poison Control Center for help.
8. Follow the directions given to you by the Poison Control Center. Depending on the poison, they may instruct you to activate EMS immediately or ask you to induce vomiting, try to prevent vomiting, or give the patient water or milk.
9. Keep the patient comfortable until medical help arrives.
10. Give empty poison containers to medical personnel and report your observations to the medical staff. **See Figure 17-27.**

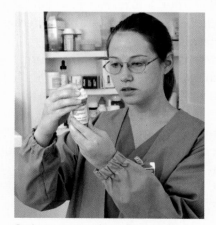

○ **Figure 17-27.** If you find a poison container, give it to your supervisor or emergency personnel.

A poison control hotline is available 24 hours a day to help you treat someone who has been poisoned. The telephone number for this hotline is usually printed on the inside cover of the phone book. The number is toll-free and will connect you with the poison control center in your area. Trained personnel will guide you through the first-aid procedures to deal with a specific poison. You must provide the following critical information:

- *Who:* age, weight, and condition of patient
- *What:* type of poison, including ingredients if known
- *How much:* quantity of poison involved
- *How:* circumstances
- *When:* approximate time taken

Procedure 17-12

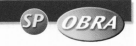

Helping an Unconscious Patient Who Has Been Poisoned

Equipment: face shield, barrier, or mask, if necessary

1. Establish unresponsiveness.
2. Call for help. Activate the EMS system.
3. Check the patient's ABCs. Maintain a clear airway.
4. Place the patient on the left side in case he or she starts to vomit.
5. Look for immediate clues to determine what type of poison was taken.
6. Call the Poison Control Center for help.
7. Perform rescue breathing or CPR only upon direction from the Poison Control Center. Some ingested poisons make it dangerous for you to perform rescue breathing.
8. Follow the directions given to you by the Poison Control Center.
9. Keep the patient comfortable until medical help arrives.

Weather Emergencies

The environment can cause a variety of serious and potentially fatal emergencies. For example, very young and very old people are at high risk for the serious health effects of extreme weather.

Heat Emergencies

Heat exhaustion is a condition caused by prolonged exposure to heat over hours to days that results in a slightly elevated body temperature and signs of dehydration. **Heat stroke** is a severe and possibly fatal condition caused by exposure to extreme heat and characterized by confusion and high fever. Heat stroke is caused by **hyperthermia**, a dangerous condition in which body temperature is elevated above the normal range.

Vital Skills MATH

Converting Temperatures

Many health care facilities use the Celsius temperature scale (°C) to record patient temperatures. On the Celsius scale, water freezes at 0° and boils at 100°. Others use the Fahrenheit scale (°F), on which water freezes at 32° and boils at 212°. Occasionally, you may need to convert from one scale to the other.

The formula to convert from °F to °C is: $°C = (5/9) \times (°F - 32)$. For example, if the temperature is 99.6° F:

$$°C = (5/9 \times (99.6 - 32)$$
$$= 5/9 \times 67.6$$
$$= 37.5$$

The formula to convert from °C to °F is: $°F = (°C \times 9/5) + 32$. For example, if the temperature is 36.8° C :

$$°F = (36.8 \times 9/5) + 32$$
$$= 66.2 + 32$$
$$= 98.2$$

Practice

Convert the following temperatures. Round your answers to the nearest tenth of a degree.
1. Convert 101.4° F to Celsius.
2. Convert 98.4° F to Celsius.
3. Convert 37.2° C to Fahrenheit.
4. Convert 38.4° C to Fahrenheit.

SAFETY FIRST

Be gentle when treating or attempting to move a hypothermic patient. The heart can be very irritable.

Signs and symptoms of heat stroke include:
- Hot, red, flushed dry skin
- High body temperature
- Rapid pulse
- Difficulty breathing
- Weakness
- Confusion or unconsciousness
- Seizure

To provide emergency care for heat stroke:
1. Establish unresponsiveness.
2. Call for help. Activate the EMS system.
3. Check the patient's ABCs. Maintain a clear airway.
4. Cool the patient by moving him or her to a shady area, removing hot clothing, and applying cool or tepid water to the skin while waiting for trained emergency medical professionals.

Cold Emergencies

Hypothermia is a condition in which the core body temperature drops below 95° F (35° C). It is caused by prolonged exposure to the cold. In addition to a low body core temperature, the signs and symptoms may include:

- Shivering
- Slow breathing
- Pale or bluish skin color
- Decreased heart rate
- Confusion leading to unconsciousness

To provide emergency care for hypothermia:

1. Establish unresponsiveness.
2. Call for help. Activate the EMS system.
3. Check the patient's ABCs. Maintain a clear airway.
4. Get the patient to a warm room or shelter.
5. If the patient is wearing wet clothing, remove it.
6. Warm the patient using dry blankets, towels, or clothing. **See Figure 17-28.**
7. Stay with the patient until help arrives. Do not try to give warm beverages to someone who is unconscious. If the patient is awake and talking, you may offer warm beverages while waiting for trained emergency medical professionals to arrive.

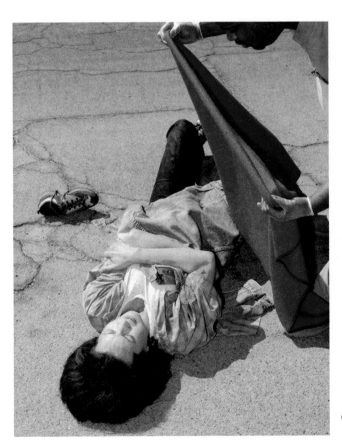

○ **Figure 17-28. Provide warmth to a person who has hypothermia.**

Chapter Summary

- Becoming certified in first aid and basic life support procedures increases the nursing assistant's skills and can help minimize the effects of injury and save lives.

- After an emergency has occurred, assess the scene for injuries and possible additional danger.

- After an emergency has occurred, activate the emergency medical services (EMS) system to summon help.

- Learn the signs and symptoms of respiratory arrest and cardiac arrest so you will know when to provide basic life support.

- The basic life support procedures for adults, children, and infants are different and must be followed according to the American Heart Association guidelines.

- The automated external defibrillator (AED) delivers an electric shock to a patient's chest to re-establish the heart's rhythm.

- Nursing assistants can learn the signs, symptoms, and emergency care procedures for assisting patients with airway obstruction, shock, stroke, hemorrhaging, seizures, burns, poisoning, heat stroke, and hypothermia.

VOCABULARY REVIEW

Directions: Match the letter of each definition in the second column with the correct vocabulary term in the first column. Write your answers on a separate sheet of paper.

Vocabulary

1. basic life support
2. cardiac arrest
3. CPR
4. emergency
5. first aid
6. Heimlich maneuver
7. hemorrhage
8. hypothermia
9. rescue breathing
10. shock
11. stroke

Definitions

A. The first care given to an injured or ill person in an emergency before medical help arrives

B. A step in basic life support, in which the rescuer forces oxygen into the patient's lungs to restore or support breathing

C. A condition in which the core body temperature drops below 95° F (35° C) caused by prolonged exposure to the cold

D. The condition that occurs when the heart and breathing suddenly stop

E. An event that calls for immediate action

F. The series of actions taken to maintain life in an emergency

G. A condition that occurs when there is damage to a blood vessel in the brain

H. A first-aid procedure for dislodging an item that is causing a person to choke

I. A condition that occurs when an inadequate blood supply is delivered to the body's tissues

J. The sudden and extreme loss of blood

K. A form of basic life support that includes activation of EMS and procedures that support both breathing and circulation

Check Your Knowledge

Review Questions: Answer each of the following questions on a separate sheet of paper.

1. What are the two goals of first aid?

2. What are the legal responsibilities of a nursing assistant when delivering emergency care?

3. Describe what is meant by checking the ABCs?

4. What makes an AED so important in the initial minutes of responding to a cardiac arrest situation?

5. List at least four signs and symptoms of airway obstruction.

6. What two groups of people is the Heimlich maneuver *not* effective for?

7. If you are concerned that a person may be in shock due to an allergic reaction, where can you look for clues?

8. How would you practice standard precautions when helping a person who is bleeding?

9. Name five possible causes of seizures.

10. What is the most important way to help a person who is having a seizure?

True or False: Read each statement carefully. Then write *True* or *False* by the statement number on a separate sheet of paper.

1. Cardiac arrest causes numbness and paralysis on one side of the body.

2. You need to be specially trained to perform basic life support.

3. Shock can be caused by heavy bleeding.

4. Blood from a damaged vein will be bright red and spurting.

5. Call the Poison Control Center if you suspect a patient is poisoned.

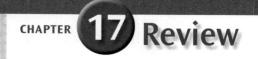
Think and Decide

Directions: Think about each of the following scenarios. Answer each question on a separate sheet of paper.

1. You arrive at the home of a patient who has fallen out of bed and cannot move the entire left side of his body. His speech is slurred, but he is able to talk to you. You are alone with the patient. What should you do?

2. You are taking care of your sister's 2-month-old baby. When you walk over to the crib to check on the baby, you notice that she is not breathing. You tap the infant's foot, and there is no response. Should you activate EMS first or start CPR first?

3. Your neighbor's power has been out of order for three days, and the temperature outside has been over 110° F (43° C). You decide to go over and check on her and you find her unconscious in her bed. Suddenly she begins to have a seizure. You immediately call 9-1-1 for help. What should you do next?

4. You walk into a long-term care resident's room and find she has a bluish color to her skin and is not breathing. After you call for help and establish unresponsiveness, you need to begin rescue breathing. What is important to remember when performing rescue breathing?

5. Mr. G., a 92-year-old long-term care resident, fell out of bed yesterday. He is now complaining of severe abdominal pain and low back pain. His pulse is fast and weak and his abdomen is swollen. He is usually alert, but he is suddenly becoming confused. Should you report these changes to the nurse? What is the possible cause of these changes?

6. Mrs. Y. is an obese 57-year-old patient on your floor at the hospital. You have served her lunch and have moved to the next bed to help Mrs. Y.'s roommate with her lunch. Suddenly, from the corner of your eye, you see Mrs. Y. clutch at her throat with both hands. What should you do?

7. You have settled your home health client, Mr. D., in the living room with a book. After telling him to call you if he needs anything, you go to the laundry room at the back of the house to fold the laundry. A few minutes later, you hear Mr. D. cry out loudly. Rushing to the front of the house, you find him in the kitchen, standing next to the stove. He is holding one hand with the other and looks as though he is in severe pain. You ask what happened, and he tells you he came to the kitchen to fix a snack and accidentally burned his hand on the stove. You examine the burn and see that it is minor. What should you do?

CNA Certification Exam Prep

Directions: This practice test contains ten questions. Each question has four suggested answers. For each question, choose the ONE that best answers the question or completes the statement. Write your answers on a separate sheet of paper.

1. Which of the following is a life-threatening situation?

   A. a victim who is conscious

   B. a victim who is asleep

   C. a victim who is not breathing

   D. a victim who is screaming

2. When is it necessary to move a victim?

   A. when the victim asks you to move him

   B. when the victim complains of cold

   C. when the scene becomes unsafe

   D. when you have stabilized the victim

3. CPR should be initiated when the victim

   A. is bleeding.

   B. is bleeding and has a pulse.

   C. is not breathing but has a pulse.

   D. is not breathing and has no pulse.

4. In most cases, where should you check for a pulse in an adult?

   A. radial artery

   B. carotid artery

   C. temporal artery

   D. brachial artery

5. In most cases, where should you check for a pulse in an infant?

   A. radial artery

   B. carotid artery

   C. temporal artery

   D. brachial artery

6. When a person is in respiratory arrest, the correct basic life support procedure is

   A. rescue breathing.

   B. CPR.

   C. Heimlich maneuver.

   D. FBAO.

7. The "A" in ABC assessment stands for

   A. airway.

   B. anatomy.

   C. AED.

   D. antibiotic.

8. The rate of CPR chest compressions for an infant or child should be

   A. about 60 compressions per minute.

   B. about 80 compressions per minute.

   C. at least 100 compressions per minute.

   D. at least 120 compressions per minute.

9. If you are administering CPR to an adult without the help of a second rescuer, the ratio of compressions to breaths should be

   A. 30 compressions, 2 breaths.

   B. 15 compressions, 2 breaths.

   C. 30 compressions, 1 breath.

   D. 15 compressions, 1 breath.

10. A person who is suspected to be in shock and does not have a spinal cord injury should be placed

    A. flat on the back.

    B. flat on the stomach.

    C. on the back with the legs raised.

    D. on the stomach with the legs raised.

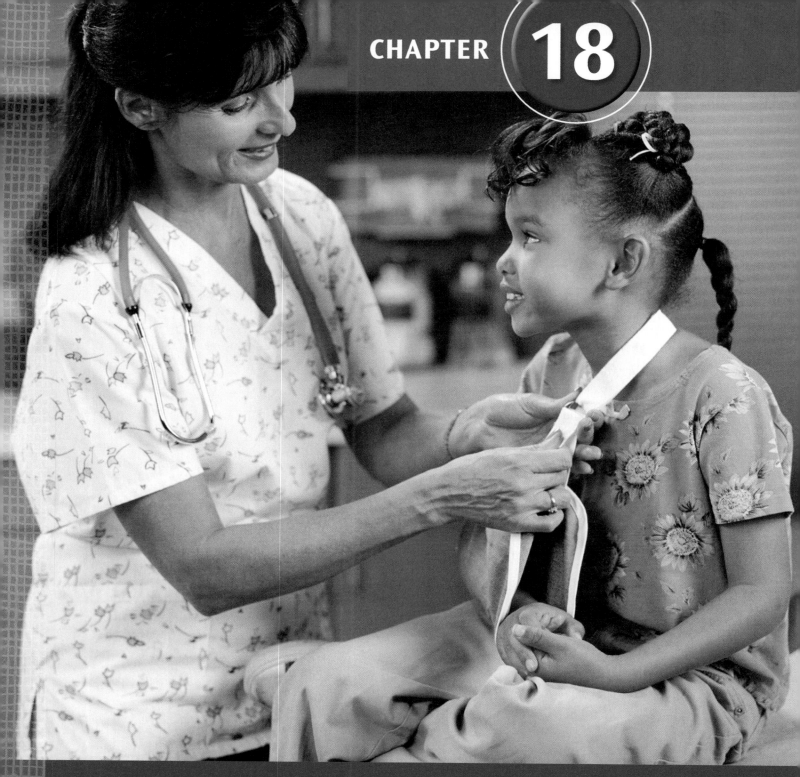

CHAPTER 18

OBJECTIVES

- Describe how to prepare and assist a patient for an examination.
- Identify the supplies and equipment that are commonly used for a physical examination.

- Describe the purposes and types of warm therapy.
- Demonstrate the safe application of warm therapy.
- Describe the purposes and types of cold therapy.
- Demonstrate the safe application of cold therapy.

- Identify the uses of bandages, dressings, and anti-embolic stockings.
- Demonstrate the application of dressings and support devices.

Examinations and Therapies

antiembolic stockings Stockings made of elastic fabric that provide support, promote blood flow, and prevent the formation of blood clots.

aquamatic pad An electric heating pad containing tubes filled with circulating water.

cold compress A cold folded and moistened cloth or towel that is placed over a small area of the body for moist cold therapy.

cold pack A dry cold treatment that is applied or wrapped around an area of the body.

cyanosis A bluish discoloration or darkening of the skin, eyelids, lips, or fingernails caused by insufficient oxygen in the blood.

elastic bandage A long strip of stretchy material that provides support and protection to extremities and joints.

phlebitis An inflammation of the veins.

postoperatively The period of time after surgery.

sitz bath A type of moist warm therapy in which the patient's perineal and anal regions are immersed in warm water in a special tub or seat.

sterile Free from microorganisms.

thrombophlebitis A condition that occurs when a blood clot causes inflammation in a vein.

warm compress A folded and moistened piece of cloth or towel that is warmed and placed over a small area of the body for moist warm therapy.

warm pack A heated moist treatment that is applied to or wrapped around an area of the body.

Assisting with Examinations

In some work situations, such as clinics and hospitals, nursing assistants escort patients to examination rooms. They may also prepare the rooms, prepare the patients, and assist in the examinations. In many long-term care facilities, where doctors visit residents in their rooms, nursing assistants prepare the residents for examinations.

Although specific duties vary depending on the facility, nursing assistants generally assist in the following ways:

- Gathering the needed draping linens and gown
- Collecting the necessary equipment
- Preparing the examination room
- Providing reassurance and support to the patient
- Helping the patient to the examination table or chair, if necessary
- Positioning and draping the patient
- Handing equipment to the examiner when requested
- Labeling specimens
- Cleaning and storing equipment after the examination

Supplies and Equipment

Preparing an examination room includes making sure the correct supplies and equipment are available. In most health care facilities, exam room supplies include cotton-tipped applicators, cotton balls, tongue depressors, alcohol wipes, disposable gloves, tissues, paper towels, slides, specimen containers, specimen labels, and emesis basins. Other items may include disposable bed protectors, bath blankets, towels, and disposable bags.

You may be responsible for laying out the equipment that the health care provider will use. This equipment could include an eye chart, a tape measure, a flashlight or penlight, and water-soluble lubricant. A sphygmomanometer, stethoscope, and thermometer will also be needed.

Some equipment is used only for specific examinations. **See Figure 18-1** to become familiar with some of these instruments, such as a tuning fork, reflex hammer, otoscope, ophthalmoscope, and vaginal speculum (for female patients).

O **Figure 18-1.** Equipment needed for a physical examination is laid out before the health care provider arrives.

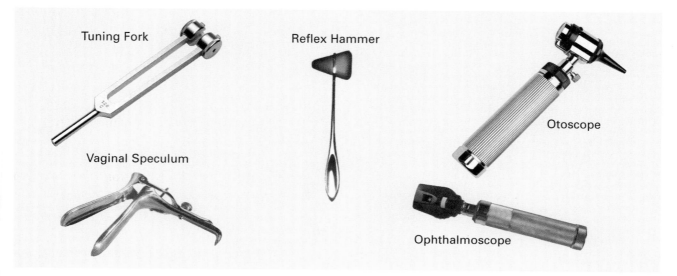

Tuning Fork

Reflex Hammer

Otoscope

Vaginal Speculum

Ophthalmoscope

If an exam will be done in a patient's room, you may be responsible for laying out the supplies and equipment needed there. You may also be responsible for maintaining a clean or aseptic field to provide infection control.

Preparing the Patient

Preparing a patient for an examination may include helping the patient undress and put on a gown. **See Figure 18-2.** You may need to assist the patient onto the examination table. You would then explain what position the patient needs to assume and assist if necessary.

Some patients are anxious before an examination. You can help reassure and support the patient in the following ways:

- Be sensitive to the patient's feelings.
- Explain to the patient what you are about to do.
- Provide as much privacy as possible with draping.
- Between procedures, ask how the patient is feeling.
- Help the patient get on the examination table. Have a seat or stool available for the examiner.
- Tell the patient what procedure is coming next. (The doctor or nurse will explain the procedure to the patient.)
- Constantly make sure that the patient is not in danger of falling, either from a standing position or off the bed or examining table.
- Protect the patient from becoming chilled during the examination. An extra bath blanket should be nearby.

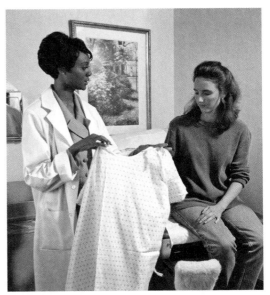

O **Figure 18-2.** The nursing assistant explains to the patient how to put on the gown.

Procedure 18-1

Assisting in an Examination

Equipment: disposable gloves

1. Wash your hands and put on gloves.
2. Identify the patient, check the ID bracelet against the chart, and call the patient by name.
3. Introduce yourself.
4. Provide privacy.
5. When the examiner lets you know the position he or she wants the patient to assume, explain the position to the patient.
6. Help the patient get into the position if necessary.
7. Hand equipment and supplies to the examiner when requested.
8. Assist with repositioning the patient when necessary.
9. When the examination is complete, assist the patient to a sitting position and offer to help the patient get dressed. Ask if the patient is dizzy or lightheaded. If so, wait a minute before asking the patient to stand. If not, help the patient to a standing position.
10. Wash your hands.
11. Transport the patient back to his or her room.
12. Clean all equipment, using gloves as needed, and return it to its storage location.
13. Remove the gloves and wash your hands.

Warm Therapy

Nursing assistants help patients when warm therapy is ordered. Heat is applied to the body to promote healing, relax muscles, ease joint pain and stiffness, and reduce tissue swelling. Heat can be applied generally or locally. Generalized applications are for the whole body. Local applications target a specific area of the body.

Applying heat locally to the skin reduces swelling and inflammation. The warmth increases blood flow to that area of the body by causing the blood vessels to dilate (become bigger). The increased blood flow sends oxygen and nutrients to the cells and tissues, promoting healing. At the same time, toxins and excess fluids can leave the area of inflammation more rapidly. **See Figure 18-3.**

When heat is applied for longer than 30 minutes, however, blood vessels tend to constrict (narrow). Therefore, prolonged application of heat will have the same effects as a cold application.

When using warm therapy on a patient, follow these guidelines to prevent accidents or injuries:

- Measure water temperature accurately. Water that is too hot (more than 110° F or 43° C) can burn the patient's skin.
- Do not spill hot water.
- Do not allow electrical devices to come in contact with water.
- Check the condition of all equipment before using it. Do not use any equipment that has a frayed cord, bent plug, or any other defect.
- At regular intervals, check the condition of the patient's skin in the area being treated. Look for redness, blisters, or irritation. Ask if the patient is experiencing any pain or numbness. If any of these signs or symptoms occurs, stop treatment and tell the nurse immediately.
- Do not apply heat for longer than 30 minutes.
- Take care around wounds and open areas on the skin. These areas are at greater risk for injury when using heat.
- Infants, young children, the elderly, and fair-skinned people are at greater risk for complications from warm applications. Their skin is fragile and can be easily burned.
- People who have decreased mental status or have decreased sensitivity from paralysis or vascular disease are also at increased risk for complications.

Moist Warm Therapy

Heat applications can be moist or dry. Moist warm therapy is a treatment that applies heat and water to the skin. Moist heat reduces drying of the skin and can penetrate deeper into the tissues. It is more effective than dry heat. Examples of moist warm applications are warm compresses and packs, soaks, tub baths, and sitz baths.

SAFETY FIRST

Be alert for burns when a patient is receiving any form of warm therapy, especially if the patient is elderly.

WARM APPLICATION

Blood Flow Is Increased

Skin's Surface

Blood Vessels

Blood vessel at normal body temperature

Blood vessel dilated by warmth

O **Figure 18-3. Applying heat to an area of the body reduces inflammation and swelling.**

Warm Compresses and Packs. A **warm compress** is a folded and moistened cloth or towel that is warmed and placed over a small area of the body for moist warm therapy. A **warm pack** is a heated treatment that is applied or wrapped around an area of the body. The compress or pack is soaked in warm water or other prescribed warmed solution. It is usually applied for about 20 to 30 minutes. A patient should never lie on a compress or pack, and it should never be placed directly on the skin. Nursing assistants should apply warm compresses or packs only under the direction of a nurse or doctor.

Warm Soaks. During a soak, some or all of the body is immersed in water. A container is filled with warm water to soak small areas of the body. A tub is used to soak a large area. Soaks typically last for about 20 minutes.

Procedure 18-2

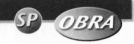

Applying a Warm Compress

Equipment: commercial compress • waterproof mattress protector • bath thermometer • towel • basin or bowl • tape, ties, or rolled gauze

1. Identify the patient, check the ID bracelet, and call the patient by name.
2. Introduce yourself.
3. Explain the procedure to the patient.
4. Wash your hands.
5. Provide privacy.
6. Place the moisture-proof mattress protector under the area of the body you will be treating.
7. Fill a basin or bowl with hot water.
8. Check the temperature of the water to make sure it is not too hot. The temperature should be between 105° F and 110° F (41° C to 43° C).
9. Open the compress.
10. Place the compress in the water to moisten, then remove it and ring out the excess water.
11. Carefully lay the compress to the site while it is still warm. **See Figure 18-4.**
12. Cover the compress with the towel. (Some facilities may recommend that a piece of plastic wrap be placed over the compress before applying the towel.)
13. You may loosely apply tape, ties, or rolled gauze over the towel to hold it in place.
14. Ask the patient if the temperature is too hot. If not, check again in 1 minute. Then

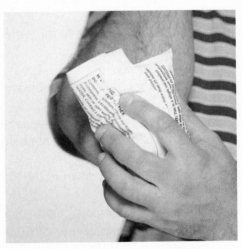

○ Figure 18-4. Be sure to apply the warm compress immediately, before it loses heat.

leave it in place for 20 to 30 minutes, but check the area every 5 minutes for signs of irritation or redness. Ask the patient if there is any pain or numbness. If there are any signs or symptoms, remove the compress and tell the nurse right away.

15. During the treatment, check to be sure the compress is still warm. If it cools, apply another warm compress.
16. After 20 minutes, remove the ties, towel, and compress.
17. Use the towel to pat dry the site.

18. Check to make sure the patient is comfortable and that the body is aligned properly.
19. Make sure the call signal is within the patient's reach.
20. Open the screen.
21. Clean the equipment and return it to storage. Place soiled towels and linens in the laundry.

22. Wash your hands.
23. Record the following and report anything unusual to the nurse:
    • Time the procedure started and ended
    • Site of the application
    • Temperature of the application
    • How the patient tolerated the procedure
    • The condition of the skin

Procedure 18-3

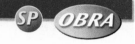

Giving a Warm Soak

Equipment: basin • bath thermometer • waterproof mattress protector • bath blanket • towel

1. Identify the patient, check the ID bracelet, and call the patient by name.
2. Introduce yourself.
3. Explain the procedure to the patient.
4. Wash your hands.
5. Provide privacy.
6. Raise the bed to a comfortable working position.
7. Place a bath blanket over the patient. Make sure the parts of the body not being treated are covered.
8. Fanfold top linens down to the foot of the bed.
9. Position the waterproof mattress protector under the part of the body that will be soaked.
10. Fill the basin one-half full with warm water. Using a bath thermometer, check the water temperature. It should be between 105° F and 110° F (41° C to 43° C).
11. Uncover the part of the body that needs treatment.
12. Position the basin so the area of the patient's body that needs treatment easily reaches the basin.
13. Slowly and gently lower the area being treated into the basin.
14. Monitor the temperature of the water in the basin every 5 minutes. When the water

loses its warmth, remove the area being treated and wrap it in a towel. Repeat Steps 10, 12, and 13.
15. During treatment, check the area every 5 minutes for signs of blistering, swelling, or redness. Ask the patient if there is any pain, burning, or numbness. If there are any signs or symptoms, remove the area from the basin and report the problems to the nurse.
16. When the treatment is finished, remove the basin and pat dry the treatment area.
17. Remove the mattress cover. Rearrange the top linens and remove the bath blanket.
18. Check to make sure the patient is comfortable and that the body is aligned properly.
19. Make sure the call signal is within the patient's reach.
20. Lower the bed.
21. Open the screen.
22. Clean the equipment and return it to storage.
23. Wash your hands.
24. Record the following and report anything unusual to the nurse:
    • Time the procedure began and ended
    • Site that was soaked
    • Temperature of the water
    • How the patient tolerated the procedure
    • The condition of the skin

Sitz Baths. A **sitz bath** is a type of moist warm therapy in which the patient's pelvic region is immersed in warm water in a special tub or seat. **See Figure 18-5.** A sitz bath lasts about 20 minutes. As with other heat therapies, a sitz bath increases blood flow to the area of the body being treated. Sitz baths are used to:

- Reduce pain in the pelvic region
- Clean *perineal* (the genital and rectal areas) wound sites
- Increase circulation
- Encourage bladder and bowel evacuation

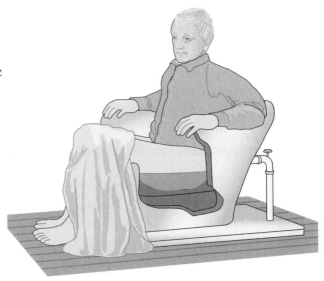

○ **Figure 18-5.** A sitz bath is given in a special tub with water above the hips. The patient's legs are out of the water.

Procedure 18-4

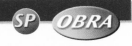

Giving a Sitz Bath

Equipment: portable sitz bath or disposable sitz bath • bath thermometer • container • bath blankets • towels • gown • disinfectant solution • wheelchair (for some patients)

1. Identify the patient, check the ID bracelet, and call the patient by name.
2. Introduce yourself.
3. Explain the procedure to the patient.
4. Wash your hands.
5. Provide privacy.
6. To prepare for the sitz bath, do one of the following:
   - If using a disposable sitz bath, position it on the toilet seat.
   - If using a portable sitz bath, position it alongside the patient's bed.
   - If using a built-in sitz bath, transport the patient by wheelchair to the room where the sitz bath is located.
7. Fill the sitz bath two-thirds full with water. The water temperature should be 105° F (41° C).
8. Place towels over metal parts of the sitz bath so no contact is made with the patient's skin. Also, place towels on the seat and front edge of the bath.
9. Help the patient raise his or her gown and tie it loosely above the waist.
10. Assist the patient to sit down on the sitz bath.
11. Cover the patient's legs and shoulders with bath blankets.
12. Make sure the patient is comfortable and that the call signal is within reach.
13. During the treatment, check the patient every 5 minutes. Ask the patient about feeling weak, dizzy, drowsy, or faint. If the patient reports any of these conditions, call for a helper and return the patient to bed.
14. After 20 minutes, help the patient stand up slowly. Assist the patient with patting dry and putting on a clean gown.
15. Help the patient get back in bed.
16. Check to make sure the patient is comfortable and that the body is aligned properly.
17. Make sure the call signal is within the patient's reach.
18. Open the screen.
19. Using disinfectant solution, clean the sitz bath. Return reusable equipment to the proper location. Put used linens in the linen hamper.

20. Wash your hands.
21. Record the following and report anything unusual to the nurse:
    - Time the procedure started and ended
    - Site of the application

- Temperature of the water
- How the patient tolerated the procedure
- Any sign of rectal bleeding
- The condition of the skin

Dry Warm Therapy

Dry warm therapy is a treatment that applies heat to the skin without water. Dry heat increases dryness of the skin but can maintain a steady temperature longer than moist heat. Heat lamps are one type of dry warm therapy. Heating pads and warm water bottles are examples of dry warm therapies that have a dry surface. They contain water, but water does not touch the patient's skin.

Aquamatic Pads. An **aquamatic pad** is an electric heating pad containing tubes filled with circulating water. The pad is attached to a separate heating unit that heats the water at a pre-set temperature and circulates it to the pad through a hose. Water flows from the pad back to the heating unit through another hose. This water reheats and flows back out to the heating pad. The heating unit should be kept level with the pad and connecting hoses. A patient should never lie on a heating pad.

Heat Lamps. Heat lamps are used to apply dry heat to a specific part of the body. A goose-neck lamp with a special bulb is placed a certain distance from the skin (usually 14 to 24 inches). The bulb is aimed at the targeted site. The bulb wattage determines the appropriate distance between the lamp and the body area being treated. Nursing assistants should use heat lamps only under the direct supervision of a nurse or doctor.

Vital Skills COMMUNICATION

Asking Questions

When you begin working, you may be expected to provide, or assist with, a range of procedures and therapies. Some of them will be familiar to you; others will not. Your employer may also ask you to perform procedures differently from the way you learned them. If you aren't sure what to do, *ask questions.*

By asking questions, you show that you are willing to learn and that you are interested in learning how to perform a task correctly. For simple questions, such as where supplies are located, you can ask a coworker. For more involved questions, ask a nurse or supervisor. For example, if you are not sure whether you can change a patient's bandage, ask your immediate supervisor.

Practice

As you read this chapter, imagine yourself participating in these activities in the hospital setting. Come up with a list of 10 questions about the procedures covered in the chapter. Indicate to whom you would direct the question: a fellow nursing assistant, the patient, or a supervisor.

Procedure 18-5

Applying a Warm Water Bottle

Equipment: warm water • warm water bottle • pitcher of hot water (115° F/46° C) • bath thermometer • hot water bottle cover • bath blanket

1. Identify the patient, check the ID bracelet, and call the patient by name.
2. Introduce yourself.
3. Explain the procedure to the patient.
4. Wash your hands.
5. Provide privacy.
6. Place a bath blanket over the patient. Make sure the parts of the body not being treated are covered.
7. Fanfold top linens down to the foot of the bed.
8. Uncover the area of the body that needs treatment.
9. Fill a pitcher with hot water. Using a bath thermometer, check the water temperature. It should be 115° F (46° C).
10. Pour the hot water into the water bottle. Stop when it is one-half full.
11. Lay the water bottle on a flat surface. Hold the neck of the bottle in an upright position to squeeze the air out. When you can see water in the neck of the bottle, the air has been squeezed out. **See Figure 18-6.**

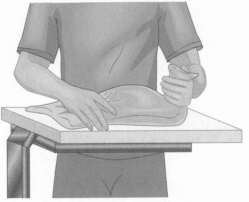

○ **Figure 18-6.** Forcing the excess air out of the water bottle. Be sure to fill the bottle with water only halfway.

12. Replace the cap, turning it tightly. Do not let the cap touch the patient's skin, because it may be hot.
13. Check the bottle for leaks.
14. Dry the bottle if it has become wet.
15. Place the bottle in its flannel cover.
16. Place the bottle on the area needing treatment. Never place the bottle under the patient.
17. During treatment, be sure the call signal is within the patient's reach. Check the area after 1 minute and then every 5 minutes for signs of blistering, swelling, or redness. Ask the patient if there is any pain, burning, or numbness. If there are any signs, remove the bottle and report the problems to the nurse.
18. When the treatment is finished, remove the bottle.
19. Rearrange the top linens and remove the bath blanket.
20. Check to make sure the patient is comfortable and that the body is aligned properly.
21. Make sure the call signal is within the patient's reach.
22. Open the screen.
23. Clean the equipment and return it to storage.
24. Wash your hands.
25. Record the following and report anything unusual to the nurse:
    - Time the procedure started and ended
    - Site of the application
    - Temperature of the water
    - How the patient tolerated the procedure
    - The condition of the skin

Applying an Aquamatic Pad

Equipment: aquamatic pad and heating unit • distilled water • cover for pad • ties or rolled gauze

1. Identify the patient, check the ID bracelet, and call the patient by name.
2. Introduce yourself.
3. Explain the procedure to the patient.
4. Wash your hands.
5. Provide privacy.
6. Uncover the area of the body that needs treatment.
7. Fanfold top linens down to the foot of the bed.
8. Place a bath blanket over the patient. Make sure the parts of the body not being treated are covered.
9. Check to be sure the pad has no leaks and that the cord and plug are in good condition. Fill the unit two-thirds full with distilled water.
10. Place the pad in its flannel cover.
11. Set the correct temperature with the key. Plug in the unit. Allow time for the water to reach the desired temperature, as instructed by the nurse.
12. Place the container on the bedside stand or overbed table.
13. Make sure the pad and hoses are level with the heating unit.
14. Gently place the pad over the treatment area. (Be sure the patient does not lie on top of the pad.) **See Figure 18-7.** Hold it in place with ties or gauze.
15. During treatment, make sure the call signal is within the patient's reach. Check the area in 1 minute and then regularly for signs of blistering, swelling, or redness. Ask the patient if there is any pain, burning, or numbness. If any signs or symptoms occur, discontinue treatment and tell the nurse right away.
16. After the specified treatment time, remove the pad.

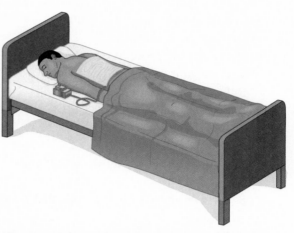

O **Figure 18-7.** An aquamatic pad heats and circulates water for dry warm therapy.

17. Check to make sure the patient is comfortable and that the body is aligned.
18. Make sure the call signal is within the patient's reach.
19. Open the screen.
20. Clean the equipment and return it to storage.
21. Wash your hands.
22. Record the following and report anything unusual to the nurse:
    - Time the procedure started and ended
    - Site of the application
    - Temperature setting used
    - How the patient tolerated the procedure
    - The condition of the skin

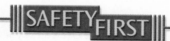

Do not use pins to hold any type of heating pad in place. These devices are electrical. Putting pins through the surface could cause electrocution.

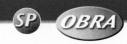

Using a Heat Lamp

Equipment: heat lamp • bath blanket • tape measure or yardstick

1. Identify the patient, check the ID bracelet, and call the patient by name.
2. Introduce yourself.
3. Explain the procedure to the patient.
4. Wash your hands.
5. Plug in the lamp first, then turn it on and give it time to warm up.
6. Provide privacy.
7. Uncover the area of the body that needs treatment.
8. Fanfold top linens down to the foot of the bed.
9. Place a bath blanket over the patient. Make sure the parts of the body not being treated are covered. Position the patient in such a way that he or she cannot accidentally roll closer to the light and risk burns.
10. Use the tape measure or yardstick to measure the distance from the bulb to the site.
11. Place the lamp an appropriate distance from the site. **See Figure 18-8.**
    - 25-watt bulb—14 inches
    - 40-watt bulb—18 inches
    - 60-watt bulb—24 inches
12. The heat lamp is normally applied for 5 to 20 minutes. Make sure the call signal is within patient's reach at all times. Check the area after 1 minute and then every 5 minutes for signs of blistering or redness. Ask the patient if there is any pain, burning, or numbness. If there are any signs or symptoms, discontinue treatment and tell the nurse right away.
13. Turn off the lamp and remove it after the prescribed number of minutes for the treatment has gone by.
14. Return the linens to their proper position and remove the bath blanket.
15. Check to make sure the patient is comfortable and that the body is aligned properly.
16. Make sure the call signal is within the patient's reach.

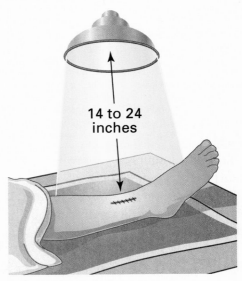

14 to 24 inches

○ **Figure 18-8.** The distance from the heat lamp to the area being treated is set by facility policy for safety. Be sure to measure accurately.

17. Open the screen.
18. Clean the equipment and return it to storage.
19. Wash your hands.
20. Record the following and report anything unusual to the nurse:
    - Time the procedure started and ended
    - Site of the application
    - Distance between the patient and the bulb
    - How the patient tolerated the procedure
    - The condition of the skin

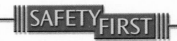

Heat lamps are not used often, because the risk of burns is very high. If you are directed to use a heat lamp, take extreme care to follow directions for safe distance and length of time. Check the condition of the skin very frequently to avoid burns. Never cover the lamp with linens—heat from the lamp could burn the linens and start a fire.

Calculating Therapy Times

A patient has an order to apply dry heat for 20 minutes 4 times a day during waking hours (8:00 AM to 8:00 PM). This task has been delegated to you as a nursing assistant. At what times would you schedule the heat therapy?

There are 12 hours between 8:00 AM and 8:00 PM, and you need to schedule 4 treatments, so divide 12 by 4 to find out how often to apply the treatments.

12 ÷ 4 = 3 hours   You will apply the treatments every 3 hours.

If you apply the first treatment at 8:30 AM, when will the other 3 treatments be scheduled?

8:30 AM + 3 hours = 11:30 AM
11:30 AM + 3 hours = 2:30 PM
2:30 PM + 3 hours = 5:30 PM

Practice

Another patient has an order to apply dry heat for 20 minutes 3 times a day during waking hours (8:00 AM to 8:00 PM). How often will you apply the treatments? Assuming you apply the first treatment at 9:00 AM, when should you schedule the other 2 treatments?

Cold Therapy

Nursing assistants also help with cold therapy. Cold is applied to the body to decrease blood flow, prevent swelling, and reduce pain. Generalized and localized applications are used. Applying cold treatments to the skin causes blood vessels to constrict. Blood flow to that area decreases. Constricted blood vessels make less oxygen available to the cells and tissues. The metabolism of the local tissues slows down. Smaller amounts of toxins are produced. **See Figure 18-9.**

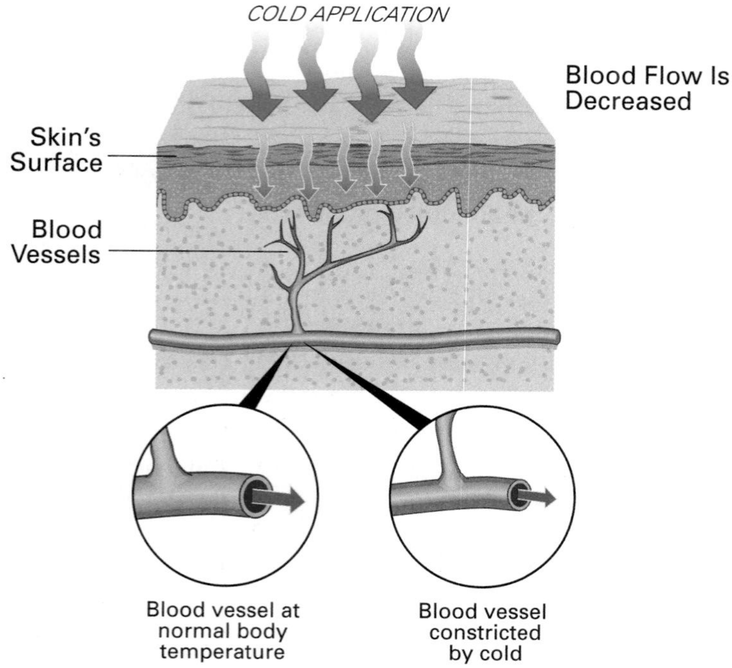

Decreased blood flow also reduces the amount of bleeding at an injury site and the likelihood of fluid buildup. In addition, cold numbs the nerve endings in the skin, so cold therapy is effective in reducing pain. It is used for the first 24 to 48 hours after an injury such as a sprain or fracture.

When cold is applied to the skin for a prolonged period of time, however, the blood vessels will dilate. Prolonged application of cold has the same effects as local warm applications. When using cold therapy on a patient, follow these guidelines to prevent accidents or injuries:

- Measure water temperature accurately. Water that is too cold can injure the patient's skin as badly as water that is too hot.
- Apply cold therapy for the exact time intervals ordered by the physician.

COLD APPLICATION

Blood Flow Is Decreased

Skin's Surface

Blood Vessels

Blood vessel at normal body temperature

Blood vessel constricted by cold

○ Figure 18-9. Applying cold locally to an area of the body decreases blood flow, prevents swelling, and reduces bleeding and pain.

Using Words and Word Parts Correctly

Many words and parts of words that you encounter in the health care setting may sound similar, but actually have very different meanings. As a nursing assistant, it is important for you to familiarize yourself with these words and become comfortable using them.

For example, the prefixes *hyper-* and *hypo-* sound alike but have opposite meanings. Someone who is hypertensive has high blood pressure. Someone who is hypotensive has low blood pressure. Note these sound-alike words and word parts:

accept/except	elicit/illicit
affect/effect	ileum/ilium
assure/ensure/insure	infra/intra
cabbage/CABG	intra/intro
cite/sight/site	metacarpal/metatarsal

mucous/mucus	pleural/plural
palpation/palpitation	super/supra
passed/past	track/tract
peritoneal/perineal/ peroneal	vial/vile
perfuse/profuse	where/were/wear/ware

Practice

1. Pick a partner and work on the list of words together. Look up the meaning of each word in the word groups.
2. Choose 10 pairs of sound-alike words or word parts from the list. Write a sentence using each word or word part. Try to write sentences that are relevant to the health care setting.

- At regular intervals, check the patient's condition. Observe for signs of **cyanosis**, a bluish discoloration or darkening of the skin, eyelids, lips, or fingernails that signals that the body is not getting enough oxygen. **See Figure 18-10.**
- Also regularly check the skin for redness, blisters, burning, or irritation. Burning and blisters tend to occur from intense cold. Ask if the patient is experiencing any pain or numbness. If any of these signs or symptoms occur, stop treatment and tell the nurse immediately.
- Infants, young children, the elderly, and fair-skinned people are at greater risk for complications from cold applications. Their skin is fragile and can be easily injured.
- Risk of injury is also increased in people with open wounds, impaired circulation, paralysis, diabetes, and decreased mental status.

Moist Cold Therapy

Like heat applications, cold therapy can be moist or dry. Examples of moist cold applications are compresses and soaks.

Cold Compresses. A **cold compress** is a cold folded and moistened cloth or towel that is placed over a small area of the body for moist cold therapy. It is left in place about 20 minutes.

Cold Soaks. Giving a cold soak is similar to giving a hot soak except for the difference in water temperature.

FOCUS ON

Heat and Cold Sensitivity

Some patients lose some of their sensitivity to heat and cold. They may feel cold even when a room is warm. When giving warm or cold therapy, check the patient often. Be sensitive to how he or she may feel. A patient receiving a cold compress on the leg may need a shawl around the shoulders or a blanket over the other leg. A patient receiving warm therapy may need a cool drink of water.

Sponge Baths. Sponge baths are a type of therapy that at one time was used for reducing a fever in adults and children. Sometimes alcohol was added to the bath water to cool the body temperature faster. Recent research has proven that sponge baths cause severe shivering, which can actually cause body temperature to rise. Sponge baths are not recommended and should be reserved for certain emergency situations, such as heat stroke, and only when close monitoring and trained emergency personnel are available. Alcohol should *never* be used in bath water.

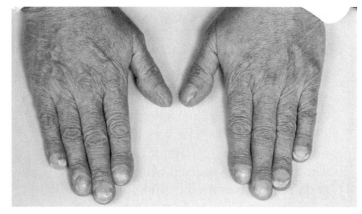

O **Figure 18-10.** When applying cold therapy, watch for signs of cyanosis, including bluish discoloration or darkening of the skin, eyelids, lips, or fingernails.

Procedure 18-8

SP OBRA

Applying a Cold Compress

Equipment: basin • washcloths, gauze, or towels (for compress) • bath thermometer • waterproof mattress pad • bath blanket • towel

1. Identify the patient, check the ID bracelet, and call the patient by name.
2. Introduce yourself.
3. Explain the procedure to the patient.
4. Wash your hands.
5. Provide privacy.
6. Fill the basin one-half full with cold water. The temperature should be between 50° F and 65° F (10° C to 18° C).
7. Put the compresses in the basin.
8. Place a bath blanket over the patient. Make sure the parts of the body not being treated are covered.
9. Fanfold top linens down to the foot of the bed.
10. Place a waterproof pad under the area being treated.
11. Uncover the area of the body that needs treatment.
12. Take a compress out of the basin and wring out the excess water.
13. Position the compress over the treatment area.
14. The cold compress can be left in place for up to 20 minutes, and the call signal should be within patient's reach. Check the area in 1 minute and then every 5 minutes for skin

discoloration and signs of blisters. Observe whether the patient is shivering or has signs of cyanosis. Ask the patient if there is any pain, burning, or numbness. If there are any signs or symptoms, remove the cold compress and tell the nurse right away.

15. When the compress is no longer cold, replace it with another cold compress.
16. After 20 minutes, remove the compress.
17. Using a towel, pat dry the skin where the compress was applied.
18. Check to make sure the patient is comfortable and that the body is aligned properly.
19. Make sure the call signal is within the patient's reach and the bed is in the correct position.
20. Open the screen.
21. Clean the equipment and return it to storage.
22. Wash your hands.
23. Record the following and report anything unusual to the nurse:
    • Time the procedure started and ended
    • Site of the application
    • Temperature of the application
    • How the patient tolerated the procedure
    • The condition of the skin

Procedure 18-9

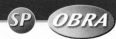

Giving a Cold Soak

Equipment: basin • bath thermometer • waterproof mattress protector • bath blanket • towel

1. Identify the patient, check the ID bracelet, and call the patient by name.
2. Introduce yourself.
3. Explain the procedure to the patient.
4. Wash your hands.
5. Provide privacy.
6. Raise the bed to a comfortable working position.
7. Place a bath blanket over the patient. Make sure the parts of the body not being treated are covered.
8. Fanfold top linens down to the foot of the bed.
9. Position the waterproof mattress protector under the area of the body that will be soaked.
10. Fill the basin one-half full with cold water. Using a bath thermometer, check the temperature. It should be between 50° F and 65° F (10° C to 18° C).
11. Uncover the area of the body that needs treatment.
12. Position the basin so the area of the patient's body that needs treatment can easily reach the basin.
13. Slowly and gently lower the area being treated into the basin.
14. Monitor the temperature of the water in the basin after 1 minute and then every 5 minutes. When the water is no longer cold, remove the area being treated and wrap in a towel. Repeat Steps 10 through 13.
15. During treatment, be sure the call signal is within the patient's reach. Check the area every 5 minutes for skin discoloration and signs of blisters. **See Figure 18-11.** Observe whether the patient is shivering or has signs of cyanosis. Ask the patient if there is any pain, burning, or numbness. If there are any signs or symptoms, remove the area from the basin and tell the nurse right away.
16. When treatment is finished, remove the basin. Pat dry the area.
17. Remove the mattress cover. Rearrange the top linens and remove the bath blanket.
18. Check to make sure the patient is comfortable and that the body is aligned properly.
19. Make sure the call signal is within the patient's reach.
20. Open the screen.
21. Clean the equipment and return it to storage.
22. Wash your hands.
23. Record the following and report anything unusual to the nurse:
    • Time the procedure started and ended
    • Site of the application
    • Temperature of the water
    • How the patient tolerated the procedure
    • The condition of the skin

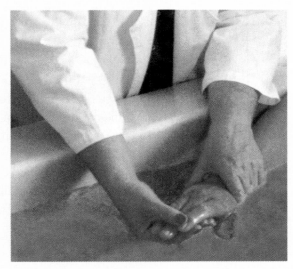

O **Figure 18-11.** While giving a cold soak, check the treatment area regularly for cyanosis or blisters. Ask the patient if there is any pain, burning, or numbness.

Making Predictions

One strategy for remembering what you read is to anticipate, or guess, what you might find in a reading selection, chapter, or book. This reading strategy is called *prediction*. Prediction helps you set a purpose for reading and allows you to focus on what you expect to learn. It also allows you to compare your ideas to what the author writes.

To make predictions about a selection, scan the chapter title and subheadings and look at the illustrations. For example, look back at Chapter 17, "Emergency Care." By looking at the headings, you can predict that the chapter covers the role of the nursing assistant in an emergency, how to help someone who is choking, and the basics of performing CPR.

As you read, update your predictions. Revise, abandon, and make new predictions. While you are reading, ask yourself continually if the text is meeting your predictions.

Practice

Before you read the "Dressings and Support Devices" section in this chapter, make a list of predictions about what you think the text will cover. As you make your predictions, note the clues that led you to each prediction. After you have read the passage, go back and analyze your predictions. Did you miss anything important? Did you think of things that were not covered in the text?

Dry Cold Therapy

Just as in dry warm therapies, in dry cold therapies, water does not touch the skin. The surface of the application is dry. Cold packs and ice bags are examples of dry cold therapies.

A **cold pack** is a cold treatment that is applied or wrapped around an area of the body. **See Figure 18-12.** A cold pack may be made by soaking a towel or cloth in cold water. There are also cold packs that are commercially available and disposable. A disposable cold pack or bag provides dry cold therapy to a local area of the body. When the disposable pack is squeezed or struck (depending on the type), a chemical reaction causes the pack to become cold. Cold packs are usually used for no more than 30 minutes.

Ice bags are also used to provide cold therapy to a local area. **See Figure 18-13.** The ice bag is filled one-half full of ice and squeezed to make sure the air is out. The cap is screwed tightly shut, and the cover is put on before applying to the area being treated. The cap should never touch the patient's skin, because it may be very cold.

Dressings and Support Devices

Nursing assistants may assist the nurse in the application of dressings and devices that enhance the patient's comfort or prevent further complications in the patient's care. Sometimes, patients need additional support to keep dressings

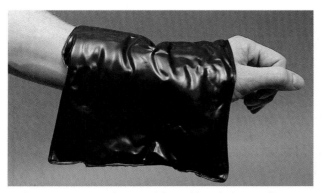

○ **Figure 18-12.** A patient receiving cold pack therapy for a wrist wound.

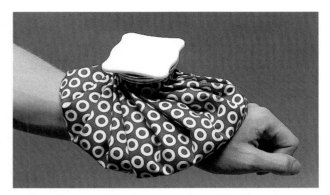

○ **Figure 18-13.** Ice bag therapy can be used in place of a commercial cold pack.

and bandages in place. They may need additional support for a part of the body that is weak or injured. Elastic bandages and special stockings are often used for these purposes.

Bandages and dressings can also be used to stop bleeding and to cover a wound. Some bandages are made of material that absorbs and protects the wound from further injury. Some dressings are very thin and are designed for protection from infection. They also facilitate healing but do not absorb excess drainage. Because an open wound places a patient at risk for infection, proper care is essential.

Procedure 18-10

SP OBRA

Applying a Cold Pack

Equipment: disposable cold pack • flannel cover • ties, tape, or rolled gauze

1. Identify the patient, check the ID bracelet, and call the patient by name.
2. Introduce yourself.
3. Explain the procedure to the patient.
4. Wash your hands.
5. Provide privacy.
6. Perform the action necessary to activate the cooling of the cold pack.
7. Place a cover or towel over the cold pack.
8. Place the covered cold pack over the site to be treated. Use ties, tape, or rolled gauze to hold the cold pack in place.
9. The cold pack can be left in place for up to 30 minutes. Make sure the call signal is within the patient's reach, and check the area every 5 minutes for skin discoloration and signs of blisters. Observe whether the patient is shivering or has signs of cyanosis.

Ask the patient if there is any pain, burning, or numbness. If there are any signs or symptoms, remove the cold pack and tell the nurse right away.

10. After 30 minutes, remove the tape (or ties or gauze), towel, and cold pack.
11. Check to make sure the patient is comfortable and that the body is aligned properly.
12. Make sure the call signal is within the patient's reach.
13. Open the screen.
14. Wash your hands.
15. Record the following and report anything unusual to the nurse:
    • Time the procedure started and ended
    • Site of the application
    • How the patient tolerated the procedure
    • The condition of the skin

Dressings

Dressings may be made of cotton gauze or synthetic material. They come in a variety of shapes and sizes. They are individually wrapped and are sterile. **See Figure 18-14.**

The nurse selects the size of the dressing based on the size of the wound. The dressing should always be larger than the wound. The dressing is secured to the patient's skin with hypoallergenic tape, plastic tape, paper tape, adhesive tape, or an elastic bandage. The kind of tape depends on what is available and whether there are any special skin considerations.

Nursing assistants are not permitted to bandage open wounds, but they may be asked to assist a nurse or to reinforce an existing dressing. **Sterile** (free from microorganisms) dressing changes are the responsibility of the nurse. Nursing assistants may sometimes be responsible for reinforcing nonsterile dressings with gauze.

Dressings must remain clean and dry in order to act as a barrier to infection. If the dressing becomes wet (due to water, wound drainage, or food spillage, for example), notify the nurse that a dressing change is needed. Report any bleeding through the dressing to the nurse right away.

If you are asked to change a patient's bandage or dressing for a wound that is not open, report the following observations:
- Swelling in the area
- Complaints of pain
- Change in color of the wound or surrounding area
- Increase or decrease in skin temperature around the wound
- Drainage from the wound

Always follow standard precautions when applying or removing a dressing, even in an emergency. You will be in direct contact with blood and body fluids. Use a clean pair of gloves to remove a dressing. After discarding the dressing, *change your gloves before applying the fresh dressing.*

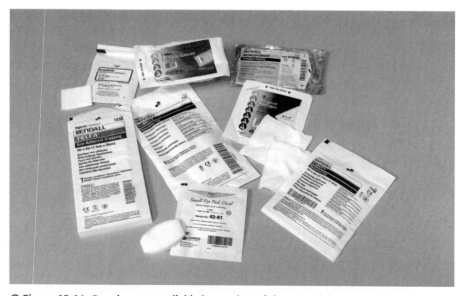

○ **Figure 18-14.** Dressings are available in a variety of shapes and sizes.

Procedure 18-11

Applying a Dressing

Equipment: sterile gauze pads, size specified by nurse • tape • disposable gloves • waste container for contaminated waste

1. Gather the supplies needed for the procedure.
2. Identify the patient, check the ID bracelet, and call the patient by name.
3. Introduce yourself.
4. Explain the procedure to the patient.
5. Open the waste container and place it within reach.
6. Wash your hands.
7. Provide privacy.
8. Wash the overbed table, including the edges where you will be placing the tape.
9. Cut pieces of tape for securing the dressing. For a 4 x 4 dressing, cut four pieces of 8-inch tape. Hang the cut tape from the overbed table.
10. Wash your hands and put on gloves.
11. Place a clean paper towel on the overbed table to provide a clean work area.
12. Open the gauze package. Do not touch the gauze. Lay the gauze package on the overbed table.
13. If there is an old dressing, remove it as follows:
    a. Pull the tape toward the wound. Be careful, especially with elderly patients whose skin is more fragile.
    b. Lift the dressing off the wound. Pull off the dressing and remaining tape. You can hold the dressing with your gloved fingertips and pull off the glove over the dressing to contain the dressing for discarding. **See Figure 18-15.**
    c. Note the color of the wound and any drainage.
    d. Place the old dressing and tape in a waste container.
    e. Remove your gloves and place them in a waste container.
    f. Wash your hands and put on clean gloves.
14. Place the clean gauze over the wound. Be careful to touch only the outer edges of the gauze.
15. Place tape over the edges of the gauze. Half of the tape should be on the gauze and half on the skin. **See Figure 18-16.**
16. Discard the gauze wrappers in a waste container.
17. Remove your gloves.
18. Open the screen.
19. Wash your hands.
20. Record the following and report anything unusual to the nurse:
    - Dressing was changed
    - Time of dressing change
    - Wound condition
    - How the patient tolerated the procedure

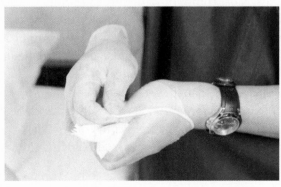

○ **Figure 18-15.** Hold the dressing with your gloved fingertips and pull off the glove over the dressing to contain the dressing for discarding.

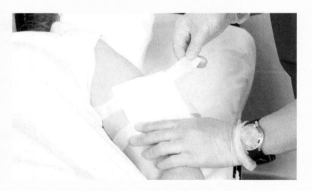

○ **Figure 18-16.** When you tape the edges of the gauze, half of the tape should be on the gauze and half on the skin.

Elastic Bandages

Elastic bandages are long strips of stretchy material that provide support and protection to extremities (hands, arms, feet, and legs) and joints (elbows, wrists, knees, and ankles). They are available in various sizes. They come in rolls and are secured with Velcro, metal clips, or tape.

Elastic bandages are used to immobilize an injured limb, such as a broken arm, and to hold dressings in place. They may also be used to protect open wounds from contaminants. They can provide muscle support after surgery or childbirth, support a strained or sprained extremity, or apply warmth to an arthritic joint. They may also be used to promote circulation in the extremities.

Follow these guidelines when applying an elastic bandage:

- Do not apply the bandage so tightly that it cuts off circulation.
- Wrap the bandage around the extremity, toward the heart. Each spiral turn should overlap the previous one in a figure-eight fashion to promote circulation. **See Figure 18-17.**
- Make sure the pressure is evenly distributed.
- Place the joint in a natural position with a slight flexion (bending).
- Keep it smooth and free of wrinkles.
- Watch for reddened areas on the skin.
- Inspect the area below (distal to) the bandage for numbness, cyanosis, swelling, and skin temperature every 1 to 2 hours or according to your facility's policy.
- Remove it every 8 hours to inspect the underlying skin.

Antiembolic Stockings

Stockings made of elastic fabric that provide support, promote blood flow, and prevent the formation of blood clots are called **antiembolic stockings**. You might also hear them called *elastic stockings*. The stockings put pressure on the veins in the legs. This pressure improves the circulation.

Antiembolic stockings are used to treat or prevent thrombophlebitis and phlebitis. **Thrombophlebitis** is a condition that occurs when a blood clot causes inflammation in a vein. **Phlebitis** is an inflammation of the veins. The stockings are usually applied **postoperatively**, or after surgery, for prevention purposes. They are also used for support when a patient has a knee or ankle sprain, heart disease, or poor circulation in the legs.

The stockings are ordered by a doctor. They come in different sizes and lengths. Most commonly, they are knee-high or thigh-high. **See Figure 18-18.** They sometimes have a hole in the foot to allow inspection and relieve pressure on the toes. It is very important to measure the patient for proper size. A nurse usually applies them the first time. When applying elastic stockings:

- Put them on before the patient gets out of bed.
- Check them frequently for wrinkles, especially around the knees.
- Check the circulation in the feet frequently.
- Remove them every 8 hours to check the underlying skin.

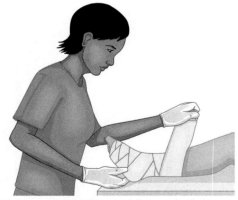

○ **Figure 18-17.** When applying an elastic bandage, wrap the bandage around the extremity, working toward the heart. Each spiral turn should overlap the previous one in a figure-eight fashion.

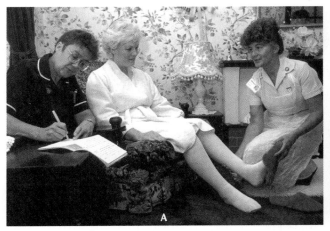
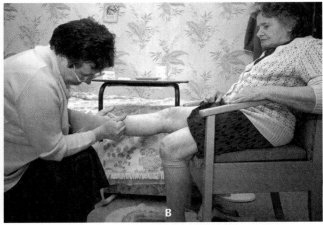

○ Figure 18-18. Antiembolic stockings are worn if ordered by a doctor. They are available in two lengths, (A) thigh-high and (B) knee-high.

Procedure 18-12

SP

Applying Antiembolic Stockings

Equipment: antiembolic stockings

1. Identify the patient, check the ID bracelet, and call the patient by name.
2. Introduce yourself.
3. Explain the procedure to the resident.
4. Wash your hands.
5. Provide privacy.
6. Make sure the antiembolic stockings are the correct size.
7. Raise the bed to a comfortable working position and lower the side rail (if appropriate).
8. Have the patient lie on his or her back. Expose one leg, keeping the rest of the body covered.
9. Turn the stocking inside out, except for the foot section.
10. Slip the foot, toes first and then the heel, over the patient's toe and heel.
11. Grasp the stocking once it is on the patient's foot and pull it up the leg, slowly and evenly as it turns right side out. **See Figure 18-19.** Avoid digging thumbs into the skin by keeping your hands flat as you work the stocking up the patient's leg.
12. The stocking should be even along the leg. Make sure to smooth all creases and wrinkles and that toes are accessible or visible.

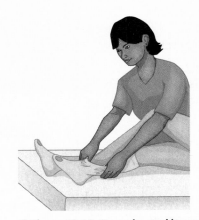

○ Figure 18-19. Grasp the stocking and pull it up the leg, slowly and evenly as it turns right side out.

13. Repeat the procedure on the other leg.
14. Cover the patient and make sure the patient is comfortable.
15. Provide for safety.
16. Open the screen.
17. Wash your hands.
18. Record the following and report anything unusual to the nurse:
    • That you have applied the stockings
    • The time the stockings were applied
    • How the patient tolerated the procedure

Chapter Summary

- Nursing assistants help prepare rooms and patients for physical examinations and may assist the health care provider in examinations.
- Nursing assistants may be responsible for laying out equipment to be used in examinations.
- Various types of warm therapy are used to promote healing, relax muscles, ease joint pain and stiffness, and reduce tissue swelling.

- Various types of cold therapy are used to decrease blood flow, prevent swelling, and reduce pain.
- Nursing assistants follow safety guidelines to prevent accidents and injuries when applying warm and cold therapies.
- Nursing assistants may apply some dressings and support devices by following instructions from a doctor or nurse.

VOCABULARY REVIEW

Directions: Match the letter of each definition in the second column with the correct vocabulary term in the first column. Write your answers on a separate sheet of paper.

Vocabulary

1. cold compress
2. cold pack
3. cyanosis
4. elastic bandage
5. phlebitis
6. postoperatively
7. sitz bath
8. sterile
9. thrombophlebitis
10. warm compress
11. warm pack

Definitions

A. A dry cold treatment that is applied or wrapped around an area of the body
B. The period of time after surgery
C. A long strip of stretchy material that provides support and protection to extremities and joints
D. A heated moist treatment that is applied or wrapped around an area of the body
E. A type of moist warm therapy in which the patient's perineal and anal regions are immersed in warm water in a special tub or seat
F. Free from microorganisms
G. A bluish discoloration or darkening of the skin, eyelids, lips, or fingernails that signals that the body is not getting enough oxygen
H. A folded and moistened cloth or towel that is warmed and placed over a small area of the body for moist warm therapy
I. A cold folded and moistened cloth or towel that is placed over a small area of the body for moist cold therapy
J. A condition that occurs when a blood clot causes inflammation in a vein
K. An inflammation of the veins

Check Your Knowledge

Review Questions: Answer each of the following questions on a separate sheet of paper.

1. Where might a doctor perform a physical examination on a long-term care resident?
2. Why should you never apply heat for longer than 30 minutes?
3. Name three methods of applying moist heat.
4. Which patients are at an increased risk for burns due to warm or cold therapy?
5. Why is a warm water bottle considered a dry warm therapy?
6. What is an aquamatic pad?
7. Why are sponge baths no longer given to reduce fever?
8. What type of dressings might a nursing assistant be responsible for reinforcing?
9. How often should you inspect the area beneath a bandage?
10. Why should antiembolic stockings be removed every 8 hours?

True or False: Read each statement carefully. Then write *True* or *False* by the statement number on a separate sheet of paper.

1. Dilated blood vessels carry more oxygen to cells and tissues for healing.
2. Antiembolic stockings are a type of warm therapy.
3. Cold therapy can be effective in reducing bleeding at an injury site.
4. Cold packs should be applied for no more than 30 minutes.
5. Nursing assistants may apply sterile dressings to open wounds.

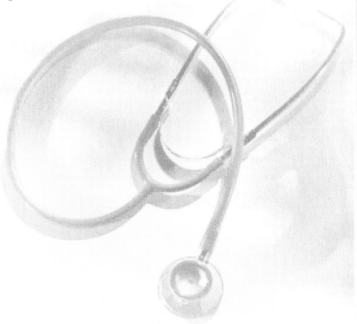

Think and Decide

Directions: Think about each of the following scenarios. Answer each question on a separate sheet of paper.

1. Clarise is a 72-year-old resident who bumped her forearm earlier this morning. The physician ordered cold packs to her forearm for 20 minutes four times a day. As you lift Clarise's arm to apply the cold pack, you notice that the bruise is now open and bleeding. What should you do prior to applying the cold pack?

2. A physician is scheduled to examine Mrs. W., a long-term care resident, at 10:00 AM. The physician has requested that the patient be draped and ready for the exam when she arrives. As the nursing assistant caring for Mrs. W., what are your responsibilities in preparing the resident for the exam? During the exam? After the exam?

3. A nurse asks you to elevate and apply a warm pack to a resident's swollen left hand for 20 minutes. How often should you check the resident's skin while the warm pack is in place? What, specifically, are you checking for?

4. While administering a cold soak to a resident's right toe, you notice the toe is becoming slightly cyanotic. What does this indicate? What should be your first action?

5. You are asked by a nurse to perform a sterile dressing change on a wound on a resident's coccyx. What action(s) should you take?

6. Mr. F. is having his scheduled sitz bath. After settling him in the bath and making sure the call signal is within his reach, you return to other duties. Five minutes later, when you return to check on him, he seems weak and can barely answer your questions. What should you do?

7. Mrs. C. almost fell in the hall this morning. To keep from falling, she grabbed a hand rail to support herself. In doing so, she twisted her right wrist. You have been asked to apply an elastic bandage to Mrs. C.'s right wrist. You wrap the bandage according to facility protocol, leaving her fingertips exposed so that you can inspect them. An hour later, when you come to check on the bandage, Mrs. C. complains that it is uncomfortable because it is too tight. You inspect the fingertips and they are cool to the touch. What should you do?

8. You have been asked to apply antiembolic stockings on Mrs. B. As you turn the first stocking inside out, you notice a flaw in the stocking. How should you proceed?

CNA Certification Exam Prep

Directions: This practice test contains ten questions. Each question has four suggested answers. For each question, choose the ONE that best answers the question or completes the statement. Write your answers on a separate sheet of paper.

1. One of the purposes of warm therapy is to
   A. decrease blood flow.
   B. reduce tissue swelling.
   C. constrict blood vessels.
   D. slow metabolism in local tissues.

2. To prevent accidents or injuries with warm therapy,
   A. measure water temperature accurately.
   B. apply heat for at least 1 hour.
   C. check the skin every 3 hours.
   D. allow the patient to apply the therapy.

3. Moist warm therapy is a treatment in which heat is applied to the skin
   A. with oil.
   B. with water.
   C. with lotion.
   D. with alcohol.

4. Which of the following is an example of dry warm therapy?
   A. warm soak
   B. sitz bath
   C. warm compress
   D. heat lamp

5. A sitz bath is a type of
   A. moist cold therapy.
   B. dry cold therapy.
   C. moist warm therapy.
   D. dry warm therapy.

6. The purpose of antiembolic stockings is to prevent
   A. wrinkles.
   B. hair growth on the legs.
   C. thrombophlebitis.
   D. postsurgical bleeding.

7. A heated moist treatment that is wrapped around an area of the body is a(n)
   A. antiembolic stocking.
   B. warm pack.
   C. warm compress.
   D. elastic bandage.

8. When applying a heat lamp with a 40-watt bulb, how far away from the patient's skin should you place the lamp?
   A. 14 inches
   B. 18 inches
   C. 24 inches
   D. 36 inches

9. What is the maximum amount of time heat should be applied in warm therapy?
   A. 10 minutes
   B. 20 minutes
   C. 30 minutes
   D. 60 minutes

10. In moist cold therapy, what should the temperature of the water be?
    A. 32° F to 42° F
    B. 50° F to 65° F
    C. 70° F to 75° F
    D. 80° F to 90° F

CHAPTER 19

OBJECTIVES

- **Describe normal urinary and bowel elimination and common problems with each.**
- **Explain the nursing assistant's role in assisting patients with elimination.**

- **Explain how to assist a patient who has a colostomy or ileostomy.**
- **Explain the procedures for collecting various kinds of urine samples.**

- **Describe different types of urine tests.**
- **Describe the procedures for the collection and testing of stool samples.**
- **Describe the collection of a sputum sample.**

Elimination and Sample Collection

abdominal distension Abnormal swelling of the abdomen.

anal incontinence The inability to control the passing of feces or gas.

bedpan A plastic container used by patients who are bedridden to urinate or defecate.

catheter A tube used to drain fluid into or out of the body.

colostomy An artificial opening from the colon (large intestine) to the abdominal wall.

condom catheter An external drainage catheter with a rubber sheath that is placed over the penis and attached to a drainage bag to assist urination.

constipation Difficulty in fecal elimination.

defecation The passing of feces from the body.

diarrhea The passage of frequent watery stools.

elimination The excretion or removal of waste from the body.

enema A liquid solution placed into the rectum to loosen stools and to remove feces.

fecal impaction A collection of hardened feces in the intestines.

fecal occult blood test (FOBT) A test used to detect the presence of hidden (occult) blood in the stool.

feces The waste material from the large intestine, or bowel.

flatulence The excessive creation and buildup of gas in the stomach and intestines.

fracture pan A type of bedpan used by patients who are unable to raise their hips high enough to sit on a regular bedpan.

hemorrhoids Distended veins surrounding the rectum.

ileostomy An artificial opening between the small intestine and the abdominal wall.

indwelling catheter A catheter that is left in the bladder over a period of time to continuously drain urine.

ostomy The surgical creation of an artificial opening in the body.

rectal tube A tube inserted into the rectum to relieve flatulence and abdominal distension.

sputum The mucous secretion from the lungs, bronchi, and trachea.

stoma An artificial opening in the body created by surgery.

stool Feces that have been excreted from the body.

suctioning The process of removing or sucking up fluid or body secretions.

suppository Semisolid medication or lubricating agent that is inserted into the rectum for absorption by the body for prevention or treatment of constipation.

urinal A special container that men use for urinating when they are bedridden.

urinary catheter A tube used to drain urine from the bladder.

urinary incontinence The inability to control the passing of urine.

urinary retention The incomplete emptying of the bladder.

urination The passing of urine from the body.

urine The waste material, or output, of the urinary system.

Elimination

Elimination is the excretion or removal of waste from the body. It includes **urination** (the passing of urine), and **defecation** (the passing of feces). Elimination is an important natural life process. The removal of bodily waste is necessary to maintain good health. Disruption in the process of elimination may be a symptom or a cause of disease.

Many factors contribute to a person's elimination habits, including:

• Age
• Illness
• Personal preference
• Medication
• Amount of salt, fiber, and fluid in the diet
• Perspiration rate
• Level of physical activity

Urinary Elimination

The urinary system removes waste and regulates the amount of water in the body. **Urine** is the output of the urinary system. It is made up of body waste and excess fluids. Urine is formed in the kidneys and flows through the ureters for storage in the bladder. When the bladder is full, urine is voluntarily eliminated through the urethra. **See Figure 19-1.** The act of emptying one's bladder is called urinating, voiding, micturition, or passing water.

It is important for good health to maintain the body's fluid balance. (See Chapter 26.) A person with low fluid intake produces less urine, so the urine tends to be concentrated. A person with high fluid intake produces more urine, which allows the urine to be more diluted. Encourage patients to drink plenty of fluids throughout the day.

Certain diseases, such as diabetes and urinary tract infections, can cause *polyuria* (frequent or excessive urination). Some people have *nocturia*, a frequent or excessive urge to urinate during the night. Older people tend to feel the urge to urinate more frequently than younger people.

The three most common problems of the urinary system are urinary tract infections, urinary incontinence, and urinary retention.

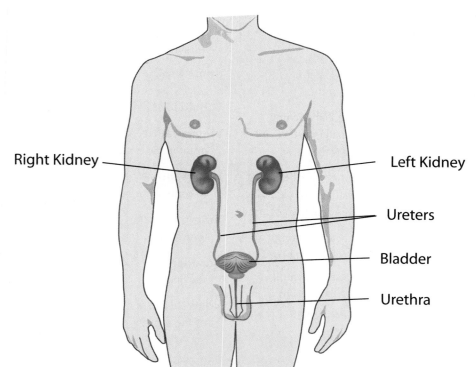

Right Kidney — Left Kidney — Ureters — Bladder — Urethra

○ **Figure 19-1. The urinary system.**

- **Urinary Tract Infection.** Anyone can get an infection in the urinary tract. Patients with urinary catheters or poor hygiene habits, however, are at greater risk. Symptoms are frequent urination, burning, urgency, pain when urinating (*dysuria*), and blood in the urine (*hematuria*). If a patient complains of any of these symptoms, or if you notice a change in the patient's urine, immediately report the situation to the nurse.

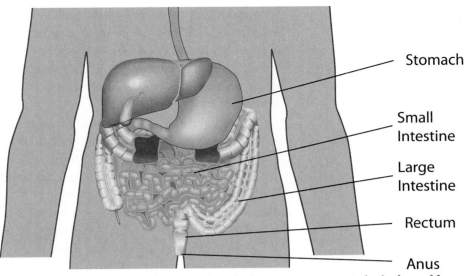

Stomach

Small Intestine

Large Intestine

Rectum

Anus

O **Figure 19-2. The lower part of the gastrointestinal system excretes waste in the form of feces.**

- **Urinary Incontinence.** The inability to control the passing of urine is **urinary incontinence**. Incontinence can be caused by disease or illness. It may be permanent or temporary. Aging can cause incontinence, because the *bladder sphincters*, which are circular muscles, lose the elasticity needed to control urination.
- **Urinary Retention.** A condition in which the bladder does not empty completely or does not empty at all is **urinary retention**. Diseases of the prostate, certain surgeries, and some medications can cause urinary retention.

Bowel Elimination

The gastrointestinal system excretes waste in the form of **feces**, the waste material of the large intestine (bowel). Partially digested foods move from the stomach to the small intestine. The small intestine further breaks down the foods, absorbs important nutrients, and moves the waste to the large intestine. Here, most of the liquid is removed and feces are formed. The body stores the feces in the rectum until they are excreted from the body. Bowel elimination is also called moving one's bowels or having a bowel movement (BM). Feces that have been excreted from the body are called **stool**. **See Figure 19-2.**

The frequency of bowel movements varies. Some people move their bowels daily, while others move their bowels every 3 to 4 days. Establishing a routine helps to maintain proper bowel function.

Bowel elimination is affected by diet, the amount of fluids ingested, exercise, and medications. Some foods and fluids (for example, rice and coffee) may interfere with regular elimination. Lack of privacy or available bathroom facilities may cause someone to ignore the urge to defecate.

Aging slows the passage of feces through the body. The slower rate causes more water to be reabsorbed by the body, resulting in harder, drier stools. If you are caring for elderly patients, encourage physical activity, offer plenty of fluids, especially water, and include high-fiber foods in the diet as directed by the dietician.

Comfortable and regular bowel movements contribute to health and well-being. The following are problems that affect normal bowel movements.

- **Flatulence.** The excessive creation and buildup of gas in the stomach and intestines is **flatulence**. If the gas is not relieved, the intestines distend, causing swelling and abdominal cramping. Flatulence is caused by gas-producing foods (for example, cabbage and bean products), constipation, medications, or surgery. The doctor may prescribe enemas, rectal tubes, or medication to help relieve flatulence.
- **Constipation.** Difficulty in fecal elimination is called **constipation**. The patient experiences hard, dry stools or no stools at all. Bowel movements become painful. Constipation is treated by eating a diet high in fiber and fluids. The patient's doctor may also prescribe a rectal suppository to soften and lubricate the stools or an enema to force the body to eliminate the feces.
- **Fecal Impaction.** A **fecal impaction** is a collection of hardened feces in the intestines. It can result from untreated constipation. A patient with fecal impaction is unable to defecate but may leak liquid stools, which seep past the impaction. Fecal impaction is treated with an oil-retention enema to soften the stools.
- **Bowel Obstruction.** A blockage in the intestine that can be related to fecal impaction. It can also be caused by a tumor or mass.
- **Hemorrhoids.** Distended veins surrounding the rectum are called **hemorrhoids**. Hemorrhoids are caused by excessive pressure on the rectum, which can occur with pregnancy or chronic constipation. Patients can experience severe pain with hemorrhoids. When you care for patients with hemorrhoids, help keep the area clean and dry, encourage adequate fluid intake, and monitor the patient's bowel movements. If any blood is seen in the stool, report the amount and color immediately to the nurse.

Vital Skills READING

Two-Column Notes

To help remember what you read, you can organize the information into columns. Two-column notes are a good way to begin. In a two-column note, you fold a piece of paper in half. The left side is Column 1; the right is Column 2. For a simple two-column note, write the main point of a passage in Column 1. In Column 2, write the supporting details for that main point.

Below is a two-column note for the preceding "Elimination" section.

Column 1	Column 2
elimination	urine or feces; remove waste; maintain health
factors affecting elimination	age, illness, medication, preference, diet, perspiration, activity
body's fluid balance	low fluid intake; high fluid intake; diseases affecting fluid balance

Practice

Choose three sections of this chapter and prepare a two-column note for each section. Place the main ideas in Column 1 and the supporting details in Column 2.

- **Diarrhea.** The passage of frequent, watery stools is **diarrhea**. The patient feels an urgency to defecate, usually accompanied by cramping. Diarrhea can be caused by medications, infection, or irritating foods. Offer the patient with diarrhea the toilet, commode, or bedpan often. Provide good skin care around the anus, because diarrhea is extremely irritating to this area.
- **Anal Incontinence.** The inability to control the passing of feces or gas is called **anal incontinence**. It can be the result of injury to the central nervous system, disease, aging, or confusion. Anal incontinence may be permanent or temporary.

Assisting with Elimination

Many patients need assistance with elimination. Certain surgeries, diseases, and conditions prevent patients from being able to perform this ADL on their own. When you help patients with elimination, you will always be expected to observe the urine and stool and report to the nurse if you see anything unusual.

When you observe and report on patients' urine, use these criteria in your description:
- **Color:** pale yellow (normal), amber, dark yellow or brown, red, or green
- **Odor:** no odor; sweet, fruity odor; foul odor; or metallic odor
- **Sediment:** some urine, especially in females, contains bits of debris
- **Clarity:** ranges from clear to very cloudy
- **Consistency:** ranges from thin to syrupy
- **Amount:** quantity of the output

When you observe and report on patients' stool, use these criteria in your description:
- **Color:** usually dark brown, but can be whitish-gray (also called *clay-colored*), beige, green, or black. Black stools are also called *tarry stools*.
- **Odor:** mild odor to foul odor. Some medications and infections cause a foul odor.
- **Consistency:** ranges from watery to hard, or can resemble tar
- **Amount:** quantity usually described as small, moderate, or large

Helping Patients Use Elimination Equipment

Some of your patients will be able to use toilet facilities by themselves. Others will need assistance getting to the toilet. Patients who cannot walk need assistance using elimination equipment that is brought to the bedside.

Helping Ambulatory Patients Use the Toilet. Some patients need help getting out of bed and walking to the toilet. Note the usual times that a patient empties the bladder, such as upon awakening in the morning, before meals, after meals, and before bedtime. Try to be available at those times to assist. Some patients may need your help to sit on the toilet and to clean themselves when they are finished. Keep in mind that using the bathroom is a private act. Give your patients plenty of privacy.

Bedside Commodes. Patients who can get out of bed but cannot walk to the bathroom use a bedside commode. A bedside commode is a portable chair with an opening in the seat and a removable container below. **See Figure 19-3.** The commode allows a patient to sit in a natural position for elimination. The container under the commode is cleaned and disinfected after the patient urinates or defecates.

The steps to help a patient use a commode are listed in Procedure 19-1. In addition to those instructions, follow these guidelines:
- Always treat the patient with respect. Using a commode can be embarrassing to a patient.
- Assist the patient with the commode as soon as requested.

Procedure 19-1

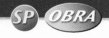

Assisting a Patient with a Bedside Commode

Equipment: bedside commode • toilet paper • blanket • robe and nonskid slippers • disposable gloves • wash basin • soap • towel • waste bag • transfer belt, if needed

1. Identify the patient and introduce yourself. Call the patient by name.
2. Explain that you are going to help the patient use the commode.
3. Provide privacy.
4. Wash your hands.
5. Bring the commode close to the patient's bed. Remove the lid of the commode.
6. Help the patient sit on the side of the bed.
7. Assist the patient in putting on a robe and nonskid slippers.
8. Assist the patient to the commode. Use a transfer belt if necessary. Make sure the patient is correctly positioned.
9. Cover the patient with the blanket.
10. Place the toilet paper and signal cord within reach. Tell the patient to signal when finished. Tell patients whose intake/output is being measured to place toilet paper in the waste bag, not the commode.
11. Wash your hands.
12. Leave the room and close the door.
13. Answer the signal immediately. Knock and pause before entering the room.
14. Wash your hands and put on gloves.
15. Help the patient with perineal care. Make sure the patient is clean.
16. Remove your gloves and wash your hands.
17. Fill the basin with warm water and assist patient with handwashing.
18. Help the patient back into the bed or chair, using the transfer belt if necessary.
19. Remove the robe and slippers, make the patient comfortable, and place the call signal within reach.
20. Put on a clean pair of gloves.
21. Cover and remove the container from the commode.
22. Take the container to the bathroom. Check urine or feces for color, odor, clarity, sediment, consistency, and amount. Measure the urine if instructed. Collect a specimen if one has been ordered. (See Procedure 19-11.) Empty the remaining contents into the toilet.
23. Clean and disinfect the container.
24. Place the container back in the commode. Clean the commode if necessary.
25. Remove your gloves.
26. Return supplies to their proper place for the next use.
27. Unscreen the patient.
28. Place dirty linens in the hamper.
29. Wash your hands.
30. Report your observations to the nurse.

- Give the patient plenty of time.
- Offer the commode at regular times, such as after meals and before bedtime. Some patients are embarrassed to ask for it.

Bedpans. A **bedpan** is a plastic device used by patients who are bedridden to urinate or defecate. **See Figure 19-4.** Some patients are able to lift themselves up to sit on the bedpan, but others need assistance. Female patients use the bedpan for urinating and defecating. Male patients use a urinal for urinating and a bedpan only for defecating.

A **fracture pan** is a type of bedpan used by patients who are unable to raise their hips high enough to sit on a regular bedpan. Patients who have had back surgery, have hip fractures, or are in traction use fracture pans. A fracture pan has a thinner rim than a bedpan and is easier to slide under a patient. **See Figure 19-5.** Like a bedpan, the fracture pan is made of plastic.

Using a bedpan can be embarrassing for the patient, especially if there is a roommate. Patients may be anxious about the noises or smells they produce. Provide as much privacy as possible. Close the curtain around the bed, lower window shades, and make the patient as comfortable as possible. Close the door to the room.

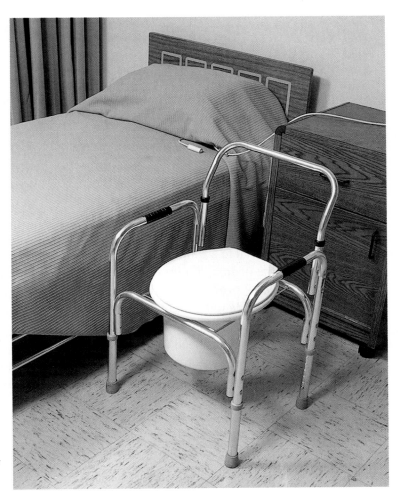

O **Figure 19-3. A bedside commode**.

Always cover the patient with a blanket after the patient is correctly positioned on the pan. Follow the same guidelines for respect and cleanliness as when providing any other toileting appliance.

After a patient uses the bedpan or fracture pan, cover the pan with its cover or a towel and take it into the bathroom. Observe the pan's contents before emptying the pan into the toilet. Then wash and disinfect it.

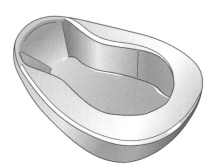

O **Figure 19-4. A bedpan**.

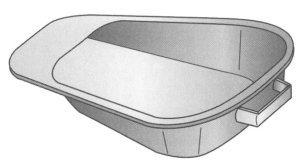

O **Figure 19-5. A fracture pan has a lower profile and a narrower rim than a bedpan**.

Procedure (19-2)

Giving a Bedpan or Fracture Pan to a Patient

Equipment: bedpan or fracture pan with cover or towel • toilet paper • wash basin • soap • towel • disposable gloves • waste bag

1. Identify the patient and introduce yourself. Call the patient by name.
2. Explain that you are going to help the patient use the bedpan (or fracture pan).
3. Provide privacy.
4. Wash your hands.
5. Raise the bed to a comfortable working level.
6. Warm the bedpan, if necessary, by running warm water over it and drying it.
7. Lower the side rail, if applicable.
8. Position the patient on his or her back. Raise the patient's head if this is permitted. The closer the patient is to a sitting position, the easier it is to use the bedpan.
9. Fold the patient's gown up and out of the way.
10. Lower the bed linens, keeping the patient's lower body covered.

For Patients Using a Bedpan:

(Note: For patients using a fracture pan, skip to Step 14.)

11. Ask the patient to flex the knees and raise the buttocks. You may need to slide your hand under the patient's back to raise the buttocks. **See Figure 19-6.**
12. Slide the bedpan under the patient. Make sure it is correctly placed. **See Figure 19-7.**
13. If the patient is unable to help in getting on the bedpan, turn the patient away from you. Lower the head of the bed. Place the bedpan against the patients' buttocks. While securely holding the bedpan, roll the patient onto his or her back. Raise the head of the bed. (Skip to Step 17.)

For Patients Using a Fracture Pan:

14. Ask the patient to raise the buttocks. You may need to slide your hand under the patient's back to help raise the buttocks.
15. Slide the fracture pan under the patient. The narrow end goes under the buttocks. Make sure it is correctly placed. **See Figure 19-8.**
16. If the patient is unable to get on the fracture pan, lower the head of the bed. Raise the buttocks with one arm and slide the fracture pan under the patient with the other arm.

For All Patients:

17. Cover the patient.
18. Raise the side rail, if applicable.
19. Place the toilet paper, waste bag, and signal cord within reach.
20. Instruct the patient to signal when finished. Tell patients whose intake/output is being measured to place the toilet paper in the waste bag, not the pan.
21. Wash your hands and leave the room.
22. Return as soon as the patient signals. Knock before you enter the room.
23. Wash your hands and put on gloves.
24. Lower the side rail, if applicable.
25. Ask the patient to raise the buttocks. Slide the bedpan out.
26. Cover the bedpan with the cover or a towel.

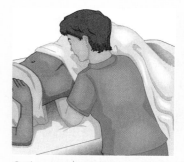

O **Figure 19-6. Help the patient raise the buttocks.**

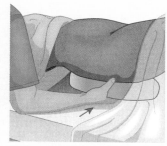

O **Figure 19-7. Position the bedpan under the patient.**

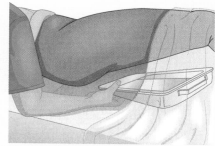

O **Figure 19-8. Correctly placing a fracture pan.**

27. Help the patient with perineal care.
28. Raise the side rail, if applicable.
29. Take the bedpan to the bathroom. Measure the urine, if instructed. Note the color, odor, clarity, sediment, consistency, and amount of urine or feces.
30. Empty the contents of the bedpan into the toilet.
31. Rinse the bedpan with cool water and clean it with a disinfectant.
32. Return the bedpan to the patient's bedside table.
33. Remove the gloves and wash your hands.
34. Fill the basin with warm water and assist the patient with handwashing.
35. Make the patient comfortable and place the signal cord within reach.
36. Unscreen the patient and wash your hands.
37. Report your observations to the nurse.

Urinals. A **urinal** is a special container that men use for urinating when they are bedridden. The urinal usually has a handle the patient can hold onto and a cap on top. A male patient can use a urinal while in bed, sitting on the side of the bed, or in a standing position. Most patients, however, prefer to stand if they are able.

As with all toileting appliances, offer the urinal at regular intervals. Empty, clean, and disinfect the urinal after each use. Replace it at the patient's bedside within reach. Never place a urinal next to the water pitcher since it may confuse the patient.

Procedure 19-3

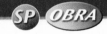

Offering a Urinal to a Male Patient

Equipment: urinal • wash basin • soap • towel

1. Identify the patient and introduce yourself. Call the patient by name.
2. Explain that you are going to help the patient use a urinal.
3. Provide privacy.
4. Wash your hands and apply gloves.
5. Help the patient to a standing position if the patient is able. If the patient cannot stand, help him lie on his back, with the bed raised at a 45° angle.
6. Place the flat side of the urinal down on the mattress. Instruct the patient to place his penis into the urinal opening. If he cannot do this himself, you should help him. Wear gloves if you need to assist.
7. Cover the patient with the linens and place the signal cord within reach.
8. Remove gloves and wash your hands.
9. Leave the room and close the door.
10. Answer the signal immediately. Knock and pause before entering the room.
11. Put on gloves and remove the urinal.
12. Make the patient comfortable and place the signal cord within reach.
13. Take the urinal into the bathroom. Observe the urine for color, odor, clarity, consistency, and amount. Measure the urine if instructed. Collect a specimen if one has been ordered. (See Procedure 19-11.)
14. Empty the contents of the urinal into the toilet.
15. Rinse the urinal with cool water, then clean and disinfect it.
16. Replace the urinal in the bedside stand or hang it on the bed within reach.
17. Remove your gloves.
18. Help the patient wash his hands using the wash basin, soap, and towel.
19. Wash your hands.
20. Make the patient comfortable and place the signal cord within reach.
21. Unscreen the patient.
22. Report your observations to the nurse.

Assisting the Incontinent Patient

Incontinence can result from spinal cord injury, central nervous system disorders, medications, reproductive system surgeries, childbirth, urinary tract infections, or stress and anxiety. It can be the result of aging or confusion.

There are many kinds of urinary incontinence.

- *Stress incontinence:* The patient dribbles urine when exercising, laughing, or coughing.
- *Urge incontinence:* The patient feels a sudden need to urinate but may not get to the toilet in time because the length of time between the urge and the opening of the urinary sphincter is decreased.
- *Functional incontinence:* The patient has bladder control but cannot feel the urge to urinate, so cannot get to the toilet in time.
- *Overflow incontinence:* The patient's bladder gets too full and leaks urine. It is sometimes the result of urinary retention.
- *Reflex incontinence:* The patient cannot feel the urge to void.
- *Mixed incontinence:* The patient has more than one type of incontinence.

Urinary and anal incontinence are embarrassing, frustrating, and uncomfortable. They can also be harmful to the patient's health. Bedsores, irritations, and infections can easily occur when a patient remains in wet or soiled clothing. Nursing assistants help patients cope with incontinence by supporting their dignity and self-esteem. They help families understand that incontinence is beyond the patient's control.

You can help the incontinent patient by:

- Offering the toilet, commode, or bedpan at regular intervals.
- Answering the call light as soon as possible.
- Showing empathy, patience, and understanding.
- Cleaning the patient immediately and providing good perineal care.

Vital Skills COMMUNICATION

Communicating with Sensitivity

For many patients, elimination issues can be an embarrassing part of being hospitalized. As a nursing assistant, it is your responsibility to be sensitive toward patients who may require assistance with elimination and to provide assistance in a professional manner.

Some important points to remember when assisting a patient with elimination:

- Respond to calls for help with elimination as quickly as possible.
- Provide privacy. Draw the curtain if the patient is bedridden. Allow the patient to be left alone if permitted but make sure the call button or signal cord is within reach.
- Refrain from commenting on the timing, odor, or appearance of the products of elimination. (However, you may need to record your observations on the patient's record.)
- Put yourself in the patient's position. Treat the patient as you would want to be treated.

Practice

With a partner, role-play the parts of a hospitalized patient who needs help with elimination and a nursing assistant. What can you do to help a patient who cannot be left alone feel more comfortable during elimination?

Pads, Briefs, and Bed Pads. Absorbent pads and briefs are available for patients with incontinence. They keep urine away from the skin to prevent bedsores and other skin problems. They also keep clothes from getting wet. Pads are worn inside the underwear. Briefs are worn instead of underwear. **See Figure 19-9.** Bed pads, or bed protectors, are absorbent pads placed over the bottom sheet to protect the linen from becoming wet or soiled. They also draw moisture away from the patient's skin. The nursing assistant is responsible for checking the patient frequently and changing the pad, brief, or bed pad when it is wet or soiled. Note that bed pads are not a substitute for toileting. Patients who are incontinent should also be toileted.

Bladder and Bowel Retraining. Bladder and bowel retraining programs may be developed for an incontinent patient. The patient's goal is to regain the ability to control the bladder or bowel. It can take many months for a patient to regain this control. Training is assessed by a nurse after a doctor gives an order. The nurse explains the training program to the patient and family members to achieve their cooperation. You may be asked to assist with the daily tasks of the training program.

When assisting a patient with bladder training:
- Offer the toilet, commode, bedpan, or urinal every two hours to start urinating.
- Provide privacy and make the patient comfortable.
- Give the patient plenty of time to void, usually about 15 to 20 minutes.
- If a catheter is used, follow the nurse's orders to clamp and unclamp the catheter for short periods.

When assisting a patient with bowel training:
- Offer the toilet, commode, or bedpan at scheduled intervals, usually after a meal, to start defecating.
- Provide privacy and make the patient comfortable.
- Give the patient plenty of time to defecate, usually about 15 to 20 minutes.
- Administer enemas as prescribed by the patient's doctor. (Information about enemas begins on page 471.)

For both bladder and bowel training, be supportive and reassuring to the patient. Never get angry if a patient has an accident. Always follow standard precautions when you are in contact with urine or feces.

Assisting with Catheters

A **catheter** is a tube used to drain fluid into or out of the body. A **urinary catheter** is a tube used to drain urine from the bladder. A nurse inserts it through the urethra into the bladder. The urine then drains into a special bag. The tubing is secured to the body with a strap or adhesive tape to keep the catheter from pulling out.

Catheters are used before and after procedures and surgery to keep the bladder empty, and for patients with urinary difficulties such as incontinence. They are also used to obtain sterile urine specimens and to accurately measure urinary output. A catheter can be used for a one-time withdrawal of urine (intermittent), or it may be in place for days or weeks.

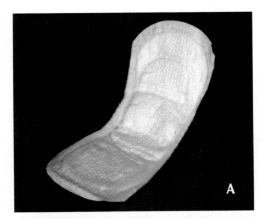

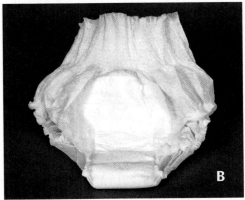

○ **Figure 19-9.** Incontinent patients may wear an incontinence pad (A) or briefs (B).

Catheters can be convenient for nursing staff when caring for patients who are incontinent. However, they are also a source for infection and should never be inserted in a patient for convenience only.

When you care for a patient with a catheter:

- Follow standard precautions.
- Check the level of urine in the drainage bag to make sure it is rising.
- Make sure there are no kinks in the catheter or tubing. Kinks would force urine back into the bladder.
- Check that the drainage bag is always lower than the patient's leg. Never attach it to a moveable part of the bed.
- Empty the drainage bag at the end of each shift or as directed by the nurse.
- Measure and record the output of the drainage bag using a graduate. A *graduate* is a transparent container with a numerical scale marked on the side for measuring fluids. All hospital patients with catheters have their intake/output measured.
- Provide perineal care and catheter care (see Procedure 19-4). Patients with catheters are at risk for urinary tract infections.
- Observe the urine for color, odor, clarity, sediment, consistency, and amount.
- Report patient complaints of pain, burning, or irritation to the nurse.
- Report to the nurse if a patient has an urge to urinate or says the bladder feels full.

Vital Skills   MATH

Averaging Hourly Urine Output

As a nursing assistant, you may be responsible for emptying and measuring urine output. Urine is measured in cubic centimeters (cc) using a graduate. Suppose the doctor has ordered a patient's output to be measured for 8 hours. The doctor wants an average hourly urine output. You measure and record the patient's urine from 0700 to 1500 hours:

0710	250 cc
0913	150 cc
1000	50 cc
1145	175 cc
1320	80 cc
1450	110 cc

To get the average hourly output, you add all of the individual outputs and then divide by the number of hours:

$250 + 150 + 50 + 175 + 80 + 110 = 815$ cc of urine in 8 hours.

815 cc $\div 8 = 101.88$ cc per hour; round to the nearest cc: 102 cc per hour.

Practice

A doctor has ordered a patient's urinary output to be measured for 12 hours, with an average hourly urine output. You measure and record the patient's urine output from 0800 to 2000 hours:

0805	200 cc
0935	170 cc
1030	75 cc
1250	150 cc
1420	75 cc
1600	150 cc
1710	250 cc
1755	50 cc

What is the total 12-hour urinary output? What is the average hourly output?

Procedure 19-4

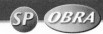

Perineal Care for the Catheterized Patient

Equipment: bath blanket • washcloths • towels • soap • basin of warm water • disposable gloves • bed protector

1. Identify the patient and introduce yourself. Call the patient by name.
2. Explain to the patient that you are going to provide catheter care.
3. Provide privacy.
4. Wash your hands.
5. Raise the bed to a comfortable working position.
6. Lower the side rail, if applicable.
7. Cover the patient with the bath blanket. Fanfold the top linens to the foot of the bed so you do not expose the patient.
8. Place the bed protector under the patient's buttocks.
9. Fill a basin with warm water between 105° and 110° F (41° and 43° C).
10. Put on gloves.
11. Perform perineal care.
    - *For a female patient:* Using a clean, wet washcloth, apply soap. Separate labia with thumb and forefinger. Gently cleanse one side of the meatus from front to back. Check for crusts or abnormal drainage. Using a clean section of washcloth, repeat on the opposite side. Rinse the washcloth and clean the catheter from the meatus down approximately 4 inches of catheter. Avoid pulling on the catheter. Rinse the washcloth with clean, warm water and repeat the procedure. Dry the perineal area with a towel.
    - *For a male patient:* If the male is uncircumcised, gently retract the foreskin. Using a clean, wet washcloth, apply soap. Begin washing the tip of the penis and meatus in a circular motion with the washcloth. Check for crusts or abnormal drainage. Repeat with a clean area of washcloth. Clean the catheter away from the penis approximately 4 inches, securing it as you clean. Avoid pulling on the catheter. **See Figure 19-10.**
12. Make sure the catheter is taped properly and the tubing is secure.
13. Remove the bed protector.
14. Clean all the equipment and store it for the next use.
15. Discard the dirty linens.
16. Remove your gloves and wash your hands.
17. Cover the patient with the bed linens and slip the bath blanket out.
18. Make the patient comfortable and place the signal cord within reach.
19. Unscreen the patient.
20. Report your observations to the nurse.

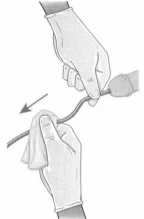

○ **Figure 19-10.** Clean the catheter, moving away from the patient's body.

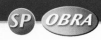
Emptying a Urine Drainage Bag and Measuring Urinary Output

Equipment: graduate • disposable gloves • paper towels • alcohol prep pad

1. Identify the patient, check the ID bracelet, and introduce yourself. Call the patient by name.
2. Explain that you are going to empty the patient's urinary drainage bag.
3. Provide privacy.
4. Wash your hands and put on gloves.
5. Place a paper towel on the floor. Place the graduate under the drain of the drainage bag on the paper towel.
6. Open the drain and let the urine run into the graduate, without touching the sides of the graduate.
7. Close the drain.
8. Wipe off with an alcohol prep pad.
9. Replace the drain in the holder.
10. Make the patient comfortable and place the signal cord within reach.
11. Unscreen the patient.
12. Measure the urinary output by placing the graduate on a level surface at eye level. Note the amount and character of the urine. If urine looks or smells unusual, report to the nurse. **See Figure 19-11.**
13. Record the amount of urine.
14. Empty urine into the toilet and flush. Discard the paper towel.
15. Wash and dry the graduate and store it for the next use.
16. Remove and dispose of your gloves.
17. Wash your hands.
18. Report the amount of urine collected and your observations to the nurse.

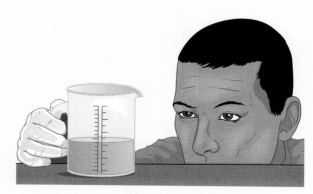

○ **Figure 19-11.** Measure the urine in the graduate.

Indwelling Catheters. A catheter that is left in the bladder over a period of time to continuously drain urine is an **indwelling catheter**. It is also called a *retention* or *Foley catheter*. It has a balloon at its tip that is inflated after the catheter is inserted into the bladder. The balloon prevents the catheter from slipping out.

The drainage tube of the indwelling catheter empties into a drainage bag. The drainage bag is attached to the patient's bed frame at a position that is lower than the body to take advantage of gravity and to keep urine from flowing back into the bladder. **See Figure 19-12.** For ambulatory patients, the tubing is connected to a leg bag, which is taped to the patient's lower leg. **See Figure 19-13.** The catheter system itself remains closed and sterile. Only the drainage bag is opened for emptying at regular intervals.

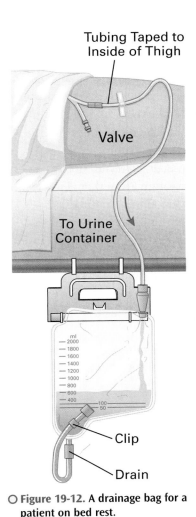

Figure 19-12. A drainage bag for a patient on bed rest.

Tubing Taped to Inside of Thigh

Valve

To Urine Container

Clip

Drain

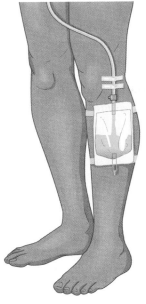

○ Figure 19-13. Secure the bag below the level of the bladder.

SAFETY FIRST

Leg bags should be used only when the patient is out of bed. If the patient lies down, the urine could flow from the leg bag back into the bladder. Be sure to change back to the bedside drainage bag when it is time for the patient to be in bed.

Nurses insert and remove indwelling catheters. Nursing assistants empty the drainage bags, provide catheter and perineal care, observe for abnormalities, and measure urine output.

Condom Catheters. A **condom catheter** is an external drainage catheter with a rubber sheath that is placed over the penis and attached to a drainage bag to assist in urination. **See Figure 19-14.** You may also hear this called a *Texas catheter*®. Many male patients find this more comfortable than an indwelling catheter. The condom is connected to tubing that drains into a drainage bag or leg bag.

Patients with condom catheters receive a new catheter each day. Some facilities require a new catheter at the change of each shift. The used one is discarded. Before a new catheter is applied, the genitals are washed, rinsed, and dried. Some patients are able to take care of their catheters and cleanup themselves. In this case, make sure that the genitals are clean and dry, and that the urine is flowing properly.

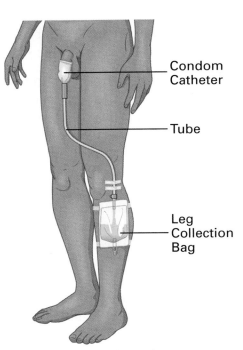

Condom Catheter

Tube

Leg Collection Bag

○ Figure 19-14. A condom catheter.

Inserting Rectal Tubes and Suppositories

A **rectal tube** is a tube inserted into the rectum to relieve flatulence and abnormal swelling of the abdomen. This swelling is called **abdominal distension**. When the rectal tube is inserted into the rectum, it allows *flatus* (gas) to pass into an attached flatus bag. The tube typically remains in the rectum for 20 minutes. Patients usually experience relief after one treatment. The rectal tube and bag come in a disposable kit that is used once and discarded. In some facilities, nursing assistants only assist in the procedure of inserting a rectal tube.

A **suppository** is a semisolid medication or lubricating agent that is inserted into the rectum for absorption by the body at the direction of a nurse. Suppositories are used to prevent or treat constipation by softening the stool. They are shaped like a cylinder and made of a waxy material, which melts inside the body. The suppository stimulates a bowel movement about 30 minutes after insertion. In some states, suppositories are administered by nurses, but you may be asked to assist the nurse during the insertion. You will place the patient in the left Sims' position and encourage the patient to hold the suppository for at least 20 minutes.

Suppositories that contain no medication may be given to patients with constipation. They are used for lubrication purposes only. A few states permit nursing assistants to administer these nonmedicated suppositories, if they have received special training.

Procedure 19-6

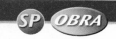

Inserting a Rectal Tube

Equipment: waterproof bed protector • disposable rectal tube with flatus bag • water-soluble lubricant • adhesive tape • disposable gloves

1. Identify the patient and introduce yourself. Call the patient by name.
2. Explain that you are going to insert a rectal tube to help relieve gas. Explain the procedure.
3. Provide privacy.
4. Wash your hands.
5. Raise the bed to a comfortable working level.
6. Lower the side rail, if appropriate.
7. Position the patient in the left Sims' position. Place the waterproof bed protector under the patient's buttocks.
8. Put on gloves.
9. Lubricate 2 to 4 inches of the tip of the rectal tube. **See Figure 19-15.**
10. Expose the anal area by lifting the edge of the bed linens.
11. Lift the upper buttock to expose the anus.
12. Ask the patient to take a deep breath.

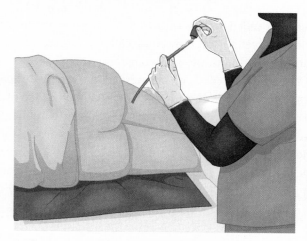

○ **Figure 19-15.** Lubricate the tip of the rectal tube.

13. As the patient exhales, gently insert the rectal tube 2 to 4 inches into the rectum. Stop if the patient complains of pain.
14. Tape the tubing to the lower buttock to hold it in place.
15. Position the flatus bag so it is on the bed behind the patient on the waterproof bed protector.
16. Remove your gloves and cover the patient.
17. Wash your hands.
18. Make the patient comfortable and place the signal cord within reach. Tell the patient the tube will remain in place for 20 minutes.
19. Leave the room.
20. Return 20 minutes after inserting the tube and put on gloves.
21. Remove the tube and flatus bag and discard them according to the facility's biohazard procedures.
22. Help the patient wipe the anal area.
23. Remove the gloves and wash your hands.
24. Make the patient comfortable and place the signal cord within reach.
25. Unscreen the patient and wash your hands.
26. Report your observations to the nurse.

Giving Enemas

An **enema** is a liquid solution placed into the rectum to loosen stools and to remove feces. A doctor orders enemas to relieve constipation and fecal impactions. In some states, nursing assistants are not permitted to give enemas. Be sure to check the law in your state.

Specific types of enemas are ordered for different purposes. A *cleansing enema* is used to clean out feces and flatus in the lower intestine. A patient may need a cleansing enema before surgery, diagnostic tests, or childbirth. There are three types of cleansing enemas: tap water, soapsuds, and saline. A *tap water enema* (TWE) uses only warm tap water. A *soapsuds enema* (SSE) has 5 mL of castile soap mixed into the warm tap water. A *saline enema* has 2 teaspoons of salt mixed into the warm tap water. The patient is encouraged to hold the cleansing enema until he or she feels the urge to defecate.

An *oil-retention enema* is given to soften feces for relief of constipation and fecal impaction. The oil is retained for a specified time, usually 30 to 60 minutes. The doctor specifies how long the patient should hold the enema.

Many facilities use *commercial enemas*, which are prepackaged in a plastic bottle with easy-to-follow instructions. The nursing assistant inserts the tip of the bottle into the patient's rectum and squeezes the bottle until the solution is out. Commercial enemas are discarded after one use.

Allow the patient to urinate before giving the enema to increase the patient's comfort. Make sure a bathroom, bedpan, or other toileting facility is available. The patient needs the toileting facility immediately after feeling the urge to defecate.

SP OBRA

Giving a Cleansing Enema

Equipment: bedpan, commode, or toileting facilities • disposable enema kit including enema bag, tubing, and clamp • graduate • bath thermometer • bed protector • lubricating jelly • disposable gloves • enema solution as ordered by a doctor • toilet paper • bath blanket • IV pole

1. Identify the patient, check the ID bracelet, and introduce yourself. Call the patient by name.
2. Explain that you are going to give the patient an enema. Explain the procedure.
3. Provide privacy.
4. Wash your hands.
5. Raise the bed to a comfortable working level.
6. Lower the side rail, if applicable.
7. Place the bed protector under the patient's buttocks.
8. Cover the patient with the bath blanket. Fanfold the top linens to the foot of the bed.
9. Place the IV pole next to the bed. Adjust the pole so the enema bag will be 12 inches above the anus or 18 inches above the mattress.
10. Place the bedpan or commode within reach.
11. Raise the side rail (if appropriate) and go to the patient's bathroom.
12. Open the disposable enema kit. Attach the tubing to the enema bag. Close the clamp on the tubing.

13. Fill the graduate with the prescribed amount of solution. Add ingredients as ordered by the patient's doctor. If soap is ordered, add castile soap last to avoid foaming.
14. Measure the temperature of the solution using the bath thermometer. The solution should be 105° F (41° C).
15. Pour the solution into the enema bag. Shake the solution gently to mix it.
16. Open the clamp and run a small amount of the solution into the sink. Reclamp. This removes air from the tubing.
17. Return to the patient and hang the enema bag on the IV pole. **See Figure 19-16.**
18. Lower the side rail, if appropriate.
19. Place the patient in the left Sims' position.
20. Put on gloves and expose the patient's anal area by lifting the top buttock.
21. Lubricate 2 to 4 inches of the tip of the enema tubing with the lubricant.
22. Ask the patient to take a deep breath.
23. Gently insert the tip of the tubing 2 to 4 inches into the rectum as the patient exhales (½ inch for infants, 1 to 1½ inches for children). Stop if you feel resistance or the patient complains of pain.
24. Unclamp the tubing and slowly administer the enema. Hold the enema tube in place as you administer the solution. Clamp the tubing to stop the enema if the patient experiences cramping. Resume when the cramping stops.
25. Clamp the tubing if the patient has the urge to defecate.
26. When most of the solution has flowed into the rectum, close the clamp.
27. Slowly withdraw the tubing from the rectum. Wrap the tip of the tubing with toilet paper and discard it according to facility policy.

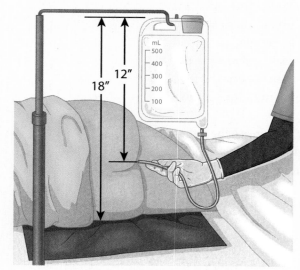

O **Figure 19-16.** Be sure the enema bag hangs at the proper height from the IV pole.

28. Encourage the patient to hold the solution as long as possible. Help hold the buttocks together if necessary.
29. When the patient is ready to defecate, help him or her to the toilet or assist with the bedpan or commode. Remind the patient not to flush the toilet.
30. Place the signal cord and toilet paper within reach.
31. Remove your gloves and wash your hands.
32. Leave the room if the patient can be alone.
33. Return immediately when the patient signals. Knock before entering the room.
34. Wash your hands and put on your gloves.
35. Observe the feces for amount, odor, color, and consistency.
36. Remove the bedpan or assist the patient back to bed.
37. Provide perineal care as necessary.
38. Cover the patient with the top linens and remove the bath blanket. Remove the bed protector.
39. Make the patient comfortable and place the signal cord within reach.
40. Empty, clean, and disinfect the bedpan or commode. Flush the toilet after the nurse looks at the output.
41. Store equipment for the next use.
42. Remove your gloves.
43. Help the patient wash his or her hands.
44. Unscreen the patient.
45. Place soiled linen in the hamper.
46. Wash your hands.
47. Report to the nurse the type of enema used, amount of solution taken, characteristics of the stool, and how the patient tolerated the procedure.

Procedure 19-8

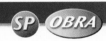

Giving a Commercial Enema

Equipment: commercial enema, either cleansing or oil • bath blanket • bed protector • lubricating jelly • bedpan, commode, or toilet facilities • toilet paper • disposable gloves

1. Identify the patient, check the ID bracelet, and introduce yourself. Call the patient by name.
2. Explain that you are going to give the patient an enema. Explain the procedure.
3. Provide privacy.
4. Wash your hands.
5. Raise the bed to a comfortable working level.
6. Lower the side rail, if appropriate.
7. Place the bed protector under the patient's buttocks.
8. Cover the patient with the bath blanket. Fanfold the top linens to the foot of the bed.
9. Place the bedpan or commode within reach.
10. Position the patient in the left Sims' position.
11. Put on gloves.
12. Expose the patient's anal area by lifting the top buttock.
13. Remove the cap from the enema bottle. Lubricate the tip with lubricating jelly if it is not prelubricated.
14. Ask the patient to take a deep breath while you perform the next step.
15. Gently insert the tip of the bottle 2 inches into the rectum as the patient exhales. Stop if you feel resistance or the patient complains of pain.
16. Squeeze and roll the plastic bottle gently until all the solution enters the rectum.
17. Remove the tip from the rectum and dispose of the bottle following facility policy for handling infectious wastes.

18. When giving an oil-retention enema, encourage the patient to hold the solution for the specified time, usually 30 to 60 minutes, before defecating. When giving a cleansing enema, encourage the patient to hold the solution until he or she feels the urge to defecate. Help hold the buttocks together, if necessary.

19. When the patient is ready to defecate, help him or her to the toilet or assist with the bedpan or commode. Remind the patient not to flush the toilet.

20. Place the signal cord and toilet paper within reach.

21. Remove your gloves and wash your hands.

22. Leave the room if the patient can be alone.

23. Return immediately when the patient signals. Knock before entering the room.

24. Wash your hands and put on gloves.

25. Observe the feces for amount, odor, color, and consistency. Save it if the nurse has asked to look at it.

26. Remove the bedpan or assist the patient back to bed.

27. Provide perineal care as necessary.

28. Cover the patient with the top linens and remove the bath blanket. Remove the bed protector.

29. Make the patient comfortable and place the signal cord within reach.

30. Empty, clean, and disinfect the bedpan or commode. Flush the toilet.

31. Store equipment for next use.

32. Remove your gloves.

33. Help the patient wash his or her hands.

34. Unscreen the patient.

35. Place soiled linen in the hamper.

36. Wash your hands.

37. Report your observations to the nurse.

Assisting with Ostomies

An **ostomy** is the surgical creation of an artificial opening in the body. The opening is called a **stoma**. Patients who have had part of their intestines surgically removed may have an artificial opening from the intestines. The opening goes through the abdominal wall to the outside of the body.

Some common reasons for intestinal surgery are colon cancer, diseases of the bowel such as diverticulitis, and trauma to the bowel. Patients with this type of ostomy may find it difficult to accept this dramatic change in their daily body functions. When caring for a patient with an ostomy, be supportive and encouraging.

Colostomy. A **colostomy** is an artificial opening from the large intestine (colon) to the abdominal wall. A diseased or injured part of the colon is removed or temporarily bypassed. The healthy part is rerouted through the abdomen and out of the body. The site of the colostomy depends on what part of the colon is diseased or injured. A colostomy can be permanent or temporary. If it is temporary, a surgeon reattaches the colon after the injured or diseased bowel heals.

The consistency of the stool passed through the stoma ranges from liquid to formed, depending on the colostomy site. The closer the colostomy is to the end of the digestive tract, the more formed the stools will be. A colostomy at the beginning of the colon results in liquid stools.

The colostomy patient eliminates stools through the stoma into a colostomy appliance, which is a plastic bag attached over the stoma. The bags are disposable. The colostomy patient must wear a colostomy appliance all the time. The appliance can be secured by a belt around the patient's body or attached with a karaya seal. (Karaya gum is a natural adhesive.)

Many patients are able to manage the care of their colostomies without any assistance. You will need to assist those who cannot. Assisting includes managing leakage around the appliance, keeping the skin clean and reducing skin irritation, and controlling odors. When assisting a colostomy patient:

- Change the colostomy appliance each time it is soiled.
- Help the patient clean the stoma and surrounding areas. Stools irritate the skin. Good skin care and personal hygiene are essential.
- Control odors by placing a special deodorant in the appliance before attaching it to the patient. If you do not have access to the special deodorant, add a tablespoon of baking soda, or chlorophyll or charcoal tablets, according to facility policy.

Procedure 19-9

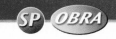

Changing a Colostomy Appliance

Equipment: bedpan with cover • bed protector • bath blanket • toilet paper • clean colostomy appliance • clean colostomy belt • bath thermometer • wash basin • washcloth • towel • soap or cleaning agent • karaya powder, ring, or other barrier • deodorant for appliance • waste bag • paper towels • disposable gloves

1. Identify the patient, check the ID bracelet, and introduce yourself. Call the patient by name.
2. Explain that you are going to change the patient's colostomy appliance. Explain the procedure.
3. Provide privacy.
4. Wash your hands.
5. Raise the bed to a comfortable working level.
6. Lower the side rail, if appropriate.
7. Place the bed protector under the patient's buttocks.
8. Cover the patient with the bath blanket. Fanfold the top linens to the foot of the bed.
9. Put on gloves.
10. Unfasten the belt and gently disconnect the appliance from the patient. Place the appliance in a bedpan.
11. Wipe around the stoma with toilet paper. Remove any feces or drainage. Discard the toilet paper in a bedpan or waste bag.

12. Cover the bedpan and take it to the patient's bathroom.
13. Note the color, odor, amount, and consistency of the feces. Empty the bedpan into the toilet. Discard the appliance in the waste bag.
14. Fill the wash basin with warm water, about 105° F (41° C). Place it on the overbed table.
15. Clean the skin around the stoma with warm water. **See Figure 19-17.** Use soap or a cleansing agent, according to facility policy. Rinse well and dry.

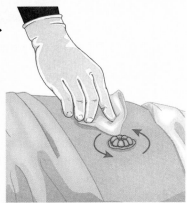

○ **Figure 19-17. Clean the skin around the stoma.**

16. Apply the karaya powder, ring, or other skin barrier.
17. Place the deodorant in the appliance.
18. Remove the backing on the new appliance. Center it over the stoma and seal it to the skin. **See Figure 19-18.** You can press gently to make sure it is sealed.
19. Refasten the belt to the appliance.
20. Remove the bed protector.
21. Discard the waste bag.
22. Remove your gloves.
23. Make the patient comfortable and place the signal cord within reach.
24. Unscreen the patient.
25. Clean and disinfect the equipment and store it for the next use.

26. Wash your hands.
27. Report your observations to the nurse.

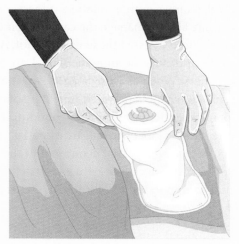

O **Figure 19-18.** Seal the appliance to the skin.

Ileostomy. An **ileostomy** is an artificial opening between the small intestine and the abdominal wall. Usually, patients with an ileostomy have had their entire large intestine removed. The stoma is created before partially digested food would enter the large intestine. Water is not yet removed from the feces, so liquid feces constantly drain from the stoma. The feces are extremely irritating to the skin because they are full of digestive juices.

Ileostomy appliances are similar to colostomy appliances. The appliance is sealed to the skin around the stoma so it fits properly to prevent feces from touching the skin. The bags are either disposable or reusable, depending on the doctor's recommendation. The bag must be emptied every 4 to 6 hours. It is replaced with a new bag or washed and replaced with a clean bag.

Procedure 19-10

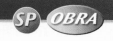

Cleaning an Ileostomy Appliance

Equipment: solvent • medicine dropper • clean ileostomy appliance • clean ileostomy belt • clamp • gauze • washcloth • towels • cotton balls • soap or cleaning agent • karaya ring • deodorant • soft brush • toilet paper • disposable gloves

1. Identify the patient, check the ID bracelet, and introduce yourself. Call the patient by name.
2. Explain that you are going to clean the patient's ileostomy appliance. Explain the procedure.

3. Provide privacy and arrange the equipment in the bathroom.
4. Wash your hands.
5. Help the patient out of bed, into the bathroom, and onto the toilet.
6. Put on gloves.

7. Direct the appliance into the toilet and remove the clamp. This empties the contents of the appliance into the toilet. **See Figure 19-19.**
8. Wipe the end of the appliance with toilet paper. (Some patients can do this themselves.)
9. Note the color, odor, amount, and consistency of the feces.
10. Place a few drops of the solvent in the medicine dropper and apply it to the skin around the appliance. The appliance will loosen.
11. Gently remove the appliance.
12. Cover the stoma with the gauze.
13. Wet a cotton ball with the solvent and wipe around the stoma.
14. Clean the skin around the stoma with water. Some facilities also use soap or a cleansing agent. Rinse well and dry.
15. Remove the gauze.
16. Place the karaya ring around the stoma.
17. Put the deodorant in the clean appliance.
18. Clamp the bottom of the clean appliance and attach the appliance to the karaya ring.

19. Remove the gloves and wash your hands.
20. Help the patient wash his or her hands.
21. Make the patient comfortable and place the signal cord within reach.
22. Unscreen the patient.
23. Put on clean gloves and clean the used appliance with the soft brush.
24. Allow the used appliance to dry.
25. Remove the gloves.
26. Store equipment for the next use.
27. Wash your hands.
28. Report your observations to the nurse.

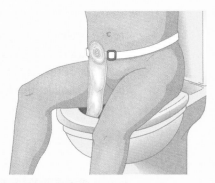

O **Figure 19-19. Empty the ileostomy appliance into the toilet.**

Collecting and Testing Urine Samples

Urine samples, or specimens, are collected for laboratory examination to help a physician diagnose an illness or evaluate treatment. A doctor orders a specific type of urine specimen:

- To diagnose a urinary tract infection or kidney disorder.
- To identify drugs in the urine.
- To determine if glucose is present in the urine in patients with known or suspected diabetes.
- During pregnancy.

Nursing assistants are often responsible for collecting urine specimens and for some urine testing. Many urine tests come in kits with easy-to-follow instructions. Other urine specimens require more complicated tests and are sent to a laboratory with a lab requisition slip. The nurse completes the lab requisition slip before the nursing assistant collects the urine specimen.

Specimens are collected in a specimen container, which is a small plastic cup with a lid. Another type of collection device is a receptacle that fits under the toilet seat and is used to collect urine and stool specimens. It is used by patients who are able to eliminate on the toilet. Patients whose intake and output are being measured, as well as patients who need to produce a stool sample, can use this device.

Collecting Urine Samples

When collecting any type of urine sample, follow these guidelines:

- Treat every patient with respect and dignity. Providing specimens can be embarrassing for patients.
- Always follow standard precautions.
- Wash your hands before and after collection.
- Help the patient wash his or her hands after collection.
- Use a separate, clean specimen container for each sample.
- Clearly label the container with the patient's name, location, date, and time of collection.
- Do not touch the inside of the container. Instruct the patient not to touch the inside of the container.
- Place the specimen container in a plastic bag and seal the bag.
- Remind female patients not to have a bowel movement at the same time the sample is being taken, and not to throw toilet paper into the collection container. The sample must be free from feces and toilet paper.

Routine Urine Sample. A routine or random urine sample is collected from every patient who enters a hospital or health care facility. It can be collected at any time of the day with no special preparation. Patients who are able to use the toilet can collect the specimen themselves after you explain the procedure to them.

Procedure 19-11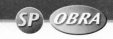

Collecting a Routine Urine Sample

Equipment: bedpan and cover, urinal, or other collection device • specimen container with a lid • graduate used to measure urine, if ordered • label and marking pen • disposable gloves • laboratory requisition form • plastic bag • waste bag

1. Identify the patient, check the ID bracelet, and introduce yourself. Call the patient by name.
2. Explain to the patient that you are going to collect a urine sample.
3. Provide privacy.
4. Wash your hands.
5. Prepare the label on the specimen container with the patient's information. **See Figure 19-20.**
6. Ask the patient to urinate in the bedpan, urinal, or other collection device. If the patient is able, he or she can go to the bathroom to provide a sample in the specimen container.

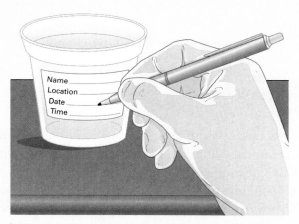

○ **Figure 19-20.** Prepare the label for a urine specimen container. Be sure to write the information clearly.

7. Remind the patient not to place toilet paper in the collection device or the specimen container. Provide a waste bag for dirty paper.
8. Put on gloves.
9. Help the patient clean the perineal area, if necessary.
10. Take the collection device to the bathroom.
11. If the patient's intake/output is being measured, measure and record the amount of urine.
12. Pour the urine into the specimen container. The container should be ¾ full.
13. Place the lid on the specimen container. Place the container into a plastic bag and seal the bag to prevent leaks.
14. Pour the remaining urine into the toilet.
15. Clean and disinfect the equipment and store for the next use.
16. Discard the waste bag.
17. Remove your gloves and wash your hands.
18. Help the patient wash his or her hands.
19. Make the patient comfortable and place the signal cord within reach.
20. Unscreen the patient.
21. Take the urine specimen to the nurse's station or the lab. Be sure to take the lab requisition slip with the specimen.
22. Wash your hands.
23. Report your observations to the nurse.

Clean-Catch Sample. A clean-catch, or midstream, sample is collected after the perineal area is thoroughly cleaned according to facility policy. Cleaning reduces the number of microorganisms from the urethral area included in the sample. Clean-catch urine kits come prepackaged.

Procedure 19-12

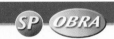

Collecting a Clean-Catch (Midstream) Sample

Equipment: clean-catch specimen kit • bedpan and cover, urinal, or other collection device • specimen container with a lid • graduate used to measure urine, if ordered • label and marking pen • disposable gloves • laboratory requisition form • plastic bag

1. Identify the patient, check the ID bracelet, and introduce yourself. Call the patient by name.
2. Explain the procedure to the patient.
3. Provide privacy.
4. Wash your hands.
5. Prepare the label on the specimen container with the patient's information.
6. Help the patient to the bathroom if the patient is able. Otherwise, perform the procedure while the patient is in bed.
7. Open the clean-catch urine kit. Remove the towelettes and the specimen container.
8. Put on gloves.
9. Perform perineal care using the towelettes.

Patients who are able can do this themselves. Remind the patient that each towelette should be used for only one wipe and should be wiped from front to back. Women should keep their labia separated until the specimen is collected. An uncircumcised male should keep the foreskin retracted until the specimen is collected.
10. Ask the patient to urinate in the collection device or the toilet.
11. Ask the patient to stop the stream of urine.
12. Hold the specimen container under the patient. Patients who are able can do this themselves.
13. Ask the patient to start urinating again.

14. Ask the patient to stop urinating when the container is about ¾ full.
15. Remove the container and ask the patient to finish urinating.
16. Place the lid on the specimen container with your clean hand. Place the container in a plastic bag and seal the bag.
17. Help the patient clean the perineal area.
18. Take the collection device to the bathroom.
19. If the patient's intake/output is being measured, measure and record the amount of urine. Make sure you include the urine in the specimen container in your calculations.
20. Pour the remaining urine into the toilet.
21. Clean the equipment and store for the next use.
22. Remove your gloves and wash your hands.
23. Help the patient wash his or her hands.
24. Make the patient comfortable and place the signal cord within reach.
25. Unscreen the patient.
26. Take the urine specimen to the nurse's station or the lab. Be sure to take the lab requisition slip with the specimen.
27. Wash your hands.
28. Report your observations to the nurse.

24-Hour Sample. A 24-hour urine sample is a collection of all the urine a patient produces in a 24-hour period. A preservative is added to the collection container to prevent the growth of microorganisms.

The patient voids first thing in the morning before the test begins, so he or she can begin the sample with an empty bladder. This voiding is discarded. All urine voided in the next 24 hours is added to the collection container. If some urine spills or is accidentally discarded, the collection must start over.

Signs must be posted near the bed and in the bathroom above the toilet to alert everyone working with the patient that a 24-hour urine sample is being collected. It is written in the patient's medical record, too, and reported to each change of shift. In addition, the patient must completely understand the procedure. Once the test is completed, the labeled container is placed in a biohazard bag for safety. The bag is then transported to a laboratory.

Procedure 19-13

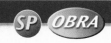

Collecting a 24-Hour Urine Specimen

Equipment: container for 24-hour collection • preservative and bucket of ice or refrigerator • two labels for 24-hour urine collection • funnel • bedpan, urinal, commode, or other collection device • disposable gloves • lab requisition slip

1. Find out from the nurse how the urine will be stored. It is usually stored with a preservative on ice or in a refrigerator.
2. Identify the patient, check the ID bracelet, and introduce yourself. Call the patient by name.
3. Explain to the patient that you are setting up a 24-hour urine specimen. Thoroughly explain the procedure.
4. Provide privacy.
5. Wash your hands.
6. Place the equipment in the patient's bathroom.

7. Write the patient's information on the urine collection container.

8. Place one of the 24-hour urine collection labels in the patient's bathroom. Place the other label near the bed.

9. Offer the patient the collection device or help the patient to the bathroom. Wear gloves if you need to help the patient.

10. Ask the patient to urinate. Discard this specimen. The 24-hour period begins after the patient urinates.

11. Write the time the test began and the time it will end on the labels and the specimen container.

12. Explain to the patient that he or she will use the collection device each time he or she urinates for the next 24 hours. Remind the patient not to have a bowel movement and urinate at the same time.

13. After the patient urinates, pour the urine into the urine collection container using the funnel. Be careful not to spill any urine. Replace the container on ice or in the refrigerator.

14. At the end of the 24-hour period, ask the patient to urinate. Add the urine to the collection container and seal the container in a biohazard bag. **See Figure 19-21.**

15. Remove the gloves.

16. Make the patient comfortable and place the signal cord within reach.

17. Clean and disinfect all the equipment and store it for the next use.

18. Remove the labels from the bed and bathroom.

19. Thank the patient for his or her cooperation.

20. Wash your hands.

21. Take the urine collection container to the nurse's station or the lab. Be sure to take the lab requisition slip with the specimen.

22. Wash your hands.

23. Report your observations to the nurse.

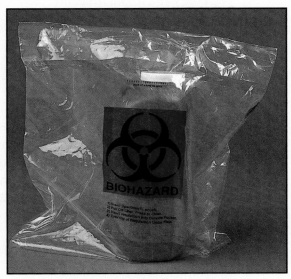

O **Figure 19-21.** Place the 24-hour urine collection container in a biohazard bag for safe transport to a laboratory.

Urine Samples from Infants and Toddlers. Children who wear diapers have not acquired bladder control. Unlike older children and adults, they are unable to urinate into a toileting device to produce a sample. To obtain a specimen, place a collection bag over the child's urethra. Diaper the child in the usual way. Periodically check the infant to see if he or she has voided. Then, pour the contents of the collection bag into a specimen container for testing.

Procedure 19-14

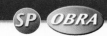

Collecting Urine from an Infant or Toddler

Equipment: disposable urine collector • specimen container and lid • label and marking pen • wash basin • sterile cotton balls • bath towel • two diapers • disposable gloves • lab requisition slip • plastic bag

1. Identify the child, check the ID bracelet, and introduce yourself. Call the child by name.
2. Explain to the child and parents that you are going to collect a urine sample. Explain the procedure.
3. Provide privacy.
4. Prepare the label on the specimen container with the patient's information.
5. Wash your hands and put on gloves.
6. Remove the child's diaper.
7. Clean the perineal area with water and sterile cotton balls. Dry the area.
8. Place the child on his or her back, with the knees flexed.
9. Remove the backing from the urine collector. Place the bag over the boy's penis or the girl's vulva. Do not cover the anus. Press the adhesive gently on the child's skin so the collector stays in place. **See Figure 19-22.**
10. Diaper the child as usual.
11. Remove the gloves.
12. Make the child comfortable and provide for safety.
13. Unscreen the child.
14. Wash your hands.
15. Return periodically to check whether the child has urinated.
16. Once the child has urinated, provide privacy. Put on gloves.
17. Remove the diaper and the urine collector.
18. Pour the contents into the specimen container. Cover it with the lid using your clean hand.
19. Discard the urine collector.
20. Provide perineal care and put a clean diaper on the child.
21. Make the child comfortable and place the signal cord within reach.
22. Remove the gloves and wash your hands.
23. Unscreen the child.
24. Place the label on the specimen container. Place the container in the plastic bag and seal.
25. Discard disposable items.
26. Take the urine specimen to the nurse's station or the lab. Be sure to take the lab requisition slip with the specimen.
27. Wash your hands.
28. Report your observations to the nurse.

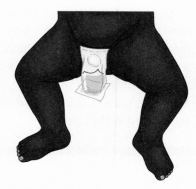

O **Figure 19-22.** Collecting urine from an infant.

Urine Samples from a Closed Urinary Drainage System. Sterile urine samples can be obtained from an indwelling catheter using a sterile needle and syringe through a drainage port in the catheter tubing. This is a procedure that should not be done by a nursing assistant. It is usually done by a nurse.

Testing Urine

Nursing assistants may test the urine of patients with diabetes, although many facilities send the samples to be tested by laboratory personnel. This testing may help the doctor regulate the patient's diet and insulin medication. If urine tests are ordered by the doctor, perform them accurately and report the results to the nurse.

Diabetic patients' urine is tested for the presence of glucose or ketones. *Glucose* is an important sugar used in the body's metabolism. It is not normally present in urine. *Ketones* are a by-product of fat metabolism. When a person no longer has glucose circulating in the blood for use by the body, the body begins to break down fat. The by-product of the fat is collected into the urine as ketones.

The products in **Table 19-1** are specific commercial products that you may hear about or use on the job. They are used when collecting and testing urine or stool samples.

○ **Table 19-1. Common Commercial Collection and Testing Products**

Product	Use
Tes-Tape®	Urine test for glucose
Clinitest®	Urine test for glucose
Acetest®	Urine test for ketones
Keto-Diastix®	Urine test for ketones
Hemoccult®	Fecal occult blood test
Specipan®	Collection device that is used on a toilet

Procedure 19-15

Testing a Urine Sample

Equipment: bedpan and cover, urinal, commode, or other collection device • specimen containers • urine testing equipment • disposable gloves

1. Identify the patient and introduce yourself.
2. Explain that you are going to test the patient's urine. Explain the procedure.
3. Provide privacy.
4. Wash your hands and put on gloves.
5. Follow Procedure 19-11 to collect a routine urine sample.
6. Test the sample, following the directions for the type of testing equipment your facility uses.
7. Clean equipment and store for the next use.
8. Remove the gloves.
9. Wash your hands.
10. Report the results and your observations to the nurse.

Straining Urine

Stones, or *calculi*, can form in the kidneys, ureters, or bladder. They may form when certain substances in the urine become very concentrated. Stones can cause intense pain as well as damage by blocking openings in the urinary system. Some stones are passed out of the body through the urine. Others must be surgically removed. The procedure of straining for stones collects the stones, crystals, and particles that are passed in urine. They are then analyzed. Analyzing the stones can sometimes determine their cause, such as excessive uric acid, excessive calcium, or other types of salts or minerals.

Procedure 19-16

Straining Urine for Stones

Equipment: disposable strainer or 4 × 4 gauze • specimen container and label • labels for the room and bathroom • bedpan and cover, urinal, commode, or other collection device • disposable gloves • lab requisition slip • plastic bag

1. Identify the patient and introduce yourself. Call the patient by name.
2. Explain to the patient that you are going to collect and strain urine to look for the presence of stones.
3. Provide privacy.
4. Place labels above the patient's bed and above the toilet in the bathroom indicating that all urine is to be strained.
5. Wash your hands and put on gloves.
6. Offer the bedpan, urinal, or bedside commode, or assist the patient to the toilet to use the collection device.
7. After the patient has voided, remove and cover the bedpan, urinal, or bedside commode.
8. Assist the patient with perineal care. If the patient was able to use the toilet, assist with perineal care and help the patient back to the room.
9. Help the patient with handwashing.
10. Make the patient comfortable.
11. Place the signal cord within reach.
12. Take the urine into the patient's bathroom.
13. Place the strainer or gauze over a specimen container.
14. Pour the urine into the strainer or gauze. **See Figure 19-23.** Any stones, crystals, or particles will remain in the strainer or on the gauze.
15. Discard the urine.

16. Place the gauze or contents of the strainer in the specimen container. Cover the container.
17. Remove the gloves and wash your hands.
18. Label the container, place it in the plastic bag, and seal.
19. Clean and store equipment for the next use.
20. Unscreen the patient.
21. Take the specimen container to the nurse's station or the lab. Be sure to take the lab requisition slip with the specimen.
22. Wash your hands.
23. Report your observations to the nurse.

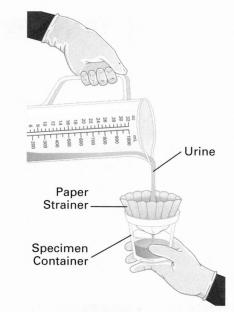

○ Figure 19-23. Straining urine for stones.

Vital Skills (WRITING)

Using Spell-Checkers

More and more hospitals are moving toward computerized medical records. That means you will record patient information on a computer. Most word processing programs have spell-check programs that can help you with your spelling. Basically, a spell-checker looks over your text and points out possible spelling errors.

Spell-check programs can be useful, but they aren't always foolproof. They cannot recognize a correctly spelled word that is used incorrectly. For instance, if you write "Mrs. Anderson asked for to aspirin" (using the word *to* instead of *two*), the spell-checker will not flag the word *to* because it is spelled correctly.

Sometimes a word will not be in the spell-check program's dictionary. If you have a question about the spelling of a word that isn't included, use a dictionary to check the spelling. (Most spell-check programs allow you to add new words, so once you have checked the spelling of a word, you can add it to the spell-check program.)

Practice

Enter the following text into a document using your computer's word processing program. Edit the paragraph with the help of your computer's spell-check program. (Note: The patient's name is correctly spelled "Wright.") What incorrectly spelled words did the spell-check miss? Were there any words you had to look up in a dictionary?

Mrs. Wright said she did not feel well this mourning. She complains of nausea and nocturia. She reports urnating 4 times between midnight and 6:00 AM. She reports an episode of diarhea at approximnately 12:30 last night. She eat halve of her brakefast. Mrs. Write asked for gingerale at 10:30 AM. She drank approximately 150 ccs of it. At 10:45 AM, her vitals sighs were 100.8-67-19-120/90.

Collecting and Testing Stool Samples

Stool samples are tested in the laboratory for the presence of blood, fat, microorganisms, worms, and other abnormal contents. Like urine, stool is an end point of the body's waste systems and can carry clues to illness and disease. Doctors might order a stool specimen for illnesses such as diarrhea, internal bleeding, or cancer, and for patients with food absorption and digestion problems. A **fecal occult blood test (FOBT)** is used to detect the presence of hidden (occult) blood in the stool.

Nursing assistants may be asked to collect stool specimens from patients. Keep in mind that this can be embarrassing to patients. Patients are asked to defecate in a bedpan, bedside commode, or a collection device that is put under the seat of a toilet. The nursing assistant takes some of the stool from the collection device and places it in the specimen container or the testing kit. The rest of the stool is emptied into the toilet. Patients who are able usually prefer to collect the samples themselves. Patients on bed rest need assistance.

Some specimens, such as those for parasites and their ova (eggs), require warm stool to ensure accurate results. You must take these samples to the lab immediately after collection.

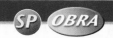

Collecting a Stool Sample

Equipment: bedpan and cover, commode, or other collection device • specimen container with lid • label and marking pen • wooden blade • waste bag • disposable gloves • toilet paper • lab requisition slip • plastic bag

1. Identify the patient, check the ID bracelet, and introduce yourself. Call the patient by name.
2. Explain to the patient that you are going to collect a stool sample. Explain the procedure.
3. Provide privacy.
4. Complete the specimen label with the patient's name, location, date, and time of collection.
5. Wash your hands and put on gloves.
6. Offer the bedpan or other collection device for the patient to urinate in before producing a stool sample. Remove the bedpan and clean it.
7. Help the patient with toileting. Offer a different bedpan or collection device.
8. Remind the patient to put used toilet paper in the waste bag.
9. Place the toilet paper and signal cord within reach and tell the patient to signal when finished.
10. Remove the gloves, wash your hands, and leave the room.
11. Return to the room as soon as the patient signals. Knock before entering.
12. Put on gloves.
13. Remove the bedpan from the patient and cover it.
14. Assist the patient with perineal care.
15. Take the bedpan into the patient's bathroom.
16. Using the wooden blade, collect about 2 tablespoons of feces and place in the specimen container. **See Figure 19-24.**
17. Put the lid on the container without touching the inside.
18. Cover the wooden blade with toilet paper and discard according to the facility's biohazard procedure.
19. Empty and clean the bedpan and store it for next use.

20. Remove the gloves.
21. Help the patient with handwashing.
22. Make the patient comfortable and place the signal cord within reach.
23. Place a label on the specimen container.
24. Place the specimen container in a plastic bag and seal.
25. Wash your hands.
26. Unscreen the patient.
27. Take the stool specimen to the nurse's station or the lab. Be sure to take the lab requisition slip with the specimen.
28. Wash your hands.
29. Report your observations to the nurse.

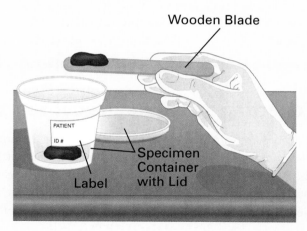

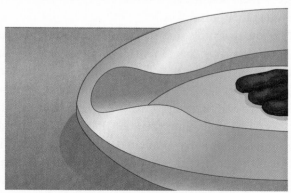

O Figure 19-24. Collecting a stool sample.

Procedure 19-18

Collecting a Fecal Occult Blood Slide

Equipment: stool sample • fecal occult blood test (FOBT) package • wooden blade • developer • disposable gloves

1. Identify the patient and introduce yourself. Call the patient by name.
2. Explain that you are going to check the patient's stool for blood. Explain the procedure.
3. Provide privacy.
4. Wash your hands.
5. Place the equipment in the patient's bathroom.
6. Follow Procedure 19-17 to collect the stool sample.
7. Put on gloves.
8. Open the back of the FOBT packet. There are two paper squares labeled A and B. The packet is designed so that you never directly touch the stool specimen.
9. Use the wooden blade to pick up a small amount of stool. Smear a small amount on the square labeled A. **See Figure 19-25.**
10. Turn the wooden blade around and pick up another small amount of stool from a different part of the specimen. Smear a small amount on the square labeled B.
11. Close the packet.
12. Turn the packet over and open it. There will be two paper areas with stool under the paper. One test area is marked positive (+), and the other is marked negative (–).
13. Open the developer and place one drop on the positive area and one drop on the negative area.
14. Wait 10 seconds.
15. The positive test area should turn blue. This indicates that the test is working.
16. Place 2 more drops of developer on the positive and negative areas. Replace the cap on the developer.

17. Read the results in 1 minute.
18. If there is no color change, the stool contains no occult blood. If the color on the negative area turns blue, the stool does contain occult blood.
19. Save the test packet to show the nurse the results.
20. Flush the remaining stool specimen down the toilet.
21. Cover the wooden blade with toilet paper and discard according to the facility's biohazard procedure.
22. Clean and disinfect the equipment.
23. Remove the gloves and wash your hands.
24. Store equipment for the next use. Return the developer to the nurse's station.
25. Make the patient comfortable and place the signal cord within reach.
26. Note the test results on the patient's chart.
27. Report the results and any observations to the nurse.

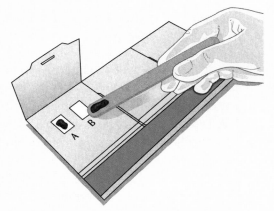

O **Figure 19-25.** Testing for occult (hidden) blood in the stool.

Collecting Other Specimens

It is important to know which collection procedures are approved for nursing assistants in your state. For example, drawing blood specimens is not a responsibility of a nursing assistant. However, you may need to assist a patient during this procedure by holding the arm or repositioning the patient if needed. Ask your supervisor if you are unsure of your responsibilities when obtaining specimens.

Collecting Sputum Samples

Nursing assistants may collect sputum samples. **Sputum** is the mucous secretion from the lungs, bronchi, and trachea. It is expelled through the mouth, but it is not the same as saliva. Respiratory problems can be diagnosed by testing a patient's sputum. It is studied for the presence of blood, microorganisms, and abnormal cells. To collect a sputum sample, the patient must cough up the sputum from the bronchi and trachea. This can be difficult and painful. It may also be unpleasant and embarrassing for the patient.

Follow these guidelines when helping a patient produce a sputum sample:

- Collect the sample as soon as the patient wakes up. There is more sputum in the lungs first thing in the morning, so it is easier for the patient to cough up.
- Do not let the patient use mouthwash or toothpaste before obtaining a sputum sample. These substances may destroy some of the microorganisms.
- Provide for privacy.
- Immediately cover the sputum sample and place it in a paper bag.
- Always follow standard precautions when in contact with body fluids.

Procedure 19-19

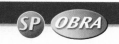

Collecting and Preserving a Sputum Sample

Equipment: sputum specimen container with lid • tissues • label and marker • waste bag • disposable gloves • lab requisition slip • plastic bag

1. Identify the patient, check the ID bracelet, and introduce yourself. Call the patient by name.
2. Explain to the patient that you are going to collect a sputum sample. Explain the procedure.
3. Prepare the label on the specimen container with the patient's information.
4. Provide privacy.
5. Wash your hands and put on gloves.
6. If the patient has eaten recently, ask the patient to rinse out the mouth with water.
7. Place the label on the container, open the lid, and give the patient the specimen container.

8. Instruct the patient to take several deep breaths and then cough deeply from the lungs to bring up sputum. The patient should cover his or her mouth and nose with a tissue while coughing.
9. The patient may need to cough several times to bring up enough sputum. You will need 1 to 2 tablespoons of sputum for the specimen.
10. Instruct the patient to expel the sputum directly into the specimen container.
11. Put the lid on the container immediately after collection.
12. Place the container in a plastic bag and seal.

13. Remove the gloves and wash your hands.
14. Make the patient comfortable and place the signal cord within reach.
15. Unscreen the patient.
16. Take the sputum specimen to the nurse's station or the lab. Be sure to take the lab requisition slip with the specimen.
17. Wash your hands.
18. Report to the nurse the date and time of sputum collection, the appearance of the sputum, the time the specimen was sent to the lab, and observations of anything unusual.

Suctioning a Patient

Some respiratory illnesses cause the upper airway to fill with fluid. If a patient cannot clear the airway by coughing, the fluids interfere with normal breathing. **Suctioning** is the process of removing or sucking up fluid or body secretions. The areas that most commonly need suctioning are the upper airway, the stomach, and surgical wounds. A doctor orders suctioning to remove excess fluid. In most states, suctioning is not performed by nursing assistants. It is performed by a nurse or respiratory therapist.

The equipment used to suction a patient includes a wall suction unit, a portable suction machine, or a disposable suction apparatus, each connected to tubing. The other end of the tubing is inserted into the body part. The suctioned materials are collected in a container. Nursing assistants do not perform suctioning procedures, but they may be asked to care for patients who require suctioning.

To suction the upper airway, a nurse places the suction tubing into the mouth (*oral suctioning*) or nose, or into the back of the throat (*tonsillar suctioning*). Secretions further down the upper airways may be in the trachea (*tracheal suctioning*).

You should be alert to signs and symptoms that a patient may need upper airway suctioning. Report them immediately to the nurse:

- Difficult or labored breathing
- Restlessness and/or anxiety
- Cyanosis
- Rapid breathing
- Gurgling or moist-sounding breathing

If you are taking care of a patient who is receiving suctioning, report any of the following observations to the nurse:

- A leakage in the tubing or suction system
- A leveling in the amount of fluid in the collection container
- A rapid increase of fluid in the collection container
- A change in color or consistency of the fluid

Chapter Summary

- Elimination is an important natural life process that varies from person to person.

- The nursing assistant helps patients with normal urination and bowel movements as well as those with commonly occurring problems.

- Incontinence is a problem for many patients for a variety of reasons. Supporting a person's dignity and self-esteem and demonstrating patience, empathy, and understanding are part of the nursing assistant's role.

- Caring for patients with catheters involves emptying and changing drainage bags, providing catheter care, observing and reporting abnormalities, and measuring urinary output.

- Enemas may be ordered to loosen stools or remove feces and flatus. The nursing assistant should follow the specific directions for each type of enema given.

- Patients with a colostomy or an ileostomy may need assistance with emptying or changing the appliance.

- Nursing assistants are responsible for collecting urine samples, for some urine testing, and for straining urine for stones.

- Nursing assistants are responsible for collecting and testing some stool samples.

- Sputum samples are best collected first thing in the morning and require the patient to cough up sputum.

VOCABULARY REVIEW

Directions: Match the letter of each definition in the second column with the correct vocabulary term in the first column. Write your answers on a separate sheet of paper.

Vocabulary
1. abdominal distension
2. catheter
3. colostomy
4. constipation
5. defecation
6. diarrhea
7. enema
8. fecal impaction
9. flatulence
10. hemorrhoids
11. ileostomy
12. rectal tube
13. sputum
14. stoma
15. suppository

Definitions
A. Difficulty in fecal elimination
B. A liquid solution placed into the rectum to loosen stools and to remove feces
C. Semisolid medication or lubricating agent that is inserted into the rectum for absorption by the body
D. A tube inserted into the rectum to relieve flatulence and abdominal distension
E. An artificial opening from the colon to the abdominal wall
F. A collection of hardened feces in the intestines
G. Distended veins surrounding the rectum
H. The passage of frequent watery stools
I. An artificial opening in the body created by surgery
J. Abnormal swelling of the abdomen
K. The mucous secretion from the lungs, bronchi, and trachea
L. An artificial opening between the small intestine and the abdominal wall
M. A tube used to drain fluid into or out of the body
N. The excessive creation and buildup of gas in the stomach and intestines
O. The passing of feces from the body

Check Your Knowledge

Review Questions: Answer each of the following questions on a separate sheet of paper.

1. List five factors that contribute to problems with elimination.

2. When would it be appropriate for a patient to use a commode?

3. What is a fracture pan?

4. What is the goal of bladder and bowel retraining programs?

5. What is an indwelling catheter?

6. Why might a patient be given a suppository?

7. What should you do if the patient experiences abdominal cramping while you are administering an enema?

8. Explain the purpose of a fecal occult blood test.

9. When is the best time to collect a sputum sample?

10. What signs and symptoms indicate that a patient's upper airway may need suctioning?

True or False: Read each statement carefully. Then write *True* or *False* by the statement number on a separate sheet of paper.

1. The frequency of urination may depend upon the amount of fluid ingested.

2. Observation of the color of a patient's stool is not a responsibility of the nursing assistant.

3. A patient who cannot raise the hips high enough to sit on a fracture pan should be provided with a regular bedpan.

4. When assisting a patient with bladder training, offer the toilet, commode, bedpan, or urinal every two hours to start voiding.

5. It is not important to wash the genitals prior to applying a new condom catheter.

Think and Decide

Directions: Think about each of the following scenarios. Answer each question on a separate sheet of paper.

1. Latoia is a 66-year-old female patient in your care at the long-term care facility. Her doctor has ordered an indwelling catheter. When you bathe this patient in the future, what are your responsibilities in addition to the basic bath and perineal care?

2. You arrive at the home of an elderly couple, the Andersons. Mr. Anderson is lying in bed with a condom catheter in place. When you walk over to inspect the urine output, you notice that the catheter has disconnected from the tubing. The patient and his bed are wet with urine. Mrs. Anderson is visibly upset about it and is crying softly. What should you do?

3. A 24-hour urine sample has been ordered for B.N., a patient on the surgical floor. The nurse hands you the container and a basin of ice and tells you to begin the collection. When you ask B.N. to urinate so that you can begin the collection, she tells you that she has just urinated and can't produce any more right now. What should you do?

4. R.U. is a patient who has had a colostomy for 10 years. He tells you that the appliance he has does not fit properly. His skin has become very irritated. What action should you take?

5. G.S., a patient with a large amount of secretions in his mouth, suddenly experiences difficulty breathing. You hear moist gurgling when he breathes, and you notice that he has become restless. Aside from keeping him calm, should you take any other action?

6. Brent is a 46-year-old patient on the surgical floor. He had major abdominal surgery a few days ago. He complains to you that he is in pain because he "has gas." You observe that his abdomen is severely extended. What should you do?

7. Mrs. R. is 83 years old. She has been a resident at the long-term care facility for several months. Her physician orders a few basic tests to be performed once a month, including a routine urine test. One morning, as you are collecting the routine urine sample, you notice a distinct pinkish tinge to the urine. What should you do?

8. You are providing colostomy care to C.V., a long-term resident in your care. When you disconnect the appliance, you notice that the skin around the stoma is red and inflamed. What should you do?

CNA Certification Exam Prep

Directions: This practice test contains ten questions. Each question has four suggested answers. For each question, choose the ONE that best answers the question or completes the statement. Write your answers on a separate sheet of paper.

1. A patient that cannot control his or her bladder has
   A. urinary retention.
   B. urinary incontinence.
   C. anal retention.
   D. anal incontinence.

2. Which of the following is a factor that may cause constipation?
   A. elevated cholesterol
   B. excessive exercise
   C. poor diet
   D. flatus buildup

3. A patient who has distended veins in the rectum has
   A. fecal impaction.
   B. flatus.
   C. hemorrhoids.
   D. anal incontinence.

4. Lubricating suppositories are given to relieve
   A. constipation.
   B. diarrhea.
   C. fecal impaction.
   D. urinary retention.

5. Excessive or frequent urination is known as
   A. nocturia.
   B. hematuria.
   C. dysuria.
   D. polyuria.

6. The type of incontinence in which a patient feels a sudden urge to urinate but cannot get to the toilet in time is
   A. stress incontinence.
   B. reflex incontinence.
   C. urge incontinence.
   D. overflow incontinence.

7. The transparent container in which urine and other fluids can be measured is a
   A. graduate.
   B. syringe.
   C. collection cup.
   D. catheter.

8. Another common term for an indwelling catheter is
   A. intermittent catheter.
   B. condom catheter.
   C. Texas® catheter.
   D. Foley catheter.

9. An enema used to soften feces for relief of constipation and fecal impaction is a(n)
   A. cleansing enema.
   B. oil-retention enema.
   C. soapsuds enema.
   D. saline enema.

10. Feces from an ileostomy are most likely to be
    A. liquid feces.
    B. semisolid feces.
    C. fully formed feces.
    D. a mixture of liquid and formed feces.

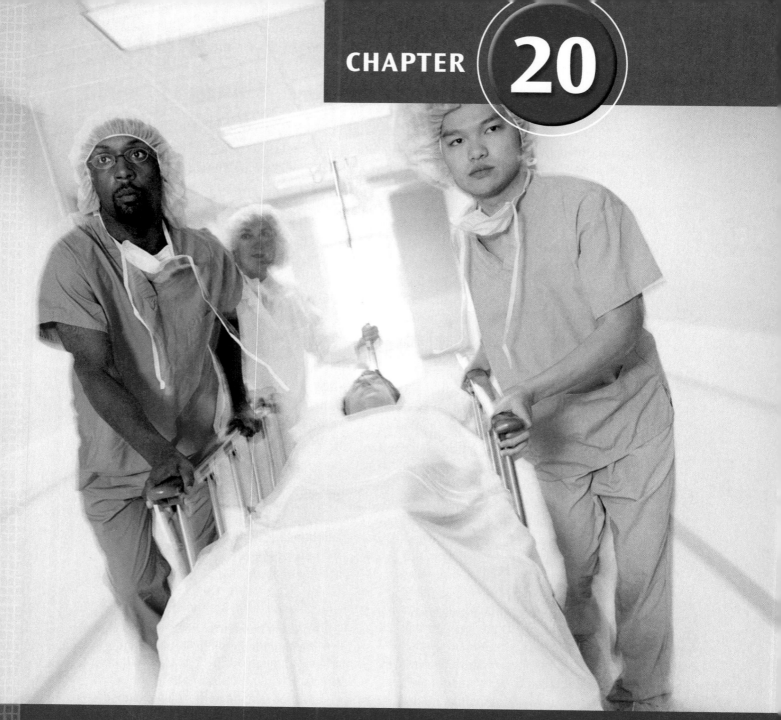

CHAPTER 20

OBJECTIVES

- Explain the importance of educating patients about surgery.
- List the nursing assistant's tasks in preparing patients for surgery.
- Demonstrate how to prep a patient's skin for surgery.

- Explain how to prepare a patient's postoperative room.
- Identify the effects of the primary types of anesthesia used for surgery.
- Describe the general care the nursing assistant provides to postoperative patients.

- Demonstrate how to assist the patient with respiratory and circulatory functions after surgery.
- Identify ways in which nursing assistants help ambulatory surgery patients.

Caring for the Surgical Patient

VOCABULARY

ambulatory surgery Surgery that does not require a hospital stay.

anesthesia The loss of sensation or the ability to feel pain.

anesthetic A drug or an agent given to patients to produce a loss of sensation.

atelectasis The collapse of a lung or part of a lung; one of the possible complications of surgery.

embolism An obstruction in a blood vessel caused by an embolus.

embolus A blood clot or other matter that has broken away and travels through the bloodstream.

incentive spirometer A device used to promote and measure maximum effort of deep breathing to prevent atelectasis.

intermittent pneumatic compression device A device that is wrapped around the legs and connected to a pump that inflates and deflates to promote circulation and help prevent blood clots.

postoperative period The time after surgery that begins when the patient is transported from the operating room to the recovery room.

preoperative period The time when the patient is admitted to the hospital until the patient goes to surgery.

surgery The use of manual procedures to diagnose and treat diseases, injuries, or deformities.

thrombus A blood clot that stays at the site where it formed.

Caring for the Preoperative Patient

Surgery is the use of manual procedures to diagnose and treat diseases, injuries, or deformities. Surgery is also called an *operation*. Some patients have elective surgery—surgery that it is optional and scheduled in advance. Cosmetic surgeries and surgeries to relieve pain and discomfort are usually considered elective. Other patients come to the emergency room because of sudden illness or accident and need emergency surgery to save their lives. Most "general" surgeries, however, are planned and are medically necessary.

All surgical patients need to be physically prepared, or prepped, for the procedure. Some will be fearful and may need help handling their fears and concerns. The **preoperative period** is the time when the patient is admitted to the hospital or surgical center until the patient goes to surgery. During this period, the health care team prepares patients physically, spiritually, and psychologically.

Educating the Patient

The nurse or doctor is responsible for educating the patient about the surgery, including each step of the surgical experience, so the patient understands the process. **See Figure 20-1.** The patient has a right to understand what will happen. Explanations also help lessen the patient's fears. The nurse or doctor provides the following information before the surgery:

- A detailed explanation of the surgical procedure, including risks and possible complications
- When the surgery will take place and approximately how long it will take
- Preoperative tests, procedures, and medications
- Skin preparation
- An explanation of "nothing by mouth" (NPO) before surgery

Vital Skills READING

Identifying Confusing Parts

As you read, you may come across ideas in the text that are confusing to you. Try to identify these confusing parts as you encounter them. You can keep track of them by making a list. On a separate piece of paper, write down the page number and a few words to remind yourself of what and where the confusing text is.

For example, while reading this chapter, you might be confused about the different devices and ways to assist with circulation. On a separate sheet of paper, you can write a note such as "Page 508, circulation." Also note any specific questions you have. For instance, "Which patients might need help with circulation?"

As you continue reading, your confusion might be cleared up, and your questions answered. If not, go back and re-read the confusing sections to try to understand the information or discuss the sections with another student or the instructor.

Practice

As you read this chapter, list the confusing parts of the text and any questions you might have. Break into groups of three or four students. See if you and your classmates can clear up the confusion and answer each other's questions about what you have read.

- What happens the morning of surgery
- What type of anesthesia will be administered
- What to expect after arriving in the operating room
- The routine of the recovery room
- Catheters, IVs, and other equipment that may be used before and after surgery
- How much pain to expect and what type of medication will be available after surgery
- How to perform postoperative exercises, such as deep breathing and leg exercises
- A recovery plan

Patients must give their consent for a surgical procedure to be performed. The doctor or nurse fully explains the surgical procedures to the patient and family members. After the patient's questions are answered, the doctor or nurse asks the patient to sign a surgical consent form. **See Figure 20-2.** No surgical procedures can be performed without this signed form. A parent or guardian signs the surgical consent form when the patient is a minor.

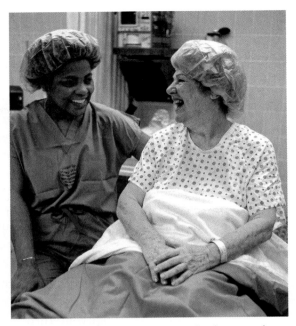

O Figure 20-1. Before any operation, the doctor or the nurse explains the surgical procedure to the patient.

Townsend General Hospital
Acknowledgement of Informed Consent

1. My physician, _____, has explained my medical condition to my satisfaction.
2. All of my questions concerning this procedure have been answered.
3. I understand that, during the procedure, additional or different procedures may be required due to unforeseen circumstances. I request that my physician perform those procedures as necessary in his or her professional judgment.
4. I agree to observation by medical students and other health care professionals in training during my procedure for the purpose of advancing their medical education.
5. I understand that any tissue removed from my body will be examined and then disposed of properly by hospital personnel.
6. I certify that I have had nothing to eat or drink, including water, since _____ AM / PM.

I further agree to the following: (Check all that apply.)
   ❑ Administration of anesthesia or intravenous sedation
   ❑ Administration of intravenous therapy
   ❑ Administration of blood products, chemotherapy, or antibiotics, as ordered by my physician
   ❑ Photography or videotaping during the procedure for the purpose of advancing medical education
   ❑ I have been given patient information sheets on _____ and have had my questions answered.

Proposed Medical Procedure: _____
_____
_____

_____   _____   _____   _____
Patient Signature   Date   Signature Witnessed By   Date

_____   _____
Signature of Legal Guardian   Date

O Figure 20-2. The patient must sign a consent form before surgery can take place.

Easing the Patient's Fears

A patient who comes to the hospital for surgery may have many fears and concerns. Emotional responses to surgery depend on past experience. Has the patient had surgery before? Does the patient have a friend who underwent the same surgery successfully? Did someone close to the patient die during surgery? You can answer general questions about surgery and be supportive emotionally, but you must direct all specific questions to the patient's nurse or surgeon.

Patients deal with fear in different ways. Some may cry or talk constantly. Others may sulk or be withdrawn. Some patients may be unusually cheerful, covering up their fear. Patients may experience fear of:
- Death, complications, disfigurement, or pain.
- The surgery's outcome or of confirming a diagnosis, such as cancer.
- Being "under the knife."
- Needles, tubes, and medical equipment.

Patients have concerns about who will take care of their homes, finances, spouse, children, pets, and work while they are in the hospital. Many patients are concerned about the costs of surgery and recuperation. These are normal and valid concerns. You can help the preoperative patient in the following ways:
- Listen to the patient.
- Explain procedures before you perform them.
- Use verbal and nonverbal communication skills. A gentle hand on the shoulder shows that you care.
- Attend to the patient's needs efficiently and gently.
- Let the nurse know if the patient has questions about the surgery.
- Report the patient's fear and anxiety to the nurse.
- Report the patient's request to see a member of the clergy or to visit the hospital's chapel.
- Reassure the patient that he or she will not be alone; someone will be there at all times.

General Physical Preparation

The nursing assistant is often asked to physically prepare the patient for surgery. These tasks include the personal care you would provide to any patient. You may be asked to:
- Help admit the patient to the preoperative nursing unit.
- Introduce the patient to the environment, including the call signal.
- Ask if the patient has a latex allergy.
- Measure and record the patient's vital signs.
- Collect a urine specimen.
- Measure the patient's height and weight. The amount of anesthetic a patient receives is determined by the patient's weight.
- Assist the patient in bathing and oral hygiene. *Note:* NPO patients must not swallow any water.
- Provide catheter care if necessary.
- Administer rectal treatments, such as an enema, if the doctor has ordered one.
- Make the patient comfortable so he or she can rest.
- Wash and shave the surgical area.
- Prepare the patient to be transported to surgery.

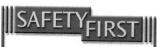

Hospitals and operating rooms contain latex equipment and products, such as gloves, drapes, IV tubing, catheters, drains, and tubes. Most surgical areas screen all patients to learn whether they are at risk for latex allergies.

A preoperative checklist is part of the patient's medical record. **See Figure 20-3.** You may be asked to perform some of the tasks on the checklist under the supervision of the nurse, who then makes sure the list is complete. After completing a task, you will initial the checklist to indicate the task is complete. In this way, the facility staff makes sure that the patient is properly prepared for surgery.

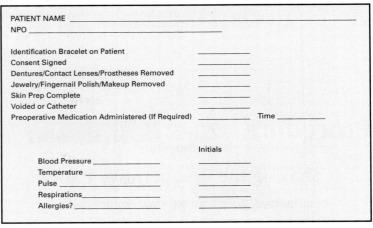

○ **Figure 20-3. The nurse is responsible for making sure the preoperative checklist is complete. The nursing assistant may be asked to perform some of the tasks on the list.**

Prepping the Skin

Preparing the patient's surgical site is an important part of preoperative care. The skin around the site must be thoroughly cleaned and shaved. Skin and hair carry microorganisms that can enter the incision if not removed. Infections can result. They are a serious complication of surgery.

The process of cleaning and shaving the surgical site is called "skin prep" or "shave prep." In most hospitals, the skin prep is performed the night before or the morning of surgery. Some surgeons prefer to supervise the skin prep, which is then performed in the operating room just before surgery. If the skin prep is performed in the patient's room, you may be asked to clean and shave the patient. The nurse will tell you which area to clean and shave. The area is determined by the type of surgery and what the doctor has ordered. **See Figure 20-4.**

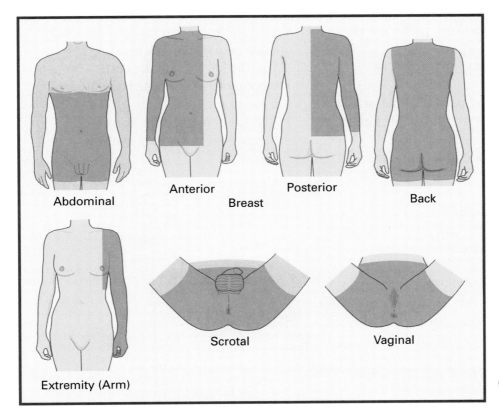

Abdominal

Anterior Breast

Posterior

Back

Extremity (Arm)

Scrotal

Vaginal

○ **Figure 20-4. Skin preparation sites for surgery.**

Some facilities use a prepackaged prep kit, which includes a disposable razor, sponge with soap, wash basin, drape, and towel. If your facility does not use kits, you will need to assemble your equipment.

Procedure 20-1

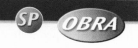

Shaving the Preoperative Patient

Equipment: bath blanket • waterproof pad • disposable prep kit • warm water • towel • disposable gloves • bath thermometer

1. Find out from the nurse the exact area you are to prep.
2. Identify the patient, check the ID bracelet, and introduce yourself. Call the patient by name.
3. Explain the procedure to the patient. The patient may want to know exactly what area you will be shaving.
4. Provide privacy.
5. Wash your hands.
6. Make sure the lighting is adequate.
7. Raise the bed to the highest level.
8. Place the bath blanket over the patient and then fanfold the top linens to the foot of the bed.
9. Position the patient so the area to be shaved is in reach.
10. Place the waterproof pad under the patient.
11. Open the prep kit. Place the supplies on the overbed table.
12. Drape the patient with the disposable drape.
13. Put on gloves.
14. Dip the sponge in water that is from 105° to 110° F (41° to 43° C). Apply soap to the skin with the sponge and work up a good lather.
15. Hold the skin taut.
16. Shave in the direction the hair grows. Hold the razor at a 45° angle. Use short strokes, rinsing the razor often. Shave very carefully so you do not nick or cut the skin. **See Figure 20-5.**
17. Wash the area with fresh soap and water. Pat dry.

18. Make sure the area is free from any hair growth.
19. Remove the drape and waterproof pad.
20. Remove your gloves.
21. Cover the patient with the bed linens and remove the bath blanket.
22. Lower the bed.
23. Make the patient comfortable and place the signal cord within reach.
24. Discard the used equipment. Place soiled linen in the hamper.
25. Open the screen.
26. Wash your hands.
27. Record on the preoperative checklist that the skin prep was completed.
28. Report the following to the nurse:
   • Procedure was completed and the area prepped
   • Any cuts or nicks on the skin
   • Observation of anything unusual

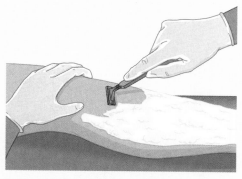

○ **Figure 20-5.** When prepping the skin, shave in the direction the hair grows and use short strokes. Hold the razor at a 45° angle.

Transporting the Patient to Surgery

You may be asked to transport the patient to the operating room. When the operating room staff calls to tell you they are ready for the patient, push the stretcher into the patient's room and raise the bed to the highest level. You may need help transferring the patient to the stretcher, especially if the patient has been medicated. Make sure other coworkers are available. Family members may accompany the patient, depending on facility policy. (See Chapter 16 for more information about safely transferring and transporting patients by stretcher.) Follow these guidelines:

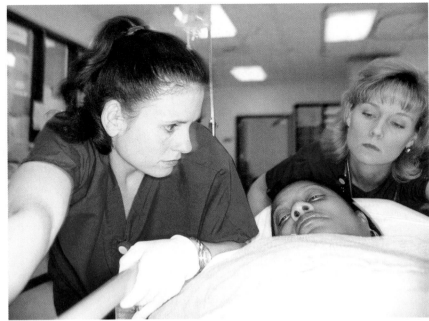

○ **Figure 20-6.** Walk slowly when transporting a patient on a stretcher to surgery.

- Transfer the patient to the stretcher.
- Secure the patient with the straps and raise the side rails.
- Cover the patient with a blanket for warmth.
- Take the patient's medical record with you if required.
- When pushing the stretcher to the surgical area, stand by the patient's head.
- Push the stretcher, feet first, slowly and carefully. **See Figure 20-6.**
- Speak gently to the patient if he or she is still awake. Be reassuring and comforting, since this is a stressful time for the patient.

When you arrive at the operating room waiting area, an attendant will take the patient from you. At this time, you can direct family members to a comfortable waiting area. Explain to them where the patient will be after surgery and about how long it will be until they can see the patient again.

Preparing the Patient's Room

Some patients will return to the same room after surgery. However, some may be sent to an intensive care unit or a coronary care unit until they have recuperated enough to return to a regular patient room.

The postoperative room must be prepared as soon as the patient is transported to the operating room. The nursing assistant prepares the room. The nurse will tell you what special supplies and equipment you need. Prepare the room as follows:

- Change the linens and fanfold the clean linens to one side so the patient can be quickly transferred from the stretcher and covered.
- Place an IV pole against the wall near the bed.
- Raise the bed to the highest level. Leave the side rails down if applicable.
- Move furniture and the overbed table to make room so the stretcher can be wheeled into the room and against the bed.
- Place the following supplies in the room: thermometer, stethoscope, sphygmomanometer, pulse oximeter, emesis basin, tissues, waterproof bed protector, vital signs flow sheet, and intake/output sheet.

Vital Skills COMMUNICATION

Taking Telephone Messages

On surgical floors, nursing assistants are often responsible for answering the telephone and taking messages. Try to answer the phone by the second or third ring. Speak in a clear voice directly into the mouthpiece. Do not eat or chew gum while you are answering the phone. Your employer may have a specific telephone answering protocol for you to follow. Generally, identify yourself by giving your name, title, and the area in which you are working. For example, you might say "Hello, Marie Smith, nursing assistant, fourth floor. May I help you?"

If the person with whom the caller would like to speak is not available, take a message. Every message should include:

- The name of the caller.
- The time of the call.
- The nature of the call.
- Whether the caller expects a return phone call.
- The caller's phone number.

Remember to be polite. If you can't answer the caller's questions, reassure the caller that someone will get back to him or her. Before hanging up, ask the caller if there is anything more you can do to help. Thank the person for calling, and say goodbye.

Practice

With a partner, take turns role-playing the following scenarios.
1. A doctor calls, looking for a nurse who just went to lunch.
2. An irate family member calls, demanding to speak with the doctor taking care of his wife. The doctor is in but doesn't want to be disturbed.
3. A coworker calls and wants you to check her schedule, which is posted in the break room. You are busy with a patient at the moment.

Caring for the Postoperative Patient

The **postoperative period** is the time after surgery that begins when the patient is transported from the operating room to the recovery room. In the recovery room, nurses monitor the patient until all vital signs are stable and the effects of anesthesia begin to wear off. The recovery room staff helps to orient the patient by asking the patient his or her name and the day of the week, and to wiggle the toes or squeeze the nurse's hand. The patient's responses tell the staff whether the patient can hear, understand, and follow easy commands.

The patient usually remains in the recovery room until vital signs are stable and the patient is fairly alert. When the patient is ready to go to the postoperative room, the recovery room nurse calls the nursing unit to say the patient is on the way. A recovery room nurse accompanies the patient to the nursing unit.

The postoperative care you give begins when the patient returns to the nursing unit. You may be asked to help transfer the patient from the stretcher to the bed. The bed is lowered and the side rails are raised. Provide extra blankets if the patient is cold. **See Figure 20-7.**

The Effects of Anesthesia

Anesthesia is the loss of sensation or the ability to feel pain. An **anesthetic** is a drug or an agent given to patients to produce this loss of sensation. It also prevents pain and induces forgetfulness and unconsciousness during surgery. Anesthetics are administered by licensed doctors called *anesthesiologists* or by *nurse anesthetists*. They are nurses who have had extensive special training and who are licensed to administer anesthetics under the supervision of an anesthesiologist.

There are three primary types of anesthesia used during surgery: general, spinal, and local. The patient's condition during the postoperative period can depend on which type of anesthesia was induced.

General Anesthesia. The patient is put under general anesthesia for lengthy or complicated surgery. A general anesthetic puts the patient to sleep and causes loss of sensation throughout the entire body. General anesthesia is administered by an IV or in a gas the patient breathes.

After general anesthesia, patients are very sleepy. They can answer questions but usually keep their eyes closed. Some patients feel nauseated and vomit during the first few hours after surgery. Within 24 hours, they become more alert.

Spinal Anesthesia. This type of anesthesia is used for male genital surgery, back surgery, and for some women in labor. A spinal anesthetic is injected into the spinal canal to create a loss of sensation from the injection point to the toes. The "spinal" blocks nerve impulses from the spinal cord to the brain. The brain does not register the feeling of pain.

The patient with a spinal remains awake and alert, although the lower extremities are numb. Patients who have received a spinal must remain supine until it wears off. The patient is alert, however, and is able to eat and drink.

Local Anesthesia. This type of anesthesia is induced to suture wounds and to perform biopsies and minor surgeries. A local anesthetic is injected directly into the surgical site to block sensation in that area. The patient remains awake during the procedure, though the doctor may give a mild sedative, a calming medication, to help the patient relax.

A local anesthetic wears off within two to three hours after surgery. The patient may begin to feel pain and request pain medication. Patients are alert after local anesthesia. A patient who also has received a mild sedative may not become alert for an hour or so.

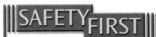

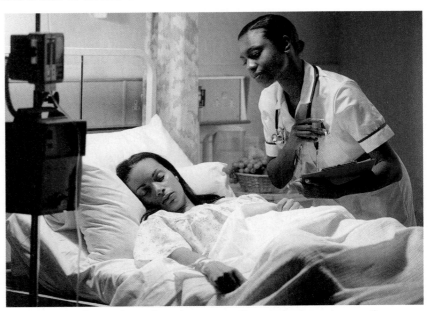

○ **Figure 20-7.** The nursing assistant's postoperative care begins as soon as the patient returns to the nursing unit.

Providing General Care

The nurse is responsible for the initial patient assessment, including taking vital signs and checking dressings, tubes, catheters, IVs, and drainage from wounds. The family is allowed into the room after the patient is made comfortable. After the nurse's initial assessment, you may be asked to provide the following ongoing patient care:

- Taking vital signs every 15 minutes for the first hour
- Taking vital signs every hour thereafter or based on the nurse's orders
- Assisting the patient with elimination needs, including recording the first voiding after surgery
- Providing liquids when permitted. The patient may be NPO or be allowed only crushed ice for several hours.
- Helping the patient eat
- Bathing the patient
- Providing skin care
- Checking catheter drainage
- Checking wound drainage
- Helping the patient with deep-breathing and coughing exercises
- Repositioning the patient every 2 hours
- Assisting the patient with leg exercises

Observing the Patient. A patient must be carefully observed after surgery. If you observe any of the following signs or symptoms, immediately report them to the nurse:

- A change in blood pressure or in pulse rate, or a weak or irregular pulse
- Labored or rapid respirations
- A change in body temperature
- Pale or cyanotic skin, lips, or fingernails
- Cold, moist, pale, or clammy skin
- Restlessness
- A change in the IV flow rate
- Increased drainage or bleeding from the wound
- Excessive thirst or pain
- Nausea, vomiting, or choking
- Any other sudden change

Psychological Needs. The postoperative patient has different psychological needs from the preoperative patient. Patients may be relieved that surgery is over, but they may be anxious about their limitations and disabilities. For example, someone who has had a limb amputated will understandably be concerned about how to perform daily activities. The patient may also have self-image problems and become depressed.

You can help your patients by being supportive and understanding. Some patients have long and slow recuperations. They need a great deal of encouragement. Always listen to your patients' concerns. Report their concerns and anxieties to the nurse.

Positioning and Turning the Patient

Postoperative patients need to change position at least every 2 hours to:
- Promote comfort.
- Prevent respiratory and circulatory complications.
- Prevent pressure sores.

The nurse will tell you how to position the patient and how often to reposition. Postoperative patients are usually positioned on their sides. When repositioned, they are turned to the other side. You must move patients slowly and carefully. Use a logrolling technique to protect the incision site and to maintain patient comfort. When positioning the patient, do not put any stress or strain on the incision. You can provide support with pillows. **See Figure 20-8.**

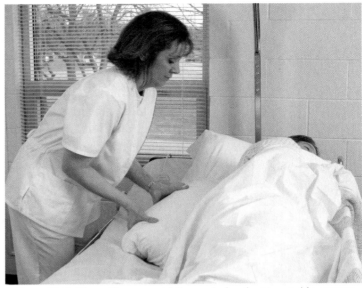

○ **Figure 20-8.** Place pillows around the surgical patient to provide support.

A turning schedule is kept to show at what times a patient should be turned. This ensures that the health care team is consistent and provides the best care for the patient.

Procedure 20-2

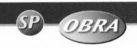

Positioning the Postoperative Patient

Equipment: pillows

1. Identify the patient, check the ID bracelet, and introduce yourself. Call the patient by name.
2. Explain that you are going to help change the patient's position.
3. Provide privacy.
4. Wash your hands.
5. Raise the bed to the highest level.
6. Go to one side of the patient's bed. Your helper should stand on the other side.
7. Remove the existing supporting pillows.
8. The patient can hold a pillow over the incision for support if able.
9. Lower the side rails if applicable.
10. Both you and your helper should place one hand near the patient's shoulder and the other hand on the buttocks. **See Figure 20-9.**
11. Gently roll the patient onto the back.
12. Place your hands on the shoulders and buttocks or hips.

13. Gently roll the patient onto the other side.
14. Provide support with extra pillows.
15. Lower the bed.
16. Make the patient comfortable and place the signal cord within reach.
17. Wash your hands.
18. Open the screen.
19. Report your observations to the nurse.

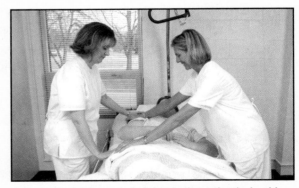

○ **Figure 20-9.** Place one hand near the patient's shoulder and the other hand on the buttocks to roll the patient onto the back.

Respiratory Care

Respiratory complications can result after surgery. One complication is pneumonia, an infection in the lung. Another complication is **atelectasis**, the collapse of a lung or part of a lung. Deep breathing and coughing help prevent these complications by:

- Expanding the lungs.
- Preventing buildup of lung secretions.
- Helping remove mucus from the lungs.

The nurse explains to the patient how important these exercises are. The nursing assistant is often asked to help patients perform deep-breathing and coughing exercises. The nurse will tell you how often the exercises should be performed and how many repetitions of each exercise the patient requires. You then teach the patient how to perform the exercise.

Coughing and deep breathing may be painful, especially if a patient has had abdominal or chest surgery. The patient is also tired, making the idea of any kind of exercise unpleasant. The patient may be afraid of opening up the incision. If the patient is taking pain medication, the exercises can be done after the medication takes effect. You can help by reassuring and encouraging the patient and by providing positive feedback.

Procedure 20-3

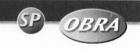

Assisting the Patient with Deep-Breathing and Coughing Exercises

Equipment: pillow • disposable gloves • tissues

1. Identify the patient and introduce yourself. Call the patient by name.
2. Explain to the patient that you are going to help with deep-breathing and coughing exercises.
3. Provide privacy.
4. Wash your hands.
5. Help the patient into a semi-Fowler's position.
6. A patient who has had abdominal surgery can hold a pillow over the abdomen to splint (protect) the incision and to provide support.
7. Put on your gloves.
8. Ask the patient to place his or her hands on the sides of the rib cage or over the incision site.
9. Ask the patient to take a slow, deep breath and hold it for 3 to 5 seconds, then slowly exhale through pursed lips. **See Figure 20-10.**

10. Repeat the exercise until the patient reaches the number the nurse specified. Report to the nurse if the patient is too exhausted to complete the specified number.

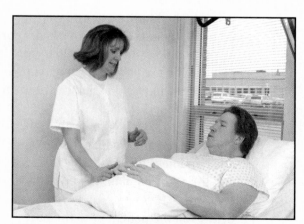

○ Figure 20-10. Coach the patient to exhale slowly through pursed lips.

11. Help the patient cough. Ask the patient to interlace the fingers over the incision, or to hold a pillow against the incision.
12. Ask the patient to take a deep breath and cough forcefully 2 times.
13. Pass the patient tissues if any secretions come up with the coughs.
14. Help the patient into a new, comfortable position.
15. Make the patient comfortable and place the signal cord within reach.
16. Discard used tissues according to facility policy. Store the pillow for next use.
17. Open the screen.
18. Remove your gloves.
19. Wash your hands.
20. Report the following to the nurse:
    - The number of times the patient performed each exercise
    - How the patient tolerated the procedure
    - Type and amount of sputum coughed up

An **incentive spirometer** is a device used to promote and measure maximum effort of deep breathing to prevent atelectasis. The physician orders the use of the device. The nurse or a respiratory therapist will teach the patient how to use it. The patient is usually encouraged to use the incentive spirometer at regular intervals, such as every 1 to 2 hours while awake. The nurse will determine how often the patient should use the device. The nursing assistant may help the patient use the device if directed by the nurse.

Procedure 20-4

Assisting the Patient with an Incentive Spirometer

Equipment: incentive spirometer

1. Identify the patient, check the ID bracelet, and introduce yourself. Call the patient by name.
2. Explain that you are going to help the patient use the incentive spirometer.
3. Provide privacy.
4. Wash your hands.
5. Help the patient to a semi-Fowler's or high-Fowler's position.
6. Instruct the patient to seal the lips tightly around the mouthpiece.
7. Instruct the patient to breathe in slowly and as deeply as possible to achieve the pre-set goal mark. (The nurse or respiratory therapist usually tests the patient and adjusts the goal as needed.) **See Figure 20-11.**
8. Tell the patient to hold the breath as long as possible (at least 2 to 3 seconds) and then to exhale slowly.
9. Encourage the patient to breathe normally and rest for a few seconds. Repeat Steps 6 through 10 as many times as instructed by the nurse.
10. After the patient completes these exercises, encourage the patient to practice coughing as described in Procedure 20-3.

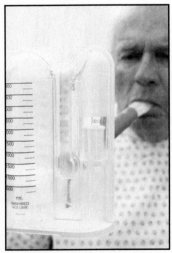

○ **Figure 20-11. A patient using an incentive spirometer.**

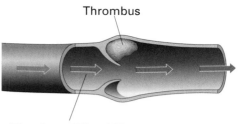

Thrombus

Direction of Blood Flow

○ **Figure 20-12. A thrombus is a stationary blood clot that forms in a vein.**

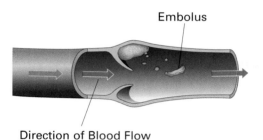

Embolus

Direction of Blood Flow

○ **Figure 20-13. An embolus is a thrombus that has broken away from the wall of the vein and moves through the circulatory system.**

Postoperative patients with increased respiratory secretions from pneumonia, cystic fibrosis, or atelectasis may need additional therapy. *Vibropercussion* is the delivery of vibrations and tapping to the exterior chest wall to loosen respiratory secretions. The vibrations are delivered with a vibrating device. The percussion is delivered with the hands. This technique is usually done by a respiratory therapist or a skilled nurse trained in this procedure. The nursing assistant helps by repositioning the patient and providing physical and psychological support during the procedure.

Assisting Circulation

Blood clots in the veins are a potential complication of surgery. A blood clot is also called a **thrombus** (plural: *thrombi*). **See Figure 20-12.** A thrombus has the potential to decrease circulation through the vein. It may also break away and travel through the bloodstream as an **embolus. See Figure 20-13.** An **embolism** is an obstruction in a blood vessel caused by an embolus.

Improved circulation helps prevent blood clots. A doctor may order a patient to wear antiembolic stockings after surgery. These stockings support the leg veins and encourage blood flow back to the heart. (Chapter 18 discusses antiembolic stockings).

The **intermittent pneumatic compression device** also improves circulation and helps prevent blood clots. This device is wrapped around the legs and connected to a pump that inflates and deflates. The constant compression prevents blood clots from forming. **See Figure 20-14.** Antiembolic stockings are typically worn underneath the device to improve its effectiveness. You may be asked to remove the intermittent pneumatic compression device when the patient gets up to use the bathroom or sit in a chair. Always check with the nurse before removing or replacing the device.

Leg exercises also stimulate circulation by increasing the flow of blood back to the heart. They are easy to perform, though you may need to help a weak patient. The exercises are usually performed every 2 hours. Each exercise is repeated 3 to 5 times.

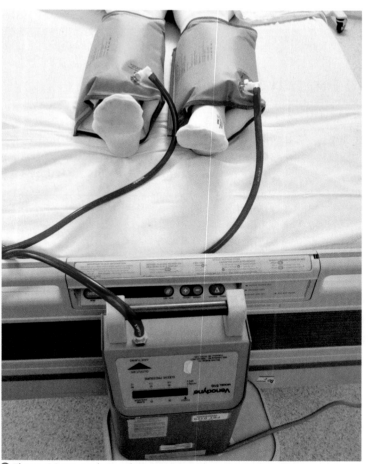

○ **Figure 20-14. An intermittent pneumatic compression device wraps around a patient's legs to prevent blood clots after surgery.**

Procedure 20-5

Helping the Patient Perform Leg Exercises

Equipment: bath blanket

1. Identify the patient, check the ID bracelet, and introduce yourself. Call the patient by name.
2. Explain that you are going to help the patient perform leg exercises.
3. Provide privacy.
4. Wash your hands.
5. Raise the bed to a comfortable working height.
6. Cover the patient's abdomen with a bath blanket and fanfold the top linens to the foot of the bed.
7. Help the patient to lie on the back, with the head supported with a pillow.

8. Instruct the patient to hold a pillow over the incision site to splint it.
9. Instruct the patient to do the following exercises. A weak patient may need your help. The patient should perform each exercise 3 to 5 repetitions.
10. Rotate each ankle in circular movements. **See Figure 20-15.**
11. Flex the toes up toward the knee, then point each foot. **See Figure 20-16.**
12. Bend and extend each knee. **See Figure 20-17.**

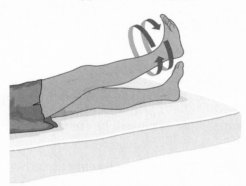

○ **Figure 20-15.** Rotate each ankle the specified number of times in each direction.

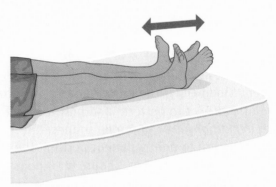

○ **Figure 20-16.** Flexing the toes up toward the knees and then pointing (extending) the toes.

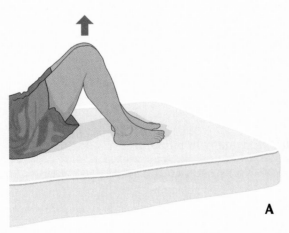

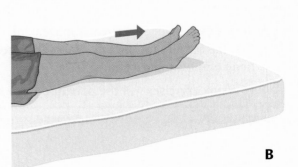

A

B

○ **Figure 20-17.** (A) Bending (flexing) and (B) extending the knees.

13. Bend each leg from the hip.
    See Figure 20-18.
14. Cover the patient and remove the bath blanket.
15. Lower the bed.
16. Make the patient comfortable and place the signal cord within reach.
17. Wash your hands.
18. Report the following to the nurse:
    - The number of completed repetitions of each exercise
    - How the patient tolerated the procedure

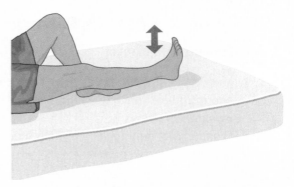

○ **Figure 20-18.** Raise each leg straight up, bending the leg at the hip. *Note:* Some physicians may order the legs to be moved laterally (toward the side of the bed) instead of straight up.

Vital Skills MATH

Calculating Exercise Repetitions

Leg exercises stimulate circulation and help prevent blood clots. The nurse will tell you what kind of exercises to perform and how many of each (*repetitions*). For example, suppose the nurse tells you to help a patient perform the following leg exercises every 2 hours for 8 hours:

- Rotate each ankle in a circular movement.
- Flex the toes up towards the knee; then point each foot.

- Bend and extend each knee.
- Bend and extend each hip.

Each type of exercise is to be repeated 5 times. How many exercises will be completed in 2 hours? How many will be completed in 8 hours?

4 types of exercises × 5 repetitions each = 4 × 5 = 20 exercises

4 sets of exercises (1 set every 2 hours) × 20 exercises = 80 exercises

Practice

The nurse has asked you to help a patient perform the following exercises once every hour for 6 hours. Each type of exercise is to be repeated 6 times.

- Rotate each ankle in a circular movement.
- Flex the toes up towards the knee; then point each foot.
- Bend and extend each knee.

How many exercises will the patient do in 1 hour? How many in 6 hours?

Vital Skills (WRITING)

Brainstorming Essay Topics

Sometimes even the best writers have trouble coming up with new ideas. One technique for generating ideas is *brainstorming*. When you brainstorm, you try to generate a lot of ideas in a short period of time. Don't edit yourself when you brainstorm—just let your ideas flow and list them. You can sort the good ideas from the not-so-good ideas later.

There are many methods for brainstorming. In the "ABC" method, you try to think of an idea or word for every letter of the alphabet. For example, if you were brainstorming about body parts using the ABC method, you might come up with *ankle, brain, colon, duodenum,* and so on. If you get stuck on a letter, skip it and try to come back to it later.

Practice

Write a five-paragraph essay about the nursing assistant's role in caring for a specific surgical patient. Follow the patient from preoperative prep through discharge. Brainstorm ideas you might include in your essay.

Ambulatory Surgery

Ambulatory surgery is surgery that does not require a hospital stay. It is also called *outpatient* or *same-day surgery*. Minor surgeries and some major surgeries are done as ambulatory surgery. Patients are admitted to the facility for surgery and go home the same day. Some ambulatory surgery centers are located within hospitals. Some are in separate facilities. This type of surgery eliminates costly hospital stays and allows patients to recover at home, sometimes with the help of a home health care aide.

Nursing assistants in ambulatory surgery units perform these tasks:
- Greeting patients and assisting with the admitting process
- Preparing the patient's bed
- Helping the patient undress
- Collecting a urine sample if needed
- Making the patient comfortable
- Transporting the patient to surgery
- Assisting the patient to the bathroom after surgery
- Helping the patient dress to go home

The nursing assistant may also perform the following tasks. In some states, advanced training is required.
- Helping a patient get out of bed to sit in a chair or walk
- Taking postoperative vital signs
- Teaching the patient how to use crutches, walkers, or other assistive devices
- Phoning patients the day after surgery to see how they feel

FOCUS ON

Surgical Techniques

Some surgical techniques minimize the cutting or invasiveness of surgery. Surgeries that used to require a large incision are now performed with laser devices or other technologies through a very small incision. Small incisions usually mean quicker recovery and less pain. These surgeries are often performed as outpatient surgery. Health insurers support these techniques because they result in shorter hospital stays and, sometimes, lower costs.

Chapter Summary

- Doctors and nurses are responsible for preoperatively educating patients about surgery.

- The nursing assistant can help preoperative patients by easing their fears.

- The nursing assistant helps with the tasks listed on the preoperative checklist to make sure the patient is ready for surgery.

- The nursing assistant may prep the patient's skin before surgery.

- Transporting the patient to surgery and preparing the patient's postoperative room may be the responsibility of the nursing assistant.

- Patients need special care when recovering from anesthesia after surgery.

- The nursing assistant helps patients avoid postoperative complications by positioning them properly and helping them with respiratory and circulatory functions.

- Nursing assistants may perform a variety of tasks in ambulatory surgery units.

VOCABULARY REVIEW

Directions: Match the letter of each definition in the second column with the correct vocabulary term in the first column. Write your answers on a separate sheet of paper.

Vocabulary
1. ambulatory surgery
2. anesthesia
3. anesthetic
4. atelectasis
5. embolus
6. incentive spirometer
7. intermittent pneumatic compression device
8. postoperative period
9. preoperative period
10. surgery
11. thrombus

Definitions
A. A drug or an agent given to patients to produce a loss of sensation
B. A device that is wrapped around the legs and connected to a pump that inflates and deflates to promote circulation and help prevent blood clots
C. A device used to promote and measure maximum effort of deep breathing to prevent atelectasis
D. A blood clot that stays at the site where it formed
E. Surgery that does not require a hospital stay
F. The time after surgery that begins when the patient is transported from the operating room to the recovery room
G. The collapse of a lung or part of a lung
H. The use of manual procedures to diagnose and treat diseases, injuries, or deformities
I. The loss of sensation or the ability to feel pain
J. The time when the patient is admitted to the hospital until the patient goes to surgery
K. A blood clot or other matter that has broken away and travels through the bloodstream

Check Your Knowledge

Review Questions: Answer each of the following questions on a separate sheet of paper.

1. What is a surgical consent form?

2. List common fears that patients may experience prior to surgery.

3. Why must the patient's skin be prepped before surgery?

4. How can you help the family when you are asked to transport a patient to surgery?

5. When does the postoperative period begin?

6. Name the three primary types of anesthesia used for surgeries.

7. Why must postoperative patients change position every 2 hours?

8. How do deep-breathing and coughing exercises prevent pneumonia and atelectasis?

9. What is the purpose of an intermittent pneumatic compression device?

10. How do leg exercises help prevent blood clots?

True or False: Read each statement carefully. Then write *True* or *False* by the statement number on a separate sheet of paper.

1. Elective surgery is usually an emergency.

2. It is normal for patients to be fearful preoperatively.

3. The nursing assistant is responsible for the tasks listed on the preoperative checklist.

4. Deep-breathing and coughing exercises are performed to remove mucus from the lungs.

5. The patient who has surgery in an ambulatory surgery center usually goes home the same day.

Think and Decide

Directions: Think about each of the following scenarios. Answer each question on a separate sheet of paper.

1. Mr. R., a patient that you are caring for, is about to have surgery to diagnose possible stomach cancer. You have been asked to transfer him to the operating room. When you arrive in his room with the stretcher, he tells you he is afraid and has decided not to have the surgery after all. What should you do? Should you take him to the operating room as you were instructed to do? Why or why not?

2. The health unit secretary asks you to bring the surgical consent form into Mrs. M.'s room and have her sign the consent form immediately. Her surgery is an emergency, but a consent form must still be signed before the surgery can take place. What is the proper way to handle this?

3. Mr. B., a 72-year-old diabetic patient, had surgery yesterday to repair his right hip. When you enter his room to check his vital signs, you notice that his lips are pale and his breathing is labored. What should you do next?

4. C.W., a postoperative patient, has been lying on her back for 4 hours because of incisional pain. She says she does not want to be repositioned because it hurts too much. Should you encourage the patient to change positions? Why or why not?

5. Mrs. P. had a hysterectomy 4 hours ago and received general anesthesia. When you come to her room to check her vital signs, she falls asleep while you are talking to her. What can you do to provide safety for Mrs. P. during her early postoperative period?

6. V.B. is a 14-year-old male in your care. He has been admitted to the hospital for abdominal surgery. You have been asked to shave the surgical area according to protocol. When you explain the procedure to V.B. and his parents, V.B. becomes extremely embarrassed. How should you proceed?

7. B.J. has been admitted to the hospital for a hysterectomy. After the nurse has explained the procedure to her and she has signed the surgical consent form, you go in to do her skin prep. She seems very frightened. She tells you that the nurse says they will do the hysterectomy using spinal anesthesia. This scares B.J. for two reasons: First, she doesn't want anyone "messing with" her spine. Second, she doesn't think she wants to be awake during the procedure. She says she didn't voice her fears to the nurse because she was afraid they would cancel her surgery. What should you do?

CNA Certification Exam Prep

Directions: This practice test contains ten questions. Each question has four suggested answers. For each question, choose the ONE that best answers the question or completes the statement. Write your answers on a separate sheet of paper.

1. For which of the following tasks is the nursing assistant responsible?
   A. preparing the patient's room
   B. signing the surgical consent form
   C. explaining the type of anesthesia
   D. completing the preoperative checklist

2. Elective surgery is
   A. usually an emergency.
   B. performed by an anesthesiologist.
   C. optional and planned.
   D. not stressful.

3. A surgical consent form allows
   A. the patient to leave the hospital.
   B. people to visit the patient.
   C. the surgeon to perform the surgery.
   D. the patient to choose the date of surgery.

4. Which of the following procedures is most likely to be done under local anesthesia?
   A. cesarean section
   B. skin biopsy
   C. ileostomy
   D. appendectomy

5. An incentive spirometer is a device that helps prevent
   A. blood clots.
   B. constipation.
   C. muscle atrophy.
   D. atelectasis.

6. Which of the following is included in preoperative care?
   A. coughing exercises
   B. incentive spirometry
   C. surgical skin prep
   D. leg exercises

7. Which of the following might you discuss with a surgical patient?
   A. details of the surgery
   B. procedures you are performing
   C. possible surgical outcomes
   D. the surgery's success rate

8. When shaving a patient before surgery, you should shave
   A. just the area you think necessary.
   B. the point of incision only.
   C. the entire body.
   D. the area that the doctor orders.

9. Skin prep is performed to
   A. sterilize the skin.
   B. show the surgeon where to cut.
   C. reduce microorganisms on the skin.
   D. make a smooth incision site.

10. In postoperative care, how often should you check the vital signs during the first hour?
    A. every 5 minutes
    B. every 10 minutes
    C. every 15 minutes
    D. every 20 minutes

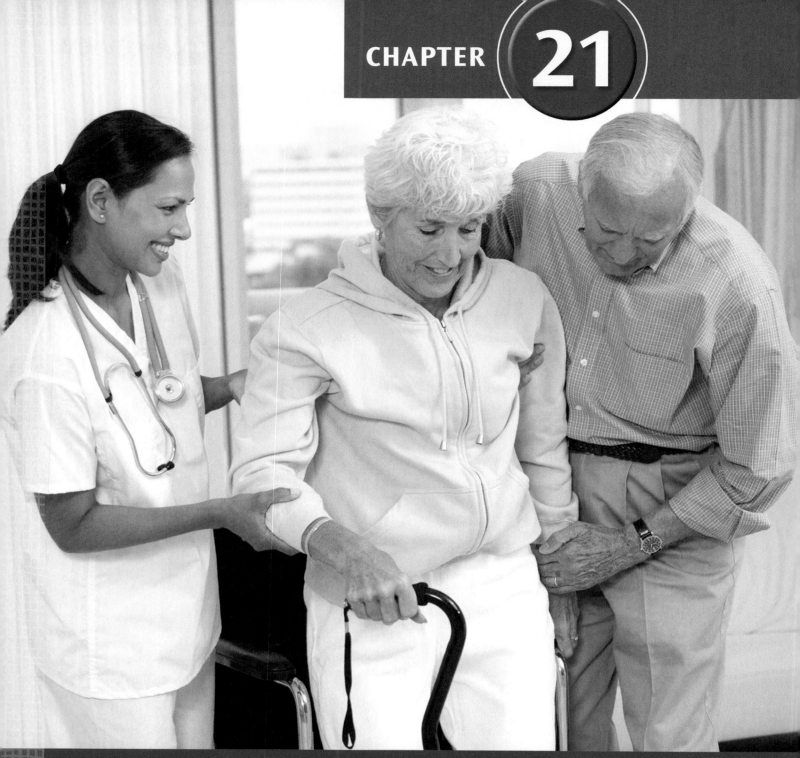

CHAPTER 21

OBJECTIVES

- Explain the goals of rehabilitation.
- Identify the members of the rehabilitation health care team.

- Describe the nursing assistant's role in patient rehabilitation.
- Assist patients with range-of-motion exercises.
- Demonstrate how to help a patient walk.

- Demonstrate how to help a patient who is falling.
- Describe the purpose and care of orthotic devices.
- Explain how to help a patient in traction.
- Explain how to care for a patient with a prosthesis.

Patient Rehabilitation

disability An impairment of function.

fracture A broken bone.

immobilize To restrict movement.

orthotic device A device applied to the body to immobilize a bone, joint, or muscles in order to restore or improve function, or prevent deformity of the body part.

prosthesis An artificial replacement of a body part.

range of motion (ROM) A joint's complete, normal range of movement.

range-of-motion exercises Special exercises designed to move all muscles and joints through their complete range of motion and to build muscle.

rehabilitation The process of restoring patients to their highest possible physical, psychological, and social functioning after an injury or illness.

rehabilitation program A structured series of activities designed to promote a patient's recovery.

restorative care The everyday process of restoring patients to their highest possible physical, psychological, and social functioning on a long-term basis.

traction A process of drawing or pulling used to promote and maintain proper bone alignment. A system of ropes, weights, and pulleys is used.

trapeze bar A triangular device that hangs above a bed to help patients transfer and position themselves.

walking aid An assistive device that helps support the body while walking.

The Rehabilitation Program

Some of your patients may be disabled. A **disability** is an impairment of function. Disabilities can be *physiological* (related to body functions), *psychological* (related to the mind and behavior), or *cognitive* (related to knowing, thinking, and reasoning). A disability can result from traumatic injury, illness, the progression of an existing disease, aging, or a birth defect. A disability might also be called a *deficit*.

Rehabilitation Goals

Rehabilitation is the process of restoring patients to their highest possible physical, psychological, and social functioning after an injury or illness. A patient in rehabilitation learns or relearns activities such as walking, dressing, speaking, or swallowing. When the relearning or restoring process happens on a daily basis, it is called **restorative care**.

If a disability is temporary, the focus of care is to return the patient to the previous level of functioning. If a disability is permanent, the focus of care is to enhance or improve the ability to function as independently as possible. One patient's goal may be to return to the workforce. Another patient's goal may be to independently engage in activities of daily living (ADLs). Still another patient's goal may be to walk again. In all cases, the patient's *potential* (what is possible) for improvement is considered.

The Rehabilitation Team

Each patient has a team of health care professionals to manage rehabilitation. The team includes doctors, therapists, nurses, nursing assistants, the patient, and the patient's family. It may include a physical therapist, occupational therapist, speech therapist, dietitian, psychologist, social worker, and a member of the clergy. **See Figure 21-1.**

To help the patient return to independence, the team develops a rehabilitation program. A **rehabilitation program** is a structured series of activities designed to promote the patient's recovery. The team meets on a regular basis to evaluate the patient's progress. It modifies the rehabilitation program and sets new goals as necessary.

The Role of the Nursing Assistant

Nursing assistants play an important role in the rehabilitation program. Although specific responsibilities will vary depending on the facility, the following guidelines apply to the nursing assistant's tasks:

- Learn about the use of special equipment in the patient's rehabilitation exercises.
- Assist in repositioning to maintain body alignment or to perform a specific activity.
- Assist the patient in performing prescribed exercises.

O **Figure 21-1.** Family members play an important role in the patient's rehabilitation, providing encouragement and support. They sometimes assist with exercises.

- Promote independence by encouraging the patient to perform all of the ADLs that he or she can. The more the patient can do, the better the quality of life.
- Regularly check the patient's condition, especially during rehabilitation activities.
- Report any problems and changes to the nurse immediately.

Nursing assistants also provide psychological care. A patient may have severe emotional reactions to the loss of body function, such as anger, fear, denial, or depression. The patient may also feel frustrated if progress seems slow. Your qualities of patience, empathy, hopefulness, and sensitivity will support and reassure the patient.

- Encourage the patient to complete the rehabilitation activities.
- Suggest that the patient measure progress over a longer time, such as monthly, instead of daily or weekly.
- Praise the patient for what he or she can do, even when there is little progress.
- Do not express sorrow or pity or say anything that could discourage the patient.

Self-esteem and relationships can be affected by a disability. The patient may not be able to return to a previous job. The patient's role in personal relationships may change. For instance, someone who is used to being the "strong one" may resent assistance. Changes in appearance and function can make a patient feel depressed, angry, or hopeless. Depression and anger, in turn, can interfere with recovery. Successful rehabilitation depends on the patient's attitude about the disability and the motivation to actively participate in a rehabilitation program.

Vital Skills   COMMUNICATION

Being Observant

Be aware of the subtle cues a patient may provide during rehabilitation. Suppose you are helping a woman who has had hip replacement surgery through her daily ROM exercises. She seems to be making progress. On her third day post-surgery, you notice that she seems to be experiencing more pain than the day before. That observation should be noted, either by charting or by notifying the nurse.

Observations of the patient's psychological and emotional progress are also important. For example, suppose you are caring for a patient who was in a car accident. At first, the patient was determined to get well and eagerly participated in the rehabilitation process. You notice that he now gets discouraged more easily. This morning as you were helping him with ROM exercises, he said, "Why should I bother with this? I'm never going to get better." That observation is an important indicator of the patient's psychological state and should be noted, either by charting or reporting to the nurse.

Practice

With a group of three or four students, discuss how it might feel to undergo rehabilitation. Consider the following scenarios:

- A young girl who has suffered a traumatic brain injury after a car accident
- An elderly man who has had a knee replacement and is expected to make a full recovery

What concerns might these patients or their families have? What cues should you watch for as you care for these patients?

Restoring Range of Motion

A joint's complete, normal range of movement is called its **range of motion**. Patients whose illnesses require lengthy bed rest need to perform **range-of-motion (ROM) exercises**. These exercises are designed to move all muscles and joints through their complete range of motion. These exercises help maintain or restore muscle and joint function and help prevent complications caused by immobility. They may also relieve the patient's discomfort.

Nursing assistants may be asked to help patients perform ROM exercises. Most facilities specify the number of times per day a group of exercises is to be performed. **Table 21-1** shows the basic actions involved in ROM exercises.

Patients may need more or less assistance, depending on their abilities. There are three levels of ROM exercises:

- **Active.** The patient is able to move the limbs without assistance.
- **Active assist.** The patient has limited ability to move the limbs and needs some assistance or prompting.
- **Passive.** The patient is unable to move the limbs, so the nursing assistant moves the limbs for the patient.

○ **Table 21-1. Range-of-Motion Actions**

Action	Description
Abduction	Moving away from the body (as of the shoulder)
Adduction	Moving toward the body (as of the shoulder)
Flexion	Bending (used for hinge joints, such as the knee)
Dorsiflexion	Bending backward
Extension	Straightening (used for hinge joints)
Plantar flexion	Extending the foot down
Hyperextension	Excessive straightening
Eversion	Moving toward the outside (as of the foot)
Inversion	Moving toward the inside (as of the foot)
Pronation	Turning downward (as of the wrist)
Supination	Turning upward (as of the wrist)
Rotation	Turning from side to side
Internal rotation	Turning inward
External rotation	Turning outward

Follow these guidelines when asked to help patients complete ROM exercises:

- Exercise only the joints the nurse tells you to exercise.
- Begin the exercises with the head or the feet. Work toward the other end of the body.
- Use proper body mechanics.
- Encourage the patient to do as much as possible without assistance.
- Move the patient's limbs gently, slowly, and smoothly.
- Do not attempt to move the limb or joint beyond its present range of motion.
- Observe for signs of discomfort or pain and report them to the nurse.

Procedure 21-1

Assisting with Range-of-Motion Exercises

Equipment: bath blanket

Repeat each exercise the number of times indicated by your supervisor.

1. Identify the patient, check the ID bracelet, and call the patient by name.
2. Introduce yourself and explain the procedure to the patient.
3. Wash your hands.
4. Provide privacy.
5. Raise the bed to a position that allows for proper body mechanics and lower both side rails.
6. Place the patient in a supine position and remove the pillow if the patient's condition allows.
7. Fanfold top linens down to the foot of the bed. Cover the patient with a bath blanket.
8. Exercise the patient's toes. **See Figure 21-2.**
   a. Flex and extend the toes.
   b. Abduct and adduct the toes (spread them apart and pull them together).
9. Exercise the patient's foot. **See Figure 21-3.**
   a. Turn the inside of the foot down and the outside of the foot up (eversion).
   b. Turn the inside of the foot up and the outside of the foot down (inversion).
10. Exercise the patient's ankle. **See Figure 21-4.**
    a. Position one hand under the foot and another under the ankle.
    b. At the same time, pull the foot forward and push the heel down (dorsiflexion).
    c. Point the toes forward or turn the foot down (plantar flexion).
11. Exercise the patient's knee. **See Figure 21-5.**
    a. Position one hand under the knee and the other under the ankle.
    b. Bend the leg to the chest (flexion).
    c. Straighten the leg back onto the bed (extension).

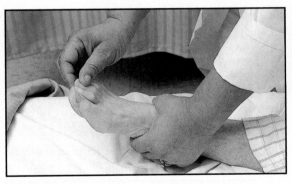

○ **Figure 21-2.** Support the foot with one hand while exercising the toes with the other.

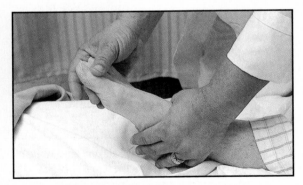

○ **Figure 21-4.** Support the ankle while moving the toes forward and down to stretch the ankle.

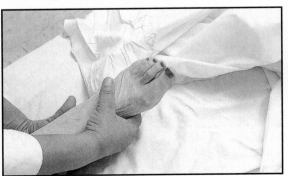

○ **Figure 21-3.** Support the heel with one hand while moving the foot with the other.

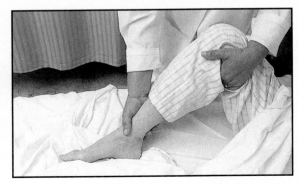

○ **Figure 21-5.** Support the ankle and knee while moving the bottom portion of the leg to exercise the knee.

12. Exercise the patient's hip. **See Figure 21-6.**
    a. Position one hand under the knee and the other under the ankle.
    b. Raise and then straighten the leg (extension).
    c. Move the leg out to the side (abduction) and then move it back to touch across the other leg (adduction).
    d. Return the leg to the bed.
    e. Turn the leg outward (external rotation) and then turn the leg inward (internal rotation).
13. Exercise the patient's fingers. **See Figure 21-7.**
    a. Keeping the fingers straight, abduct and adduct the fingers and thumb.
    b. Straighten the fingers out (extension) and then make a fist (flexion).
    c. Touch the tip of each finger to its base (flexion) and then straighten it (extension).
14. Exercise the patient's thumb. **See Figure 21-8.**
    a. With one hand, hold the patient's hand. With your other hand, hold the thumb.

    b. Move the thumb away from the index finger (abduction) and then move the thumb toward the index finger (adduction).
    c. Bend the thumb in toward the palm of the hand (flexion) and then move the thumb out to the side of the fingers (extension).
    d. Move the thumb to touch the tip of each finger (opposition).
15. Exercise the patient's wrist. **See Figure 21-9.**
    a. Hold the wrist with both of your hands.
    b. Move one of your hands forward and bend the patient's hand downward (flexion) and then straighten out the hand (extension).
    c. Bend the hand back (dorsiflexion).
    d. Turn the wrist and hand toward the thumb (radial flexion).
    e. Turn the wrist and hand toward the pinky finger (ulnar flexion).

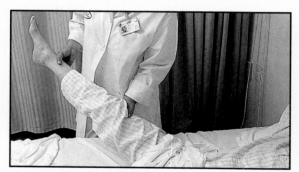

○ **Figure 21-6.** Support the ankle and knee while moving the entire leg to exercise the hip.

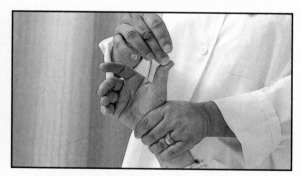

○ **Figure 21-8.** The thumb is exercised separately from the fingers.

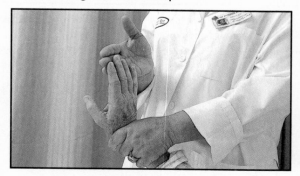

○ **Figure 21-7.** Support the wrist with one hand and move the fingers with the other.

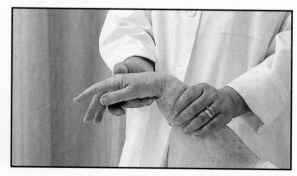

○ **Figure 21-9.** Move the wrist while holding the forearm.

16. Exercise the patient's forearm. **See Figure 21-10.**
    a. Turn the hand so the palm faces down (pronation).
    b. Turn the hand so the palm faces up (supination).
17. Exercise the patient's elbow. **See Figure 21-11.**
    a. Hold the wrist with one hand and the elbow along the body with your other hand.
    b. Bend the arm so the hand touches the shoulder on the same side of the body (flexion) and then straighten the arm (extension).
18. Exercise the patient's shoulder. **See Figure 21-12.**
    a. Hold the wrist with one hand and the elbow with your other hand.
    b. Raise the arm out straight in front of the body and up over the head (flexion) and then lower the arm down to the patient's side (extension).
    c. If the patient is standing or sitting in a chair, move the arm behind the body (hyperextension).
    d. Move the straight arm away from the side of the body (abduction) and then move the straight arm down to the side of the body (adduction).

    e. Bend the elbow and position it at shoulder height. Supporting the elbow and wrist, move the forearm down and toward the body with the palm down (internal rotation). Then move the forearm toward the head with the palm up (external rotation).
19. Go to the other side of the bed or chair and repeat Steps 8 through 18 for the limbs and joints on the other side of the patient's body.

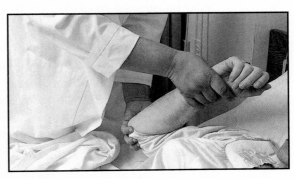

O **Figure 21-11.** Support the elbow and wrist to move the arm and exercise the elbow.

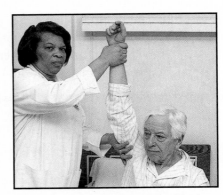

O **Figure 21-12.** Exercise the shoulder by moving the patient's arm.

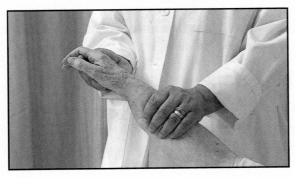

O **Figure 21-10.** Exercise the forearm by turning the palm downward and then upward.

20. Exercise the patient's neck. **See Figure 21-13.**

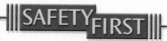

Use extreme caution when performing ROM exercises on a patient's neck. If possible, clients should do neck ROM exercises for themselves.

a. Position your hands on the patient's head. Move the head forward until the chin touches the chest (flexion), then back to the neutral position.

b. Move the head backward so that the chin points upward (extension), then back to the neutral position. Do not hyperextend the head. Doing so could interrupt blood flow to the brain and cause the patient to lose consciousness.

c. Rotate the head to the right side, chin to shoulder, and back to the neutral position. Then rotate to the left side, chin to shoulder, and back to the neutral position (right/left rotation).

d. Move the head, right ear to right shoulder, and back to the neutral position. Then move the head, left ear to left shoulder, and back to the neutral position (right/left lateral flexion).

21. Make sure the patient is comfortable and that the body is aligned properly.

22. Unfold the top linens and cover the patient. Straighten the bed linens.

23. Remove the bath blanket and replace the pillow.

24. Make sure the signal light is within the patient's reach.

25. Raise the side rails of the bed if necessary and lower the bed.

26. Open the screen.

27. Wash your hands.

28. Report and record the time of the exercises, the joints exercised and the number of times, any complaints of pain, and the degree to which the patient participated.

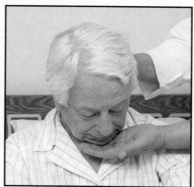

○ **Figure 21-13.** Head motions keep the neck loose and exercise its muscles. Here, the nursing assistant helps the patient perform flexion.

Helping a Patient Walk

Patients recovering from illness, injury, or surgery must regain mobility if possible. They will need to practice *ambulation* (walking). Bed rest and some complications can cause patients to be weak or unsteady. They may experience dizziness or feel faint. These patients will need help when they first begin walking. You can assist by:

• Making sure the patient sits and stands slowly.
• Making sure the patient uses hand rails in hallways and other areas.
• Clearing the pathway of objects.
• Asking for a helper if needed.
• Using a transfer, or gait, belt to help the patient walk.
• Making sure the patient's posture and gait (manner of walking) are correct.

Vital Skills · MATH

Procedure 21-2

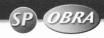

Using a Transfer Belt to Help a Patient Walk

Equipment: transfer belt • robe • nonskid slippers or shoes

1. Identify the patient, check the patient's ID band, and call the patient by name.
2. Introduce yourself and explain the procedure to the patient.
3. Wash your hands.
4. Provide privacy.
5. Help the patient move to a sitting position in bed, following all safety guidelines.
6. Put on the patient's nonskid slippers or shoes and help the patient put on the robe.
7. Place the transfer belt around the patient's waist, over the patient's clothes.
8. Position the buckle off center in the front or to the side, but never at the back.
9. Tighten the belt snugly around the patient's waist. It should not interfere with breathing or comfort. Two of your fingers should fit comfortably under the belt.
10. Help the patient move to a standing position:
    a. Position yourself in front of the patient.
    b. The patient may put his or her hands flat on the bed and push off, or have the patient put his or her hands on your shoulders. Do not let the patient put hands around your neck—you could injure yourself or the patient.
    c. Grasp both sides of the transfer belt.
    d. To brace the patient, block the knees with your knees and feet with your feet.
    e. On the count of three, straighten your knees and raise the patient to a standing position.
11. Hold the transfer belt at the side and the back. Stand slightly behind so you can help if the patient starts to fall. Do not leave the patient alone.
12. Ask the patient to stand in a position that represents good body posture, with the head held up and the back straight.
13. Position yourself on the patient's left side unless the patient has right-sided weakness. Help the patient walk. Stay at the patient's side and provide support by grasping the transfer belt. Coordinate your stride with the patient's. For example, as the patient steps forward with the left foot, step forward with your left foot. **See Figure 21-14.**

14. Observe the patient's gait. If the patient does not appear to be walking properly (e.g., shuffling instead of picking the feet up), give the patient specific suggestions: "Lift the left foot; straighten your toes; put your heel down; put the front of your foot down," etc.

15. Encourage the patient to walk the distance ordered by the nurse or therapist. Do not rush the patient. If the patient cannot complete the entire distance, do not force it.

16. When the walk is finished, assist the patient with returning to bed:

    a. Ask the patient to stand against the side of the bed.

    b. Turn the patient's body a quarter turn so that the backs of both knees are touching the bed.

    c. Ask the patient to place both hands on the mattress or on your shoulders, not around your neck.

    d. Hold on to both sides of the transfer belt.

    e. Gently lower the patient onto the bed, bending your knees as you do so.

    f. Remove the transfer belt.

    g. Remove the patient's robe and slippers or shoes.

    h. Help the patient lie down in bed.

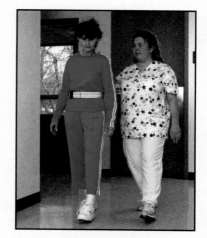

O **Figure 21-14.** Coordinate your stride with the patient's stride.

17. Lower the head of the bed to a comfortable position for the patient.

18. Make sure the patient is comfortable and that body alignment is correct.

19. Straighten the bed linens and make sure the signal light is within the patient's reach.

20. Raise the side rail on the side of the bed closest to you if necessary.

21. Unscreen the patient.

22. Wash your hands.

23. Report and record the following:
    • The distance walked
    • How the patient tolerated the procedure

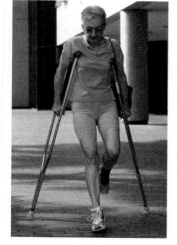

O **Figure 21-15.** A patient using axillary crutches. Prompt the patient to bear weight on the hand grips rather than in the axillary areas.

Walking Aids

Some patients need to use a **walking aid,** an assistive device that helps support the body during ambulation. Crutches, canes, and walkers are walking aids.

The patient is measured and fitted for a specific walking aid by a nurse or physical therapist. The aid must be an appropriate type and height. The physical therapist will instruct the patient about the proper way to use the walking aid and the proper gait to use. You can assist the patient by following these safety guidelines:
• Before giving a walking aid to the patient, make sure it has been fitted properly.
• Replace a walking aid that has cracks, bends, worn tips, or loose bolts.
• Make sure the patient is wearing flat shoes with nonskid soles.
• Make sure the patient maintains proper posture to avoid straining back and neck muscles.

Crutches. These are walking aids used for patients who are unable to use one leg or who need to gain strength in both legs. They are made of either wood or aluminum. The type of crutches used depends on the patient's mobility needs.
• The *axillary crutch* has a curved surface on which to rest the axilla (underarm). **See Figure 21-15.**

- The *forearm crutch* is made of aluminum and equipped with a cuff that is placed around the forearm to stabilize the wrist. **See Figure 21-16.**

Canes. A cane is a walking aid that provides balance and support for a patient with weakness on one side of the body. The patient holds the cane on the stronger side of the body. The top of the cane should reach the patient's hip. The tip, or point, should be positioned about 6 to 10 inches from the side of the foot. Patients who need little support use a single-point cane. Patients who need maximum support use a three- or four-point cane.

Walkers. A walker is a walking aid made of a lightweight yet sturdy material, such as aluminum, that has four points at the bottom to provide stability. It is used when a patient needs more support than a cane or crutches can provide. If the patient needs to carry items while walking, a bag attachment can be added to the front of the walker. Patients should not carry any items in their hands when using a walker, because both hands must be free to hold on to the walker for support.

In some cases, patients are able to use walkers that have front wheels instead of the two front legs (front-wheeled walkers). The basic procedure for using a front-wheeled walker is almost the same as for a nonwheeled walker. However, the patient must be instructed to make sure the back feet are solidly on the ground before putting any weight on the walker.

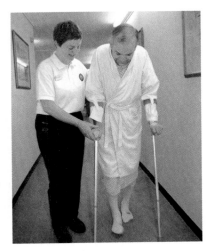

○ **Figure 21-16. A patient using forearm crutches.**

Vital Skills — WRITING

Deleting Unnecessary Words

The secret to good writing is "pared-down prose." Good writers eliminate unnecessary words—the "extra" words that don't contribute to understanding. Read the following sentences:

- Allison went down to Mrs. Johnson's room in order to help her get out of her bed.
- Allison went to Mrs. Johnson's room to help her out of bed.

In the second sentence, four words have been eliminated. As a result, the sentence is more concise while retaining its meaning.

You might have to rearrange a sentence to eliminate unnecessary words. Read the following sentences:

- All patients who are staying on the fourth floor should be getting their linens changed today.

- All fourth floor patients should have their linens changed today.

The second sentence was rearranged to make it more concise.

When you write, make deletion your last step. Eliminate as many words as possible.

Practice
Write a five-paragraph essay on living with a disability. Exchange your essay with a partner. Start deleting! Delete as many words as possible from your partner's text without changing the meaning.

Procedure 21-3

Helping a Patient Walk with a Cane

Equipment: transfer belt • cane • nonskid footwear • robe

1. Identify the patient, check the ID bracelet, and call the patient by name.
2. Introduce yourself and explain the procedure to the patient.
3. Wash your hands.
4. Provide privacy.
5. Put on the patient's nonskid slippers or shoes and help the patient put on a bathrobe.
6. Help the patient to a standing position using the transfer belt as described in Procedure 21-2, Using a Transfer Belt to Help a Patient Walk.
7. Place the cane in the patient's hand on the patient's strong side, while you support the patient's weak side using the transfer belt.
8. Assist with the gait pattern ordered or tell the patient to move the cane forward 6 to 10 inches before taking a step. The patient will move the weak leg forward even with the cane. Next, the patient will move the stronger leg forward and slightly ahead of the cane and the weak leg. **See Figure 21-17.**
9. Remind the patient to use good posture, with eyes straight ahead, and to walk without dragging the weak foot.
10. When going down stairs, assist the patient to move one step at a time, putting the cane and the weak side first, then the strong side.
11. When going up stairs, assist the patient to move one step at a time, with the strong side first, and then the cane and the weak side.
12. Observe the patient's walking and how the patient tolerates walking with a cane.
13. Encourage the patient to walk the distance ordered.
14. When the patient is ready to rest, assist the patient to return to bed or a chair.
    a. Ask the patient to stand against the side of the bed or a chair.
    b. Turn the patient's body a quarter turn so that the backs of both knees are against the bed or chair.
    c. Ask the patient to place both hands on the arms of the chair, on the mattress, or on your shoulders (not around your neck).
    d. Hold on to both sides of the transfer belt.
    e. Gently lower the patient onto the bed or chair, bending your knees as you do so.
15. Remove the transfer belt and the patient's bathrobe and slippers or shoes.
16. Place the signal light within the patient's reach.
17. Make sure the patient is comfortable and that body alignment is correct.
18. Raise the side rail on the side of the bed closest to you if necessary.
19. Store the cane as appropriate.
20. Wash hands.
21. Record and report the following:
    • The distance walked
    • How the patient tolerated the procedure

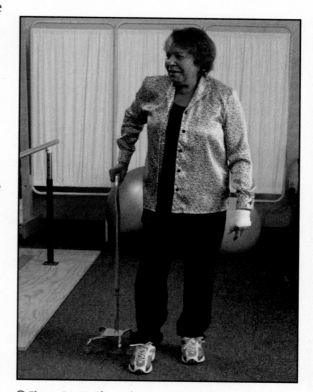

○ **Figure 21-17.** The patient moves the stronger leg in front of the cane.

Procedure 21-4

Assisting a Patient with a Walker

Equipment: transfer belt • walker • nonskid footwear • robe

1. Identify the patient, check the ID bracelet, and call the patient by name.
2. Introduce yourself and explain the procedure to the patient.
3. Wash your hands.
4. Provide privacy.
5. Place the patient's nonskid slippers or shoes on the feet and help the patient put on a bathrobe.
6. Help the patient to a standing position using the transfer belt as described in Procedure 21-2, Using a Transfer Belt to Help a Patient Walk.
7. Position the walker in front of the patient.
8. Assist the patient to grasp the hand rests and move into the walker.
9. Grasp the transfer belt to provide support on the patient's weak side and stand slightly behind the patient.
10. Remind the patient to use good posture and keep eyes looking straight ahead.
11. Instruct the patient to lift the walker off the floor and place it approximately 6 inches ahead of the feet or until the back legs of the walker are even with the toes. Cue the patient to take 2 steps forward toward the walker, one at a time. Repeat. **See Figure 21-18.**
12. Encourage the patient to walk the distance ordered.
13. When the patient is ready to rest, assist the patient to return to bed or a chair.
    a. Ask the patient to stand against the side of the bed or a chair.
    b. Turn the patient's body a quarter turn so that the backs of both knees are against the bed or chair.
    c. Ask the patient to place both hands on the arms of the chair, on the mattress, or on your shoulders (not around your neck).
    d. Hold on to both sides of the transfer belt.
    e. Gently lower the patient onto the bed or chair, bending your knees as you do so.
14. Remove the transfer belt and the patient's bathrobe and slippers or shoes.
15. Place the signal light within the patient's reach.
16. Make sure the patient is comfortable and that body alignment is correct.
17. Raise the side rail on the side of the bed closest to you if necessary.
18. Store the walker as appropriate.
19. Wash hands.
20. Record and report the following:
    • The distance walked
    • How the patient tolerated the procedure

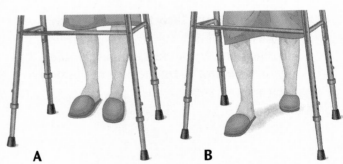

A   B

○ **Figure 21-18.** (A) First, the patient places the walker about 6 inches in front of the feet. (B) Then the patient moves the feet, one at a time, up to the walker.

Falling

If you are with a patient who begins to fall, do not try to prevent the fall. Injuries may be worse if you do. Instead, slowly guide the patient to the floor. Direct the patient away from objects that could cause injury. Protect the patient's head from coming into contact with any hard surface, such as the floor. Stay with the patient and give reassurance.

Patients who are at risk for falls should wear a transfer belt and should be attended by a nursing assistant or other health care worker trained to use it. The transfer belt provides a way to support the patient who may be starting to fall.

Procedure 21-5

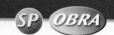

Helping a Patient Who Is Falling

Equipment: none

1. Position your body in a way that offers a firm base of support. Move your feet a comfortable distance apart and straighten your back. Use proper body mechanics.
2. If the patient is wearing a transfer belt, grasp the belt. If not, put your arms around the patient's waist or under the arms. Pull the patient's body toward your body. **See Figure 21-19.**
3. Position one of your legs as a rest for the patient's buttocks. Let the patient's buttocks rest on your knee.

4. Gently lower the patient to the floor by letting him or her slide down your leg. As you lower the patient, bend your knees and hips. **See Figure 21-20.**
5. Have a charge nurse check the patient's condition.
6. Transfer the patient back to bed. Ask several helpers to assist if necessary.
7. Put the signal light within easy reach of the patient.
8. Wash your hands.
9. Make a report of the incident, including the following in your report:
   - The date and time of the incident
   - An objective account of the fall
   - The patient's reaction to the incident

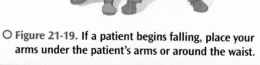

O **Figure 21-19.** If a patient begins falling, place your arms under the patient's arms or around the waist.

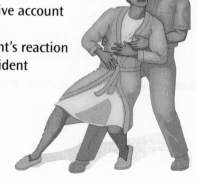

O **Figure 21-20.** Lower the patient to the floor.

Orthopedic Care

Orthopedics is the area of medicine that deals with the prevention and correction of musculoskeletal disorders. Treatment may involve ways to **immobilize** (restrict from movement) bones, joints, or muscles in order to heal. For instance, a **fracture** (broken bone) may need to be immobilized to promote proper bone alignment. Orthotic devices and traction are used for this purpose.

Orthotic Devices

An **orthotic device** is applied to the body to immobilize a bone, joint, or muscles in order to restore or improve function, or prevent deformity of the body part.

There are three primary types of orthotic device: braces, splints, and casts. A *brace* is an orthotic device that supports a specific part of the body to correct deformities or to prevent the movement of a body part. There are back braces, neck braces, and braces to support the ankle, knee, or wrist. For example, an ankle-foot orthotic is a brace that limits or controls movement in the foot and ankle. **See Figure 21-21.** Braces are made of plastic, metal, or leather. They include padding to protect the skin.

A *splint* is a temporary device used to immobilize a fractured or sprained part of the body, such as an arm or finger. It is used for a short time to promote healing. A splint can be a piece of metal or wood taped around a body part. An arm in a cast might be held in place with a cloth splint. **Figure 21-22** shows a leg splint.

A *cast* is a support molded around the affected body part to immobilize it during the healing process. Casts are made of plaster, plastic, or fiberglass. Plaster casts are applied with gauze and wet plaster, so care must be taken while the cast dries. Follow these guidelines for cast care:

- As the cast is drying, do not cover it with any material, including blankets. A cast gives off heat as it dries. If the heat cannot escape, the patient's skin could be burned. However, do not allow the patient to become chilled. Cover other (noncasted) body parts and use a bed cradle if necessary to keep drafts away.
- The patient should be turned regularly to allow all areas of the cast to dry.
- Before the cast dries, avoid making indentations by pressing with your fingers or hands.
- Use pillows to support the entire length of a wet cast. If pillows are plastic lined, place 3 to 5 towels or a folded blanket between the pillow and the cast to prevent burns until the cast is dry.
- Elevate the cast extremity with pillows to decrease and prevent swelling.
- Keep the cast dry.
- Protect the skin from rough edges of the cast.

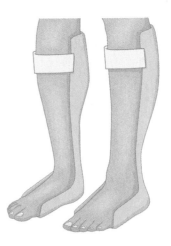

○ **Figure 21-21.** An ankle-foot orthotic.

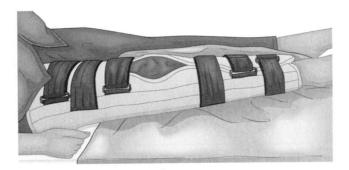

○ **Figure 21-22.** A removable leg splint.

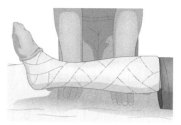

○ **Figure 21-23.** Support a cast with the palms of the hands when lifting.

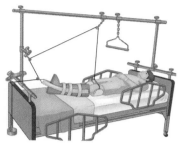

○ **Figure 21-24.** A patient in traction.

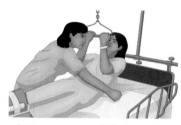

○ **Figure 21-25.** While the nursing assistant makes the bed, the patient uses the trapeze bar to lift the buttocks off the bed.

• When lifting an extremity in a cast, always support the cast with the palms of your hands. **See Figure 21-23.**
• Do not allow the patient to insert objects into the cast.

If a patient with an orthotic device has any of the following signs or symptoms, immediately report them to the nurse:

• Pain: indication of a pressure sore, decreased circulation, or damage to nerves
• Swelling and tightness around the device: possible decreased circulation
• Pale, cyanotic, or cold skin: possible decreased circulation
• Odor or very warm skin around the device: possible infection
• Drainage on or under the cast, chills, fever, nausea, or vomiting: possible infection
• Inability to move the fingers or toes, numbness, or tingling: indication that the device is too tight or is pressing on a nerve, and that circulation is decreased

Traction

Traction is a process of drawing or pulling used to promote and maintain proper bone alignment. A system of ropes, weights, and pulleys is used. **See Figure 21-24.** Traction is used to:

• Reduce and immobilize fractures.
• Treat muscle spasms.
• Correct or prevent deformities.

Traction can be applied to the arms, legs, neck, or pelvis. *External traction* (or *skin traction*) involves attaching weights to material that is attached to the skin. *Internal traction* (or *skeletal traction*) requires inserting a pin directly into the bone. Mechanical devices are attached to the pin, and weights are attached to these devices. *Continuous traction* is traction that is always in use. *Intermittent traction* can be removed for brief periods, as indicated by the doctor.

Some patients in traction use an overhead frame with a **trapeze bar**. This triangular device, which hangs above the bed, helps patients transfer and position themselves. It encourages the patient to assist in self-care and rehabilitation. **See Figure 21-25.**

Vital Skills (READING)

Identifying Key Concepts

One strategy to help you remember what you read is to pick out the key concepts. *Key concepts* are the main ideas of the text. By identifying the key concepts, you can make the most of your reading and studying time.

You can identify key concepts by looking at the structure of the text. The title of the chapter and the subtitles (or headings) usually identify key concepts. Supportive graphics and visuals usually focus on key concepts, too.

Practice

From your library or the Internet, find material about patient rehabilitation. The material should be four or five pages long. As you read, write the key concepts on a separate piece of paper. Then paraphrase them. Write a summary paragraph of the key concepts you found.

Follow these guidelines when providing special care to patients in traction:
- Make sure the patient is properly positioned in bed. If the patient is not in the right position, traction can be ineffective or even cause harm.
- Never adjust the ropes, weights, or pulleys.
- Keep the weights off the floor.
- Assist the patient with the activity plan, including ROM exercises.
- Assist the patient with ADLs as necessary.
- Provide the fracture pan for elimination.
- Provide frequent skin care.
- If the patient has skeletal traction, observe the pin site for changes.
- When making the patient's bed, place the bottom linens on the bed from the top down. The patient who is able can use a trapeze bar to lift the buttocks off the bed.
- Get a nurse or physical therapist if the patient has questions about the traction.

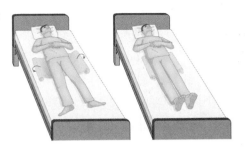

O **Figure 21-26.** A trochanter roll keeps the hip in proper alignment.

Hip Fractures and Replacements

Hip fractures are common among the elderly population, often due to falls. Surgery may be done to repair a hip fracture instead of casting or traction. This enables the patient to ambulate sooner and prevents the complications of bed rest. The orthopedic surgeon may replace the broken hip with an artificial hip made of synthetic material. This surgery is called *total hip replacement*. Some patients have a total hip replacement to treat severe arthritis.

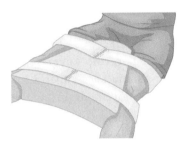

O **Figure 21-27.** A hip abduction wedge keeps the leg abducted.

Two types of devices are used to keep the leg abducted when treating these patients. Trochanter rolls are rolled-up material (such as a towel) placed against the hip to prevent the hip or leg from turning outward. **See Figure 21-26.** Hip abduction pillows or wedges are foam wedges, sand bags, or any item that will stabilize the hip. **See Figure 21-27.**

When caring for a patient who has a hip fracture or total hip replacement, the nursing assistant should remember to:
- Keep the affected leg abducted at all times to prevent external rotation of the hip.
- Provide a straight-backed chair with arm rests when the person is to be seated.
- When turning the patient, use the logrolling technique.
- Follow the lifting plan and activity plan created by the rehabilitation team.
- Provide excellent skin care.

Assisting with a Prosthesis

A **prosthesis** is an artificial device that replaces a lost body part, such as an arm or leg. **See Figure 21-28.** Using a prosthesis can help the patient return to a previous level of functioning. It enables the patient to improve mobility and can also help improve body image. When caring for a patient with a prosthesis, the nursing assistant should:
- Inspect the skin that comes in contact with the prosthesis and report signs or symptoms of redness, irritation, pain, or numbness.
- Assist the patient daily to remove the prosthesis and clean the limb with soap and warm water.
- Allow the limb to dry before reapplying the prosthesis.
- Avoid the use of lotions, powders, or oils on the limb unless instructed by the nurse.
- Assist the patient with prescribed ROM exercises.

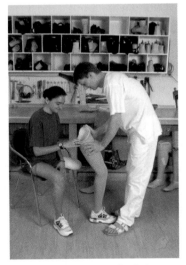

O **Figure 21-28.** A prosthesis for an amputated leg.

Chapter Summary

- Each patient has an individual rehabilitation program with specific goals.

- Each patient has a team of health care professionals to manage rehabilitation.

- The nursing assistant's role in rehabilitation is to provide physical, psychological, and emotional care.

- Range-of-motion exercises are one way the nursing assistant helps patients maintain muscle strength and movement during the rehabilitation process.

- As soon as a patient is able, walking becomes an important activity in the rehabilitation program. When patients first begin to walk, however, they need extra care and attention.

- Patients may need a walking aid, such as crutches, a cane, or a walker.

- If a patient begins to fall, try to gently guide the patient to the floor.

- Orthotic devices are used to immobilize an affected body part during healing.

- Traction is used to treat fractures and other orthopedic conditions.

- Patients with a prosthesis require extra care and concern to help restore their highest level of functioning.

VOCABULARY REVIEW

Directions: Match the letter of each definition in the second column with the correct vocabulary term in the first column. Write your answers on a separate sheet of paper.

Vocabulary

1. disability
2. fracture
3. immobilize
4. orthotic device
5. prosthesis
6. range of motion
7. range-of-motion exercises
8. rehabilitation
9. rehabilitation program
10. restorative care
11. traction
12. trapeze bar
13. walking aid

Definitions

A. An artificial replacement of a body part
B. Special exercises designed to move all muscles and joints through their complete range of motion and to build muscle
C. A triangular device that hangs above a bed to help patients transfer and position themselves
D. A broken bone
E. A structured series of activities designed to promote a patient's recovery
F. A device applied to the body to immobilize a bone, joint, or muscles in order to restore or improve function, or prevent deformity of the body part
G. A process of drawing or pulling used to promote and maintain proper bone alignment
H. An impairment of function
I. An assistive device that helps support the body during ambulation
J. The process of restoring patients to their highest possible physical, psychological, and social functioning after an injury or illness
K. A joint's complete, normal range of movement
L. To restrict movement
M. The everyday process of restoring patients to their highest possible physical, psychological, and social functioning on a long-term basis

Check Your Knowledge

Review Questions: Answer each of the following questions on a separate sheet of paper.

1. Name five people that may be involved in a patient's rehabilitation program.

2. List three reasons for performing ROM exercises.

3. A nurse instructs you to assist a patient with range-of-motion exercises. What questions should you ask the nurse before beginning?

4. When a patient has been on bed rest for 3 to 4 days, what are some problems that may occur when you assist the patient to walk?

5. What is a forearm crutch?

6. On which side of the body should the patient use a cane? Why?

7. List five significant patient signs and symptoms that the nursing assistant should report to the nurse when caring for a patient with an orthotic device.

8. Why should you never place a new cast on pillows lined with plastic?

9. What is internal traction?

10. What is a trochanter roll?

True or False: Read each statement carefully. Then write *True* or *False* by the statement number on a separate sheet of paper.

1. A patient who is unable to move the limbs must do active assist ROM exercises.

2. Crutches are used when a patient cannot use one leg or when both legs need to gain strength.

3. It is important to observe the skin around a cast for signs of irritation.

4. When caring for a patient in traction, it is the nursing assistant's responsibility to adjust the ropes, pulleys, and weights.

5. When caring for a patient with a prosthesis, apply lotion only if the patient asks for it.

Think and Decide

Directions: Think about each of the following scenarios. Answer each question on a separate sheet of paper.

1. You are assisting Mr. V., a 45-year-old rehabilitation patient, with passive range-of-motion exercises. He is expressing frustration about his overall abilities. He tells you that he is fearful about going home because he doesn't know if he can take care of himself. How could you best respond to his concerns?

2. Mr. C.J., an 85-year-old resident, is up and walking for the first time after being in bed for a week with pneumonia. What can you do while walking with him to help prevent him from falling?

3. A 13-year-old patient on the pediatric unit fractured her lower leg and is in traction until she has surgery later in the day. When you enter the room, you discover that the weights are sitting on the floor. What should you do?

4. Mr. W. is a long-term care resident who had a stroke 3 weeks ago. The stroke affected his right side. While you are helping Mr. W. bathe, you are providing passive range of motion to his right arm. He grimaces when you flex and extend his hand and wrist. Aside from recording the time of the exercises and the resident's response, should you take any other action?

5. After breaking her hip, Mrs. A. was transported to the hospital for treatment. When she returned to the long-term care facility, her physician wanted her to sit and dangle for a few days, but to be walking by the end of the week. Mrs. A. was willing to sit and dangle, but she is now refusing to stand, even with the help of a walker. She says she doesn't want to break her hip again. What might you do?

6. Calin is a 23-year-old patient who was in an automobile accident. His left arm is in a cast from above the elbow to just above the fingertips. While you are checking Calin's vital signs, you notice that the fingers on his left arm are cold and bluish-white. What should you do?

7. You are providing care for Mr. G., a long-term care resident whose leg was amputated above the knee several years ago. Mr. G. has a prosthetic leg. When you inspect the part of his skin that comes in contact with the prosthesis, you notice that it looks red and irritated. Mr. G. tells you that it has been itching and asks if you will put some powder on it before replacing the prosthesis. What should you do?

CNA Certification Exam Prep

Directions: This practice test contains ten questions. Each question has four suggested answers. For each question, choose the ONE that best answers the question or completes the statement. Write your answers on a separate sheet of paper.

1. ROM exercises the patient does with help from the nursing assistant are done at the
   A. active level.
   B. active assist level.
   C. passive level.
   D. participative level.

2. Pronation means
   A. turning downward.
   B. turning from side to side.
   C. bending backward.
   D. turning upward.

3. Which of the following is a guideline to follow when assisting patients with ROM?
   A. do everything for the patient
   B. move the limb as far back as possible
   C. encourage the patient to help
   D. exercise all extremities daily

4. Which is an example of an assistive device?
   A. walker
   B. cast
   C. prosthesis
   D. traction

5. When helping a patient with rehabilitation exercises, a nursing assistant should
   A. encourage the patient to do as little as possible.
   B. express sorrow over the patient's limitations.
   C. provide emotional support for the patient.
   D. decide how many times an exercise should be done.

6. Abduction means
   A. bending backward.
   B. moving toward the body.
   C. moving away from the body.
   D. straightening.

7. Internal traction is also known as
   A. intermittent traction.
   B. muscular traction.
   C. skeletal traction.
   D. continuous traction.

8. Pale or bluish skin observed around the edge of a cast may be a sign of
   A. decreased circulation.
   B. an infection.
   C. a pressure sore.
   D. hypertension.

9. If a patient begins to fall, the nursing assistant should
   A. push a wheelchair under the patient.
   B. slowly guide the patient to the floor.
   C. try to prevent the fall.
   D. pull the patient back up by one arm.

10. When helping a patient use a walker correctly, the first step is to have the patient place the walker approximately how far ahead of the feet?
    A. 6 inches
    B. 12 inches
    C. 18 inches
    D. 24 inches

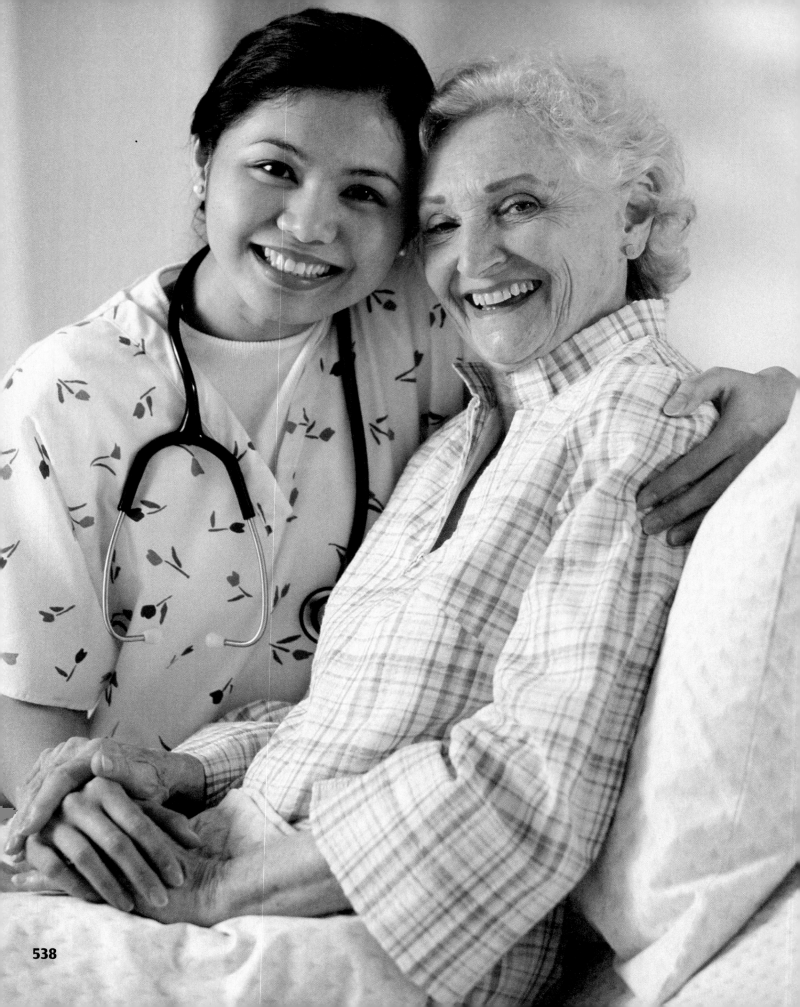

UNIT 5

Long-Term Care

Chapter 22 Personal Care in a Long-Term Care Facility

Chapter 23 Caring for Patients with Chronic Illnesses

Chapter 24 Assisting the Elderly in Long-Term Care

Unit 5 presents information about long-term care facilities and the special needs of the people who live in these facilities. Chapter 22 details the personal care needs of residents and explains how to meet these needs. Chapter 23 discusses the needs of residents who have chronic, or long-term, illnesses. Finally, Chapter 24 focuses on the special needs of elderly residents.

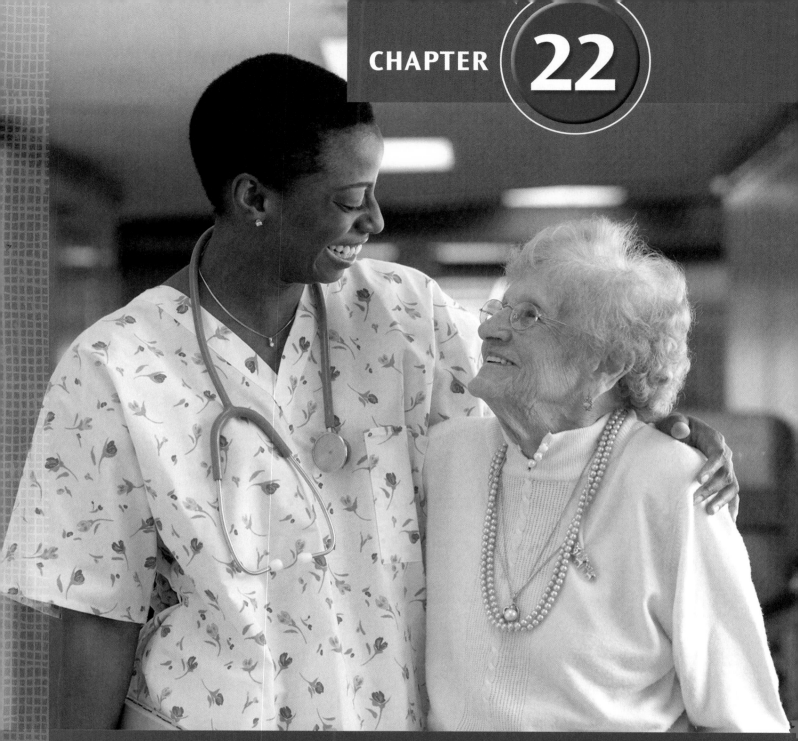

CHAPTER 22

OBJECTIVES

- **Explain the importance of hygiene and grooming for residents in long-term care facilities.**
- **Describe how nursing assistants help residents with personal hygiene and grooming tasks.**

- **Describe oral hygiene practices for conscious and unconscious residents.**
- **List signs and symptoms to report after assisting with oral care.**
- **Demonstrate procedures for assisting residents with hair care, bathing, perineal care,**

nail care, massage, shaving, and dressing.
- **Identify risk factors, stages, and prevention methods for pressure sores.**
- **Describe the proper care of assistive devices such as eye appliances and hearing aids.**

Personal Care in a Long-Term Care Facility

VOCABULARY

atrophic skin Skin that has become thinner, fragile, and less elastic due to aging.

dandruff White flakes on the hair and scalp accompanied by itching.

decubitus ulcer An area of the skin that has broken down because of constant pressure or friction.

dentifrice An oral cleaning agent, such as a paste, gel, powder, or liquid.

dentures False teeth.

dermatitis An irritation or inflammation usually seen as an itchy, red rash.

excoriations Surface skin problems, such as scratches or scrapes.

grooming Making the appearance neat.

halitosis Bad breath.

hemiparesis Paralysis or numbness on only one side of the body.

hygiene The condition of cleanliness and health.

lesion A break in the skin or mucous membranes.

oral hygiene The practices that clean and maintain the mouth, teeth, and dentures.

oral swab A disposable, soft foam swab used in oral care. Some contain a dentifrice.

paresis Partial paralysis.

pediculosis A parasitic infestation of head lice.

perineal care The care given to the genital and rectal areas.

perineum The genital and rectal areas.

periodontal disease Disease that affects the supporting structures of the teeth and gums, and can lead to decay and eventually loss of teeth.

pressure sore An area of the skin that has broken down because of constant pressure or friction.

scales Small, dry flakes of skin.

Helping Residents with Hygiene

Most residents of long-term care facilities are elderly people with one or more serious health conditions. Others are children and adults with injuries, mental or cognitive disabilities, or severe physical disabilities. These conditions make it difficult for people to care for themselves at home. Many residents need assistance with activities of daily living (ADLs), such as personal hygiene tasks.

Hygiene is the condition of cleanliness and health. Personal hygiene tasks include the cleaning and body care we perform daily. **Grooming** is making the appearance neat, such as combing the hair. **See Figure 22-1.** Nursing assistants help residents perform these tasks to keep residents safe, clean, refreshed, and healthy. Grooming also helps prevent body odors, promotes self-esteem, increases stimulation, and promotes relaxation.

Residents have personal care routines that have been developed to suit their specific needs. For example, some may need special bathing procedures or specific skin products. Many personal hygiene procedures are performed early in the day. Some personal hygiene, however, is provided throughout the day, according to a resident's needs. Some tasks are performed at bedtime.

Nursing assistants encourage residents to help with their personal care. Even a little independence can build self-esteem. As the condition improves, the resident may become more independent. For example, a bedridden resident may be able to brush the teeth if the equipment is placed on the overbed table.

Some residents are too ill or weak to perform their own personal hygiene tasks. Nursing assistants help these residents. Some residents are unconscious. Nursing assistants provide their total hygiene care. Depending on the needs of the resident and the facility's policy, you may be asked to provide total personal care or partial care during your shift.

Oral Hygiene

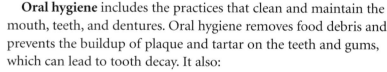

Oral hygiene includes the practices that clean and maintain the mouth, teeth, and dentures. Oral hygiene removes food debris and prevents the buildup of plaque and tartar on the teeth and gums, which can lead to tooth decay. It also:

- Prevents mouth odor caused by food, beverages, tobacco, and some illnesses.
- Prevents infection. Infections can cause swelling, redness, a whitish coating on the tongue and lips, and a bad taste.
- Prevents **periodontal disease**. This disease affects the supporting structures of the teeth and gums, and can lead to decay and eventually loss of teeth.
- Prevents dental cavities (caries).
- Keeps mouth tissues moist and comfortable. Older people produce less saliva, creating dryness in the mouth. Oxygen therapy, dehydration, tobacco use, medication side effects, radiation therapy, anxiety, and stress also cause dry mouth.
- Improves nutrition. Oral hygiene improves the taste of food, which can increase the appetite.

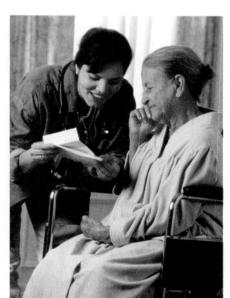

○ **Figure 22-1.** All residents in long-term care facilities have the right to be clean and well groomed.

Oral hygiene equipment should be individualized to the resident's special needs. **See Figure 22-2.**

- A soft-bristle toothbrush minimizes inflammation and prevents bleeding. Hard-bristle toothbrushes should never be used, because they can injure the gums.
- A **dentifrice** is an oral cleaning agent, such as a paste, gel, powder, or liquid.
- An **oral swab** is a disposable, soft foam swab used for oral care. Some oral swabs contain a dentifrice.
- Dental floss removes food from between the teeth, and plaque and tartar from the teeth and gums.

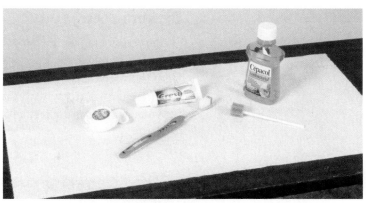

○ **Figure 22-2.** A soft toothbrush, dentifrice, oral swabs, dental floss, and mouthwash may be used for general oral hygiene.

- Mouthwash may used by some residents. It should be diluted to prevent drying of the oral cavity for the elderly or those with dry mucous membranes due to illness.
- Padded tongue blades hold the mouth open for dependent residents.
- A denture cup, cleaning solution, and a denture brush are used for residents with dentures. **Dentures** are false teeth.

Ideally, oral hygiene is performed when the resident wakes up in the morning, after each meal, and at bedtime. Most facilities order oral hygiene to be performed at least twice a day. Some residents prefer to perform oral care more often. Residents must receive more frequent or special oral care if they have conditions or disorders such as:

- Infections or lesions. *Thrush* is a fungal infection that occurs in the mouth and creates a white coating over the tongue. Residents with thrush may require additional and more frequent cleaning of the tongue and oral mucous membranes. A **lesion** is a break in the skin or mucous membranes.
- Bleeding disorders or the use of *anticoagulants* (medications that are given to prevent the blood from clotting). Use a soft toothbrush or oral swab to clean and stimulate the oral cavity while taking care not to cause further bleeding.
- Periodontal disease. Inflammation and bleeding can be minimized by stimulating and cleaning the oral cavity with a soft toothbrush and oral swabs. Special and more frequent oral care help prevent **halitosis**, or bad breath, caused by disease.

Some residents require oral care every two hours. They include residents who are NPO (nothing by mouth), have a nasogastric tube in place (see Chapter 26), have an elevated temperature, are receiving oxygen therapy, or are dying. Oral care keeps the lips, tongue, and mucous membranes of the mouth moist.

After oral care, observe and report the following conditions to the supervisor:

- Discoloration, irritation, redness, bleeding, swelling, sores, lesions, white patches, or cracks of the mouth, gums, tongue, or lips
- Bad breath that does not improve after oral hygiene
- Complaints of pain or discomfort
- Loose, broken, damaged, or decaying teeth
- Changes in the resident's ability to tolerate or participate in oral hygiene

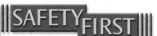

Always follow standard precautions when performing oral hygiene. The resident's gums may bleed, or there may be open lesions or infections in the mouth.

Brushing the Teeth

Some residents are able to get out of bed, walk to the sink, and perform oral care. Others may need help assembling the supplies but are able to brush their teeth themselves. When you assist an ambulatory resident to brush the teeth, provide safety and stay with the resident according to facility policy. If necessary, provide a chair for the resident to lean on at the sink.

Procedure 22-1

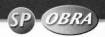

Helping a Resident on Bed Rest Brush the Teeth

Equipment: toothbrush • dentifrice • cup of cool water and straw • mouthwash • emesis basin • towels • paper towels • disposable gloves

1. Identify yourself, check the ID bracelet, and call the resident by name.
2. Wash your hands and put on gloves.
3. Explain that you are going to provide oral care.
4. Provide privacy for the resident.
5. Position the overbed table at a comfortable working height. Place the paper towels on top of the table. Arrange the equipment on the table.
6. Raise the head of the bed to a comfortable, upright position for the resident.
7. Place a towel across the resident's chest to protect the gown and bed linens.
8. Moisten the toothbrush and help the resident apply dentifrice.
9. Move the overbed table so the resident can brush easily.
10. Assist the resident in brushing the teeth and massaging the gums. First clean the upper teeth, then the lower teeth. **See Figure 22-3.**
11. Help the resident rinse the mouth and expectorate into the emesis basin.
12. When the resident is finished brushing, offer cool tap water. Instruct the resident to rinse and to expectorate the water in the emesis basin.
13. If the resident requests mouthwash, pour a small amount of mouthwash in a clean cup. Dilute the mouthwash with water.

The resident swishes the mouthwash and expectorates it into the emesis basin.
14. Wipe the resident's mouth.
15. Make the resident comfortable and provide for safety.
16. Clean and put away equipment. Wipe the table and return it to its original position.
17. Unscreen the resident.
18. Wash your hands.
19. Report unusual observations to the supervisor.

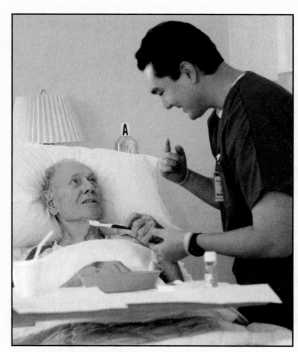

○ **Figure 22-3.** Help the bedridden resident brush the teeth and massage the gums.

Flossing the Teeth

Flossing helps remove food from between the teeth, and plaque and tartar from the teeth and gums. Flossing is usually done after meals and at bedtime. Some people floss before they brush their teeth, and some after. Depending on the facility's policy, you may perform flossing for a resident who cannot floss. Always use standard precautions when flossing teeth because the gums may bleed. Do not floss the teeth of residents who:

- Receive anticoagulant therapy.
- Have frequent seizures.
- May bite.
- Are unconscious.

Procedure 22-2

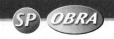

Flossing a Dependent Resident's Teeth

Equipment: dental floss • glass of water and straw • mouthwash • emesis basin • towels • paper towels • disposable gloves

1. Identify yourself, check the ID bracelet, and call the resident by name.
2. Wash your hands.
3. Explain that you are going to floss the resident's teeth.
4. Provide privacy for the resident.
5. Position the overbed table at a comfortable working height. Place the paper towels on top of the table. Arrange the equipment on the table.
6. Raise the head of the bed to a comfortable, upright position for the resident.
7. Place a towel across the resident's chest to protect the gown and bed linens.
8. Put on gloves.
9. Break off an 18-inch length of dental floss. Hold the dental floss between the thumb and index finger of each hand. Stretch it tight. Gently move the floss up and down between the resident's teeth. **See Figure 22-4.** Then pull the floss out through the front (instead of the top) to avoid loosening fillings. Change the position of the floss for each tooth. Do not force the dental floss below the gum line.

10. Offer the resident water or diluted mouthwash periodically to swish in the mouth to loosen debris. Hold the emesis basin under the chin so the resident can expectorate.
11. Wipe the resident's mouth with a towel.
12. Make the resident comfortable. Provide for safety.
13. Clean and put away the equipment. Wipe the table and return it to its original position.
14. Remove your gloves.
15. Unscreen the resident.
16. Wash your hands.
17. Report unusual observations to the supervisor.

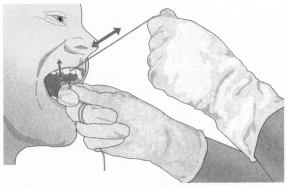

○ **Figure 22-4.** Gently move the floss up and down between the teeth.

Denture Care

Dentures must be cleaned the same way natural teeth are cleaned. When you are caring for a resident who wears dentures:

- Clean dentures as often as you would natural teeth.
- Handle dentures with care. They break or chip easily, especially if they are dropped on a hard surface such as a sink or the floor. They are the resident's property and are difficult and expensive to replace.
- Use cold or lukewarm water. Hot water can warp dentures and harden protein material that may have adhered.
- When the resident is not wearing them, store dentures in a denture cup with cool water in a safe place. Clearly label the denture cup with the resident's name.
- Provide privacy when removing, cleaning, or replacing dentures to avoid causing the resident embarrassment.

After completing denture care, observe and report oral problems to the supervisor, including:

- Resident complaints of pain or discomfort relating to the dentures.
- Broken, damaged, or poorly fitting dentures.
- Changes in the resident's ability to tolerate or participate in denture care.
- Any visible gum inflammation or areas of bleeding.

Procedure 22-3

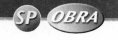

Caring for Dentures

Equipment: denture cup labeled with resident's name • denture brush or toothbrush • denture cleanser • dental soaking agent, if specified • emesis basin • towels or washcloth • gauze squares or tissues • soft toothbrush • mouthwash • disposable gloves

1. Identify yourself, check the ID bracelet, and call the resident by name.
2. Wash your hands.
3. Explain to the resident that you are going to provide denture and oral care.
4. Provide privacy for the resident.
5. Assist the resident to a sitting position, if possible.
6. Place a towel across the resident's chest.
7. Ask the resident to remove the dentures and place them in the emesis basin with a washcloth on the bottom. If the resident is unable to remove the dentures, you will need to remove them. Put on gloves. Use a gauze square to grasp the upper denture.

Pull it slightly downward to break the suction. Gently remove the denture once the seal is broken. Place it in the emesis basin. Remove the bottom denture by grasping with a gauze square and pulling slightly upward. Place it in the emesis basin.

8. Make the resident comfortable. Provide for safety. Explain that you will be right back.
9. Take the emesis basin, denture cup, denture brush, and cleaner to the sink.
10. Line the bottom of the sink with paper towels or a washcloth, place the emesis basin in the sink, and fill the sink with water one-third full to cushion a falling denture. Be careful not to contaminate your gloves.

11. Place one of the dentures in the palm of your hand and rinse in cold water. If you prefer, you can grasp the denture securely between your thumb and two fingers. Brush with denture cleanser or toothpaste until all surfaces are clean. Brush dentures up and down, holding them securely to avoid dropping them. Repeat for the other denture. **See Figure 22-5.** Dentures may also be soaked in a denture cleaning solution.

12. Rinse the dentures in cool water, fill the denture cup with cool water, and place the dentures in the denture cup. Use a dental soaking agent in the cup if specified. Rinse the emesis basin. Take the denture cup to the resident's bedside.

13. At this time, you can help the resident brush the gums with a soft toothbrush and offer diluted mouthwash to refresh the mouth.

14. Offer the resident the dentures. If the resident does not want them, leave them in the denture cup. Store it in a safe place. If the resident wants the dentures, supervise or assist the resident in replacing them in the mouth. Ask if a denture adhesive is used before inserting them.

15. To insert dentures, grasp the upper denture with one hand. Raise the upper lip with the other hand and insert the denture. Gently press on the denture to make sure it is securely in place. Grasp the lower denture with one hand. Lower the bottom lip with the other hand and insert the denture. Gently press on the denture to make sure it is securely in place.

16. Offer the resident a washcloth to clean the face or assist as needed.

17. Remove the gloves.

18. Make the resident comfortable, reposition as needed, and provide for safety.

19. Clean and store the equipment for the next use.

20. Unscreen the resident.

21. Wash your hands.

22. Report unusual observations to the supervisor.

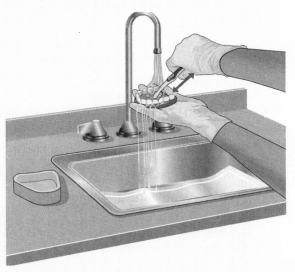

○ **Figure 22-5. Cleaning dentures.**

Oral Hygiene for Dependent Residents

Residents who are unconscious also need oral care. Use an oral swab and a padded tongue blade to clean the mouth of an unconscious resident. A padded tongue blade is used to hold the mouth open. Be sure the resident is turned on the side with the head turned to prevent choking or gagging. This position also helps prevent aspiration. Do not put too much fluid in the mouth, because unconscious residents usually cannot swallow and may choke. Remember that even if the resident seems to be unconscious, he or she may still be able to hear. You can provide important comfort and security by talking to the resident before and while you are providing oral hygiene.

After completing oral care, observe and report oral problems to your supervisor. Include changes in the resident's ability to tolerate the procedure, such as problems with gagging, choking, drooling, and swallowing.

Procedure 22-4

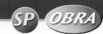

Performing Oral Care for an Unconscious Resident

Equipment: soft toothbrush • padded tongue blades • applicator sticks • gauze squares or oral swabs per facility policy • mouthwash or cleaning agent • emesis basin • paper towels • washcloth • towels • lubricant (glycerin or petroleum jelly) • disposable gloves

1. Identify yourself, check ID bracelet, and call the resident by name.
2. Explain to the resident what you are about to do. Do not speak louder than usual.
3. Wash your hands and put on gloves.
4. Provide privacy.
5. Position the overbed table at a comfortable working height. Place the paper towels on top of the table. Arrange the equipment on the table.
6. Raise the bed to a comfortable working position and lower the side rail if necessary.
7. Position the resident in a side-lying position, facing you, to help avoid choking and aspiration. Place a towel over the pillow and one over the cheek to protect clothing.
8. Place an emesis basin near the mouth.

9. Moisten the toothbrush or oral swab with water and dip in cleaning solutions (mouthwash, toothpaste, or other cleaning agent). Eliminate excess liquid.
10. Open the mouth by separating the upper and lower teeth with a tongue blade. Suction toothbrushes are sometimes used to prevent aspiration of food and fluid.
11. Clean the gums, teeth, tongue, and the inside of the mouth gently and thoroughly. **See Figure 22-6.** Rinse the toothbrush or oral swab as needed.
12. Use water on an oral swab to rinse the mouth.
13. Wash the face and mouth with a warm washcloth.
14. Dry the resident's face and mouth with a towel.
15. Lubricate the lips with glycerin or petroleum jelly, if instructed in the care plan. Use a water-soluble lubricant, according to facility policy, when oxygen is in use.
16. Make the resident comfortable and provide for safety. Reposition the resident as needed.
17. Return the bed to its lowest position.
18. Clean and put away the equipment. Wipe the table and return it to its original position.
19. Remove your gloves.
20. Unscreen the resident.
21. Wash your hands.
22. Report unusual observations to the supervisor.

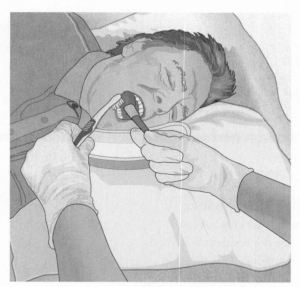

○ **Figure 22-6. Dependent residents require help with dental hygiene.**

Hair Care

Good hygiene includes keeping the hair neat and clean. An attractive hairstyle adds to a resident's feelings of well-being and self-esteem. When hair and scalp are dirty, the resident may feel uncomfortable, and the scalp may itch or have an odor.

Nursing assistants help residents with hair care as requested or needed while encouraging independence when possible. An ill or disabled resident may be unable to maintain his or her hair.

Brushing and Combing Hair

Brushing or combing hair stimulates circulation and distributes oil along the hair shaft. Brush or comb the resident's hair every morning. Long hair tangles easily and may need to be combed or brushed several times during the day to keep it from becoming matted. A resident may request hair care before visiting hours or for a special occasion. Style the hair according to the resident's preference. Ethnic background, culture, weather, and age all contribute to how a resident styles his or her hair.

To safely care for a resident's hair:
- Use a comb that does not have sharp edges that could injure the scalp.
- Use a wide-toothed comb for residents with curly, thick, or coarse hair.
- Always brush the hair from scalp to hair ends, taking a small section at a time.
- Avoid pulling the hair while combing or brushing.
- Braid a resident's hair only with permission.
- Never cut a resident's hair, even if it is tangled and you are unable to brush it through. Report the problem to your supervisor.

When assisting a person with hair care, you may notice **dandruff**, white flakes on the hair and scalp accompanied by itching. Dandruff falls easily from the hair shaft and can be treated with a commercial shampoo. **Pediculosis** is a condition that may look like dandruff but is a common parasitic infestation of lice on the scalp. This condition is treated with a special shampoo formulated to kill the live insects. The egg sacs, or *nits*, seen on the hair shaft do not fall off easily and require a special comb for removal. Report either of these conditions to the nurse so a treatment plan can be ordered for the resident.

Procedure 22-5

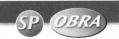

Brushing or Combing a Resident's Hair

Equipment: brush or comb • mirror

1. Identify yourself, check the ID bracelet, and call the resident by name.
2. Wash your hands.
3. Explain to the resident that you are going to comb and brush his or her hair.
4. Provide privacy.
5. Assist the resident to a sitting or Fowler's position.
6. If hair is smooth and tangle free, brush or comb hair from scalp to hair ends.

7. If hair is tangled, separate small locks of hair. Grasp each section firmly in one hand to prevent pulling on the scalp, and begin brushing or combing from the bottom section toward the scalp as tangles are removed. **See Figure 22-7.**

8. If hair is kinky or very curly, use a wide-toothed or pick-style comb to gently comb hair.

9. Arrange hair in the style preferred by the resident.

10. Clean the brush or comb and return to the appropriate place.

11. Make the resident comfortable and provide for safety.

12. Wash hands.

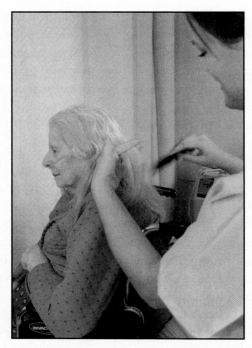

○ **Figure 22-7.** Gently comb small sections from the bottom to untangle the hair.

Shampooing Hair

Shampooing hair removes oils and dirt. The frequency of shampooing varies. Some people like to shampoo every day and some once a week. Hair products and conditioners also vary. When possible, follow the resident's personal choice. Residents of different ethnic backgrounds usually select products based on their hair type and texture.

Residents who are able to shower or bathe usually prefer to shampoo in the shower or tub. A handheld nozzle can be used to shampoo in a tub or shower. If a resident can sit in a chair, you can shampoo the hair in a sink. If a resident is bedridden, hair can be shampooed in bed.

Procedure 22-6

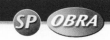

Shampooing a Bedridden Resident's Hair

Equipment: shampoo • conditioner, if desired • face towel or washcloth • two large towels • bed protector • water basin or pail • water supply (large pitcher or shampoo nozzle attached to faucet) • water trough • bath thermometer • comb • hair dryer • mirror

1. Identify yourself, check the ID bracelet, and call the resident by name.

2. Wash your hands.

3. Explain to the resident that you are going to shampoo his or her hair.

4. Provide privacy for the resident.

5. Position the overbed tray at a comfortable working height. Assemble equipment.

6. Raise the bed to a comfortable working height.

7. Remove the pillow and place the waterproof bed protector under the resident's head. Place a towel over the resident's chest to protect the gown and bed linens.

8. Place the water trough under the resident's head and pad under the neck with a towel. Position the basin or pail on a chair under the trough to catch the water that drains from the hose. **See Figure 22-8.**

9. Loosen the resident's gown and fold it over at the neck.

10. Comb the hair to loosen oils.

11. Run the water until it is warm, from 105° to 110° F (41° to 43° C).

12. Wet the hair thoroughly. Apply a small amount of shampoo. You can cover the resident's eyes with a washcloth to protect them.

13. Work up a lather using both hands. Work from the hairline to the back of the scalp.

14. Use your fingertips to gently massage the scalp.

15. Rinse the hair with warm water. Apply more shampoo and repeat if requested or needed.

16. Apply a small amount of conditioner if the resident requests it. Massage conditioner through the hair.

17. Rinse the hair thoroughly with warm water.

18. Gently pat dry the resident's face and forehead with a towel.

19. Wrap the hair with a large towel. Remove the water trough. Remove all other equipment from the bed.

20. Change the resident's gown if necessary.

21. Comb the hair.

22. Use a hair dryer on a low setting to dry the hair. Style the hair according to the resident's request. Hold up the mirror so the resident can see the results.

23. Make the resident comfortable and provide for safety.

24. Clean and store the equipment for the next use. Discard disposable equipment.

25. Unscreen the resident.

26. Wash your hands.

27. Report unusual observations to the supervisor.

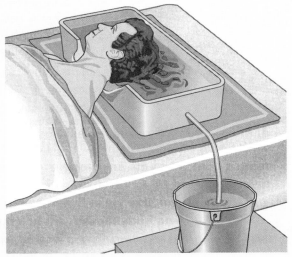

O **Figure 22-8. Giving an in-bed shampoo.**

Bathing and Showering

A bath is an important part of resident care. Bathing:
- Removes dirt from the body.
- Helps eliminate body odors.
- Stimulates circulation and prevents skin breakdown.
- Exercises muscles that might otherwise be unused.
- Relaxes and refreshes the resident.
- Enhances self-esteem.
- Gives the nursing assistant an opportunity to observe skin problems and to communicate with the resident.

Communicating with Visitors

If you work in a long-term care facility, you will probably get to know residents' family members and friends. Your responsibilities may include greeting and interacting with visitors. Keep these tips in mind:

- Greet visitors as they come in the door or when you pass them in the hall. Make eye contact and say hello. They are visiting the home of a loved one. Make them feel welcome.
- If visitors look lost, ask if you can direct them to a room.
- Address visitors and residents formally (using Mr. or Ms.) unless you have been told otherwise.
- Protect residents' privacy. Do not share their medical information or discuss them with visitors.

Practice

In groups of three or four, role-play a nursing assistant and visitors. Practice communicating clearly and kindly. Switch roles so that every student has a chance to be the nursing assistant.

Baths are usually given as part of after-breakfast care. Some residents prefer a bath later in the day or in the evening. Whenever possible, the resident's request should be granted.

Personal choice, weather, illness, and physical activity level dictate how often a resident bathes. Some residents bathe daily, while others prefer bathing once or twice a week. Very sick and incontinent residents need to be bathed often. Most long-term care facilities require a resident to bathe at least twice a week.

Safety Rules for Bathing

Observe these rules when preparing for a resident's bath or shower:
- Eliminate drafts in the bathing room by closing doors and windows.
- Follow the doctor's or nurse's orders for the type of bath the resident is to receive. For example, whirlpool baths may not be permitted for residents with certain medical conditions.
- Collect equipment and the resident's personal supplies before beginning the bath.
- Check the temperature of the water to prevent burns or chills. Water should be between 105° and 110° F (41° and 43° C).
- Use a bath mitt when bathing a resident. It will help retain heat and water more effectively to keep the resident warm.
- When giving a bed bath, keep the resident covered except for the area you are washing. This helps maintain privacy and keeps the resident warm.
- Protect the resident from falling. Place nonskid floor mats in tubs and showers. Encourage the resident to use hand rails. If the resident can be left alone, show the resident the signal cord. Help the resident in and out of the shower or bath.
- Keep the bathroom door unlocked in case you need help. Follow your facility's policy about leaving the resident alone in the shower or tub.
- Wash from the cleanest areas to the dirtiest areas to prevent infecting clean areas.
- Rinse the skin thoroughly to remove all the soap. Soap can dry the skin.
- Gently pat the skin dry to decrease friction and prevent skin breakdown.
- Wash the skin if urine or feces touch it. Rinse well and pat dry.
- Follow standard precautions when bathing or helping bathe a resident.

Observations When Bathing

When bathing or helping bathe a resident, you have the opportunity to observe the resident's body. Observe and report any of the following signs to the charge nurse:

- Skin changes, such as color (areas of redness or paleness), cyanosis, rashes, bruises, broken skin, dryness, bleeding or drainage, unusual odors, skin temperature, and complaints of pain or itching
- Yellow or thickened fingernails or toenails
- New hair loss, nits, or flaking, itchy, or sore scalp
- Redness or yellowing of the eyes
- Apparent changes in mental or cognitive status
- Changes in the resident's ability to tolerate the bathing procedure

Bathing Methods

A resident may have a tub bath or shower, a partial or complete bed bath, or a whirlpool bath. The type of bath depends on the resident's condition, personal choice, and the ability to provide self-care. A doctor may prescribe a special kind of bath or special cleaning agents. Always respect the resident's privacy during bathing.

Tub Bath. A tub bath is a relaxing way for a resident to bathe. When needed, the nursing assistant helps the resident wash body areas that are difficult to reach. Some residents take tub baths when they are able to bathe alone but cannot stand for long periods. A resident's doctor may order a bath for therapeutic reasons. The supervisor will tell you if you need to add special oils or medication to the bath water.

Protect the resident from falls when getting into and out of a tub. A bath should not last for more than 20 minutes. Never leave a resident alone in a bathtub.

Shower. Showers are for residents who are strong enough to get out of bed, walk, and stand for a longer period. Shower chairs are usually available if a resident wants to take a shower but is too weak to stand. You can wheel the shower chair into the shower, and the resident can perform personal care while seated.

Residents need to be protected from falling when in the shower. Health facilities have hand rails in the shower stalls. Encourage residents to use them getting in and out of the shower. Also, without intruding on the resident's privacy, remain near the shower area in case the resident needs help with soaping or rinsing.

Bed Bath. Some residents are well enough to assist in personal care but not well enough to be transported to a bath or shower. They may receive a partial bed bath, which means washing the face, hands, axillae, and perineum. The resident is given the bathing supplies and asked to wash as much of the body as possible. The nursing assistant helps the resident clean areas that are hard to reach. **See Figure 22-9.**

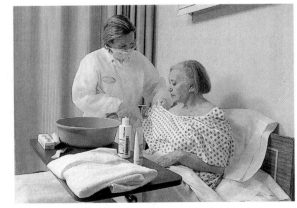

○ **Figure 22-9. Getting a resident ready for a partial bath. Note that gown and gloves are not always necessary for a partial bath. Follow your facility's policy.**

A complete bed bath is given to a resident who is too weak or otherwise unable to leave the bed. A complete bed bath cleans the resident's entire body. The resident may be able to provide little to no self-care. The charge nurse will tell you if the resident is able to assist with the bath and will also explain the resident's specific limitations and problems.

Before you begin the procedure, explain to the resident that you are going to provide a bed bath. Many people have never had a bed bath. They may feel embarrassed about having another person bathe them.

Whirlpool Bath. A whirlpool bath is a special bathtub used for residents who need extra stimulation to their skin, muscles, and joints. The whirlpool water contains soap to cleanse the resident.

Procedure 22-7

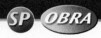

Helping an Ambulatory Resident Bathe or Shower

Equipment: shower chair • soap and soap dish or wall-mounted soap dispenser • washcloth • two bath towels • bath blanket • bath thermometer • bathrobe and slippers • shower cap • clean gown, pajamas, or street clothes • deodorant or antiperspirant • other personal care items as requested

1. Assemble supplies in the bathing area.
2. Wash the tub or shower. Place a rubber bathmat on the tub or shower floor.
3. Place a bathmat on the floor outside the tub or shower.
4. Go to the resident's room. Wash your hands.
5. Identify yourself, check the ID bracelet, and call the resident by name.
6. Explain to the resident that you are going to assist with a bath or shower.
7. Provide privacy for the resident. Help the resident undress and put on a bathrobe and slippers.
8. Assist the resident out of bed and to the bathing area. Use a shower chair, if necessary.
9. Have the resident sit on a chair while you prepare the water. For a bath, fill the tub halfway with water and use a bath thermometer to check the temperature. The temperature should be between 105° and 110° F (41° and 43° C). For a shower, turn on the water, and adjust the temperature until the water is comfortable. Test the water temperature with your elbow or the inner part of your wrist.

10. Help the resident remove the bathrobe and slippers and put on a shower cap if desired. Assist the resident into the tub or shower. Wheel the shower chair into the shower if the resident needs to sit. **See Figure 22-10.**
11. In most facilities, policy does not allow a resident to be left alone in a tub or shower. If facility policy does permit the resident to be left alone, explain how to use the signal cord. Ask the resident to signal when bathing is complete. Place the bathing supplies within reach.

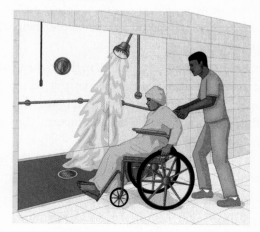

○ Figure 22-10. A resident who cannot stand for long can enjoy a shower sitting in a shower chair.

12. Place a bath towel on the chair. Leave the room if the resident is strong enough to be left alone, but stay nearby. Follow the rules for your facility. Many facilities require a nursing assistant to remain near the room while residents bathe or shower.
13. Wash your hands.
14. Check the resident every 5 minutes. A resident should not remain in the tub or shower for more than 20 minutes.
15. Return when the resident signals. Knock before entering.
16. Help the resident out of the tub or shower and onto the chair.
17. Wrap the bath towels around the resident. Help the resident pat dry.

18. Help the resident apply deodorant or anti-perspirant and other personal care products requested, such as lotions.
19. Provide a back massage.
20. Help the resident into clean clothes.
21. Help the resident return to his or her room.
22. Make the resident comfortable and provide for safety.
23. Gather and place soiled linen in the dirty laundry hamper.
24. Clean, replace, and store equipment for the next use. Discard disposable items.
25. Unscreen the resident.
26. Clean the bathing area. Wash your hands.
27. Report unusual observations to the nurse.

Procedure 22-8

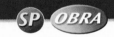

Giving a Complete Bed Bath

Equipment: soap and soap dish • bath basin • bath thermometer • washcloths • face towel • bath towel • bath blanket • clean gown • orange stick and emery board for nail care • oral hygiene equipment • body lotion • body powder if allowed or desired • deodorant or antiperspirant • comb or brush • paper towels • other toilet articles as requested • bedpan or urinal • clean linens if necessary • disposable gloves

1. Identify yourself, check the ID bracelet, and call the resident by name.
2. Wash your hands.
3. Explain to the resident that you are going to give a complete bed bath.
4. Provide privacy for the resident.
5. Line the overbed table with paper towels. Place the supplies on it. Adjust the table to a comfortable working height.
6. Offer the bedpan or urinal. (Wear gloves when in contact with bodily fluids.)
7. Put on clean gloves if the resident has any open lesions or wounds.
8. Raise the bed to a comfortable working height and make sure side rails are raised.
9. Assist the resident with oral hygiene.

10. Remove the top linens while covering the resident with a bath blanket. Protect the resident's privacy.
11. Lower the head of the bed so the resident is lying flat. Give the resident at least one pillow to raise the head slightly.
12. Slip the resident's gown or pajamas off underneath the blanket. Place the soiled clothing in a dirty linen hamper.
13. Fill the wash basin with warm water that is between 105° and 110° F (41° and 43° C). Place the basin on the overbed table.
14. Lower the side rail on the side nearest you.
15. Place a face towel over the resident's chest to keep the bath blanket dry.

16. Form a mitt around your hand with one of the washcloths. **See Figure 22-11.**

17. Wet the mitt. Wash the resident's eyes with water only. Wipe eyes from the inside corner toward the outside corner, using a different corner of the mitt for each eye.

18. Ask the resident if you should use soap on the face. If the resident is unconscious or cannot tell you, do not use soap on the face.

19. Rinse the washcloth and apply soap, if requested. Wash the face, ears, and neck.

20. Pat dry the skin using the towel on the resident's chest.

21. Place a bath towel under the resident's far arm. Wash, rinse, and pat dry the arm, shoulder, axilla, and hand. Raise the side rail.

22. Repeat for the other arm.

23. Apply deodorant or antiperspirant if requested.

24. Apply body lotion and powder as needed or requested.

25. Care for the hands and nails if necessary. Place the hands in a wash basin to soak.

26. Place a bath towel over the resident's chest. Fold the bath blanket underneath down to the resident's waist.

27. Reach under the bath towel to wash, rinse, and pat dry the chest area. Observe under a female resident's breasts for redness.

28. Fold the bath blanket down to the pubic area. Wash, rinse, and pat dry the abdomen.

29. Pull the bath blanket over the resident's body. Slide the towel from under the blanket.

30. Change the water if it is cool or soapy. Raise the side rail before you leave the resident to change the water.

31. Lower the side rail. Fold the bath blanket up to expose one entire leg. Place a bath towel under the leg.

32. Flex the knee. Wash the leg with long strokes. **See Figure 22-12.** Put the bath basin on the towel and place the resident's foot in the basin. Use the orange stick to clean under the toenails.

33. Remove the basin and pat dry the leg, foot, and toes. Dry between the toes. Cover the leg. Raise the side rail.

34. Repeat for the other leg.

35. Change the bath water. Raise the side rail before you leave the resident.

36. Lower the side rail. Turn the resident onto the side away from you. Help the resident move his or her back close to you. Place a bath towel on the bed along the resident's back.

37. Wash the resident's back and buttocks with long, firm strokes. Rinse and pat dry. *Note:* In elderly residents, the skin can be quite fragile. Do not use strokes so firm that you injure the skin.

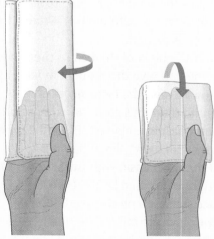

O **Figure 22-11.** Making a bath mitt with a washcloth. Fold the washcloth around your hand and then over your palm. Then fold the top down and tuck it under.

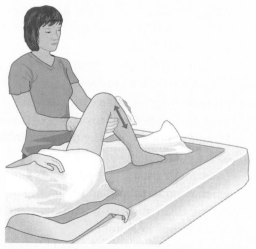

O **Figure 22-12.** Washing the leg with long strokes during a complete bed bath.

38. Using a clean washcloth, allow the resident to wash the perineal area. Adjust the overbed table so the resident can comfortably reach the supplies. Place the signal cord in the resident's reach. Tell the resident to call when finished. Answer the call promptly.

39. If the resident is unable to clean the perineal area, you will assist or do so. See Procedure 22-10.

40. Give the resident a back rub. Perform range-of-motion exercises as ordered.

41. Apply lotion as appropriate, taking care not to rub over areas that are reddened.

42. Put a clean gown, pajamas, or street clothes on the resident.

43. Place a towel over the pillow. Comb or brush the resident's hair.

44. Make the bed and change the linens if the bedding is wet.

45. Lower the bed and raise the side rails, if ordered.

46. Make the resident comfortable and provide for safety.

47. Gather and place soiled linen in the dirty laundry hamper.

48. Clean, replace, and store equipment for the next use. Discard disposable items.

49. Wipe off the overbed table with the paper towels. Discard them.

50. Remove your gloves.

51. Unscreen the resident.

52. Wash your hands.

53. Report unusual observations to the supervisor.

Procedure 22-9

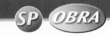

Giving a Whirlpool Bath

Equipment: whirlpool • whirlpool chair • bath thermometer • liquid soap • washcloth • bath towels • bath blanket • body lotion • deodorant or antiperspirant • resident's clothing or gown • disposable gloves

1. Prepare the tub before bringing the resident to the whirlpool area. Wash your hands. Make sure the tub is clean. Fill the tub with water to about 8 inches from the top. The water should be between 105° and 110° F (41° and 43° C).

2. Make sure the room is warm.

3. Add one capful of liquid soap (or follow the directions accompanying the tub).

4. Assemble the equipment.

5. Wash your hands.

6. Get a whirlpool chair. Take the chair and bath blanket to the resident.

7. Identify yourself, check the ID bracelet, and call the resident by name.

8. Wash your hands.

9. Explain to the resident that you are going to help with a whirlpool bath. Escort the resident to the bath area.

10. Provide privacy for the resident.

11. Help the resident undress. Cover him or her with a bath blanket.

12. Position the resident in a whirlpool chair. Secure the straps. Take the resident to the tub.

13. Place the bath towels over the resident. Remove and fold the bath blanket.

14. Some whirlpool baths open on the side so the resident sits as if in a chair. Others have lifts with slings. Step on the "up" pedal to engage the chair. Make sure that both pins are locked into the arm slots. Secure the safety latches.

15. Raise the seat to maximum height. Rotate the seat 90° so the resident faces you. Guide the chair to the tub edge so the resident is over the edge, parallel to the tub.

16. Guide the resident's feet over the tub edge and toward the bottom of the tub.

17. Lower the resident into the tub by gently pressing down on the pedal or electronic control. The water should reach the resident's chest.

18. Press the turbine button to turn on the whirlpool. **See Figure 22-13.** The whirlpool should run for 5 minutes.

19. After the whirlpool stops, apply gloves and assist the resident with washing the face and upper and lower body.

20. Step on the "up" pedal until the resident's feet are level with the whirlpool. Dry the upper body.

21. Raise the seat to the maximum height. Pull the chair and the resident toward you, as you lift the resident's feet out of the tub.

22. Dry the legs and feet.

23. Cover the resident with a bath blanket.

24. Lift the safety latch on the whirlpool chair.

25. Slowly lower the lift until the whirlpool chair is flat on the floor.

26. Remove your gloves. Help the resident dress. Gather and place soiled linen in the dirty linen hamper.

27. Return the resident to the room. Help with grooming.

28. Make the bed and change linens, if necessary.

29. Make the resident comfortable and provide for safety.

30. Unscreen the resident.

31. Wash your hands.

32. Return to the tub room and clean the tub according to the manufacturer's directions.

33. Clean, replace, and store equipment for the next use. Discard disposable items.

34. Report unusual observations to the supervisor.

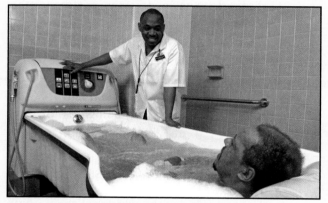

○ **Figure 22-13.** Always follow safety instructions when using a whirlpool bath or chair.

Perineal Care

The **perineum**, or *perineal area*, consists of the genital and rectal areas. **Perineal care** is the care given to the genital and rectal areas. These areas are warm and moist and provide an excellent environment for microorganisms to grow. The perineum must be kept clean to avoid discomfort and infection. Perineal care is performed at least once a day, usually as part of the daily bath routine. However, you must wash incontinent residents each time urine or feces touch the skin.

Residents are encouraged to wash the perineum. If they are unable to do so, you will need to assist them. Some facilities use premoistened cloths or special solutions for this care. Wash from the cleaner to the dirtier area. Wash women from the vagina toward the anus. Rinse the area thoroughly because soap residue can cause dryness and irritation. Dry the area well.

Procedure 22-10

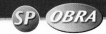

Cleaning the Perineal Area

Equipment: soap or perineal wash solution and soap dish • bath thermometer • washcloth or disposable wipes • bath towel • bath blanket • bed protector • basin of water • disposable gloves

1. Identify yourself, check the ID bracelet, and call the resident by name.
2. Wash your hands.
3. Explain to the resident that you are going to clean the perineal area.
4. Provide privacy for the resident.
5. Lower the side rail on the side you will be working, if applicable.
6. Drape the resident with the bath blanket. Fanfold top linens to the foot of the bed.
7. Position the resident on the back. Place the bed protector under the hips.
8. Ask the resident whether he or she is able to clean the perineal area.
9. Fill the basin with warm water, from 105° to 110° F (41° to 43° C). Place the basin on the overbed table, with the soap or perineal wash, washcloth or disposable wipes, and the towel.
10. Undrape only the area between the resident's legs.
11. If the resident is able to clean himself or herself, place the signal cord within reach and leave the room. Return in a couple of minutes.
12. If the resident is unable to clean himself or herself, raise the bed to a comfortable working height. Help the resident flex the knees and spread the legs with feet flat on the bed.

13. **For a female resident:** Put on gloves. Wet the washcloth and make a mitt around your hand. Use soap or a perineal wash solution. Use one gloved hand to separate the vulva. With the other gloved hand, wipe the perineum area from the front to the back using single strokes. **See Figure 22-14.** Wipe down the center first, then wipe each side, using a clean section of the washcloth with each stroke. Rinse the washcloth often. Wipe the inner labia. Rinse the washcloth. Clean and rinse the inner part of the vulva.
14. **For a male resident:** Put on gloves. Wet the washcloth and make a mitt around your hand. Use one gloved hand to retract the foreskin if the resident is uncircumcised. Grasp the penis. Wash the penis using a circular motion from the urethral opening and work outward and downward, using a clean section of the washcloth with each stroke. Rinse the washcloth often. Rinse the area. Pat dry and return the foreskin to its natural position. Clean the shaft of the penis using downward strokes. **See Figure 22-15.** Rinse the area. Clean the scrotum, pubic, and groin areas.
15. Rinse and dry the area thoroughly.
16. Fold the bath blanket between the legs, help lower the legs, and turn the resident away from you. Clean the buttocks. Expose

○ **Figure 22-14.** When performing female perineal care, always wash from front to back.

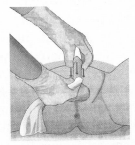

○ **Figure 22-15.** When performing male perineal care, use downward strokes to clean the penis.

and clean the anal area from front to back. Rinse the washcloth often. Continue wiping until the area is clean.

17. Rinse and pat dry the buttocks and anal area.
18. Return the resident to the back.
19. Remove the bath blanket. Remove and dispose of the bed protector.
20. Cover the resident with the bed sheet.

21. Make the resident comfortable and provide for safety.
22. Empty the dirty water into the toilet. Place the dirty linens in the dirty linen hamper. Clean and store equipment for the next use.
23. Remove your gloves. Wash your hands.
24. Unscreen the resident.
25. Report unusual observations to the supervisor.

Nail Care

Nail care for the hands and feet is part of grooming. It is a right of every resident receiving personal care. Nicely manicured hands add to a resident's self-esteem. Nail care is also performed to prevent infection, odors, and injury from scratching. It is performed as often as needed. Care of the hands and feet is included in the daily bath.

Nails, especially if they are brittle, are easier to cut if they are soaked first in warm water for 10 to 20 minutes. Fingernails are cut straight across, without damaging the skin, or according to facility policy. They can then be filed and shaped according to the resident's preference. Female residents may have personal nail care supplies. They may ask you to apply nail polish after performing nail care.

Vital Skills — MATH

Bath Temperatures

When you give a resident a bath or shower, the temperature of the bath water should be between 105° F and 110° F. Don't guess. Use a bath thermometer to test the water.

Example: Suppose you check the water temperature and the thermometer shows a temperature of 135.6°. By how many degrees does the water temperature need to be adjusted?

Answer: You must bring the temperature down to at least 110° F. Subtract 110 from 135.6 to find out how many degrees lower the temperature should be: 135.6 − 110.0 = 25.6° F.

Practice

1. Suppose you check the water and the thermometer shows a temperature of 124.8° F. By how much would you need to lower the water temperature?
2. Suppose you check the water and the thermometer shows a temperature of 62.4° F. By how much would you need to raise the water temperature at a minimum?

Toenails are of special concern for some residents because they can easily become infected. Nursing assistants do not usually cut toenails, so check your facility policy. Nail care should never be performed by a nursing assistant for residents with the following:

• Diabetes
• Anticoagulation therapy
• Severe cardiovascular disease
• Poor circulation to hands and feet
• Extremely thick nails or ingrown toenails

Report observations of dryness, redness, tenderness, or very cold or hot hands or feet to the supervisor.

Procedure 22-11

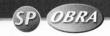

Cleaning and Trimming Nails

Equipment: bath basin • towel or bathmat • paper towels • washcloth • soap • bath thermometer • nail clipper • orange sticks • emery board • lotion • towels • disposable gloves • optional: nail polish • nail polish remover • cotton balls

Note: The basic steps of this procedure may be used to cut the toenails of residents who are not diabetic and have no conditions affecting toenails.

1. Identify yourself, check the ID bracelet, and call the resident by name.
2. Wash your hands.
3. Explain to the resident that you are going to provide nail care.
4. Provide privacy for the resident.
5. Position the overbed table so it is at a comfortable working height. Assemble your equipment.
6. Assist the resident to a sitting position or to a bedside chair. Place the signal cord within reach.
7. If a resident is wearing nail polish and wants it changed, remove the nail polish. Put a small amount of nail polish remover on a cotton ball and gently rub each nail.
8. Place a towel or bathmat on the floor under the resident's feet. Adjust the overbed table to a comfortable height in front of the resident.
9. Line the overbed table with paper towels. Place the bath basin on the table. Fill the basin with warm water, from 105° to 110° F (41° to 43° C). Assist the resident to wash the hands.
10. Let the hands soak for 10 to 20 minutes if nails are brittle, 5 to 10 minutes if they are not. Get more warm water if necessary. Begin working first on the hand that is done soaking.
11. Remove the resident's hands from the basin. Dry them thoroughly with the towel.
12. Apply gloves.
13. Use the orange stick or a towel to push back the cuticles, if this is facility policy. (Pushing the cuticles back is now avoided in many facilities). Use the orange stick to gently clean under each nail.
14. Clip fingernails straight across. Do not cut too close to the skin.
15. File and shape nails with round corners using the emery board. Wash the resident's hands to remove debris.
16. Massage the resident's hands with lotion. Apply nail polish if the resident desires.
17. Refill the bath basin with warm water and place it on the floor under the resident's feet. Soak the feet for 10 minutes.
18. Remove the feet from the basin and dry thoroughly with the towel.
19. Use a new orange stick to clean under the toenails.

20. Clip toenails straight across using care not to cut too close to the skin.
21. File and smooth the nails with the emery board.
22. Use a washcloth to scrub calloused areas of the feet.
23. Apply lotion to feet.
24. Help the resident return to bed if necessary.

25. Make the resident comfortable and provide for safety.
26. Clean and store the equipment for the next use. Discard disposable equipment.
27. Remove soiled linens.
28. Unscreen the resident.
29. Remove gloves.
30. Wash your hands.
31. Report any abnormalities to the supervisor.

The Role of Massage

Massage helps stimulate circulation and relieve tension. Nursing assistants give massages, or back rubs, to residents:

- After a bath or shower. If it is not possible to give a resident a bath before giving a back rub, wash the back first if it is moist from perspiration.
- Before bedtime to residents who need to feel relaxed.
- After repositioning bedridden residents to stimulate circulation.

Some residents should not receive back rubs because the pressure on the back could complicate an illness or injury. Always check with the supervisor or the resident's chart before giving a back rub.

It is easiest to give a back rub while the resident is prone. If this is not possible, position the resident on the strong side. Use lotion to lessen the friction between your skin and the resident's skin. With long, firm strokes, work your hands up and down the back and shoulders. Your hands should always remain in contact with the resident's skin. *Note:* In elderly residents, the skin can be quite fragile. Do not use strokes so firm that you injure the skin.

Procedure 22-12

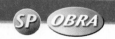

Giving a Back Rub

Equipment: bath blanket • bath towel • lotion • disposable gloves, if needed

1. Identify yourself, check the ID bracelet, and call the resident by name.
2. Wash your hands.
3. Explain to the resident that you are going to give a back rub.
4. Provide privacy for the resident.
5. Raise the bed to a comfortable working height. Lower the side rail on your side.
6. Position the resident flat on the bed in a prone position, or in a side-lying position with the back toward you.

7. Expose the back, shoulders, and the top of the buttocks. Cover the rest of the body with the bath blanket.
8. Wear gloves only if the skin is not intact. Gloves tend to tear fragile skin.
9. Warm the lotion under warm running water or rub a small amount of lotion between your hands. Explain to the resident that the lotion may feel wet and cool.
10. Make long strokes with both hands. Always keep at least one hand on the resident's

back during the back rub. Apply more lotion as needed.

11. Begin at the base of the spine. Stroke in an upward motion, up the spine to the neck, then in an upward motion toward the shoulders. Complete a circle at the shoulders and massage the upper arms. Bring your hands back down at the back, one hand on each side, in a circular motion using long, soothing strokes. Complete a circle at the buttocks and repeat the cycle for 3 to 5 minutes. **See Figure 22-16.**

12. Massage bony areas and pressure spots using a circular motion with the finger. Never rub any reddened areas. Instead, note areas of redness, rashes, sores, or cuts to the nurse immediately.

13. Make long, firm strokes to end the back rub. Tell the resident you are finishing.

14. Gently pat dry excess lotion with the bath towel.

15. Refasten the resident's gown. Remove the bath blanket and cover the resident.

16. Raise the side rail and make the resident comfortable. Provide for safety.

17. Store lotion for the next use. Remove soiled linens.

18. Unscreen the resident.

19. Remove gloves if worn. Wash your hands.

20. Report unusual observations to the supervisor.

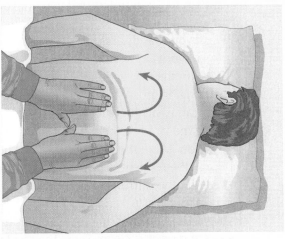

○ **Figure 22-16.** Use circular motions when giving a back rub.

Shaving

Shaving is part of most men's daily grooming. Being clean-shaven contributes to a feeling of general comfort and self-esteem. Some men grow beards or style facial hair according to personal preference, ethnic background, or religious beliefs. Ask the resident how he likes to be shaved.

Never shave a resident unless instructed to do so. Some men are not permitted to shave because of skin conditions or the need to prevent infections from nicks or scratches. Some men do not shave during certain weeks of the year for religious reasons. Others choose to be shaved only by family members.

You can shave residents with electric razors or disposable safety razors, depending on the resident's preference or facility policy. Electric razors are used for residents with bleeding precautions. Never use an electric razor to shave a resident who is receiving oxygen therapy due to the risk of electric shock. Use standard precautions when shaving a resident. The razor may nick the resident's skin and cause bleeding.

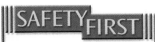

SAFETY FIRST

When you use an electric razor, practice the appropriate safety precautions for using electrical appliances. Make sure that plugs are grounded and no wires are frayed. Do not use the razor near water.

Procedure 22-13

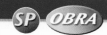

Helping a Nonambulatory Resident Shave

Equipment: towels • washcloths • electric or disposable razor • basin of warm water • bath thermometer • mirror • shaving cream or gel • gauze pads • aftershave lotion if the resident desires • disposable gloves

1. Identify yourself, check the ID bracelet, and call the resident by name.
2. Explain to the resident that you are going to help him shave.
3. Wash your hands and put on gloves.
4. Provide privacy for the resident.
5. Position the overbed table at a comfortable working height. Assemble the equipment so it can easily be reached.
6. Raise the head of the bed to the highest position. Make the resident comfortable.
7. Drape the resident's chest with a large towel.
8. Position the mirror so the resident can see his face.
9. If the resident uses an electric razor, make sure the razor is clean. Show the resident how to hold the razor and how to turn it on and off. Stay with the resident as he shaves. Make sure the resident does not miss any areas.
10. If a resident is using a disposable razor, fill the wash basin with warm water, from 105° to 110° F (41° to 43° C). Use a warm washcloth to dampen the face and soften the hair. Help the resident apply the shaving cream or gel.
11. Help the resident shave himself. Clean the razor in the wash basin whenever hair or shaving cream accumulates. Never leave a resident alone when he is shaving.
12. When the resident is done shaving, provide a clean, warm washcloth so he can wipe his face. Dry his face thoroughly.
13. If the skin gets nicked, apply pressure directly over the spot with a gauze pad. Report the incident to the supervisor.
14. Help the resident apply aftershave lotion if he wishes.
15. Dispose of the razor in the sharps container.
16. Clean the supplies and store them for the next use.
17. Place dirty linens in a dirty linen hamper.
18. Remove your gloves.
19. Make the resident comfortable and provide for safety.
20. Unscreen the resident.
21. Wash your hands.
22. Report unusual observations to the supervisor.

Procedure 22-14

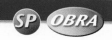

Shaving a Dependent Resident

Equipment: towels • washcloths • electric or disposable razor • basin of warm water • bath thermometer • mirror • shaving cream or gel • gauze pads • aftershave lotion if resident desires • disposable gloves

1. Identify yourself, check the ID bracelet, and call the resident by name.
2. Explain to the resident that you are going to shave him.
3. Wash your hands. Put on gloves.
4. Provide privacy for the resident.
5. Position the overbed table at a comfortable working height. Assemble the equipment so it can easily be reached.
6. Raise the head of the bed to the highest position. Make the resident comfortable.
7. Drape the resident's chest with a large towel.

8. Position the mirror so the resident can see his face.
9. If the resident uses an electric razor, make sure the razor is clean. Shave the face, including the chin and neck area.
10. If the resident uses a disposable razor, fill the wash basin with warm water, from 105° to 110° F (41° to 43° C). Use a washcloth to dampen the face and neck.
11. Apply the shaving cream or gel on the face, including the neck area.
12. Start in front of one ear. Hold the skin tight to prevent nicks and cuts. Bring the razor down the cheek toward the chin. **See Figure 22-17.** Repeat until the shaving cream lather is gone.
13. Shave the area between the nose and upper lip by moving the razor in short downward strokes. Clean the razor in the wash basin often.
14. Ask the resident to raise his chin. Shave the neck area by bringing the razor up toward the chin.
15. Use a clean, warm washcloth to wash the face and neck. Dry thoroughly.
16. Apply aftershave lotion, if he wishes.

17. If the skin has been nicked, apply direct pressure over the spot with a gauze pad. Report the incident to the charge nurse.
18. Dispose of the razor in the sharps container.
19. Clean the supplies and store them for the next use.
20. Place dirty linens in a dirty linen hamper.
21. Remove your gloves.
22. Make the resident comfortable and provide safety.
23. Unscreen the resident.
24. Wash your hands.
25. Report unusual observations to the supervisor and, to protect yourself, document the report on the back of the ADL flow sheet. Have the supervisor or charge nurse initial your report.

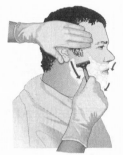

O **Figure 22-17.** Shaving follows the direction of hair growth.

Vital Skills READING

Reading Aloud to Residents

Reading aloud is a great way to connect with residents. Reading can be informal. For example, you can read parts of the newspaper to residents in the morning as they eat. Reading can also be a regularly scheduled activity. Residents can gather to hear the next chapter of a book and then discuss it.

When you read to people who are hearing impaired, speak in a normal voice and use lower tones. Many people can hear lower-pitched sounds better than higher-pitched sounds. Speak clearly and let the residents see your mouth to lip-read. If you are reading to visually impaired residents, describe photos or graphics that are included.

Be creative. For example, have residents pick foreign countries they would like to learn about. Spend one reading session each week on a different country.

Practice

Brainstorm for ideas about a reading program for residents. Consider magazines, newspapers, books, or poetry. Choose a single idea to present to your classmates. Present it by reading the material you selected aloud to them. (Pick a passage that lasts about 5 minutes.)

Dressing

Residents living in long-term care facilities usually wear street clothes during the day, although some wear a hospital gown. The nursing assistant helps dress and undress the resident in clothes that the resident chooses. Encourage residents to make choices whenever possible.

Give residents as much independence in dressing or undressing as they are physically able to manage. Residents who have had a stroke that resulted in **paresis** (partial paralysis) or **hemiparesis** (paralysis or numbness on only one side of the body) may need assistance with dressing. However, residents who are limited physically may be able to dress themselves if they have:

- Loose-fitting clothing.
- Clothing with hooks and loop fasteners instead of buttons and snaps.
- Clothing storage that is easily accessible.

As strength and mobility improve, encourage the resident to do more and, even if not feeling well, to get dressed in the morning. A resident may need to change clothes during the day if clothes become soiled or the resident becomes uncomfortable.

When undressing a resident, remove clothes in the opposite order of dressing. Do not leave the resident uncovered.

Procedure 22-15

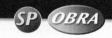

Dressing a Resident Who Has Limited Use of Limbs

Equipment: resident's clothes

1. Identify yourself, check the ID bracelet, and call the resident by name.
2. Explain to the resident that you are going to change his or her clothing.
3. Wash your hands.
4. Raise the bed to a comfortable working height.
5. Check the resident's clothing to make sure it is clean and in good repair.
6. Throughout the procedure, allow the resident to do as much as possible for him- or herself.
7. Remove the clothing the resident is wearing.
8. First help the resident put on underwear. To put on underpants, position the resident on the back. Guide the feet through the leg openings. Pull the underpants up the legs and position the elastic at waist level.
9. Use the same technique to dress a resident in slacks or panty hose by gathering the leg of the garment and pulling it up the leg, one leg at a time. First do the leg further from you. Roll the resident from side to side or lift the buttocks to pull garment up. Fasten pants if applicable.
10. Put on each sock. Make sure the toes are correctly aligned and the heel of the sock is positioned correctly on the foot.
11. Put on the resident's shoes or slippers, as the resident requests.
12. Put a bra on female residents. Slide her arms through the bra straps. Adjust the cups to fit over the breasts and adjust the shoulder straps.
13. Turn the resident to her side to close the hooks in back as required. You can put the bra on backwards, then close the hooks in front and rotate the bra around the body if you find it easier. Then guide her arms through the straps.
14. Put on the resident's shirt and/or undershirt. If the resident chooses a pullover-type shirt, ask the resident to raise the arms. Help pull the garment over the head. Place the weak arm through the sleeve first, then the stronger arm.

15. If the resident chooses a shirt that opens in the front, gather the sleeve, grasp the weaker arm at the wrist, and slide the sleeve over the arm. **See Figure 22-18.**
16. Ask the resident to roll toward you and tuck the shirt beneath the back. Ask the resident to roll away from you and pull the garment through toward you.
17. Gather the other sleeve and slide it over the other arm.
18. If a female resident chooses to wear a dress, place the dress over her head. Place her arms through each sleeve.
19. Adjust the garment to fit the body. Fasten the garment.

20. Make the resident comfortable and provide for safety.
21. Place the dirty clothes in a dirty linen hamper.
22. Wash your hands.
23. Report unusual observations to the supervisor.

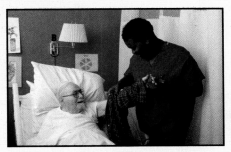

○ **Figure 22-18.** Remember to slide the sleeve over the resident's weaker arm first.

Providing Skin Care

Skin care is an important part of daily grooming. Healthy skin can be maintained by bathing the resident as needed. Pat the skin dry after bathing. Apply lotions to prevent moisture loss and skin-care products according to the resident's need and personal preference. Massage the skin often. Encourage residents to eat a well-balanced diet and drink plenty of fluids.

As you care for the resident's skin, observe for dryness and changes in color or temperature. Look for the following problems as well:
- **Excoriations**, which are surface skin problems, such as scratches or scrapes
- **Dermatitis**, an irritation or inflammation usually seen as an itchy, red rash
- **Scales**, which are small, dry flakes of skin. Very dry skin may be caused by certain medications or diseases, although some shedding of the skin is normal.
- Skin infections, sometimes caused by fungi, especially if the resident has a weakened immune system (in diseases such as AIDS). A fungal infection can often begin under the resident's toenails.

Pressure Sores

A **pressure sore** is an area of the skin that has broken down because of constant pressure or friction. The skin becomes injured from lack of circulation, which destroys the tissue. Pressure sores are also called **decubitus ulcers**, *bedsores*, and *pressure ulcers*. They are the most serious skin problems for residents.

Several factors can put a resident at risk for pressure sores:
- Immobility and limited activity. The weight of the body exerts pressure on the skin. Constant pressure reduces circulation and promotes pressure sore formation.
- Moisture, particularly when due to incontinence or poor hygiene
- Poor nutrition and hydration
- Friction and shearing force, as described in Chapter 16
- Loss of sensory perception. Residents with circulation problems or cognitive impairment may not recognize pain or discomfort.
- **Atrophic skin.** As skin ages, it becomes thinner, fragile, and less elastic.
- Residents who are paralyzed, diabetic, unconscious, obese, or very thin

Bony areas are the most common sites for pressure sores. Check the areas around the shoulder blades, elbows, knees, heels, ankles, the back of the head, ears, hips, and the lower spine. These areas normally are covered with thinner skin. You may also see pressure sores on breasts or on male genitals.

Pressure sores that are not treated become large and painful. A pressure sore begins as either pale or reddened skin. The resident may complain of pain, burning, or tingling. Do not rub an area that is pale or reddened from pressure. Massage or rubbing could damage underlying skin and blood vessels. If the skin breaks, a pressure sore has formed. The wound must be kept extremely clean, since it provides a portal of entry into a susceptible host. Use standard precautions when treating a resident who has a pressure sore.

The Stages of Pressure Sores

Pressure sores are classified into four stages, depending on the degree of tissue damage observed. **See Figure 22-19.** The four stages are:

- **Stage I:** Skin remains intact, but there has been a color change to either extreme whiteness or redness.
- **Stage II:** Skin is broken or cracked through the epidermis, dermis, or both. The sore is considered superficial and may look like a blister or a tear in the skin.
- **Stage III:** The sore includes the fatty tissue and is considered full thickness.
- **Stage IV:** The sore involves the full thickness of the tissue into muscle, bone, or other supporting structures such as tendons.

Preventing Pressure Sores

Once a pressure sore has formed, it is difficult to cure. It is best to prevent them in the first place. Cleanliness, frequent position changes, and good skin care are essential for preventing pressure sores. Specifically, you should:

- Turn and reposition the resident every two hours.
- Avoid tearing or shearing skin by lifting instead of pulling when repositioning residents. Use a mechanical lifting device if possible.
- Give a back rub each time you reposition the resident.
- Do not let a resident sit on a bedpan longer than 5 minutes. The pressure from the rim can cause a pressure sore.
- Keep linens clean, dry, and free of wrinkles, crumbs, or foreign objects. Even a small wrinkle can cause enough pressure to create a pressure sore.
- Keep the skin clean and dry. Thoroughly rinse off soap when bathing. Keep skin free of urine, feces, and perspiration. Provide perineal care after each occurrence of incontinence. Use a disposable bed protector. If feces become dried on the skin, dampen a washcloth with baby oil to loosen and remove them.
- Apply body lotion to dry areas often. Use moisture barriers as appropriate for residents who are incontinent. Never use powders in skin folds.
- Use pillows and towels to prevent skin from touching skin. Place a pillow between the resident's legs so the inner thigh area, knees, and ankles do not become irritated.
- Use pillows, supports, and other prevention devices to cushion at-risk areas. Put a foam rubber or gel-filled cushion on the resident's wheelchair seat. To reduce direct pressure over bony areas such as elbows and heels, use special protectors shaped to fit these areas. **See Figure 22-20.** Sheepskins in many

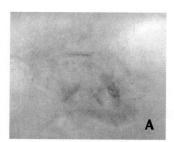
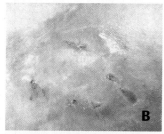
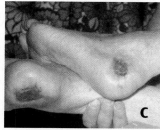
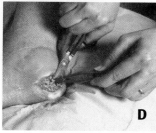

○ **Figure 22-19.** Stages of pressure sores: (A) Stage I; (B) Stage II; (C) Stage III; (D) Stage IV.

sizes and shapes can help reduce pressure on body parts. "Egg crate" wheelchair cushions and mattresses redistribute pressure and allow for air circulation. **See Figure 22-21.** Air or water flotation mattresses and advanced technology beds help prevent pressure sores over areas of the body that are pressure points. **See Figure 22-22.** Note that devices approved for use in long-term care facilities vary by state. Use only those devices that are approved in your state.

• Report the first signs of a pressure sore to your supervisor so that treatment can begin immediately to prevent further damage.

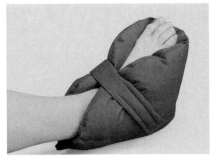

O **Figure 22-20.** Heel protectors help prevent this resident's skin from rubbing against linens and hard surfaces that may cause pressure sores.

Caring for Eye Appliances

Eye care includes keeping the resident's eyes clean and caring for eye appliances. Encourage residents to wash the face and encrustation from the eye area every morning. Eyes must be kept clean to avoid infection and injury. **See Figure 22-23.** Report to the supervisor if you observe redness or swelling around the eye, drainage at the corners, or yellowing of the eye. Be sure to wear gloves, especially if eye drainage is noted, and wash your hands. This type of eye discharge can be infectious. Do not allow the eye drainage to touch the unaffected eye. Instruct the resident to avoid rubbing the eyes.

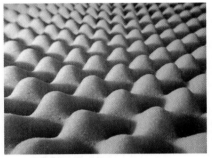

O **Figure 22-21.** Egg crate wheelchair cushions slightly redistribute pressure and allow for air circulation.

Eyeglasses

Many people wear glasses to correct vision problems and sunglasses to shield the eyes from harsh light. Clean eyeglasses give the resident a clear field of vision. Dirty glasses can limit vision, affecting safety and making the resident uncomfortable.

Eyeglasses should be kept in a safe place when not being worn. They should be labeled with the resident's name and stored carefully in an eyeglass case. Never place glasses with the lenses down on the furniture. Never touch the lens when handling glasses. Instead, hold them by the frames. Report broken glasses or resident complaints of discomfort or vision problems to the supervisor.

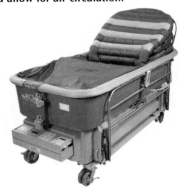

O **Figure 22-22.** Specialty beds use advanced technology to prevent pressure sores or to relieve areas that already have skin breakdown.

Contact Lenses

Contact lenses are plastic discs that fit directly on the pupil of the eye. The type of lenses a resident wears determines when they should be removed. Most are worn for 12 to 14 hours per day and then removed at night. Some people wear extended-wear lenses for up to one month without removal. Observe eyes for redness, swelling, irritation, or discharge when a resident has contact lenses in place.

To remove a lens, wash your hands and then pinch the lens between the pads of your index finger and thumb, pulling it from the eye. Follow specific cleaning instructions for the type of lens worn. Store the lenses in a case that separates the right and left lenses.

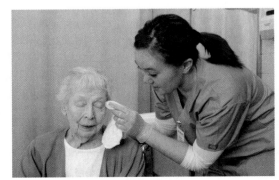

O **Figure 22-23.** Cleaning around the resident's eyes.

Artificial Eyes

A resident who has lost an eye from injury or illness may wear an artificial eye. Artificial eyes are made from plastic materials or a special type of glass. They are individually made for each resident to match the eye the resident lost.

Your supervisor may ask you to assist a resident in caring for an artificial eye. The artificial eye must be properly cared for to avoid infection in the eye socket and to keep the eye clean. Artificial eyes are cleaned according to the resident's routine eye care practices. Follow your facility's policies for providing care for the artificial eye. Watch for and report redness of the surrounding tissue, drainage from the eye socket, or crusting of eyelashes. These signs may indicate an infection.

Procedure 22-16

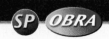

Caring for a Resident's Eyeglasses

Equipment: eyeglasses • cleaning solution • water • lint-free cloth

1. Identify yourself, check the ID bracelet, and call the resident by name.
2. Wash your hands.
3. Explain to the resident that you are going to clean his or her eyeglasses.
4. Provide privacy for the resident.
5. Carefully remove the glasses from the resident, touching only the frames.
6. Clean the glasses with cool running water and rinse with a cleaning solution.
7. Dry them with a cloth (lint-free, if available). Paper products scratch plastic lenses.
8. Place the eyeglasses in an eyeglass case or return them to the resident.
9. Make the resident comfortable and provide for safety.
10. Unscreen the resident.
11. Wash your hands.

Vital Skills — WRITING

The Six-Step Writing Process

You can break down the writing process into six steps. These steps work whether you're writing an essay, a short story, or a poem.

1. *Prewriting* is preparing to write. It might include brainstorming for ideas about a topic or for the content of your work. Research is done in this step.
2. *Drafting* is the writing step, also called the rough draft. Get your thoughts on paper without worrying about style or sentence construction.
3. *Edit and revise* what you've written. Clarify parts that don't make sense and tighten up your sentences by eliminating unnecessary words. Remember to change some passive verbs to action verbs.
4. *Proofread* your work when you're satisfied with your revisions. Correct grammar, spelling, and format errors. Ask a friend to read your work to catch errors you've missed.
5. *Prepare the final copy.* Incorporate all the changes from the editing and proofreading stages. Read through your work one last time to make sure there are no errors.
6. *Publish* your work. This step may take the form of a formal presentation or publication or simply turning in your work to the instructor.

Practice
Using the steps listed, write an essay on what you imagine life in a long-term care facility would be like.

Caring for a Hearing Aid

A hearing aid amplifies and directs sound into the ear. A hearing aid can help residents hear better but cannot fully restore hearing. **See Figure 22-24.** Most hearing aids include a microphone, an amplifier, an ear mold, a cord, and an on/off switch. Newer types contain computer chips that automatically adjust the volume. Hearing aids are fragile and expensive. The following tips will keep a hearing aid in good working order.

- Do not wash a hearing aid. Follow manufacturer's instructions for cleaning the ear mold. Use clean gauze to wipe off the exterior, but do not use soap, water, alcohol, or any other fluid for cleaning. Complete cleaning must be done by the dealer. Remove the hearing aid before the resident bathes or showers.
- Handle the hearing aid gently and do not drop it.
- Do not expose a hearing aid to heat or moisture.
- Do not get lotions, sprays, or shampoos on the hearing aid. They can clog the mechanism.
- Do not let the resident wear a hearing aid while sleeping.
- Check the batteries before inserting a hearing aid. The battery case should close easily. If it does not, the batteries could be the wrong size.
- Test the batteries by turning the hearing aid on. Turn up the volume control. When you put the hearing aid next to your ear, you should hear a whistle.
- Check the batteries if the resident cannot hear properly.

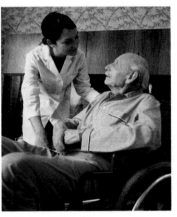

○ **Figure 22-24.** When speaking to a resident wearing a hearing aid, look directly at the resident and speak clearly.

Procedure 22-17

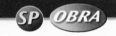

Inserting and Removing a Hearing Aid

Equipment: disposable gloves

1. Identify yourself and the resident. Call the resident by name.
2. Wash your hands.
3. Explain to the resident that you are going to insert or remove his or her hearing aid.
4. Provide privacy for the resident.

Inserting the hearing aid:

5. Put on gloves. Check the resident's ear for wax buildup or anything unusual. Turn the hearing aid off.
6. Allow the resident to insert the hearing aid if able.
7. If you are inserting the hearing aid, place the hearing aid over the resident's ear, if appropriate, with the ear mold piece hanging free.
8. Adjust the hearing aid behind the ear.
9. Gently insert the ear mold into the ear canal. Gently twist the ear mold into the curve of the ear. Push up and in with one hand. Use your other hand to pull gently on the earlobe.

10. Turn the hearing aid on and adjust the volume to a comfortable level.
11. If the resident complains that the hearing aid is uncomfortable, it may need to be refitted. Report this to the supervisor.

Removing and storing the hearing aid:

12. Turn off the hearing aid.
13. Gently pull on the upper ear to loosen the outer portion of the hearing aid.
14. Lift the ear mold up and out.
15. Remove the batteries before storing the hearing aid in its case in a safe place. Make sure the case is labeled with the resident's name.
16. Make the resident comfortable and provide for safety. Place the call signal within the resident's reach.
17. Unscreen the resident.
18. Remove gloves and wash your hands.
19. Report unusual observations to the supervisor.

Chapter Summary

- Hygiene and grooming are important factors in maintaining residents' health and well-being.

- Nursing assistants help residents perform personal hygiene while encouraging them to participate in their care as much as possible.

- Oral hygiene care includes providing individualized cleaning of the mouth, teeth, and dentures for conscious and unconscious residents.

- Hair care, bathing, perineal care, nail care, massage, shaving, and dressing are part of a resident's regular hygiene and grooming.

- Many factors put residents at risk for pressure sores. Nursing assistants should be aware of the stages of pressure sores and ways to prevent skin breakdown.

- Nursing assistants may help residents care for assistive devices such as eyeglasses, contact lenses, artificial eyes, and hearing aids.

VOCABULARY REVIEW

Directions: Match the letter of each definition in the second column with the correct vocabulary term in the first column. Write your answers on a separate sheet of paper.

Vocabulary

1. atrophic skin
2. dandruff
3. dermatitis
4. excoriations
5. halitosis
6. hemiparesis
7. hygiene
8. lesion
9. paresis
10. pediculosis
11. perineal care
12. periodontal disease
13. pressure sore
14. scales

Definitions

A. A break in the skin or mucous membranes

B. Partial paralysis

C. The care given to the genital and rectal areas

D. Bad breath

E. An area of the skin that has broken down because of constant pressure or friction

F. Disease that affects the supporting structures of the teeth and gums, and can lead to decay and eventually loss of teeth

G. White flakes on the hair and scalp accompanied by itching

H. Skin that has become thinner, fragile, and less elastic due to aging

I. Paralysis or numbness to only one side of the body

J. Surface skin problems, such as scratches or scrapes

K. A parasitic infestation of head lice

L. Small, dry flakes of skin

M. An irritation or inflammation usually seen as an itchy, red rash

N. The condition of cleanliness and health

Check Your Knowledge

Review Questions: Answer each of the following questions on a separate sheet of paper.

1. Why is it important for residents to practice personal hygiene?

2. Why should a nursing assistant wear gloves when assisting a resident with oral hygiene?

3. When bathing a resident, what signs and symptoms on the skin should you report to your supervisor?

4. For whom would a doctor order a whirlpool bath?

5. Nursing assistants do not perform nail care for residents with certain conditions or therapies. What are they?

6. How should you position a resident for a back rub?

7. When dressing a resident who has hemiparesis, which arm goes in first when putting on a shirt?

8. Which stage of a pressure sore does not involve a break in the skin?

9. Why should bed linens be kept free of wrinkles?

10. List three types of eye appliances you may be asked to care for.

True or False: Read each statement carefully. Then write *True* or *False* by the statement number on a separate sheet of paper.

1. Medications can cause a white coating to form on the tongue.

2. Never allow a resident to remove dentures, even if he or she is able.

3. When a resident is bathing, close doors and windows to avoid drafts.

4. Perform perineal care once a day for an incontinent resident.

5. A resident should wear a hearing aid while sleeping for safety reasons.

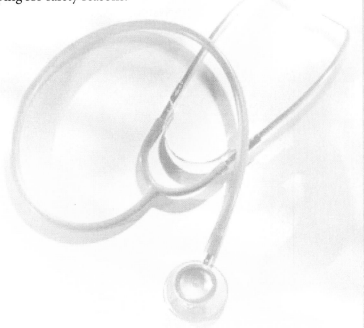

Think and Decide

Directions: Think about each of the following scenarios. Answer each question on a separate sheet of paper.

1. Mrs. M. is a long-term care resident who has been unconscious for more than a week following a stroke. At the beginning of your shift, you enter the room to perform Mrs. M.'s oral care. You notice a white coating on her tongue. What action(s) should you take?

2. Ms. H. is a new resident at the long-term care facility. She has been living alone and has been unable to care for herself properly for several weeks due to extreme weakness. While combing her hair, you notice white flakes on her scalp and hair. Is this something you should report? Why or why not?

3. Mr. E. is an elderly resident who has been placed on bleeding precautions because he is on a blood-thinning medication. When you come to his room this morning, he says he wants you to help him shave his facial hair. What action should you take?

4. J.W. is a 99-year-old resident who was recently admitted to the long-term care facility where you work. He has a hearing aid, but he is having difficulty hearing. The battery has recently been changed. However, the hearing aid appears to be very dirty. He asks you to clean the hearing aid for him. What should you do?

5. Mr. B. is on bed rest after suffering a major stroke. To prevent pressure sores, the physician orders an air bed for Mr. B. Aside from that, what can the nursing assistant do to assist in preventing the development of pressure sores?

6. Mrs. T. is a 74-year-old resident who has worn dentures for many years. Her dentures were old and, over the years, had become ill-fitting. However, she was used to them and managed quite well. A few weeks ago, her daughter arranged to have new dentures made for her. Since then, Mrs. T. has stopped eating anything that requires much chewing. She eats only soft foods such as applesauce and puddings. When you ask her if something is wrong, she tells you that the new dentures hurt when she bites down. She didn't want to complain because her daughter spent a great deal of money to get them for her. What should you do?

7. Ms. K. has diabetes. During her morning personal care, Ms. K. shows you her right hand. Two of the fingernails are torn and rough. She says she accidentally tore them while trying to get the plastic wrapper off a magazine her son brought her. She asks you to trim the nails for her, because she doesn't have a nail clipper. What should you do?

CNA Certification Exam Prep

Directions: This practice test contains ten questions. Each question has four suggested answers. For each question, choose the ONE that best answers the question or completes the statement. Write your answers on a separate sheet of paper.

1. When you were brushing Mrs. Taylor's teeth, you noticed a white coating on her tongue. This is a fungal infection called
   A. thrush.
   B. halitosis.
   C. periodontosis.
   D. lesions.

2. When brushing hair, you should brush
   A. from the end of the hair to the scalp.
   B. from the scalp to the end of the hair.
   C. from the left side to the right side.
   D. from the right side to the left side.

3. When shaving a man's facial hair, you should hold the skin
   A. taut and shave upward.
   B. loosely and shave upward.
   C. taut and shave downward.
   D. loosely and shave downward.

4. When dressing a person with a weakness on the left side, you should
   A. apply clothing on the strong side first.
   B. apply clothing on the weak side first.
   C. let the resident dress herself.
   D. get help from another nursing assistant.

5. What measure can you take to prevent pressure sores on a resident with limited mobility?
   A. frequent position changes
   B. rub the area briskly
   C. withhold certain foods
   D. keep the resident bedridden

6. Before beginning any personal care procedure, you should
   A. tell the resident not to worry.
   B. identify the resident.
   C. put on a gown and mask.
   D. put up the side rail.

7. Oral hygiene cleans the
   A. mouth.
   B. face.
   C. perineal area.
   D. eyes.

8. When providing perineal care, always wipe
   A. from back to front.
   B. from front to back.
   C. from side to side.
   D. in all directions.

9. A back rub should last about
   A. 1 to 2 minutes.
   B. 3 to 5 minutes.
   C. 15 to 20 minutes.
   D. 30 to 45 minutes.

10. Another name for a pressure sore is
    A. skin rash.
    B. cyanosis.
    C. meningitis.
    D. decubitus ulcer.

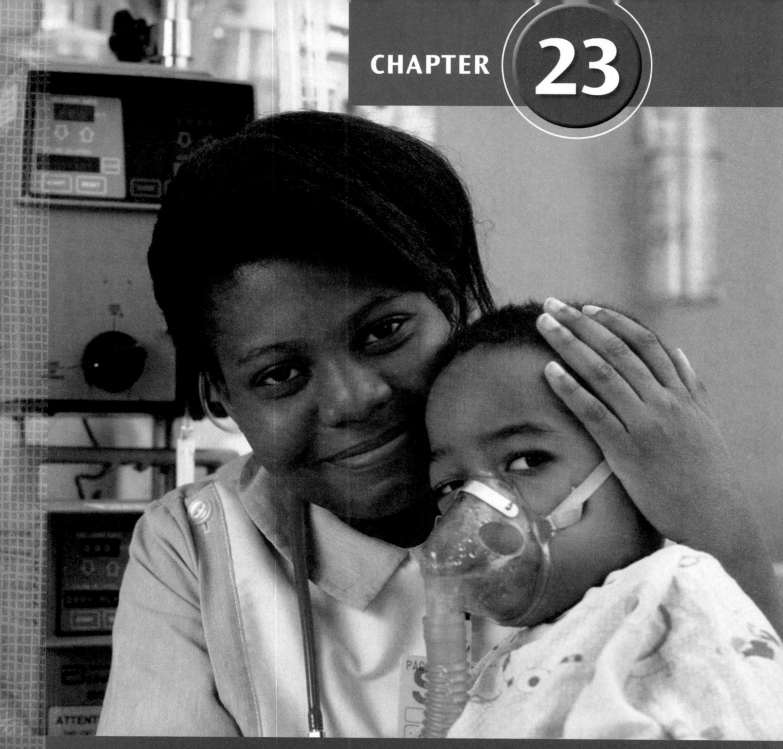

CHAPTER 23

OBJECTIVES

- Discuss the challenges of dealing with chronic illness.
- Identify causes and symptoms of various chronic illnesses.
- Describe the nursing assistant's role in caring for patients with diabetes mellitus.

- Demonstrate how to test a patient's blood glucose level.
- Describe the nursing assistant's role in caring for patients with cardiovascular, respiratory, or neurological disorder.

- Describe the nursing assistant's role in caring for patients with cancer, AIDS, or kidney failure.

Caring for Patients with Chronic Illnesses

VOCABULARY

acquired immunodeficiency syndrome (AIDS) A syndrome caused by the human immunodeficiency virus that attacks the immune system and affects the body's ability to fight other diseases.

angina pectoris Severe pain or pressure in the chest caused by reduced blood flow and an inadequate oxygen supply to the heart muscle.

aphasia The inability or impaired ability to communicate through speech, writing, or signs.

asthma A respiratory disease caused by narrowing and inflammation of the airways in response to triggers.

atherosclerosis A condition in which fat deposits build up on the inner walls of blood vessels.

cancer A malignant (harmful), uncontrolled growth of abnormal cells. Cancer generally invades healthy tissue and stops normal body functioning.

cerebrovascular accident (CVA) A sudden interruption in the blood supply to the brain; a stroke.

chemotherapy A therapy that uses drugs to destroy or slow the growth of cancer cells.

chronic Lasting a long time (as of an illness or condition).

chronic bronchitis Inflammation in the lungs, with increased mucus production and a chronic productive cough that is present for at least three months in two successive years.

chronic obstructive pulmonary disease (COPD) A group of chronic, progressive lung diseases characterized by airway obstruction and a loss of elasticity of the lungs.

congestive heart failure (CHF) The heart's inability to pump effectively, which can result in a buildup of excess fluid in the lungs.

emphysema A condition in which the air spaces in the lungs become enlarged and overinflated, resulting in the loss of elasticity.

gangrene The death of tissue, usually caused by poor blood circulation.

human immunodeficiency virus (HIV) A virus that is transmitted through blood and body fluid contact and causes AIDS.

hyperglycemia A condition that occurs when the blood glucose level is abnormally high.

hypoglycemia A condition that occurs when the blood glucose level is abnormally low.

insulin A hormone produced by the pancreas that the body uses to convert glucose into energy.

kidney dialysis A process in which a machine is attached to a patient's circulatory system, by a catheter or some other device, to remove waste products from the blood.

kidney (renal) failure A chronic condition that involves gradual, progressive, and irreversible damage to the kidneys.

multiple sclerosis (MS) A progressive disease of the nervous system that affects how nerve impulses are sent to and from the brain.

Parkinson's disease A progressive disease that affects the part of the brain that handles muscular control and function.

radiation therapy A therapy that uses x-rays to destroy cancer cells.

stroke A sudden interruption in the blood supply to the brain.

syndrome A group of signs and symptoms that occur together.

transient ischemic attack (TIA) A small stroke that temporarily reduces blood flow to the brain but results in less damage than a stroke; a ministroke.

Chronic Illness

Unlike sudden illnesses, such as a cold or the flu, **chronic** (lasting a long time) illnesses occur gradually and last a long time, usually more than three months. Some conditions are not severe, and a patient can live with the chronic condition in relative comfort. For example, someone with diabetes that is under control may have little difficulty with daily activities. But on occasion, the condition flares up, interrupting the patient's life and requiring medical attention. Some illnesses are progressive—the person becomes worse over time.

Chronic illnesses often have a severe impact on patients, such as restricting breathing or movement. They affect the activities of daily living. They also affect patients emotionally. Someone whose lifestyle is changed in important ways may be depressed, anxious about the future, or easily upset.

Caring for patients with chronic illnesses poses a challenge to health care workers. Your role is to help patients lead as full a life as possible. Remember that they may be trying to cope with a condition that never permits them to feel completely well. Most chronic diseases have national and local support groups to help patients and their families understand their conditions and how to deal with them effectively. Support groups are also available to health care workers who care for people with chronic illnesses. These groups can help you work through your own emotions and concerns in caring for chronically ill patients. **See Figure 23-1.**

Through technology and medical advancements, more and more people are living longer with many different diseases and illnesses. Nursing assistants care for many people with one or more chronic illnesses. The more you understand about chronic illness, the better you will be able to care for patients' physical and psychological needs. The goal is to help your patients be as independent as possible.

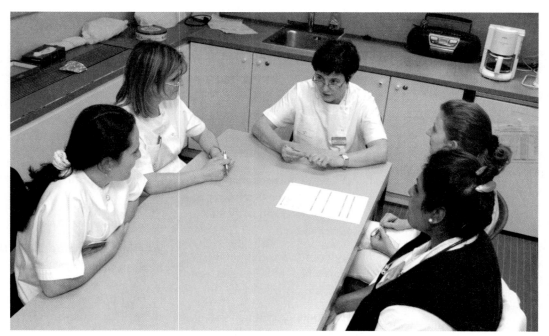

O **Figure 23-1.** Meeting with a support group can provide emotional support as well as technical information you may need about the disease.

Vital Skills — WRITING

Using Active Verbs

Generally, using the active form of verbs is a good way to improve your writing. While it isn't possible (or desirable) to make every verb active, your writing will be more direct, concise, and emphatic when you use active verbs.

How can you tell the active form from the passive? In an *active* sentence, the subject performs the action that the verb describes. In a *passive* sentence, the subject receives the action that the verb describes.

Read the following examples:

• I walked the dog.
• The dog was walked by me.

In the first sentence, the subject ("I") is doing the walking. It is an active sentence.

The second sentence is wordier and less direct.

Practice

Research a chronic illness and write a five-paragraph essay about it. Highlight each passive verb you used. See how many you can change to the active form. Save your research. You will use the same work for an oral presentation in the Vital Skills: Communication activity in this chapter.

Patients with Diabetes Mellitus

Diabetes mellitus (DM) is a disease of the endocrine system. It results when the body cannot change carbohydrates—starches and sugar—into energy. Normally, when carbohydrates are eaten and digested, the amount of sugar (glucose) in the blood rises. In reaction, the pancreas, a gland of the endocrine system, produces insulin. **Insulin** is a hormone the body uses to convert glucose into energy.

A person who has diabetes either does not produce enough insulin or is unable to use the insulin effectively. The excess glucose remains in the blood. This dangerous condition can cause the following signs and symptoms:

• Fatigue
• Weight loss
• Muscle cramps
• Blurred vision
• Polydipsia (excessive thirst)
• Polyphagia (excessive hunger)
• Polyuria (frequent urination)

If diabetes is not controlled, other complications may develop. These include damage to the kidneys and nerves. Changes in the retina can occur and may lead to blindness. Circulation may decrease, causing slow healing, increased fatigue, and pain and loss of sensation in the fingers and toes. Diabetes mellitus complications are the leading cause of blindness and of amputations not resulting from trauma.

Types of Diabetes Mellitus

There are two primary types of diabetes mellitus. Type 1 DM usually occurs abruptly in people under 30. It is also called *insulin-dependent diabetes* (formerly *juvenile-onset diabetes*). In this case, the pancreas does not produce enough insulin. Children and adults who have type 1 DM can become severely ill.

Type 2 DM usually occurs in middle age. It is also called *noninsulin-dependent diabetes* (formerly *adult-onset diabetes*). In this case, the pancreas does not produce enough insulin, or the body has enough insulin but the cells do not respond to the insulin properly. This is called *insulin resistance*. Type 2 DM is usually related to obesity or inactivity. Many people who have type 2 DM experience a gradual onset of the disease. They may be unaware of their condition for years. The disease may be discovered during a routine physical examination.

Controlling Diabetes

People with type 1 DM control the condition with insulin injections, diet, and exercise. Type 2 DM can be controlled by a combination of diet and exercise, oral medication, and sometimes insulin injections. The health care team, including the patient's doctor and a dietitian, provides education for the patient and family about diabetes and its treatment.

Diet and Exercise. Losing weight and balancing types of food are important in controlling diabetes. Some patients can control type 2 DM by weight reduction alone. Chapter 26 discusses food groupings and exchange lists that keep blood glucose levels in balance. Exercise is important for both losing weight and improving circulation.

Drugs. Treatment may also include medication. Some patients with type 2 DM may take oral drugs to keep levels of blood sugar low. The doctor decides whether the patient should also receive insulin. People who are unable to produce enough insulin will require delivery of insulin. Some long-term care residents receive insulin through injections, either from a nurse or by self-injection. Home health care clients may be able to administer their own insulin. **See Figure 23-2.**

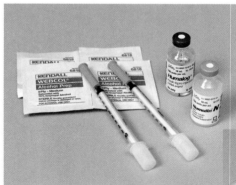

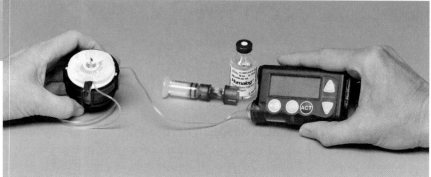

O **Figure 23-2. Insulin can be delivered using a syringe or an insulin pump.**

Vital Skills (MATH)

Percentage of Meals Eaten

Residents with diabetes must usually follow a special diet to help control their blood sugar. It is important that they eat at regular intervals and eat all of their food. Therefore, you may be asked to record the percentage of each meal a resident has eaten. To find a percentage, divide the amount the person ate by the original amount on the plate and then multiply by 100.

Example: Lunch includes 3 oz of meat, and the resident ate 2 oz.

$2 \div 3 = .66$

$.66 \times 100 = 66\%$ of the meat

Practice

The menu for a resident's lunch is shown in the first column of **Table A**. The amount the resident ate is shown in the second column. Copy the table to a separate sheet of paper and fill in the third column with the percentage of each food the resident ate.

○ Table A.

Lunch Item	Amount Eaten	Percent Eaten
4 oz broiled chicken	1 oz broiled chicken	?
1 cup broccoli	¾ cup broccoli	?
1 cup fruit	1 cup fruit	?
1 glass milk	½ glass milk	?
1 cup tea	¼ cup tea	?

Monitoring Glucose

A quick blood test using capillary blood from a finger stick may be done to test a patient's blood for glucose. This type of glucose testing is recommended by the American Diabetes Association (ADA). It is the accepted practice for hospital and long-term care, and home use. Testing is usually done four times a day, but the nurse will tell you when and how often to test. Nurses, nursing assistants, or patients themselves, especially those in home care, conduct the test once training has been achieved successfully. The blood test is more precise than a urine test, because the test measures the amount of glucose, not just whether it is present.

Pricking the patient's finger produces a drop of blood. The blood is then placed on a test strip and compared to a color chart. A meter can also be used to perform the color-match test. In this case, the test strip is fed into the meter and the test results are immediately available. Normal blood glucose should be between 70 to 110 mg/dl (milligrams to deciliters). However, it is not the nursing assistant's responsibility to interpret and make decisions once the results are obtained. The results of the glucose testing should always be reported to the nurse, whether they are within normal range or not.

Procedure 23-1

Testing Capillary Blood Glucose

Equipment: blood glucose meter • reagent strip • lancet or lancet injector • alcohol swabs • cotton balls • paper towels • disposable gloves

Note: Check with your facility to be sure this procedure is within the nursing assistant's scope of practice.

1. Identify the patient, check the ID bracelet, and call the patient by name.
2. Introduce yourself. Explain the procedure to the patient. Ask the patient to perform hand hygiene.
3. Wash your hands and put on gloves.
4. Provide privacy.
5. Position the patient in a semi-Fowler's or sitting position.
6. Lower the side rail, if appropriate.
7. Calibrate the meter and perform a control test following manufacturer's instructions. (Every manufacturer requires a control test to ensure accurate results.)
8. Prepare the lancet device, if appropriate.
9. Remove the reagent strip from the container and place it on the paper towel. Place the lid back on the container.
10. Select and prepare a finger for the puncture. The side of an adult's finger is the preferred site instead of the center portion of the finger.
11. Massage the base of the finger gently to increase blood flow to fingertip.
12. Clean the side of the selected finger with an alcohol swab and allow the site to dry completely.
13. Remove the cover from the lancet.
14. Place the lancet against the side of the finger and activate the needle, puncturing the skin. **See Figure 23-3.**
15. Wipe the first drop of blood with the cotton ball.
16. Gently squeeze the finger to produce a large drop of blood.
17. Holding the test strip, touch the reagent strip to the drop of blood on the test pad or tip, depending on the manufacturer's instructions.
18. Measure the blood glucose by either inserting the reagent strip into the meter or pressing the timer. Wait the designated time for the glucose meter to indicate that the reagent strip should be placed in the meter. (Refer to the manufacturer's directions for specifics of this step.)
19. Read glucose results on the meter display. (Monitors will vary.) **See Figure 23-4.**
20. Turn the meter off.
21. Dispose of the strip and lancet in an appropriate receptacle.
22. Remove gloves and properly dispose of them.
23. Report the following to your supervisor:
    • That the test is complete
    • Your findings
    • Any unusual observations

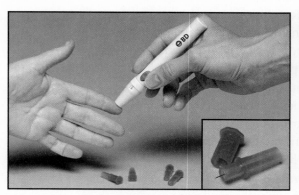

○ **Figure 23-3.** Puncture the skin with the lancet to draw blood.

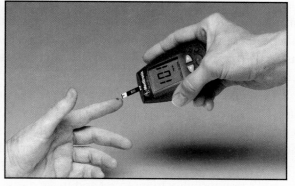

○ **Figure 23-4.** Read the results on the meter display.

Hypoglycemia. A condition called **hypoglycemia** occurs when the blood glucose level is abnormally low. This may occur if a patient has skipped a meal or taken too much insulin. Hypoglycemia can cause dizziness, weakness, shakiness, a feeling of hunger, headaches, trembling, slurred speech, blurred vision, confusion, disorientation, and cool, clammy skin. It can also contribute to infections or poor healing. *Tachycardia* (rapid heart beat) and *tachypnea* (rapid respirations) may occur. Report any or all of these signs and symptoms immediately to the nurse.

Blood glucose testing will confirm low blood sugar or no sugar in the bloodstream. When a patient who is alert and awake experiences hypoglycemia, give 4 to 6 ounces of orange juice, 2 packets of sugar, several pieces of hard candy, or 1 tablespoon of honey or grape jelly. This may provide enough sugar to raise the blood glucose level.

In a severe condition of hypoglycemia, a diabetic patient may go into hypoglycemic or *insulin shock* and have a seizure. The patient could also go into a *diabetic coma*, a state of unconsciousness resulting from extremely low or extremely high blood glucose levels. It is a serious and potentially fatal condition. Call for help or call 9-1-1. The doctor, nurse, or emergency personnel will treat an unconscious patient with a medication administered intravenously to quickly raise the blood sugar level.

Hyperglycemia. A condition called **hyperglycemia** occurs when the blood glucose level is abnormally high. This condition may occur when a patient with diabetes has forgotten to take medication, is injured, dehydrated, or ill with an infection and fever. The patient may be confused, tired, or groggy and have hot, dry skin or low blood pressure. Respirations may become very deep. A sweet or fruity smelling mouth odor may be detected. Blood glucose testing will verify high sugar levels. If the glucose imbalance is not treated, diabetic coma can occur. If you observe any of these signs in a patient, tell your supervisor immediately. In this case, coma is treated with insulin administered with an IV and with the delivery of fluids to the system.

Special Care. A nursing assistant can assist patients with diabetes in the following ways to help control the condition and prevent the onset of hypoglycemia or hyperglycemia.

- Monitor the diet. Diabetic patients must follow a special diet recommended by the ADA. Report a change in appetite, an inability to eat a meal, and uneaten food. Be sure the patient eats only what is ordered and limits sugar intake. Make sure meals and snacks are served on time. These patients should never skip meals.
- Make sure patients take medications as ordered.
- Report changes in exercise, complaints of pain, or mood changes and changes in mental status. The doctor may need to alter the insulin dosage to compensate for these changes.
- Observe for signs and symptoms of hypoglycemia or hyperglycemia. Especially in home health care, you should be ready to assist by providing a conscious patient with some type of easily consumed sugar. Follow your facility's procedure for diabetic emergencies and report the situation immediately to the supervisor.

Special Care for Circulation Problems

Poor circulation can result in the loss of sensation in fingers and toes, and in slow healing. For people with diabetes mellitus, small cuts and bruises can become major problems. Because of numbness, they may not be aware of injury to their feet and hands. Once damaged, skin is slow to heal. **See Figure 23-5.** If blood cannot reach an extremity, the patient may develop **gangrene** (death of tissue, usually caused by poor blood circulation). **See Figure 23-6.** The diseased area may have to be *amputated*, or surgically removed. To minimize risk, follow these special care requirements for patients with diabetes:

- Protect the patient from scrapes and cuts. Patients should always wear shoes, but they should also avoid tight socks, garters, or hose. Examine the feet daily, watching for bruises, red spots, or breaks in the skin.
- Avoid skin problems by keeping the patient's skin dry and clean. Pat skin dry rather than rubbing it after bathing, and use skin lotion to soften dry areas. Make sure to dry the area between the toes.
- Avoid hot baths or heating pads. Patients with impaired circulation and sensation cannot feel heat and are at great risk for burns.
- Monitor feet and toenails. When the patient's toenails need to be cut, tell your supervisor. Only a licensed health care provider can provide nail care for patients with diabetes.
- Keep clothing and bed linens loose to allow for good circulation.
- Encourage exercise to improve circulation.

Patients with Cardiovascular Disease

Cardiovascular disease includes chronic problems of the circulatory system. These problems may occur in the heart muscle or the blood vessels or both. Cardiovascular disease is the leading cause of death in the United States. Those at risk for developing cardiovascular disease include the elderly (men until age 60, and then the risk is equal between men and women), African-Americans, and people who smoke. Also at risk are people with hypertension, high cholesterol, obesity, inactivity, stress, or a family history of heart disease.

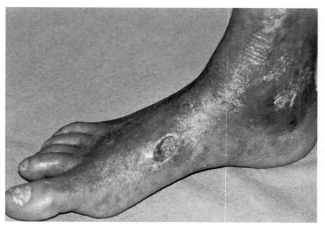

○ **Figure 23-5.** A patient with diabetes may have sores, particularly on the feet and legs, that do not heal well due to poor blood circulation.

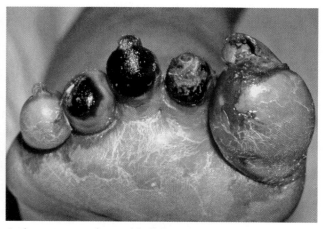

○ **Figure 23-6.** Patients with diabetes are at risk for developing gangrene in the extremities, which can require amputation.

Hypertension

Patients with hypertension (abnormally high blood pressure) may not be aware of their condition until blood pressure is measured. Hypertension is a risk factor for many other diseases, including coronary artery disease, congestive heart failure, stroke, and kidney failure. As a result, medications may be ordered to lower the blood pressure. Lifestyle changes are often needed, too. For example, exercising, reducing stress, reducing weight, reducing the amount of salt in the diet, and not smoking can help lower blood pressure.

Atherosclerosis

Atherosclerosis is a condition in which fat deposits build up on the inner walls of blood vessels. Blood vessels may become totally blocked, which impedes the flow of blood and oxygen to the body's systems. If blockage occurs in the coronary arteries, the person is at risk for coronary artery disease, such as angina pectoris. Some patients may undergo surgical treatment to reopen arteries. Risk factors include high cholesterol, diabetes mellitus, hypertension, sedentary or stressful lifestyle, and obesity. Treating and controlling these factors is necessary to avoid further disease.

Angina Pectoris

Severe pain or pressure in the chest caused by reduced blood flow and an inadequate oxygen supply to the heart muscle is called **angina pectoris**. Some patients feel referred pain in other areas, such as the neck, jaw, shoulders, or arms, typically on the left side. Attacks generally occur after increased exertion, a very large meal, cold weather exposure, or stress. During an attack, a patient may feel faint or nauseated or may perspire or vomit. With rest, the pain may subside in a few minutes.

The drug nitroglycerin relieves the pain of an angina attack. Many patients in long-term care facilities or home care administer their own nitroglycerin and keep track of their dosage. In other cases, the nurse in charge administers a tablet or a spray, which is delivered under the tongue. The expiration date of tablets should be checked regularly, because the drug loses strength over time.

The goal of caregivers is to help the patient with angina pectoris to be as independent as possible while avoiding painful attacks. Remind patients to relax and breathe slowly when they feel chest pain. Make sure patients always keep their nitroglycerin nearby.

Congestive Heart Failure

The condition known as **congestive heart failure (CHF)** is the heart's inability to pump effectively, which can result in a buildup of excess fluid in the lungs. Blood flow to the heart is insufficient. Blood pressure may rise, and the patient may have a buildup (congestion) of fluid. CHF is often the result of hypertension or a previous heart attack.

When the congestion is on the left side of the heart, fluid backs up in the lungs and respiratory congestion occurs. When the congestion is on the right side of the heart, *edema*, or swelling, occurs in the feet and ankles, neck veins bulge, and liver function decreases. **See Figure 23-7.**

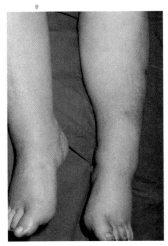

○ **Figure 23-7.** Congestive heart failure, which causes edema, can result in life-threatening complications.

With this condition, various organs do not receive enough oxygen from the blood. For example, the kidneys may react by removing fewer wastes. Too little blood to the brain causes dizziness or confusion. When CHF goes undetected or untreated, the patient can develop *pulmonary edema*, a potentially fatal condition in which the lungs fill with fluid.

CHF is often a condition of the elderly, so long-term care patients may need help with breathing and controlling fluids. A number of drugs are used to strengthen the heart and reduce fluid buildup. More frequent urination is a side effect of these medications. You may be asked to measure and record patient intake and output daily to make sure fluids are being removed. You should also offer toileting assistance frequently. Report leg and finger cramping to the supervisor. Cramping may indicate an electrolyte imbalance that needs to be carefully monitored. In addition, you can make patients more comfortable by:

- Providing rest periods often as you help with daily activities. CHF patients become tired after little effort, even eating a meal or washing up.
- Helping patients sit in a Fowler's position with the feet and legs elevated.
- Helping patients sleep in a Fowler's position or with pillows supporting the head and back, and legs elevated.

Myocardial Infarction

After a patient recovers from myocardial infarction (heart attack), rehabilitation begins. Gradually, patients who are otherwise healthy often become active again. Medications and other treatments help the patient avoid another heart attack. Therapies often include lifestyle changes, such as an exercise program, stress reduction program, and dietary adjustments.

When providing care for patients with chronic heart disease, however, be alert for the signs of myocardial infarction. When a patient's heart is weakened by chronic disease, heart attack is a constant threat. Be sure you know these signs and symptoms:

- Persistent chest pain described as crushing or stabbing
- Pain radiating to the left arm, hand, shoulder, neck, jaw, or back
- Difficulty breathing
- Nausea and vomiting
- Profuse sweating
- Anxious feelings

If you think a patient is having a heart attack, get help immediately. If you are caring for a client at home, activate the emergency medical system by calling 9-1-1.

Special Care Requirements

Generally, when caring for patients with cardiovascular disease, the nursing assistant provides care that focuses on circulation and fluid status. Actions for care include:

- Accurate measurement of fluid intake and output.
- Frequent and accurate measurement of vital signs.
- Daily or weekly measurement of weight.
- Application and removal of antiembolic stockings to facilitate circulation in the legs.
- Careful and frequent skin care.
- Assistance with prescribed diet and fluid restrictions if appropriate.

Patients with Respiratory Disorders

The most frequently occurring respiratory disorders are in a category called **chronic obstructive pulmonary disease (COPD)**. COPD is a group of chronic, progressive lung diseases characterized by airway obstruction and a loss of elasticity of the lungs. Examples of COPD are emphysema, chronic bronchitis, and asthma.

Emphysema and Chronic Bronchitis

Emphysema is a condition in which the air spaces in the lungs become enlarged and overinflated, resulting in the loss of elasticity. Bronchitis is inflammation of the bronchial airway's mucous membranes. **Chronic bronchitis** is inflammation in the lungs, with increased mucus production and a chronic productive cough that is present for at least three months in two successive years. A chronic productive cough is one that produces sputum. Chronic bronchitis often accompanies emphysema.

Cigarette smoking is the most common cause of emphysema and chronic bronchitis in older adults. Years of constant irritation to the lungs results in an increase in the production of mucus and stiffness of the airways. As the disease progresses, air gradually becomes trapped within the lungs. This causes a buildup of carbon dioxide and a decrease in oxygen levels.

Nursing assistants should observe for the following signs and symptoms of respiratory distress in patients with emphysema or chronic bronchitis:
- Shallow, rapid respirations with a longer expiration than inspiration
- Increased pulse and blood pressure
- Pursed lip breathing
- Pale or cyanotic skin, particularly around the lips and mouth
- Fever with acute flare-ups
- Cough with or without sputum production
- *Orthopnea* (inability to breathe easily unless sitting or standing)
- Restlessness and anxiety or a decrease in the level of consciousness

Asthma

Asthma is a respiratory disease caused by narrowing and inflammation of the airways in response to triggers (such as allergens, fumes, or chemical exposures). It begins as an acute disease. If it progresses over time, however, it is categorized as a chronic lung condition. Typical signs and symptoms of asthma include shortness of breath, wheezing, increased pulse and blood pressure, and chest tightness.

Treatments

Many patients with respiratory diseases administer their own medications if they begin to have difficulty breathing. *Bronchodilators* are medications that act to dilate or relax the muscles in the upper airways of the lungs. They help patients breathe more easily. Bronchodilators are delivered in a variety of forms, including inhalers and nebulizers.

An *inhaler* is a small, handheld device used to deliver inhaled medications. A *nebulizer* is a device that mixes humidified air with medication to create a mist or spray. The patient uses a mouthpiece to inhale the medication. **See Figure 23-8.** Both devices deliver medications quickly to ease breathing difficulty.

Many patients with COPD require oxygen therapy at least some of the time. Some use oxygen continually. Become familiar with the kind of oxygen device and the amount of oxygen your patients need. Increasing the flow rate of oxygen can be dangerous to patients with COPD. It can eliminate the drive to breathe on their own. This can result in *apnea*, or the absence of breathing. Most patients receive oxygen via a nasal cannula at low flow rates of 0.5 to 2 liters to prevent this complication.

Special Care Requirements

Respiratory disease can cause frequent episodes of anxiety in patients. Not being able to breathe is frightening. Patients may feel panic. Remain calm and act fast when a patient experiences problems with the airway or breathing.

When caring for patients with a chronic respiratory disease, assist the patient in the following ways:

- Provide or assist with frequent oral hygiene to keep mucous membranes moist and healthy.
- Encourage adequate fluid intake to make it easier for the patient to cough up sputum. Properly dispose of sputum that is coughed up.
- Observe for changes in sputum, such as color, consistency, and amount. Report these changes to the nurse immediately. They could be signs of pneumonia, a common complication of COPD. *Pneumonia* is an acute infection of the lungs, usually treated with antibiotics.
- Assist with frequent handwashing if the patient is coughing up sputum.
- Position patients by elevating the head of the bed or sitting them up in a chair when possible to allow for full expansion of the lungs.

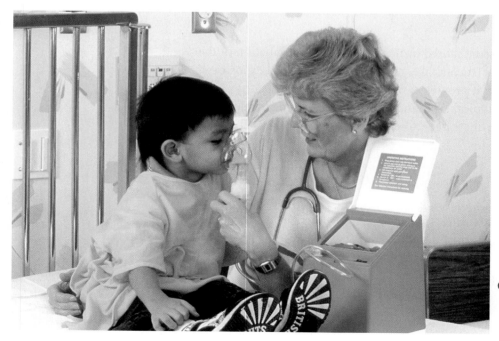

○ **Figure 23-8.** A nebulizer can be used to administer medication to patients to help with breathing difficulties.

- Clean skin around the patient's oxygen mask or cannula two to three times per day. Observe for redness or signs of skin breakdown.
- Allow plenty of time at meals, because these patients may get very tired while eating.
- Encourage exercise combined with adequate rest periods to avoid extreme fatigue and to prevent increased respiratory distress.
- Be supportive when anxiety levels increase.
- Report signs of respiratory distress immediately.
- Wash hands frequently.

Vital Skills   READING

Identifying New Words

In your reading, you may come across words you can't identify. Before you reach for a dictionary, try these strategies for identifying new words.

- Look for a *prefix* at the beginning of the word. For example, the word *intravenous* contains the prefix *intra-*, which means "within."
- Look for a suffix at the end of the word.
- Look for the root word.
- Look for context clues. Can you figure out the word's meaning by looking at the words around it?
- If you can't determine the meaning of the word, look it up in a dictionary.

  For example, can you figure out the meaning of the italicized word in the following sentence, using the above strategies?

  Mrs. Corinthos was *incapacitated* after her severe fall.

- The root of the word is *capacitate*, as in "capacity." It means "having the ability to do a task; to perform or produce."

- You have seen the prefix *in-* used before: *inability, intolerable*. It means "non" or "not."
- You can deduce from the context that being incapacitated is probably not a positive thing, since it happened as the result of a severe fall.
- So you can deduce that *incapacitated* means "not having the capacity or ability to perform."

Practice

Identify the italicized words below using the strategies provided.

1. Mrs. Wilson's total *parenteral* nutrition arrived from the pharmacy and is in the refrigerator.
2. The pathology report said her infection was caused by an *anaerobic* bacterium.
3. To cut down on the risk of infection, use an *antiseptic* soap when you wash your hands.
4. She is scheduled for a *bronchoscopy* later today.
5. After her surgery, she will need to have a *nasogastric tube* in place for three days.

Patients with Neurological Disorders

Neurological disorders affect the functioning of the brain, the spinal cord, or the peripheral nervous system. Damage to these areas can affect sensation, mobility, muscular control, coordination, balance, speech, vision, hearing, and cognitive ability. Patients may also experience great pain. Many patients need assistance or retraining in ADLs, as well as other types of rehabilitation.

Stroke

A **stroke**, also known as a **cerebrovascular accident (CVA)**, is a sudden interruption in the blood supply to the brain. It causes a sudden loss of neurological functioning. A stroke can be caused by:

- A blood clot blocking the flow of blood in a vessel.
- A blood vessel bursting in the brain.
- Cerebral hemorrhaging.

Symptoms of a stroke are weakness, loss of sensation or paralysis on one side of the body, headache, loss of hearing, poor vision, confusion, and disorientation.

Although they can happen to people of any age, strokes are more common in the elderly. Risk factors include high cholesterol levels, hypertension, diabetes mellitus, smoking, and stress.

A stroke usually results in brain damage due to the death of brain cells. The patient may have reduced functioning on the side opposite the brain damage. Damage to the left side of the brain may affect language abilities. Patients who have had a stroke may experience **aphasia**, the inability or impaired ability to communicate through speech, writing, or signs. A patient who understands the spoken word but cannot speak coherently has *expressive aphasia*. A patient who cannot speak or understand what is said has *receptive aphasia*.

Right-side brain damage may cause problems with thinking and memory loss. Communicating with a person who has suffered a stroke can be challenging for the caregiver as well as the patient and family.

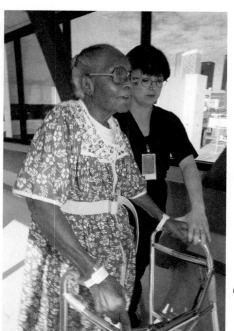

Some patients experience a **transient ischemic attack (TIA)**, also called a ministroke. These small strokes temporarily reduce blood flow to the brain but result in less damage than a stroke. However, repeated TIAs may lead to the loss of mental functioning, coordination, and muscle strength. **See Figure 23-9.** A TIA may indicate that a patient is at risk for a stroke. Thus, a TIA may alert those who provide medical care to take steps that will help the patient avoid having a stroke.

○ **Figure 23-9.** A resident who has had several TIAs may use a walker. Always stay close to such a resident to help in case of sudden weakness or falling.

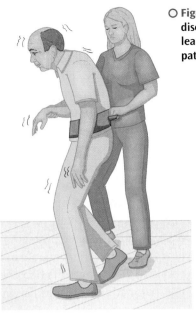

○ **Figure 23-10.** Patients with Parkinson's disease develop a shuffling gait and may lean forward when walking. Assist the patient to prevent falling.

Patients who have suffered a stroke may be faced with a great many challenges as they adapt to physical, mental, emotional, cognitive, and social changes. Symptoms of a stroke may be permanent. This may require extensive rehabilitation to help the person achieve the highest possible level of functioning.

A stroke is a medical emergency followed by a long, frustrating recovery period. To help CVA patients, first analyze how they have been affected. For example, think about which limbs are paralyzed and which ADLs have become most difficult. The care that is planned should assist with these problems. Patients should use their unaffected muscles to exercise the affected ones as much as possible.

Parkinson's Disease

Parkinson's disease is a progressive disease that affects the part of the brain that handles muscular control and function. Movements are slowed down, tremors develop, and muscles become stiff and rigid. Patients eventually lose the ability to control muscle movements. There is no cure for the disease, although there are drugs that may slow its progression and reduce symptoms. Parkinson's usually affects people over age 65.

These patients do not lose their mental abilities. It is important to keep that in mind when working with Parkinson's patients, because you may see them become depressed by the continuing loss of muscle control. Some will seek out counseling to help them cope with their physical limitations. Be sensitive to the feelings patients may have about their physical problems.

Patients with Parkinson's disease develop tremors or rigidity, poor posture, and a shuffling walk. **See Figure 23-10.** They may fall often. Lack of mobility may lead to constipation. They may drool and have great difficulty in eating, swallowing, and talking. Facial expressions may appear masklike, or frozen. Emotionally, they may be depressed or easily upset.

Loss of control over movements can be helped by focusing on safety, good nutrition, mobility, and medications. Remind the patient to try to remain calm and not to hurry, because tremors may increase when the patient is nervous or upset.

FOCUS ON

Attitude

The attitude of patients with chronic illness can make a difference in how quickly and successfully they adjust to physical and psychological changes. Caregivers can help patients maintain a positive outlook. For example, a patient who has had a stroke may appreciate words of encouragement and be able to work harder to achieve rehabilitation goals.

Multiple Sclerosis

Multiple sclerosis (MS) is a progressive disease of the nervous system that affects how nerve impulses are sent to and from the brain. The cause of the disease is not yet known, and there is no cure. The onset of the disease is gradual. Most people with MS experience their first symptoms between the ages of 20 and 40. Some people experience a slow, gradual decline over many years. Others have periods of remission in which symptoms lessen or disappear. Then symptoms will suddenly reappear and be more severe. Over time, the patient's condition usually declines, and additional care is needed.

Symptoms of MS include problems with motor function and loss of feeling in the extremities, such as weakness, numbness, and tingling. Painful muscle spasms that limit movement may become a part of daily life. As the disease progresses, the patient may begin to have gait and balance problems that require assistive devices, such as crutches or a walker. In time, patients may lose function of the legs, requiring use of a wheelchair. Some patients become partially or totally paralyzed. Blurred or double vision, dizziness, and ringing in the ears can be symptoms seen in this disease. Some patients lose their vision or hearing. Some have swallowing disorders.

Bowel and bladder function are usually affected. Patients may experience constipation. Laxatives or increased fiber may be prescribed by the doctor to minimize constipation. Bowel and bladder incontinence are common as the disease progresses. When keeping the patient clean and maintaining skin integrity become difficult, a doctor may order the insertion of an indwelling catheter.

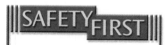

Many patients with neurological disorders are at risk for burns because they have lost sensation. Test food, beverages, bathwater, and warm applications for proper temperature when providing assistance.

Paralysis

Paralysis is the loss of voluntary muscle movement. It can affect one limb, one area of the body, or the whole body. A patient with *hemiplegia* is paralyzed on one side of the body. This condition is usually the result of a stroke. The patient is unable to move body parts on the affected side and loses the ability to feel heat, cold, pressure, and pain on that side. If the patient's face is affected, one eyelid may droop or one eye may not close. The eye can become dry and irritated because of the lack of tears. The patient is at risk for choking, because one side of the mouth does not move while chewing. Additionally, the patient may drool if one side of the mouth does not close. The patient is also at risk for burns, since the skin is not sensitive to temperature on the paralyzed side.

A patient with *paraplegia* is paralyzed from the waist down. This condition is usually the result of a spinal cord injury, such as from a car accident or a fall. These patients are prone to pressure sores, so good skin care and frequent repositioning are essential. They are also at risk for urinary tract infections. Since the lower part of the body has no sensation, particular attention must be paid to the elimination needs.

A patient with *quadriplegia* is paralyzed from the neck area down, though some quadriplegics have partial use of their upper extremities. **See Figure 23-11.** Quadriplegia is usually the result of a high spinal cord injury. These patients need assistance with all ADLs. They are at risk for respiratory and urinary tract infections and for pressure sores.

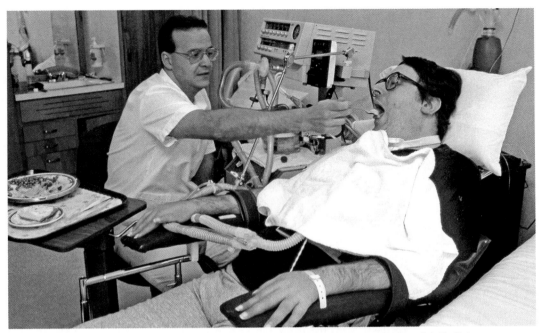

○ **Figure 23-11.** Some patients with quadriplegia need assistance with all activities of daily living.

Special Care Requirements

For all patients with neurological disorders, special care requires the nursing assistant's patience and encouragement. You can help patients in the following ways:

- Keep the patient comfortable and position the patient in correct body alignment. Support paralyzed limbs in bed. Reposition the patient as ordered, at least every two hours. Include small shifts of weight to help prevent pressure sores.
- Exercise should be encouraged whenever possible to minimize muscle atrophy and contractures and minimize constipation. Help the patient exercise according to the doctor's or physical therapist's orders, including ROM exercises.
- Encourage the patient to rest to avoid becoming overtired.
- Maintain a safe environment to protect the patient from injury. Provide safety from falling. Use side rails if ordered.
- Assist with the patient's diet to ensure good nutrition and provide plenty of fluids. Some patients may have swallowing disorders. To prevent choking, encourage small bites and slow and thorough chewing. Make sure that no food is left in the mouth after eating. Be especially observant during meals if the patient's face has been affected. If sensation has been lost on one side, place food on the unaffected side and at the back of the mouth.
- Assist the patient with all ADLs as necessary, including personal hygiene and elimination. Assist with bladder and bowel retraining and catheter care, if necessary. A diet high in fluids and fiber promotes regular bowel movement.
- Encourage the patient to be as independent as possible. Arrange the room so the patient can easily reach needed items. Include the patient in all decisions concerning care.
- Encourage the patient to use assistive devices to help with ADLs.
- Provide emotional support and encouragement. Be sensitive to the feelings patients may have about their physical problems.

Communication

Many patients with neurological disorders have difficulty communicating. Some have aphasia. Some have problems with motor skills, making it hard to write. Patients with cognitive damage may be unable to understand what is being said. To promote independence and minimize frustration for the patient, the following communication approaches should be used:

• Treat patients with respect at all times.
• Be patient and encourage patients to take their time when communicating.
• Use a normal tone when speaking.
• Pay close attention to the patient when communicating. Actively listen to the patient.
• Familiarize yourself with the patient's speech if possible.
• Do not pretend you understand the patient if you do not. Instead, try to clarify the message using other methods.
• Pay particular attention to the patient's body language.
• Use gestures to point or show the patient what you are saying.
• Provide alternative communication methods such as a white board, pictures, or flash cards for those who no longer have the motor coordination skills to write. Provide pencil and paper, a chalkboard, a picture board, an electronic talking device, or a personal computer for patients who have difficulty speaking. **See Figure 23-12.**

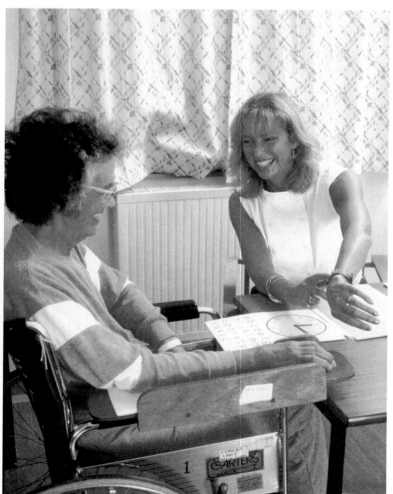

Patients with Cancer

Cancer is a malignant (harmful), uncontrolled growth of abnormal cells. Cancer generally invades healthy tissue and stops normal body functioning. This can occur in any part of the body. If the cancer cells are not controlled, they spread and move to other parts of the body. The most common cancers occur in the lungs, colon, rectum, prostate, breast, and uterus. Cancer can eventually cause death.

○ **Figure 23-12. Some patients with aphasia can communicate by using a picture board.**

Cancer Treatment

There are three general types of treatment for cancer. One type of treatment or a combination may be used, depending on the kind and location of the cancer and other factors such as the overall health of the patient.

- Surgery may be performed to remove a cancerous tumor. Surgery is often followed by radiation therapy or chemotherapy to prevent the cancer from spreading or growing again.
- **Radiation therapy** is a therapy that uses x-rays to destroy cancer cells.
- **Chemotherapy** is a therapy that uses drugs to destroy or slow the growth of cancer cells.

Both types of therapy have drawbacks. Radiation therapy causes discomfort, because the skin may be burned in the area of the treatment. Chemotherapy is hard to apply to cancer cells without damaging healthy cells at the same time. Patients can experience severe side effects from both treatments, including hair loss, loss of appetite, loss of vision or hearing, weight loss, nausea, vomiting, and diarrhea.

A typical symptom of cancer is pain. Although pain may not be pronounced at the outset, it can become severe as the disease advances. Drugs, often very powerful, are used to help patients endure their pain. These drugs may have side effects, such as constipation.

Special Care Requirements

The care of patients with cancer varies, depending on the type of cancer and the treatment provided. However, all care includes the following:

- Closely observing the patient's condition. Report any change immediately. Treatment may need to be changed to control pain or other side effects.
- Listening supportively to the patient, family, and friends. A diagnosis of cancer is very difficult for patients and their loved ones. It may cause denial, anger, fear, and anxiety. Patients must be given time to verbalize their feelings about this diagnosis. Many people believe that a hopeful, positive attitude helps patients heal. Kindness and support are valuable allies during the treatment process.
- Controlling infection. The usual treatments for cancer make a person more vulnerable to infection. Follow strict handwashing guidelines and standard precautions against infection.
- Encouraging rest. Some therapies last a long time. A patient may receive chemotherapy over the course of many weeks, for example. Patients need strength to combat the cancer and endure treatment.
- Encouraging good nutrition. Treatment often decreases the appetite of cancer patients, yet they need proper food to heal and maintain their strength. Make mealtimes as appetizing as possible. Provide smaller, more frequent meals and snacks. Radiation sometimes causes a metallic taste. Using a baking-soda mouthwash 15 minutes before eating can reduce the taste and improve the patient's appetite.
- Encouraging frequent oral hygiene and adequate fluids. This will keep mucous membranes moist and the mouth feeling fresh.
- Keeping skin and perineal areas clean and dry. Proper care minimizes discomfort and infection.
- Responding to ongoing needs. Keep the signal cord within easy reach and answer the call signal promptly.

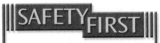

Because patients with cancer are extremely vulnerable to infection, they may be cared for in isolation rooms to protect them. Caregivers and visitors, if allowed, must always follow isolation precautions.

Patients with AIDS

Acquired immunodeficiency syndrome (AIDS) attacks the immune system and affects the body's ability to fight other diseases. AIDS is a syndrome, not a single disease. A **syndrome** is a group of signs and symptoms that occur together. The patient usually dies from infections the body cannot withstand.

People can develop AIDS after exposure to the **human immunodeficiency virus (HIV)**. HIV may be transmitted sexually, by contaminated needles and syringes, or by infected mothers to their babies. The body fluids and blood of the infected person carry the virus. The virus is not transmitted by sweat; by casual (nonsexual) touching such as holding hands, hugging, or giving a back rub; or from a drinking fountain. It can be transmitted only when infected blood or body fluids come in contact with another person's blood or mucous membranes.

Some people develop AIDS soon after infection with HIV. Others may not show signs of AIDS for many years. The only way to know if someone is infected with HIV is by performing a blood test. The virus always remains in the bloodstream.

Currently, there is no cure for AIDS. However, drugs are available to prevent a patient who is infected with HIV from developing AIDS. Patients must be made as comfortable as possible. Health care workers must also be comfortable and safe. When providing treatment that involves possible contact with blood or any body fluids, always follow standard precautions.

Symptoms of AIDS

People with AIDS have some or all of these signs and symptoms:

- Appetite and weight loss
- Fever
- Night sweats
- Diarrhea
- Weakness
- Skin rashes or purple blotches
- Swollen glands
- White spots in the mouth
- Dry cough

These symptoms are the result of the AIDS patient's damaged immune system. Patients with AIDS are unable to fight off microorganisms. Healthy people can fight these microorganisms, but they cause infections in patients with AIDS. As these infections worsen, patients with AIDS may develop pneumonia, Kaposi's sarcoma (a rare type of skin cancer), HIV wasting syndrome (loss of 10 percent or more of body weight in a short time), and other conditions, such as memory loss, paralysis, or mental disorders.

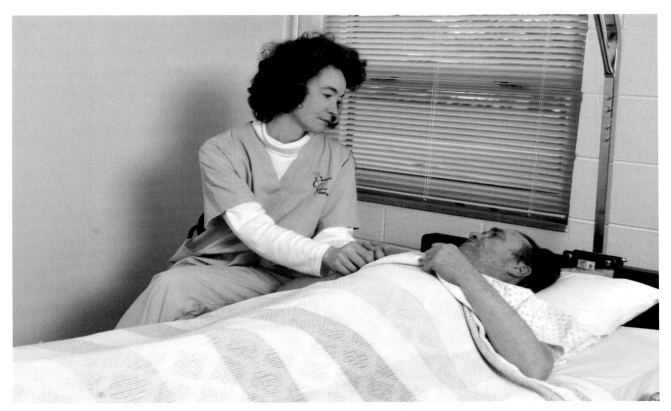

○ Figure 23-13. Many patients with AIDS feel alone and unsupported. The nursing assistant can provide emotional care as well as physical care to help these patients.

Special Care Requirements

AIDS signs and symptoms may change over time. When you care for patients with AIDS, you must observe and react to these changing conditions. Also, because AIDS is a transmittable, incurable syndrome, patients with AIDS are often isolated from their families or friends. The warm support of caregivers is important.

• Convey your concern for patients by showing respect and compassion. Listen to patients' concerns and worries. Provide emotional care by being trustworthy, positive, and dependable. **See Figure 23-13.**

• Control infection as you would with any communicable illness. Do not spread infections that could harm the patient, such as cold, chicken pox, or flu. Wash your hands frequently and handle food correctly. Remind family members and friends to follow these guidelines.

• When patients have lost weight and are bedridden for long periods, their position in bed should be changed often. Take special care of the patient's skin condition to avoid pressure sores. Maintain the patient's mobility as much as you can. Assist with ROM exercises as instructed.

• Follow normal care guidelines (remembering standard precautions) for conditions such as fever, diarrhea, mouth infection, muscle loss, mental difficulties, and chronic fatigue.

• Take extra care to ensure the patient's right to confidentiality.

Patients with Kidney Failure

Kidney failure, also called *renal failure*, is a chronic condition that involves gradual, progressive, and irreversible damage to the kidneys. It may result from a disease, an injury, or a chronic illness such as diabetes mellitus or hypertension. When a patient has kidney failure, the urinary system is no longer able to remove wastes from the body. A buildup of body wastes begins to involve many other body systems. This can quickly lead to death if not treated.

Symptoms of Kidney Failure

As waste products build up in the body, patients may have any of these signs or symptoms:
- Fatigue and weakness
- Vomiting or nausea
- Hypertension
- Muscle cramps
- Weight loss, especially from muscle mass
- Severely dry, itching skin
- An ammonia smell to the skin

People who have kidney failure often need to have kidney dialysis or a kidney transplant. **Kidney dialysis** is a process in which a machine is attached to a patient's circulatory system, by a catheter or some other device, to remove waste products from the blood. **See Figure 23-14.** There are two types of dialysis. One requires the injection of a cleansing solution through a permanent catheter inserted into the peritoneal space. The other requires the patient to have a permanent shunt in the arm or ankle that is periodically attached to a cleansing machine.

A kidney transplant is a surgery that replaces a nonfunctioning or diseased kidney with a healthy, donated kidney. Patients who have received a transplanted kidney must take drugs that suppress the immune system, so the body will not reject the new kidney. They are at high risk for infectious diseases.

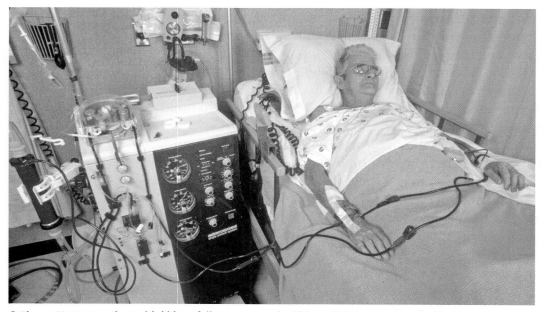

○ **Figure 23-14. A patient with kidney failure may require kidney dialysis to remove bodily wastes.**

Special Care Requirements

Patients with kidney failure often have many dietary restrictions, including the limiting of proteins. They experience extreme fatigue. Nursing assistants can provide the following care for these patients:

- Encourage plenty of rest.
- Accurately monitor all food and fluid intake. The amount of fluid patients can safely drink in a day is usually limited.
- Provide elimination assistance. Most patients on dialysis can no longer urinate normally.
- Keep the areas around permanent catheters or shunts used for the exchange of fluids clean and free of infection. These areas are checked by trained personnel for continuous and proper operation.

Vital Skills   COMMUNICATION

Giving an Oral Presentation

Your education won't end when you become a nursing assistant. Many hospitals provide continuing education and training while you are on the job. As part of that education, you may be called on to give an oral presentation.

An oral presentation does not mean that you simply read a paper to an audience. In an effective oral presentation, you speak to the audience, sharing what you know about a subject in an interesting manner.

The following guidelines can help you make an effective oral presentation:

- Be prepared. The better you know the subject matter, the more confidently you can talk about it.
- Organize your material. You can start your talk by giving a brief rundown of the topics you will cover. For example: "In this talk, I'll explain what type 2 diabetes is, who is affected, what the symptoms are, and the consequences the disease can have on a person's health."
- Make eye contact to keep the audience interested and engaged in what you are saying.
- Use visual aids, but keep them simple. Visual aids should supplement what you have to say, not serve as a replacement.
- Use a little humor. It's a good way to keep your presentation lively.
- Slow down! Some people talk faster when they get nervous. Remember to speak slowly.
- Vary your voice—don't speak in a monotone.
- Practice your presentation. Make sure it fits in the allotted time frame.
- Be confident. It may be easier said than done, but practice helps build confidence.

Practice

Prepare a five-minute oral presentation on the chronic illness you wrote about in the Vital Skills: Writing assignment in this chapter. Take turns making presentations to the class.

Chapter Summary

- Chronic illnesses cause symptoms that make daily activities difficult. Chronically ill patients often require special types of care from health care workers, family, friends, and support groups.

- Understanding the causes and symptoms of chronic illnesses helps the nursing assistant better understand how to care for patients.

- Nursing assistants provide care for patients with diabetes mellitus that includes helping them control the disease, monitor blood glucose levels, and prevent complications of poor blood circulation.

- Nursing assistants provide special care, including emotional and supportive care, to patients with chronic illness based on the nature and symptoms of the condition.

VOCABULARY REVIEW

Directions: Match the letter of each definition in the second column with the correct vocabulary term in the first column. Write your answers on a separate sheet of paper.

Vocabulary

1. angina pectoris
2. aphasia
3. asthma
4. atherosclerosis
5. cancer
6. chronic bronchitis
7. chronic obstructive pulmonary disease
8. congestive heart failure
9. emphysema
10. hyperglycemia
11. hypoglycemia
12. multiple sclerosis
13. Parkinson's disease
14. stroke

Definitions

A. A condition that occurs when the blood glucose level is abnormally low
B. A condition in which fat deposits build up on the inner walls of blood vessels
C. A condition in which the air spaces in the lungs become enlarged and overinflated, resulting in the loss of elasticity
D. Inflammation in the lungs, with increased mucus production and a chronic productive cough that is present for at least three months in two successive years
E. A progressive disease of the nervous system that affects how nerve impulses are sent to and from the brain
F. Severe pain or pressure in the chest caused by reduced blood flow and an inadequate oxygen supply to the heart muscle
G. A progressive disease that affects the part of the brain that handles muscular control and function
H. A group of chronic, progressive lung diseases characterized by airway obstruction and a loss of elasticity in the lungs
I. A malignant, uncontrolled growth of abnormal cells
J. A sudden interruption in the blood supply to the brain
K. A condition that occurs when the blood glucose level is abnormally high
L. A respiratory disease caused by narrowing and inflammation of the airways in response to triggers
M. The inability or impaired ability to communicate through speech, writing, or signs
N. The heart's inability to pump effectively, which can result in a buildup of excess fluid in the lungs

Check Your Knowledge

Review Questions: Answer each of the following questions on a separate sheet of paper.

1. How do chronic illnesses differ from other illnesses and diseases?
2. Name five symptoms of diabetes.
3. What lifestyle factors will help reduce the risk of hypertension?
4. What medication should patients with angina pectoris keep close at hand in case they experience chest pain?
5. Why is it important to monitor the intake and output of a patient with congestive heart failure?
6. What sputum changes should a nursing assistant report?
7. How can you help keep a patient with a neurological disorder from choking while eating?
8. What is the difference between radiation therapy and chemotherapy?
9. What percentage of body weight is lost before a patient is considered to have HIV wasting syndrome?
10. Describe what happens when a patient has kidney failure.

True or False: Read each statement carefully. Then write *True* or *False* by the statement number on a separate sheet of paper.

1. Some patients who have had a stroke have difficulty in speaking or in understanding speech.
2. A ministroke (TIA) may indicate that a patient is at risk for a CVA.
3. Loss of control over movement is the main symptom of patients with Parkinson's disease.
4. Treatment for cancer often reduces the patient's appetite.
5. The symptoms that patients with AIDS exhibit do not change once they have been diagnosed with the syndrome.

Think and Decide

Directions: Think about each of the following scenarios. Answer each question on a separate sheet of paper.

1. Vanessa, a 72-year-old resident in your care, is difficult to arouse for breakfast this morning. You notice when you ask her to state her name that her speech is slurred. What should you do?

2. Mr. H. has cancer of the lymph nodes. The supervisor has explained that it is very important to prevent infections because Mr. H.'s immune system is impaired. To help prevent infections for Mr. H., what types of assistance can you provide?

3. Mrs. M., a 77-year-old resident in your care, has expressive aphasia. Another nursing assistant is helping you change her bed linens and is talking about her personal home situation as though Mrs. M. cannot hear her. What is your most appropriate action?

4. Mrs. D., a long-term care resident, has had a stroke that affected the left side of her body. You are helping her eat her breakfast. Her face is affected on the right side, and she is having difficulty chewing. Where should you place the food in her mouth?

5. Mrs. N. is a 69-year-old resident who has chronic obstructive pulmonary disease. She is refusing to eat or drink fluids because she is too tired. She is receiving oxygen at 1 liter per minute. What can

you do to assist her to increase her calorie and fluid intake?

6. J.L. is a home care patient. He has diabetes, for which he takes insulin daily by mouth. Today when you arrive, you find him sitting on the floor and unable to get up. He is shaking, and when you ask him what happened, he seems disoriented and confused. On a nearby table, you see his pill organizer and notice that the insulin for tomorrow as well as that for today is missing. What may have happened? What should you do?

7. W.R. is a 63-year-old long-term care resident who has chronic kidney failure. He has had a cold, from which he is currently recovering. However, his throat is dry, and he repeatedly uses the call signal to request water. What should you do?

8. Mrs. F. is a 70-year-old long-term care resident who has emphysema. She requires oxygen continually, and her physician has ordered a flow rate of 2 liters per minute. When you bring her lunch today, she asks you to "turn up the oxygen." She believes she would be able to breathe better and enjoy her lunch more if the oxygen flow rate were higher. What should you do?

CNA Certification Exam Prep

Directions: This practice test contains ten questions. Each question has four suggested answers. For each question, choose the ONE that best answers the question or completes the statement. Write your answers on a separate sheet of paper.

1. One symptom of kidney failure is
   A. low blood pressure.
   B. dry, itchy skin.
   C. agitation.
   D. high energy.

2. Special care requirements for cancer patients include
   A. controlling infection.
   B. providing increased activity.
   C. limiting fluid intake.
   D. decreasing caloric intake.

3. One of the symptoms of AIDS is
   A. increased appetite.
   B. weight gain.
   C. constipation.
   D. night sweats.

4. What is aphasia?
   A. difficulty swallowing
   B. impaired speech
   C. difficulty breathing
   D. irregular heart rate

5. Which of the following is a symptom of myocardial infarction?
   A. excitability
   B. difficulty swallowing
   C. profuse sweating
   D. aphasia

6. Which of the following is a treatment for diabetes mellitus?
   A. group therapy
   B. diet control
   C. radiation therapy
   D. surgery

7. What is *most* likely to cause an angina pectoris attack?
   A. eating a light meal
   B. a short, slow walk
   C. sleeping
   D. emotional stress

8. HIV can be transmitted by
   A. sharing a room with an infected person.
   B. sexual contact with an infected person.
   C. tightly hugging an infected person.
   D. helping an infected person get dressed.

9. Which of the following is helpful in caring for a person with CHF?
   A. providing periods of vigorous exercise
   B. offering toileting assistance frequently
   C. helping the patient lie flat in bed
   D. offering frequent skin care

10. A CVA can be caused by
    A. a blood vessel bursting in the brain.
    B. the loss of voluntary muscle movement.
    C. narrowing of the airways.
    D. inflammation in the lungs.

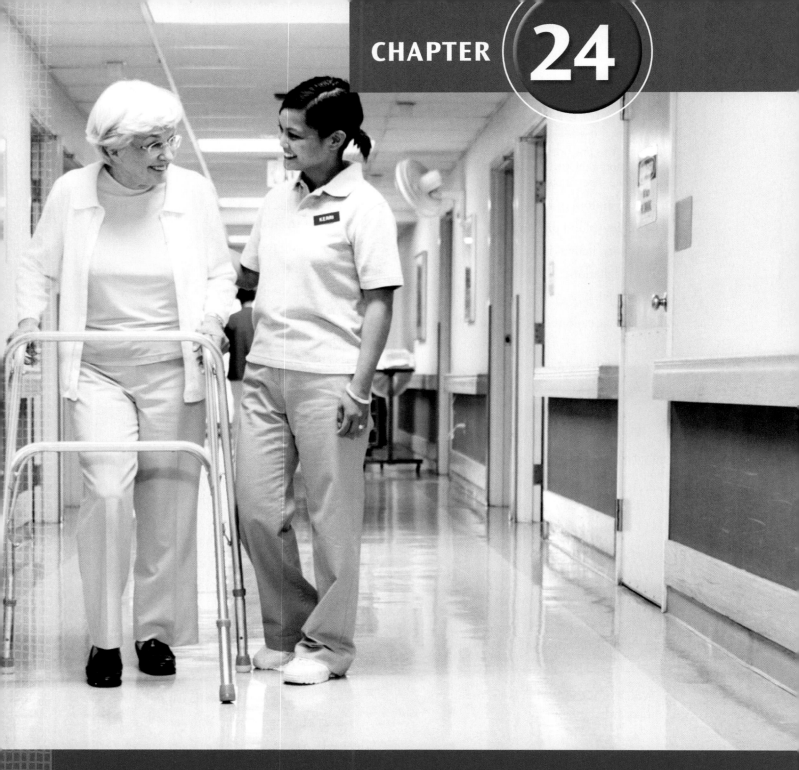

OBJECTIVES

- Practice procedures for helping residents exercise.

- Discuss the physical changes of the aging process.

- Recognize the psychological and social changes of the aging process

Assisting the Elderly in Long-Term Care

VOCABULARY

ambulate Walk and move around freely without being restricted to a bed or wheelchair.

autonomy Independence and the freedom to make one's own decisions about health care and other life issues.

bed cradle A device or frame placed on the bed at the resident's feet to keep pressure from the top linens off the feet.

bed rest Confined to bed by a doctor's order.

elderly A broad term that describes people in the later years of their lives.

foot board A device placed at the foot of a resident's mattress to prevent the plantar flexion that leads to foot drop.

foot drop A condition in which the foot falls down, or droops, at the ankle.

geriatrics A health care specialty that meets the health care needs of elderly people.

muscle atrophy A condition in which the muscles decrease in size and waste away from lack of use.

muscle contracture Deep, painful tightening and shortening of the muscles that cannot easily be relieved.

osteoporosis Loss of bone density, causing bones to become brittle and break more easily.

plantar flexion Bending of the foot downward.

strict bed rest Confined to bed by a doctor's order and not allowed to do anything for oneself, including any form of exercise, unless ordered by a doctor.

Care of the Elderly

Elderly people experience varying degrees of physical changes because of their age. Aging is a normal process—a natural part of human growth and development. It is not a disease or illness. Some changes, such as graying hair or wrinkled skin, do not affect health. Many people enter old age in reasonably good health and continue to lead active, involved lives.

Other changes, however, such as having a stroke or Alzheimer's disease, may lead to health issues or inability to care for themselves. Chronic illness often requires care in a long-term care facility or nursing home.

Autonomy

Long-term care facilities offer a wide range of living arrangements, ranging from apartments, condos, and assisted living to the traditional long-term care facility. This range of options allows elderly people more **autonomy**—independence and the freedom to make their own decisions about health care and other life issues. Residents can live independently but still use the facility's services. When the resident's health changes, he or she can move from independent living to other areas providing a greater range of services. This continuity of care appeals to many people.

Family Roles

Adult children may choose to care for aged parents when they are no longer to remain in their own homes. Safety is an issue. However, many times the grown children do not live in the same community. They still work and are raising their own families. Finances sometimes prevent the round-the-clock care their parents need. In these cases, decisions must be made. Assisted living and long-term care facilities offer appropriate options for providing the services needed by an older person who cannot be cared for in the home.

This is an emotional time, not only for the elderly, but also for their children. When a family decides to place a parent in a long-term care facility, they may need reassurance that they made the right choice. Never make a judgment. Show empathy and help the resident and the family through the changes that follow long-term placement.

Resident Exercise and Activities

Residents need exercise to maintain and improve their health and fitness. Appropriate levels of physical activity can have a positive impact on anyone's health. **See Figure 24-1.** The opposite is also true, however. A sedentary, or inactive, lifestyle can increase the probability of health complications. A sedentary resident is at risk for pressure sores, constipation, and fecal impaction, as well as blood clots, urinary tract infections, weakness, osteoporosis, depression, and pneumonia.

When muscles are not used, they may contract and become painful, limiting use. **Muscle contracture** is a deep, painful tightening and shortening of the muscles that cannot easily be relieved. These contractions can cause permanent deformity and disability, as well as loss of movement. **Muscle atrophy** occurs when the muscles decrease in size and waste away. Regular exercise helps to prevent muscle contracture and atrophy.

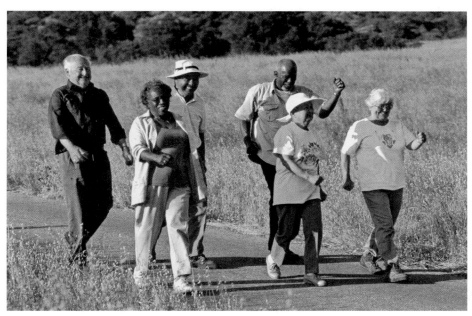

○ **Figure 24-1.** Exercise can help elderly people live a healthier life.

Benefits of Exercise

Exercise at any age is valuable. The benefits of regular exercise may include:
- Reducing the risk of developing heart disease, adult-onset diabetes, hypertension (high blood pressure), osteoporosis, and certain cancers.
- Modifying the body's cholesterol level.
- Slowing the loss of bone mass associated with aging.
- Burning calories and helping to control body weight.
- Conserving muscle.
- Managing stress.
- Providing increased energy levels.
- Promoting a sense of well-being.
- Positively affecting self-esteem.
- Helping a person sleep.
- Allowing for socialization.

Components of Exercise

A proper exercise program has four components:
- **Cardiovascular fitness** boosts the heart's ability to pump blood and deliver oxygen throughout the body.
- **Muscular fitness** strengthens the muscles. Strong muscles help maintain proper body posture and assist the circulatory system by pushing blood through the blood vessels.
- **Flexibility fitness** allows the joints to move freely and without pain through a full range of motion.
- **Body composition fitness** helps reduce the amount of fat in the body.

The Resident's Ability to Exercise

Residents in long-term care facilities have different limitations and disabilities that may limit what they can physically do. To help each resident exercise appropriately, exercise should focus on his or her abilities. The resident's health care provider will order or approve any new exercise program. Some facilities have a physical therapist, too, who is trained to design an exercise program for each resident.

To be effective, exercise should begin slowly and increase gradually as a person gains strength. For example, if you are helping someone start a walking program, pick a short goal, such as to the next room. (Check with a doctor or physical therapist to set the goal.) Help the resident walk at a reasonable pace that he or she can maintain for the distance. After a week or so, when this walk becomes comfortable, gradually increase the distance and speed.

Many long-term care facilities also have daily exercise programs. These are low-impact exercises. They are fun and residents are encouraged to exercise, within the limits of their ability.

The Resident on Bed Rest. Some residents are on **bed rest**. They are confined to bed by a doctor's order. These residents may be able to assist with the activities of daily living and may be allowed to perform stretching and lifting exercises. **See Figure 24-2.** Check the care plan about the type and frequency of exercise the resident is to receive, or discuss it with your supervisor. Residents on **strict bed rest** are not allowed to do anything for themselves and cannot do any form of exercise unless ordered by a doctor. For these patients, the nursing assistant may do passive range-of-motion exercises if ordered by the doctor.

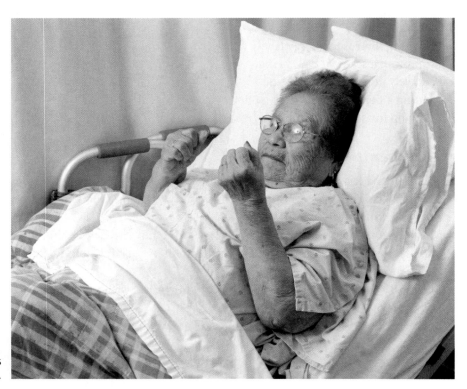

○ **Figure 24-2.** Even a resident on bed rest should exercise as much as her physician allows.

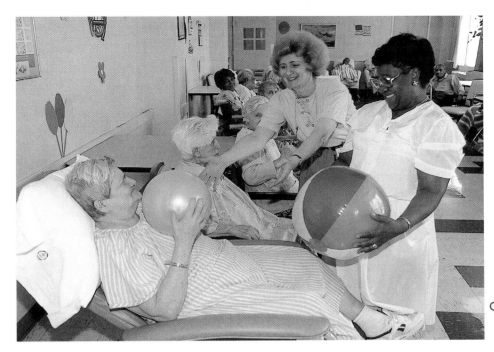

○ Figure 24-3. Nonambulatory residents can exercise while sitting.

The Resident in a Wheelchair. A resident confined to a wheelchair should be encouraged to exercise, but only if a doctor orders. The resident can stretch, lift, and perform rhythmic movements of large muscle groups, as shown in **Figure 24-3**. Residents in wheelchairs can also assist with activities of daily living and exercise the arms and hands. They can also perform small shifts of weight from side to side and back to front to relieve pressure over bony prominences and help prevent pressure sores from forming. Encourage these residents to be as independent as possible.

The Ambulatory Resident. Residents who can **ambulate** (walk and move around freely without being restricted to a bed or wheelchair) are called *ambulatory residents*. They can participate in simple stretching exercises, light weight-lifting, and cardiovascular exercise, such as swimming, dancing, and walking. Walking is an ideal exercise because it involves most of the large muscle groups. It does not require expensive equipment and can be done almost anywhere.

Encourage ambulatory residents to move as much as possible. In a health care facility, you can help a resident walk up and down the hallways or outside, when weather permits. In a client's home, you can plan a daily walk. Always allow the resident to assist with as many of the activities of daily living as possible. These activities use muscle groups, help maintain coordination, and promote independence.

Reasons to Stop Exercise

In spite of its benefits, exercise may not be appropriate for all residents. When helping a resident exercise, watch for the following signs and symptoms:
- Extreme shortness of breath
- Weakness
- Irregular heartbeat
- Pain or pressure in the chest, neck, jaw, or arms

- Dizziness, cold sweats, or fainting
- Nausea or vomiting
- Abnormally pale skin color
- Increased confusion

If you notice any of these signs or symptoms, stop the exercise and help the resident sit or lie down. Immediately contact the charge nurse or supervisor.

Recreational Activities

Recreational activities can be mentally as well as physically beneficial. Health care facilities plan recreational activities appropriate to the abilities of most of the residents. Encourage residents to participate and have a good time. Many recreational activities provide exercise as well as entertainment. These are examples of typical recreational activities at a health care or adult day-care facility:

- Musical presentations in which the residents sing, clap, and move their legs
- Plays and skits the residents rehearse and perform
- Physical activities, such as group walks or dancing
- Entertainment and sport activities, such as ball-playing, exercise classes, bingo, movies, cooking classes, knitting classes, sewing classes, resident meetings, and gardening
- Visiting with friends
- Working with others on worthwhile projects

Activities such as gardening and crafts allow residents to exercise while having fun. Many residents had hobbies before they became residents. Related activities provide a way for them to stay busy, exercise, and do something they are used to and know how to do. **See Figure 24-4.**

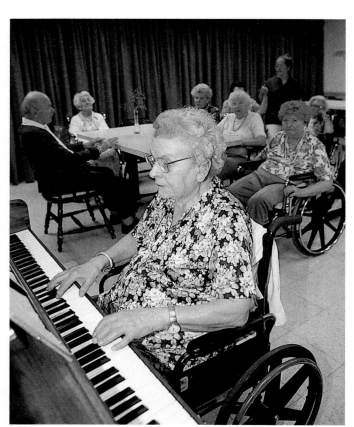

O **Figure 24-4.** This 100-year-old piano player entertains her fellow residents twice a day. The residents enjoy her music and often sing along.

Vital Skills (MATH)

Calculating Exercise Times

You are helping a resident with an individualized exercise program. The physical therapist has prepared a program that includes stretching, walking, and cool-down exercises. The plan calls for 10 minutes of stretching, ¼ mile of walking, and 15 minutes of cool-down exercises. For this resident, it takes 44 minutes to walk 1 mile. How much time should you allow for the resident to complete his exercise program?

First, you need to figure out how long it will take the resident to walk ¼ mile. You know that it takes 45 minutes to walk 1 mile. It takes 4 quarter miles to equal a mile, so you can divide 45 minutes by 4 to find out how much time it takes to walk ¼ mile:

$$44 \div 4 = 11 \text{ minutes or } 11 \text{ minutes}$$

Now you can add the times for stretching, walking, and cool-down:

$$10 + 11 + 15 = 36 \text{ minutes}$$

Practice

Another resident has a different individualized exercise program. The physical therapist has prepared a program that includes 12 minutes of stretching, ½ mile of walking, 10 minutes of "beach ball toss," and 10 minutes of cool-down exercises. This resident can walk a mile in 40 minutes. How much time should you allow for this resident to complete his exercise program?

Geriatric Care

The word **elderly** is a broad term that describes people in the later years of their lives. **Geriatrics** is a health care specialty that meets the health care needs of elderly people. A geriatric resident who lives in a long-term care facility may be advanced in age and may be suffering from one or more chronic or weakening illnesses.

The aging process is a natural progression of life that affects every person and body system at a different rate, although there are common characteristics in all elderly people. The main physical changes of aging include a slowing down of the body systems. Many changes are gradual and go unnoticed for a long time. Some aging signs affect physical appearance, such as gray hair, wrinkled skin, a slow walk, and stooped posture. These changes do not affect the individual's ability to function in society. Other changes, such as sight and hearing impairment or chronic illness, increase the person's risk of injury and pose a health threat. Safety is a major concern for elderly people whether they live at home or in a long-term care facility.

When caring for elderly patients, it is natural for you to have a variety of feelings as you watch their health decline. You are forced to deal with your own mortality and your feelings about aging. Your coworkers are experiencing similar emotions. It is usually helpful to speak with your coworkers or to the charge nurse when you have had a difficult experience with one of the residents. Coworkers can offer empathy and someone to talk to. They can help you understand what you are feeling.

Physical Changes of the Aging Process

All of the body systems are affected by the aging process. This section lists each body system and its changes related to aging. These changes may or may not occur in a given resident. When they do occur, they are experienced in varying degrees.

Cardiovascular Changes. The heart muscle may become less elastic as a person ages, and the heart may become less efficient. Arteries and veins narrow, which reduces blood flow. Therefore, less oxygen is carried throughout the body. Orthostatic hypertension can occur. In addition, injuries tend to heal at a slower rate.

Nervous System Changes. As age advances, a person has slower reaction times. Less blood is pumped to the brain, which can cause dizziness and problems with balance. Sleep patterns may change, and depression may occur.

Sensory System Changes. Elderly people often have reduced vision, increasing the risk of falls and injury. They may have slower reactions to light and glare. Their eyes may be dry due to a lower level of tear production. Reduced hearing increases the risk of accidents and injury. Nutrition may be affected as a result of decreased sense of taste and smell. Elderly people may also have a loss of thirst, resulting in a decreased intake of fluids. Their sense of touch may be reduced also, making them less likely to feel pain and more prone to accidents.

Respiratory System Changes. The lungs tend to lose elasticity as people age, causing less oxygen to be taken into the body. Breathing becomes shallow. Elderly people may also have less strength for coughing.

Musculoskeletal System Changes. Changes also occur to muscles and bones as people become older. Muscles weaken and atrophy. **Osteoporosis** (loss of bone density, causing bones to become brittle and break more easily) may occur. Joints become less flexible and can cause pain. Height decreases, and mobility may decrease as well.

Integumentary System Changes. The skin of elderly people becomes atrophic: it is dry and has lost elasticity, causing wrinkling. Brown spots, commonly called *age spots*, develop. The skin loses its subcutaneous fatty layer, so elderly people may feel colder. The skin tears and bruises more easily. Nails become thick and tough. Hair turns gray or white and may become thinner.

Digestive System Changes. The organs of the digestive system change or slow down. For example, the body produces less saliva. Teeth may be lost, making it difficult to chew. Release of various digestive enzymes and chemicals is reduced, resulting in indigestion, constipation, or fecal impaction. Absorption of vitamins and minerals becomes more difficult.

Vital Skills — READING

Setting a Purpose for Reading

Before you begin to read anything—a book, newspaper, or research article—you should set your purpose for reading. Determine what you want learn from what you are about to read. The purpose for reading may be determined by your instructor. For example, you may be asked to read this chapter and list five physical changes that occur with aging. Sometimes you will need to determine the purpose for reading on your own. You can do this by asking yourself some questions.

For example, suppose you have just found out from your doctor that you have high blood pressure. You have some questions about the condition, so on your way home, you pick up a book on high blood pressure from the library. Before you read, you can set your purpose for reading by listing some questions you would like to have answered.

- What is considered normal blood pressure?
- What can I do to lower my blood pressure?
- Will having high blood pressure affect my health?
- What are the treatments for high blood pressure?

Practice

Imagine that your grandmother is about to be placed in a long-term care facility. You want to know more about long-term care and what your grandmother may experience. You go to the library and pick up a book called *The Elderly and Long-Term Care*. Set your purpose for reading: List five questions that you would like to have answered by reading this book.

Urinary System Changes. Kidney function and filtration may be reduced in elderly people. They may have a decreased ability to empty the bladder completely, and the bladder muscles may weaken. Loss of bladder control or incontinence may occur.

Sexual Changes. Frequency of sexual activity lessens in later years for a variety of reasons. Decreases in the hormones testosterone (males) and estrogen and progesterone (females) occur. Women go through menopause (stop menstruating). After menopause, women can no longer conceive a child. Because estrogen and progesterone are needed to maintain healthy female reproductive tissue, as their levels decrease, tissues in the vagina, uterus, and genital area become dry and thin. However, many elderly people do still have an interest in sexual activity and sexual needs.

Physical Care for the Elderly Resident

When you understand the physical aspects of aging, you are better prepared to care for the geriatric resident. Geriatric residents who are in an assisted living or long-term care facility or are being cared for at home by a home health agency have a care plan. The care plan will alert you to any disabilities. The care plan also allows for continuity of care among various agencies and facilities. These are some of the ways you can assist the elderly resident:

- Observe the resident for complications of poor circulation, such as bruising, wounds that do not heal properly, and cold hands or feet. Along with observation, listen to what the resident tells you.
- Apply comfort devices as directed. For example, if a resident suffers from **foot drop** (a condition in which the foot falls down at the ankle), a **foot board** can be placed at the foot of the mattress. **See Figure 24-5.** The foot board prevents the **plantar flexion** (bending of the foot downward) that leads to foot drop. Some residents also need a **bed cradle**—a device or frame placed on the bed at the resident's feet (or other area of the body) to keep pressure from the top linens off the feet. This relieves pressure that could cause pressure sores. Special mattresses and wheelchair cushions may be required for some patients with especially delicate or easily bruised skin.
- Apply assistive devices, including eyeglasses, dentures, hearing aids, canes, walkers, and wheelchairs as directed by a physician or supervisor. These devices help the resident be more independent.
- Be aware of the resident's physical limitations. Do not allow the resident to overexert.

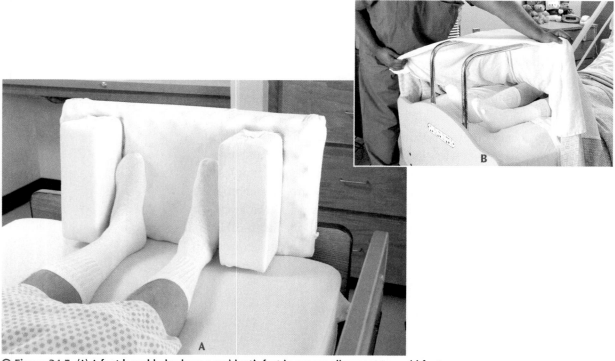

O **Figure 24-5.** (A) A foot board helps keep a resident's feet in proper alignment to avoid foot drop. (B) A bed cradle is a metal frame that keeps the top linens from putting pressure on the top of the resident's feet.

- If you are caring for a bedridden resident, change the position often to avoid pressure sores. Keep the skin of residents' perineal areas clean and dry. Provide extra blankets and sweaters to compensate for loss of body fat.
- Never tease or show anger toward a resident who is incontinent. Residents are embarrassed by incontinence. Clean them and provide personal care while maintaining their dignity and privacy.
- Give the resident plenty of time to chew food. Encourage the resident to eat fresh fruits, vegetables, and liquids to avoid constipation. A high-fiber diet encourages bowel regularity. Follow the care plan and the physician's orders.
- Provide foods that are flavorful and encourage the resident to eat. Explain what is being served. Provide liquid dietary supplements if a doctor determines that the resident is not consuming sufficient nutrition from food.
- Recognize that people of all ages are sexual beings. Give the resident privacy for a sex life if the resident requests it. Do not tease residents about love relationships. Always treat residents with respect and dignity.
- When residents need help with activities of daily living, remember that they were once able to do these things without assistance. Show kindness, patience, and acceptance as you help these residents with their basic needs.
- Permit residents to groom themselves. For women, this may include applying makeup and styling hair; for men, it may mean shaving and hair care. They will feel better about themselves and feel more attractive to others when they are nicely groomed.
- Provide for safety and prevention of falls.

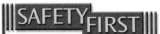

SAFETY FIRST

Always assist residents as necessary and maintain their rooms neatly to prevent falls. Falls can be very serious for elderly people because their bones are less dense and break easily.

Vital Skills WRITING

Creating an Outline

An outline is a good way to organize your thoughts before you begin writing. A good outline shows how your ideas are organized and how they relate to each other. It includes the points you will address in your paper and organizes them in a visual format. A traditional outline has three sections: an introduction, a body, and a conclusion.

For example, below is a general outline for a five-paragraph essay.

Title:
I. Introduction:
   A. general information on topic
   B. thesis statement
II. Body
   A. main idea (body paragraph 1)
     1. supporting detail
     2. supporting detail
   B. main idea (body paragraph 2)
     1. supporting detail
     2. supporting detail
   C. main idea (body paragraph3)
     1. supporting detail
     2. supporting detail
III. Conclusion
   A. restatement of supporting details
   B. final statement

Practice
Based on what you've read in this chapter, prepare an outline for a five-paragraph essay on either physical changes of the aging process or exercise and the elderly.

Discussing Levels of Long-Term Care

The type of long-term care facility in which people live depends on their income and level of independence. In general, as the level of care a person needs increases, the cost of the stay in long-term care increases. A person who is still fairly independent and has an adequate income may choose a privately run personal care home or an assisted-living facility. Those with limited financial resources may go to a state-run nursing home only when they are no longer able to live independently.

Practice

Contact a long-term care facility and ask if you can interview someone in administration about their services. Prepare your questions ahead of time. Ask about the care level the residents receive and activities they may participate in. What is the average cost per resident and are there "extra" costs (for example, for meals or personal items such as shampoo)? Does the facility accept residents with limited income? How large is the staff? Prepare a 5-minute oral presentation for class about your findings.

Psychological and Social Changes

The aging process affects psychological well-being and social environments, too. Residents must make emotional adjustments to the natural life issues involved in aging. This can be even more difficult because they may lose their peers.

All people have the same basic emotional needs:
- To feel safe and secure, both physically and financially
- To have friends and companions
- To feel worthy
- To have the opportunity to learn, achieve, and gain recognition

As they become increasingly frail, residents may need your assistance to help them make new friends and to have new opportunities for learning and social interaction.

Some natural life events and issues elderly residents face are:
- Death of a spouse
- Death of friends
- Retirement
- Change in housing
- Change in social status
- Loss of independence

- Change in self-esteem
- Change in relationships with grown children
- Fear of illness, injury, and death
- Adjustment to a new role in the family
- More leisure time and the need for new activities
- Need to form new friendships in a new environment

To help elderly residents deal with psychological and social issues, the nursing assistant can:

- Encourage residents to pursue their interests to keep the mind active. Encourage them to think, read, and otherwise challenge the mind. Word searches and crossword puzzles are good ways to exercise the mind.
- Be an understanding listener. Use therapeutic communication strategies such as reminiscing about their experiences. This technique can sometimes help the resident deal with the loss of friends or family members.
- Approach each resident as an individual. It is important to be accepting of each individual's desires and capabilities, and to support each resident's efforts—both emotionally and physically. **See Figure 24-6.**
- Encourage residents to form new relationships. Loneliness is a common problem among elderly people. Many people have lost friends and partners, and new relationships may bring happiness and fulfillment into their lives.

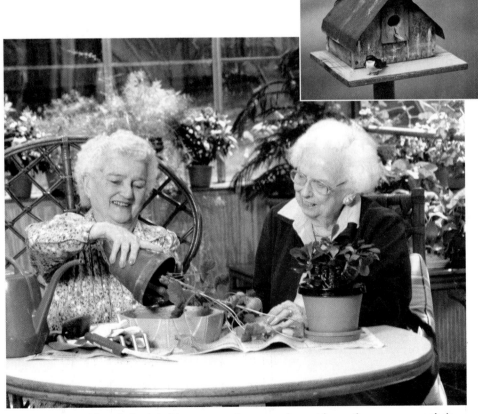

○ **Figure 24-6.** Although these residents can no longer garden outdoors, they can pursue their love of plants and birdwatching.

CHAPTER 24 Review

Chapter Summary

- Aging is a normal part of human growth and development.

- Autonomy remains important for people as they grow older.

- Exercise helps people maintain and improve their physical and psychological health throughout the life span.

- Most residents can exercise to some extent—even those who use a wheelchair or are on bed rest. Only residents on strict bed rest cannot exercise.

- As people age, physical changes occur that affect their ability to move about and care for themselves.

- Physical care of elderly people includes comfort measures and measures to prevent problems from poor circulation and lack of exercise.

- Elderly residents are dealing with many life events that can cause psychological and social changes. The role of the nursing assistant is to support, encourage, listen, and provide opportunities for them to continue to grow and make new friends within their limitations.

VOCABULARY REVIEW

Directions: Match the letter of each definition in the second column with the correct vocabulary term in the first column. Write your answers on a separate sheet of paper.

Vocabulary
1. ambulate
2. autonomy
3. bed cradle
4. bed rest
5. elderly
6. foot board
7. foot drop
8. geriatrics
9. muscle atrophy
10. muscle contracture
11. osteoporosis
12. plantar flexion
13. strict bed rest

Definitions
A. Independence and the freedom to make one's own decisions about health care and other life issues
B. Confined to bed by a doctor's order
C. Loss of bone density
D. A frame that keeps pressure from linens off a resident's feet
E. A specialty that meets the health care needs of elderly people
F. A condition in which muscles decrease in size and waste away from lack of use
G. Confined to bed by a doctor's order and not allowed to do anything for oneself
H. A device placed at the foot of a mattress to keep a resident's feet aligned properly
I. Bending of the foot downward
J. Walk and move around freely
K. Deep, painful contractions of the muscles
L. A condition in which the foot falls down at the ankle
M. A broad term that describes people in the later years of their lives

Check Your Knowledge

Review Questions: Answer each of the following questions on a separate sheet of paper.

1. Briefly describe changes in family roles as a person becomes elderly.

2. What is the best way to prevent muscle contractures and muscle atrophy?

3. List the four components of a proper exercise program.

4. What types of exercise might a resident on bed rest be allowed to perform?

5. What types of exercise are appropriate for ambulatory residents?

6. Why might blood flow be reduced in elderly people?

7. What happens to the skin as people age?

8. Briefly describe the hormonal changes in men and women as they become elderly.

9. When might a bed cradle be indicated for a resident?

10. What can a nursing assistant do to help a resident who is depressed about his loss of independence?

True or False: Read each statement carefully. Then write *True* or *False* by the statement number on a separate sheet of paper.

1. Dizziness in elderly people may be caused by less blood being pumped into the brain.

2. Elders do not have a need for friends and companions.

3. Bones in elderly people become more dense, causing them to be brittle.

4. An elderly person's heart muscle loses elasticity.

5. Dryness and lost of elasticity in the skin can cause wrinkling.

Think and Decide

Directions: Think about each of the following scenarios. Answer each question on a separate sheet of paper.

1. Mr. J. is a long-term resident who has been in your care for more than a year. He has become bored with his everyday activities and tells you he wants to begin an exercise program. What steps should be taken to begin a program for Mr. J.? How can you help?

2. Mr. F. has seen Mr. J.'s new exercise program. He has noticed how much better Mr. J. seems to feel and how much more cheerful he is with the care-givers and other residents. Mr. F. decides that he wants to exercise also. However, Mr. F. is confined to a wheelchair. What types of exercises might his doctor recommend?

3. E.S. has been exercising with a group of residents in the all-purpose room. She suddenly becomes dizzy, short of breath, and confused. What should you do?

4. Mr. Tyler was a robust man when he was younger. As he approaches his 90th birthday, he has white hair. He has lost some of his hearing and wears a hearing aid. His gait has become slower, he stoops when he walks, and he sometimes has trouble with balance. What body systems are associated with each of these changes?

5. M.J. is a long-term care resident who has always been concerned about keeping her mind active. She looks for things to do that will challenge her mind. Today, she is sitting in the all-purpose room working on a book of word search puzzles. However, she admits that she is getting a bit tired of word puzzles. What suggestions might you make for other mind-challenging activities?

6. Mrs. K. and her daughter, Mina, made a mutual decision to move Mrs. K. to a long-term care facility because her daughter had to go back to work. She can no longer meet Mrs. K.'s needs. Mrs. K. confides that every time Mina comes to see her, they both become very depressed. They both wish that Mrs. K. could have remained in Mina's home. What might you do for Mrs. K. and Mina?

7. D.W. is a fairly new resident at the long-term care facility. He has had an interesting life and usually enjoys talking about it. When you go to D.W.'s room this morning to help with his personal care, he seems quieter than usual and speaks sharply to you once or twice. When you ask if anything is wrong, he apologizes for being rude and explains that he is frustrated because he has become dependent on others—including you—for the smallest of personal services. He misses being able to care for himself. What should you do?

CNA Certification Exam Prep

Directions: This practice test contains ten questions. Each question has four suggested answers. For each question, choose the ONE that best answers the question or completes the statement. Write your answers on a separate sheet of paper.

1. Which of the following is a complication that can arise from a sedentary lifestyle?
   A. diarrhea
   B. incontinence
   C. contractures
   D. muscle bulk

2. Which of the following is a benefit of exercise?
   A. elevated cholesterol
   B. decrease in bone mass
   C. muscle atrophy
   D. sense of well-being

3. You are taking a resident for a walk. Which of the following is a reason for stopping the walk?
   A. pressure in the chest
   B. low temperature
   C. cold hands
   D. depression

4. A cardiovascular system change associated with aging is
   A. frequent bouts of incontinence.
   B. increased risk for falls.
   C. loss of interest in activities.
   D. reduced blood flow.

5. Which would you do to help the geriatric resident?
   A. discourage the use of a walker or cane
   B. encourage the pursuit of hobbies
   C. make all choices for the resident
   D. have no set routine for the resident

6. Which of the following is a natural life change a geriatric resident may face?
   A. death of a close friend
   B. increased career stress
   C. increased independence
   D. increased mobility

7. Which of the following is a sign of poor circulation in a geriatric resident?
   A. dry skin
   B. brittle bones
   C. cold feet
   D. painful joints

8. Which activities may be appropriate for a patient on bed rest?
   A. stretching
   B. walking
   C. swimming
   D. dancing

9. Which of the following devices may help a resident whose feet are being irritated by the top linens?
   A. foot board
   B. bed cradle
   C. special mattress
   D. wheelchair cushion

10. Which of the following may help meet the sexual needs of a resident?
    A. stretching
    B. eating
    C. walking
    D. grooming

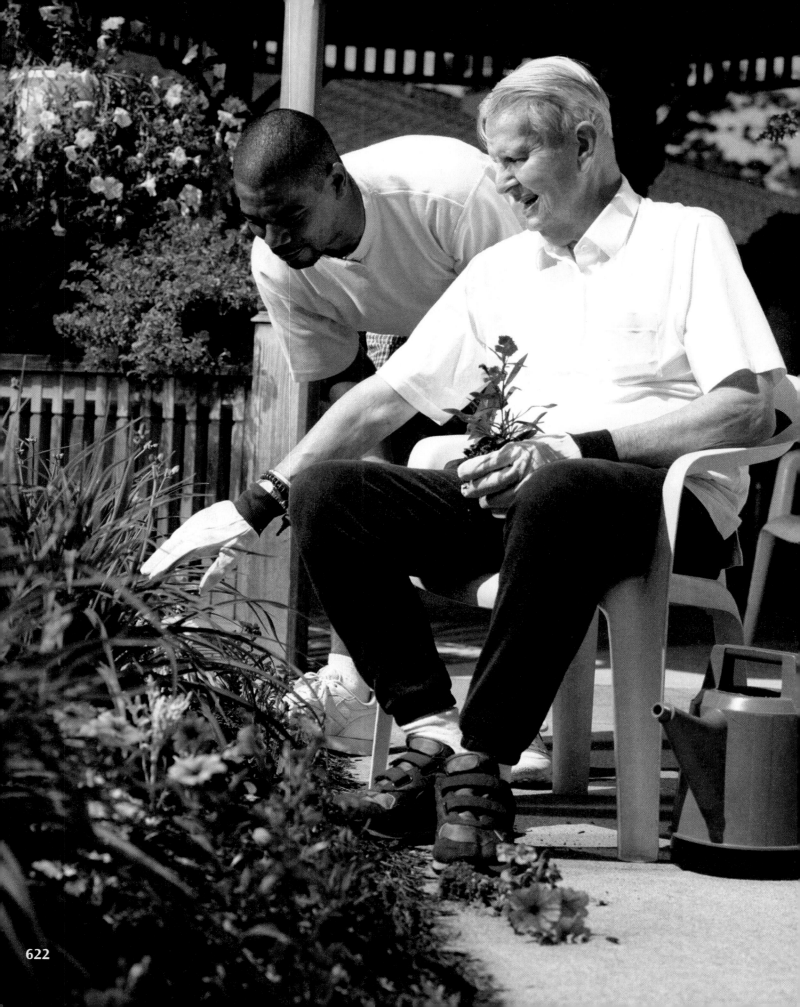

UNIT 6

Home and Special Care

Chapter 25 Home Health Care

Chapter 26 Nutrition

Chapter 27 Understanding Mental Health

Chapter 28 Nursing Assistant Specialties

Chapter 29 Care for the Terminally Ill

Chapter 30 Death and Postmortem Care

Unit 6 presents information about special situations in which nursing assistants may perform their jobs. These chapters provide an understanding of home health care, mental health care, and various other opportunities available to nursing assistants. The final two chapters describe the emotional and procedural requirements of providing care for dying patients.

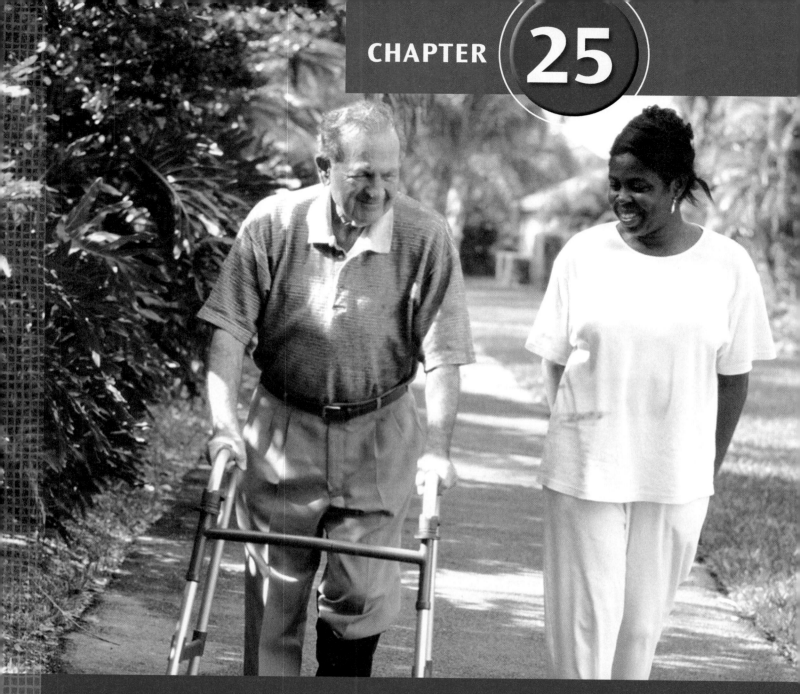

OBJECTIVES

- Identify the members of the home health care team.
- List basic responsibilities of the home health aide.
- Describe the qualities of an effective home health aide.
- Explain how the home health aide helps with the client's progress and independence.

- Describe how the home health aide interacts with the client's family.
- Identify the records and reports required in home health care.
- Describe infection control and housekeeping tasks in home health care.
- Describe how to plan and safely prepare food for a client.

- List ways to provide a safe home environment for the client.
- List ways to handle emergencies that may occur in the home.
- Explain how to recognize and report client abuse.

Home Health Care

VOCABULARY

abandonment Ending help or support without providing notice or getting the client's consent; leaving without notice.

case manager The supervising nurse in a home health care agency who plans and oversees the care of the client and provides assignments to the home health aide.

client care record A record of all the care given to a home health care client.

domestic violence The act of physically injuring, or causing to be injured, a family member or someone else who lives in the home.

home health aide A person who provides basic personal care and health-related services for a client in the client's home.

resource management Having resources on hand when they are needed and using them efficiently.

respite care Relief time for family caregivers to take care of personal needs or have time off.

time management Planning and scheduling your time to do tasks efficiently.

time/travel record A log that describes how the home health aide has spent time with the client, traveling to and from the client's home, and doing errands for the client.

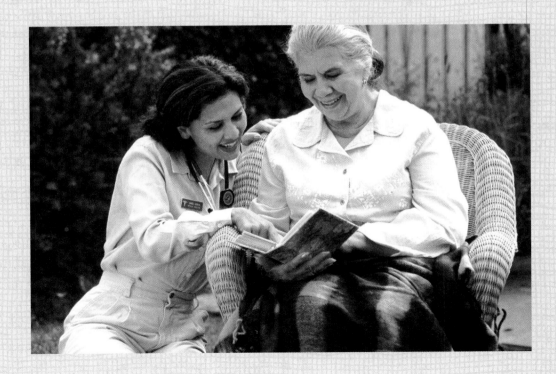

The Home Health Aide

A **home health aide** provides basic personal care and health-related services for a client in the client's home. Not all home health aides are trained as nursing assistants. However, many nursing assistants choose to work in home health care. Before becoming a home health aide, you will need to find out about the education and certifications required by your state. You may need additional training.

Some home health aides find their jobs through friends, newspaper ads, senior centers, or home care agencies. Most, however, work for home health care agencies.

Working on a Team

An agency's health care team usually includes the client and the client's family, home health aides, a supervising nurse, and the client's physician. There may also be specialists on the team, such as a physical therapist or a dietitian. The supervising nurse is responsible for the client's care. This registered nurse may be called a **case manager**.

The supervising nurse makes an initial visit to the client to assess the client's need for services and to assess the home environment. Based on this information, the team develops a care plan for the client. The care plan:

- Identifies the client's needs and how to meet those needs.
- Establishes goals and ways to measure the client's progress.
- Creates a schedule that specifies how often and for how long home health aides will visit. It also specifies how long the client might need the agency's service.

Scheduling

Based on the care plan, the home health aide is assigned a specific number of hours each day or each week. Agencies schedule assignments depending on each aide's work load. A home health aide may visit three or four clients in a day or one client for many months or even years.

Home health aides may provide the following services:

- Assist a client for short periods, such as an hour or two once a day or once a week. **See Figure 25-1.**
- Provide **respite care**, or relief time for family caregivers to take care of personal needs or have time off
- Work an 8-hour shift during the day, evening, or night
- Live in a client's home and provide 24-hour care
- Provide personal care to several clients every day
- Provide short-term help after the birth of a newborn, assisting an older person recovering from a broken bone, or caring for a client who is dying
- Assist a chronically ill or disabled person for a long period of time

Responsibilities of the Home Health Aide

Home health aides are essential members of the health care team. They see the client more often than other team members. They follow all policies and procedures for the health, safety, and well-being of the clients. Home health aides are expected to communicate clearly, follow legal and ethical guidelines, and work within the scope of practice. Infection control and standard precautions are followed at all times.

Home health aides perform many procedures similar to those provided by nursing assistants. The most common tasks include:

- Help with the client's personal care and ADLs
- Measure vital signs and record intake and output
- Assist the client with mobility and range-of-motion exercises
- Follow orders specified in the client's care plan
- Provide recreational therapy as directed by professional staff
- Promote and assist with physical and mental independence
- Transfer and position the client
- Observe, record, and report as instructed, using proper forms
- Handle emergencies
- Assist with nutrition by preparing and serving meals
- Maintain a safe, clean, organized environment for the client
- Perform agreed-upon housekeeping chores
- Change the bed linens and do the laundry
- Make medical appointments for the client. Recording what happens at these appointments is very important. For example, the doctor may order a change of medication or other form of therapy. The family and case manager must be informed in writing or verbally of changes in the treatment plan.
- Transport the client to appointments within the guidelines of agency policies. You will need a valid driver's license. If you are using your own vehicle, you will need to provide proof of insurance coverage. **See Figure 25-2.**

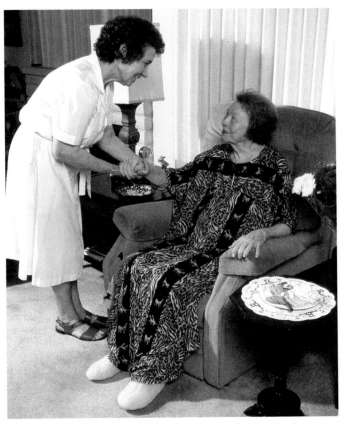

O **Figure 25-1.** The home health aide may spend only a few hours a week assisting a client.

As in any other health care facility, some procedures may be performed only by nurses. Home health aides may assist the nurse in certain procedures that aides may not do themselves. Make sure you have a written job description from the agency. If working on your own, write down your duties and confirm them with the client when you accept an assignment.

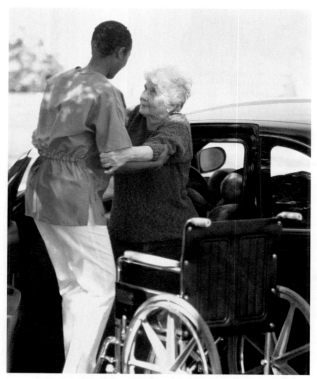
○ Figure 25-2. Home health aides sometimes transport clients to medical appointments.

Qualities of an Effective Home Health Aide

The home health aide should have the same qualities for effective nursing assistants that are described in Chapter 1. You will need to be tolerant and courteous at all times to the client and family members. As in any other health care job, respect the client's confidentiality and do not tell anyone other than team members what is going on in the home. Acting ethically, responsibly, and within the law at all times will ensure that you provide excellent client care. You will also need to recognize, discuss, and plan ways to help meet the client's expectations. The following qualities are also important for home health aides:

- **Empathy.** A home health care client needs special understanding. You may be the only person the client sees for days at a time. The client may be lonely, depressed, angry, or very excited about a new grandchild. You can show empathy for the client's situation by handling these emotions gently. You can also show empathy for the client's family members. They are going through a period of change.

- **Honesty.** The home health aide may handle the client's money and care for the client's possessions. Handle money and possessions carefully and in a trustworthy manner, and be a trusted helper to the client.

- **Dependability.** The client and the agency must know that the home health aide will arrive on time and work the full number of hours scheduled. If an aide does not show up for work or leaves early without notifying someone, the client will be left alone. This is **abandonment**, or leaving without notice.

- **Adaptability.** Home health aides may work in many types of homes, with many types of people, under many different conditions. You will need to be flexible and able to adapt, sometimes several times during the day as you go from home to home.

- **Self-discipline.** Home health aides work independently. They are usually checked on by a case manager only by telephone. Working on your own requires *self-discipline*, the ability to work without constant supervision by others. You have to complete tasks without being told and serve the client's needs without specific guidance.

The home health aide also needs to develop good management skills for time and resources. **Time management** is planning and scheduling your time to do tasks efficiently. This does not mean hurrying to get everything done. Do not sacrifice safety when managing your time. Managing time includes being able to:
- Organize your workload and client-care assignments to make good use of time
- Complete assignments accurately and in a timely manner

- Follow an established work plan with the client and family
- Select and prioritize goal-relevant activities and tasks
- Develop and follow a time schedule to complete a job assignment

Resource management is having resources on hand when they are needed and using them efficiently. Resources include money, supplies and equipment, people, technology, and information. Managing resources includes being able to:

- Make use of agency resources when planning care. For example, if you cannot transfer a client by yourself, ask to have another aide work with you at that client's home.
- Prepare and use budgets for cost-effectiveness. For instance, if you purchase food for the client, make sure you budget how much money you will need for shopping. Then make careful buying decisions so you do not go over the budget.

Vital Skills (MATH)

Calculating Weekly Earnings

Nursing assistants who work as home health aides keep track of their own hours. If they work independently, they must also keep track of how much each client owes so that they can prepare and present an invoice for payment.

Suppose you are a nursing assistant earning $9.25 per hour. You are assigned to work for three clients:

Client #1: Three times a week (M, W, F) from 8 AM to noon
Client #2: Twice a week (T, TH) from 8 AM to 4 PM
Client #3: Three times a week (M, W, F) from 1 PM to 4 PM

How many hours will you work in a week?

Monday: 4 hours + 3 hours =	7 hours
Tuesday:	8 hours
Wednesday: 4 hours + 3 hours =	7 hours
Thursday:	8 hours
Friday: 4 hours + 3 hours =	7 hours
Total:	37 hours

What is your total salary for the week?
37 hours @ $9.25 per hour = $342.25

What is your total salary from each client?
Client #1: 4 hours @ 3 times a week = 12 hours @ $9.25 = $111.00
Client #2: 8 hours @ 2 times a week = 16 hours @ $9.25 = $148.00
Client #3: 3 hours @ 3 times a week = 9 hours @ $9.25 = $83.25

Check your math by adding the totals for each client. Does the answer match the total salary for the week?

$111.00 + $148.00 + $83.25 = $342.25

Practice

Suppose you are working for the following clients, earning $9.50 per hour. Determine how many total hours you will work, your total weekly salary, and your weekly salary for each client.

Client #1: Three times a week (M, W, F) from 8 AM to 4 PM
Client #2: Twice a week (T, TH) from 8 AM to noon
Client #3: Twice a week (T, TH) from 1 PM to 5 PM

- Plan ahead for what you will need. This can mean making sure you bring your instruments, PPE, reporting forms, and cleaning supplies each day. It can also mean having plenty of gas in your car at the start of the work day, so you won't have to stop between clients.
- Store, distribute, and use materials and space efficiently. For instance, keep all of the client's bathing supplies neatly organized in a small bin near the tub.
- Keep records of resources. You might keep an inventory list of supplies that should always be on hand at the client's home.
- Substitute household items or make equipment or supplies that you need. For example, you might need to apply dry cold therapy for the client, but the client does not have an ice bag. Instead, put ice cubes in a sealable plastic bag. Make sure to wrap the bag in a towel to protect the client's skin.

Home health care offers flexible hours, independence, and the chance to build close relationships with clients. If you are considering home health care for your career, think about your interests, attitudes, aptitudes (abilities), and personality. Try to determine if you have the qualities necessary to work in this environment.

The Client's Progress

The home health aide helps the health care team meet the goals set in the care plan. Goals differ widely for different clients. You may help clients with the following goals:
- To regain all former abilities and health. This might be the goal for an elderly client with a hip replacement who expects to make a full recovery.
- To maintain independence despite the effects of illness and the normal changes brought about by aging. You can encourage and assist the client to keep or reach some level of independence.
- To maintain the client in a clean, safe, and comfortable environment. This might be the goal when there is no expectation that the client's health will improve.

Some clients are weak from long-term illness, have permanent physical or mental disabilities, or are dying. Some stages of illness represent a certain kind of progress. For example, a chronically ill client may gradually make progress accepting the illness and its effects. A terminally ill client may go through certain stages as death approaches. The progress through those stages may help ease the passage from life to death. You can encourage this kind of progress when appropriate. In these cases, the goal is to ensure the best possible outcome for the client.

You can promote progress and independence in the following ways:
- Encourage clients to make their own decisions if possible. This can include even minor decisions, such as which linens to put on the bed.

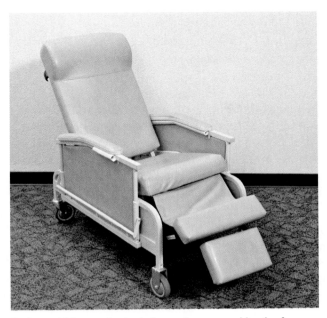

○ **Figure 25-3.** A geriatric chair may have several levels of adjustment for the client's comfort.

- Encourage clients to perform tasks that are within their ability. Even if they do tasks poorly, they will make a greater effort with your encouragement. Continued improvement builds confidence and strength. Praise the client's efforts and successes.
- Encourage clients to use assistive aids and adaptive furniture. For example, a client with limited mobility may be more independent by using a geriatric chair. It is a chair that reclines and is adjustable at several angles to provide comfort and relieve pressure. You can adjust the position of the chair as needed so the client can rest or sit up to participate in activities. **See Figure 25-3.**
- Help clients regain movement as soon as possible. Encourage the client to do prescribed exercises as ordered. Encourage walking with or without aids, if appropriate. Assist with range-of-motion exercises to increase mobility.
- Help clients participate in enjoyable activities. Some clients can do puzzles, sew or embroider, use a computer, or care for plants or pets. Some will enjoy getting out to do errands, such as shopping, or to visit friends. Most clients enjoy watching television, but encourage them to be as active as possible every day.

Vital Skills WRITING

Avoiding Plagiarism

Plagiarism means that you have taken someone else's words, thoughts, or ideas and used them in your writing without giving that person proper credit. Plagiarism is a serious offense; most schools have strict policies against plagiarism that can result in expulsion from school.

In most cases, plagiarism is easy to avoid.

- Never buy a paper or have someone else write a paper for you on which you put your name.
- Never cut and paste entire sentences and paragraphs from Web sites and put them in your paper without properly indicating that the work is someone else's (and crediting the source).
- Never use another person's ideas without giving that person credit for the ideas.

You do not need to cite a source when you are giving your own opinion, writing the results of your own research, or including generally accepted facts or common knowledge in your writing.

Some tips for avoiding plagiarism:

- Use your own thoughts, expressed in your own words.
- When you use someone else's exact words, use quotation marks and cite the source.

- If any fact that you learn while conducting your research is new to you, it is not common knowledge.
- The best way to avoid plagiarism? When in doubt, cite a source.

Practice

Below are some examples of sentences that might be included in a research paper. Read each example and decide whether you need to cite a source.
1. Every year, more than 400,000 Americans die from cigarette smoking.
2. Many experts say taking vitamins is essential for good health.
3. In my house, we try to eat a well-balanced diet containing fruits, vegetables, and whole grains.
4. Quitting smoking is difficult.
5. Smoking can lead to lung cancer, bronchitis, chronic obstructive pulmonary disease, and death from burn accidents.

Interacting with the Family

Family members can play an important role in setting and meeting the client's care and treatment goals. They can encourage the client and provide other emotional support. Their love and attention is beneficial to the client. Some family members are very closely involved in providing physical care as well and may have tips for caring for that person.

The home health aide can further assist the client by building a positive relationship with the family. They may be able to provide specific information about the client that will help give better care. If family members are difficult or challenging, be tolerant. They usually have the client's best interest at heart. Respect their involvement with the client, whether they live nearby or far away. They may wish to speak to you regularly for updates about the client and for reassurance.

Follow your agency's policies about reporting to the client's family. If you do give reports, be objective. Give simple, straightforward answers to questions. When you do not know the answer to a question or if the question is medical, refer the family to the client's doctor or the nurse. If possible, let the client answer general questions.

As the client's condition changes, family and friends may not be aware of new limitations. Loved ones may contradict a client's or doctor's wishes. You are hired to care for the client and should follow his or her instructions as long as they are not dangerous or unhealthy. If the doctor has given you specific instructions, follow them. For instance, if the doctor tells you that a client with diabetes cannot have sweets, and a relative brings the client a box of cookies, do not serve them. Use the opportunity to teach family members about the dangers of not following the doctor's instructions. If that fails, put the cookies aside so the client does not have access to them. Report this to the case manager. It may be possible to adjust the diet so that the client can enjoy this treat from loved ones once in a while.

Recording and Reporting

Part of a home health aide's job responsibility includes completing reports to the home health agency and sometimes to other medical personnel. (Aides who work on their own usually give reports only to the client's family or doctor. These reports may be informal.) Reporting observations and care is extremely important since, in many instances, the aide is the client's only outside contact for long periods.

The home health aide measures the client's progress toward goals and reports on that progress. Your reports will be used to determine whether the client needs more attention or can be discharged from home care. When creating reports:
• Provide accurate, objective information.
• Report events in the order they occurred.
• Chart or report all observations and procedures.
• Identify mental, physical, and behavioral changes.
• Include client needs if they have changed.
• Report according to your agency's chain of command.

Most agencies have a formal system of communication. There may be times when you report in person or over the phone, but you should always provide written reports, too. If you work for an agency, you will submit the report to your case manager.

A **client care record** is a record of all the care you give a specific client. It includes observations, client response to care, progress notes, and housekeeping and food tasks performed. It is sometimes called a *daily report*. It may also include places to record arrival and departure times. **See Figure 25-4.**

A care log may be kept in the home, especially for a client who needs 24-hour care. The log serves as a report for the aides on each shift, so they will know what has happened that day.

Employee Name (Print)

Client Name – Last, First

Address

Week Ending / /	SUN	MON	TUE	WED	THUR	FRI	SAT	I certify that I have worked the hours listed on this time sheet.
Service Date								
Time Start	AM PM	AM PM	AM PM	AM PM	AM PM	AM PM	AM PM	Signature _____
Time Finish	AM PM	AM PM	AM PM	AM PM	AM PM	AM PM	AM PM	Approved _____
Hours Worked								Notes Reviewed _____ RN

PERSONAL CARE	SUN	MON	TUE	WED	THUR	FRI	SAT
Bath ❑ Part							
❑ Comp							
❑ Tub							
❑ Shower							
Peri Care							
Skin Care							
Mouth Care							
Dressing							
Shampoo							
Shave ❑ Elect							
❑ Safety							
Foot Care							
Nails ❑ Clean							
❑ File							
Toilet ❑ BSC							
❑ Bedpan							
❑ Toilet							
Bowel Movement							
Other (specify)							

ACTIVITY	SUN	MON	TUE	WED	THUR	FRI	SAT
Ambulation							
Exercises							
Transfers							
Reposition							
Other (specify)							

NUTRITION	SUN	MON	TUE	WED	THUR	FRI	SAT
Meal Plan/Prep							
Marketing							
Feeding							
Intake/Output							
Other (specify)							

HOMEMAKING	SUN	MON	TUE	WED	THUR	FRI	SAT
Bed ❑ Make							
❑ Change							
Bedroom							
Bathroom							
Kitchen							
Laundry							
Shopping							
Conversation							
Activity							
Other (specify)							

SPECIAL TREATMENT	SUN	MON	TUE	WED	THUR	FRI	SAT
Temp – Oral							
Pulse							
Resp							
Weight							
Med. Reminder							
Other (specify)							

○ **Figure 25-4. The client care record of a home health aide working for an agency.**

A **time/travel record** is a log that describes how you have spent your time with the client, traveling to and from the client's home, and doing errands for the client. These forms may be daily or weekly. The form may be for one client or for all of the clients you have seen that day or that week. The log includes the names of clients visited and starting and ending times. **Figure 25-5** is a simple example of a time/travel record. These records determine how the agency gets paid and, in turn, how aides are paid. A record for logging miles traveled may also be submitted, if the aide is to be reimbursed for mileage.

DAY	DATE	TIME IN	TIME OUT	TOTAL HOURS	AUTHORIZED SIGNATURE
MON	/ /				
TUES	/ /				
WED	/ /				
THUR	/ /				
FRI	/ /				
SAT	/ /				
SUN	/ /				

CLIENT NAME (**PRINT**):

CLIENT ADDRESS:

Employee Name (Print):

Employee Signature:

Client/Employee   I acknowledge that I have read the terms and conditions on the reverse side of the time card. I agree and abide to these terms and conditions. I certify said time is correct.

Time cards must be in the office by noon Tuesday.

○ **Figure 25-5.** A simple weekly time/travel record notes time spent with the client.

Home health aides who are employed directly by clients are responsible for keeping track of their hours, expenses, mileage, and other related items. To receive your pay, you may have to submit a weekly invoice such as the one shown in **Figure 25-6**. As an independent worker, you will also have to pay your own taxes and social security.

A home health aide may be asked to shop for clothing, food, cleaning supplies, and gifts for family members. Make good choices and stay within a proposed budget. If expense money is given to you in advance, keep accurate records. Whether you work on your own or for an agency, keep all receipts to turn in with expense reports.

Invoice #2235

Date: 10/20/07

To: Mrs. Carmelita Jones
14 Sullivan Street
Chicago, IL 60610
773-555-1212

From: Angela Johnson
5757 W. Fargo Street
Chicago, IL 60657
773-555-3450
Social Security Number 001-99-1111

For: Services for Week of 10/14/07

Care Provided	Hours Worked
Measured Vital Signs	15 @ $8.50/hour
Bed Bath/Shampoo	
Catheter Care	
Laundry	
Changed Linens	
Prepared Lunch	**Total Due: $127.50**

○ **Figure 25-6.** A self-employed home health aide submits a weekly invoice to the client.

Monitoring Comprehension

As you read, you should constantly be asking yourself whether you understand the material. It might sound hard to read and question yourself at the same time, but with practice, it becomes easier. One technique is to stop at the end of each paragraph and try to sum up the paragraph in your own words. (You can do this aloud if you are reading alone at home.) If you are stuck on a section, try rereading it. Still confused? It might be time to ask a fellow student or your teacher for help.

Good readers know when they have missed an idea and must go back and reread a section, or ask someone for help. They also know when to put the book down and look up a word in the dictionary. By constantly monitoring your comprehension as you read, you can build on what you know and work on areas that aren't as clear. With practice, you'll find it's easier to move forward through a chapter when you understand the concepts that have already been covered.

Practice

As you read the "Infection Control and Housekeeping" section, write one summary sentence for each paragraph.

Infection Control and Housekeeping

Besides providing health and personal care to clients, home health aides may be asked to care for the household as well. In all cases, discuss these duties with the case manager, client, or the client's family. Follow standard precautions and all other guidelines for infection control.

General Cleaning

Some assignments involve only light housekeeping tasks. For other clients, you may clean the whole house and do all the laundry. **See Figure 25-7.** In either situation, always clean up after yourself and the client. When cleaning, disinfecting, and sanitizing, wear appropriate personal protective equipment as necessary. Be sure to follow good handwashing techniques when you are doing housework while also caring for the client.

Vacuuming. Vacuum carpeted floors once a week. If there are pets, you may have to do certain areas more frequently. Vacuuming includes getting dust out from under furniture and from corners. Be sure to empty the vacuum bag. Some bags are permanent and must be emptied into the garbage pail. Paper bags should be replaced when they are full.

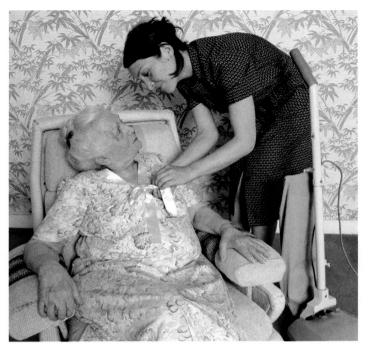

○ **Figure 25-7.** Housekeeping tasks are an important part of working in home care.

Dusting. Dust at least once a week, paying particular attention to surfaces in the client's room. Dust can be harmful for clients with breathing problems. Window blinds should be dusted or vacuumed lightly with a brush every couple of weeks.

Washing Floors. The kitchen floor may need mopping often. Depending on the type of surface, use a cleaner that allows you to damp-mop quickly. Use a bucket or, if there is a double sink, one sink can be used for rinsing and one sink can hold the cleaning solution. If you use the sinks, however, wash and disinfect them thoroughly afterwards. Bathroom floors should be washed at least once a week.

Cleaning Bathrooms. The bathroom should be cleaned at least once a week, depending on the client. If the client uses the bathroom daily, the aide may need to clean areas around the toilet daily. Most porcelain surfaces can be sanitized with a cleaner containing bleach. Scrub toilets using a brush for the bowl and a surface cleaner and paper towel or sponge for the rest. Clean sinks, tubs, and tile with a surface cleaner. Make sure to clean toothbrush and soap holders, too. Clean the bathtub or shower after each use.

Cleaning the Kitchen. Keeping the kitchen clean helps prevent infection. Scrub counters and sinks with a bleach-containing agent. A dishwasher's dry cycle sterilizes the dishes. If you only have a few dishes, rinse them thoroughly, put them in the dishwasher, and wait until it is full to run the machine. If you are not using a dishwasher, a capful of bleach in the dishwater will help keep bacteria to a minimum.

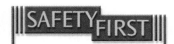
Handling Trash. Kitchen garbage should be removed daily. Empty pails and wastebaskets as needed, but at least once a week. Garbage should be put outside in cans with tight-fitting lids. You may be asked to put out the cans for garbage pickup. You may also be responsible for handling recycling of plastics, glass, cans, and paper.

Straightening Up. One of your daily tasks is to straighten up the area where you have worked or where the client has been sitting. At the end of your shift, make sure everything is in its place, so that the home is orderly and safe.

Laundry

You may be responsible for doing the client's laundry. When doing the laundry, follow the care instructions on the tags. Make sure to dry and put away all the laundry when you've finished.

You can generally make the bed with fresh linens once a week. If the client has incontinence, change the linens as soon as they become wet or soiled. Use a waterproof pad to protect the bottom sheet and save on daily changing. Wash dirty linens as soon as possible. If the client has been incontinent, the smells on the linens will fill the house with odors.

Clients may prefer to change into clean clothing every day, even if they are virtually bedridden. Generally you will be able to use your judgment about how often clothes and pajamas need washing. Always follow the client's preferences.

Clients with skin problems may need special detergents. When doing laundry for infants, use only detergents meant for infants and wash their clothes separately from the family's other laundry.

Food Preparation

Home health aides often prepare and serve meals. You may help with menu planning and purchase food for the client. Before shopping, discuss food preferences with the client.

The following list explains the basic guidelines for buying and handling food:

- Purchase only what is necessary for the client's meals and snacks. Many home health clients are on a strict budget. Use newspaper coupons and look for advertised specials to save money. Some clients may enjoy cutting coupons and marking specials.
- Check food labels to be sure the contents are appropriate for the client on a special or restricted diet. Even if not on a restricted diet, everyone needs to follow nutritional guidelines. Chapter 26 discusses nutrition and the basic food groups. Be aware of these guidelines when planning meals and choosing food for a client.
- Ask if the client has any food allergies. Check the ingredients list on food packaging to make sure the food does not contain food allergens.

- Be sensitive to cultural preferences and religious restrictions. For example, some people eat no meat. The client or the client's family will inform you of preferences and restrictions.
- Wash your hands thoroughly before each stage in preparing food.
- Prepare food in clean cooking utensils and on clean counters and other surfaces. Do not touch food once it is cooked and ready to be served. If you must taste food or try it for heat, use a clean spoon, but do not put it back in the pot.
- Be especially careful when handling raw food. For instance, raw chicken may contain *Salmonella* bacteria, which causes a serious, sometimes fatal, illness. If you touch raw chicken and then a fresh salad without washing your hands, you could transmit the bacteria. Proper handwashing techniques will prevent spreading bacteria.
- Clean all dishes and surfaces immediately after a meal. Food left on dishes and counters is a prime place for bacteria to grow.
- Store leftover foods in the refrigerator in tightly covered containers. Label the container with the date. Use these foods promptly.

FOCUS ON

Nutrition

Federal laws state that the daily values of all foods must be listed on a nutrition facts label. **Figure 25-8** shows two nutrition facts labels. One is for reduced fat (2%) milk, and the other is for nonfat milk. If a client's diet restricts the calories consumed from fat, which milk should the client choose? Which of the two contains less cholesterol?

REDUCED FAT MILK
2% Milkfat

Nutrition Facts

Serving Size 1 cup (236 mL)
Servings Per Container 1

Amount Per Serving	
Calories 120	Calories from Fat 45
	% Daily Value*
Total Fat 5g	8%
Saturated Fat 3g	15%
Trans Fat 0g	
Cholesterol 20mg	7%
Sodium 120mg	5%
Total Carbohydrate 11g	4%
Dietary Fiber 0g	0%
Sugars 11g	
Protein 9g	17%

Vitamin A 10%	•		Vitamin C 4%
Calcium 30%	• Iron 0%	•	Vitamin D 25%

*Percent Daily Values are based on a 2,000 calorie diet. Your daily values may be higher or lower depending on your calorie needs.

NONFAT MILK

Nutrition Facts

Serving Size 1 cup (236 mL)
Servings Per Container 1

Amount Per Serving	
Calories 80	Calories from Fat 0
	% Daily Value*
Total Fat 0g	0%
Saturated Fat 0g	0%
Trans Fat 0g	
Cholesterol Less than 5mg	0%
Sodium 120mg	5%
Total Carbohydrate 11g	4%
Dietary Fiber 0g	0%
Sugars 11g	
Protein 9g	17%

Vitamin A 10%	•		Vitamin C 4%
Calcium 30%	• Iron 0%	•	Vitamin D 25%

*Percent Daily Values are based on a 2,000 calorie diet. Your daily values may be higher or lower depending on your calorie needs.

O **Figure 25-8.** Compare the nutrition facts labels on these two types of milk.

Some clients have little or no appetite because of illness. Make mealtime pleasant and serve food in an appetizing way. For example, prepare foods of different colors and textures to stimulate the appetite. If the client goes to the table for meals, make sure it is set neatly and food is displayed nicely on the plate. If the client does not go to the table, prepare the food on a tray. Serve the tray to the client in a timely manner so the food is warm and tasty. The tray should be sturdy and able to fit over the client's lap, whether in bed or sitting in a chair.

Ask the client if he or she would like company while eating. Having company and conversation may help the client consume more of the meal. Take your time if you need to assist the client with eating. Allow the client to choose what to eat first. Encourage thorough chewing and swallowing.

A Safe Environment

A home assessment will be conducted before a client is enrolled with a home health care agency. The case manager will identify potential hazards. The home health aide can also conduct regular safety surveys.

- Make sure there are smoke detectors in the home and test them regularly.
- Make sure the areas around the water heater and furnace are free of trash and debris that could pose a fire hazard.
- If the client has a small personal heater, make sure it is in good working order. Turn it off and disconnect it when not in use. Keep the area around it free of clutter.
- Electrical appliances should be in good working order. Do not use them if cords are frayed. Do not use extension cords unless they are rated and approved for the appliance.
- Make sure electrical outlets are grounded. When disconnecting a cord from the wall outlet, grasp the plug and pull firmly. Do not pull the cord.
- Look for evidence of rodents and bugs. They create a health risk. If they are present, ask your case manager about methods of pest control. A professional pest-control company may need to be called.
- Keep doors and windows locked at all times.

The home health aide is responsible for keeping the client's environment safe. A client's room in the home should be maintained using the same safety guidelines as those for a resident's room in a long-term care facility. (See Chapter 6.) Keep the floors clear so the client does not trip and fall. Remove throw rugs and keep walkways clear of clutter. Furniture should be arranged so it does not create a barrier. Move items the client frequently uses to a low shelf or nearby table.

Do not allow the client to smoke in bed. If the client must smoke, make a safe smoking area in a well-ventilated part of the house. Make sure ashtrays are always nearby and empty them frequently. Do not empty ashtrays into a wastebasket. Use an empty coffee can for disposing of ashes and cigarette butts. Do not leave the client alone when smoking. Keep smoking materials and lighters in a safe place and have the client ask for them. If the client is using home oxygen, follow safety precautions. Do not let the client smoke when using oxygen. Educate the client with oxygen safety tips, stressing that it is highly flammable.

Medications in the home should be kept where the client can easily reach them, if appropriate. If there are young children in the home, or if the client is cognitively impaired, keep medicines locked up if possible. If medications need to be refrigerated, keep them on a separate shelf or compartment in the refrigerator. Keep medications neatly organized, and check for expiration dates.

Handling Emergencies

Emergencies in the home are similar to those that occur in health care facilities. However, a facility has specific, practiced procedures to follow. Emergency workers or other case managers are usually available to help. Chapters 6 and 17 explain how to prevent accidents and fires and what to do in emergencies. You can apply those same basic rules to home care situations.

Create a home safety plan with the client and family members. First, familiarize yourself with exits and list the steps to take in case of a fire or other emergency. Plan an escape route for you and your client in advance so you can remain calm if there is an actual emergency. Review the plan on a regular basis with the client and with others who provide care.

Know where emergency supplies are stored. They include flashlights, batteries, fire extinguishers, and a portable radio for other types of emergencies. **See Figure 25-9.** Post emergency telephone numbers near the phones. Know who to contact in an emergency. In most communities, you can dial 911 to activate emergency medical services.

Ask the client, the family, or the case manager if the client has any conditions that might result in an emergency medical situation. For instance, you will need to know how to assist a client with diabetes who goes into insulin shock. If your client uses an oxygen tank or a ventilator, you will need to know about supplemental supplies or alternative power sources, such as a generator or batteries, in case there is a power failure. You should also know whether the client has a DNR

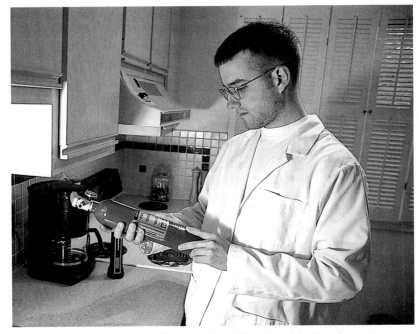

○ **Figure 25-9. Read the instructions on a home fire extinguisher in advance to prepare for an emergency.**

order. This is the medical treatment order that tells health care providers not to use CPR on a client if the heart or breathing stops.

You must also know when you are not able to handle a situation. Always call 911 in a health crisis situation, and then call your case manager. When an emergency is resolved, notify family members who have asked to be kept informed. They may wish to pay an extra visit, or they may decide that the client needs additional help for a while.

Most homes can withstand the most common types of storms. If a serious weather emergency, such as a flood, tornado or hurricane, is expected, you and the client may have to be evacuated. In such cases, follow the instructions of emergency workers. Be prepared to transport medications and documents with the client.

If there is a power failure, heat and air conditioning will stop working. Keeping the client cool or warm can avoid a health crisis, particularly for elderly clients. If the home is too hot, open windows and give overheated clients a sponge bath. Provide extra clothing and blankets to clients if the heating system shuts down.

As with any other emergency, use common sense and remain calm. Never leave a client alone when there is an emergency. If you must leave, call your case manager or emergency personnel for help.

Reporting Abuse

All clients have the right to be free of abuse, mistreatment, and neglect. However, clients are sometimes abused by health care workers. Some may be abused by family members. In particular, the elderly, the disabled, and other dependent adults may be at risk for abuse by family members, especially if they live in the same home. Family members providing constant care may experience stress and may become violent toward the client. Some family members abandon the person who is ill or disabled.

You must never abuse, neglect, or abandon a client. In addition, as a health care worker, you are legally required to report the following:

• Suspected abuse, neglect, or domestic violence. **Domestic violence** is the act of physically injuring or abusing a family member or someone else who lives in the home. See Chapter 4 for information about recognizing the signs of abuse.
• Sexual harassment
• Abandonment

If a client has bruises or other signs of abuse, carefully ask the client about them. If you notice a continuing pattern of bruises and do not get satisfactory answers, inform your case manager or the health care professional involved in the client's care.

Follow your agency's policies and procedures about reporting. If no one acts on your report, call adult protective services, an ombudsman from the local agency on aging, or an abuse hotline in your area. In a life-threatening situation, call the police. Report abandonment immediately so the client will not be left alone. Social service agencies provide protection and care in cases of abandonment.

It is important not to overreact, because reporting can lead to uncomfortable investigations and may upset the client. Use common sense. Do not report a single small bruise that will not heal. In spite of this caution, remember that your primary responsibility is to make sure the client is protected.

Vital Skills — COMMUNICATION

Conducting a Formal Meeting

Parliamentary procedure is a way for groups to organize and run meetings. It is used by many different types of groups—organizations from the U.S. Congress to the local garden club. By following some basic rules, groups can ensure that meetings are run in an organized, fair, and timely way, and that everyone in the group has a chance to participate and make their views known.

Parliamentary procedure most often follows a set of guidelines called *Robert's Rules of Order*, which were developed by General Henry M. Robert in the 1800s. Since then the rules have been revised several times. *Robert's Rules of Order Newly Revised* is the version most organizations commonly use today.

Meetings follow this general schedule:

- Meeting called to order
- Minutes of the last meeting read and approved
- Reports of committees
- Unfinished business
- New business
- Announcements
- Adjournment

The rules governing meetings are complex, but some general guidelines for parliamentary procedure include:

- The chairperson (or president) presides over the meeting.
- Members should stand to address the chairperson or group.
- A member who wishes to make a motion must be recognized by the chairperson.

- A motion must be seconded by another member (a member does not need to be recognized by the chairperson to second a motion).
- The group discusses the motion and decides on action to take (the group may decide to approve, reject, postpone, or refer to committee).
- The group votes on the action to take.
- The results of the vote are announced by the chairperson.
- Only one motion at a time is considered by the group.
- Members should not leave their seats until the chairperson adjourns the meeting.

Example: You are a member of the nursing assistants association at your school. At the next meeting, you want to suggest that the group visit a local nursing home on a regular basis to read to the residents. You introduce your idea by saying, "I move that we establish a group to visit a local nursing home to read to the residents." If someone seconds your idea, the group would discuss your idea and then vote on it. The vote may be to reject, withdraw, postpone, or refer your idea to a committee. Members vote by saying "aye" or "no."

Practice

With four or five class members, establish a group of your choice. Take turns being the chairperson to run the meeting. Have each member introduce a motion to the group, which will then be voted upon.

CHAPTER 25 Review

Chapter Summary

- The home health care team creates a care plan that includes identifying the client's needs, establishing goals, and creating a schedule.

- Home health aides provide the same caregiving tasks as nursing assistants but also assist with home care and food preparation.

- Home health aides possess personal qualities that enable them to work independently in a home environment, with clients, family members, and other team members.

- Building a positive relationship with the client's family members is important, but home health aides always put the client's instructions, well-being, and safety first.

- Certain records and reports must be completed accurately to communicate client care and the hours worked by the home health aide.

- Working in the home requires strict attention to infection control and may include housekeeping tasks.

- Home health aides provide a safe environment for clients, which includes preparing in advance to handle emergencies.

- Recognizing and reporting client abuse is an important responsibility in home health care.

VOCABULARY REVIEW

Directions: Match the letter of each definition in the second column with the correct vocabulary term in the first column. Write your answers on a separate sheet of paper.

Vocabulary

1. abandonment
2. case manager
3. client care record
4. domestic violence
5. home health aide
6. resource management
7. respite care
8. time management
9. time/travel record

Definitions

A. A record of all the care given to a home health care client

B. Having resources on hand when they are needed and using them efficiently

C. A log that describes how the home health aide has spent time with the client, traveling to and from the client's home, and doing errands for the client

D. A person who provides basic personal care and health-related services for a client in the client's home

E. Planning and scheduling your time to do tasks efficiently

F. The act of physically injuring a family member or someone else who lives in the home

G. Ending help or support without providing notice or getting the client's consent

H. Relief time for family caregivers to take care of personal needs or have time off

I. The supervising nurse in a home health care agency who is responsible for the client's care

Check Your Knowledge

Review Questions: Answer each of the following questions on a separate sheet of paper.

1. What information is included in the schedule for the client's care plan?

2. Describe three qualities of an effective home health aide.

3. List three ways the home health aide can promote a client's progress and independence.

4. What information is reported in the client care record?

5. Which type of record determines how the agency gets paid?

6. List the types of general cleaning for which a home health aide may be responsible.

7. When caring for a client with incontinence, how often should you change the bed linens?

8. Who conducts a home safety assessment before enrolling a client with an agency?

9. What should you do when there is an emergency in a client's home that you can't handle?

10. As a health care worker, what are you legally required to report about a client?

True or False: Read each statement carefully. Then write *True* or *False* by the statement number on a separate sheet of paper.

1. Home health aides help only with the client's personal care.

2. If a client hires you independently, you must pay your own taxes.

3. Trash and debris around a furnace could pose a fire hazard.

4. Food preparation should include a focus on nutrition.

5. If you think a client is being abused, ask family members what has happened.

Think and Decide

Directions: Think about each of the following scenarios. Answer each question on a separate sheet of paper.

1. Mary works independently part-time for clients. She finds the work rewarding but is often exhausted at the end of the week. She sometimes thinks she would be better off with a full-time job, but she reminds herself of her independence and the clients she is fond of. Discuss the advantages and disadvantages of working as an independent.

2. You are working in the home of Robert White, a 78-year-old COPD client on oxygen. A small fire breaks out in the utility room in the garage. The smoke alarm alerts you to the problem. What should you do?

3. You are going to the market for a client. You will be doing the shopping for meals for the next two days. You check the client's care plan to see if there are any food allergies or dietary restrictions listed and discover that the client is allergic to peanuts. Explain how to determine if specific foods at the market are safe for the client to eat.

4. Mollie Adams is recovering from a stroke. Her daughter, who lives in another city, contacted a home health agency to care for her mother. You are going to be one of her caregivers. Part of Mollie's rehabilitation program is to regain as much independence as possible. List some of the things you can do to help Mollie achieve her goals.

5. You work for a home health agency. You are interested in a short-term assignment. Justin and Anna Morgan take care of Justin's mother in their home. They need to go on a short business trip. They have contacted the agency to arrange for respite care. Explain what respite care is. If you accept this assignment, what will your duties be? How long will each shift be?

6. You have gone shopping for groceries for your home health client. The cost of the groceries came to $62.45. You paid for them out of the $80 the client gave you before you left his home. When you return with the groceries and give him the change, he says, "Oh, no, you do such a good job for me—you just keep the change." What should you do?

7. Janna is an 84-year-old home health client who is suffering from severe pancreatitis. Her physician informed the health care team last week that she has developed diabetes secondary to (as a result of) the pancreatitis. After the pancreatitis has been cleared up, the diabetes may disappear, but for now, Janna's diet must be restricted. Janna's daughter, who arrived this morning from out of town, does not know about the diabetes. She has brought her mother a gift of her favorite chocolate cake. How should you handle this situation?

CNA Certification Exam Prep

Directions: This practice test contains ten questions. Each question has four suggested answers. For each question, choose the ONE that best answers the question or completes the statement. Write your answers on a separate sheet of paper.

1. A successful home health aide is always
   A. attractive.
   B. honest.
   C. rich.
   D. a registered nurse.

2. A home health aide usually reports to a
   A. case manager.
   B. government agency.
   C. neighbor.
   D. physical therapist.

3. Home health aides are often reimbursed for
   A. mileage while working for a client.
   B. the clothing they wear on the job.
   C. personal long-distance telephone calls.
   D. trips to the mall on their day off.

4. A home health aide's housekeeping duties may include
   A. cleaning the gutters.
   B. painting the walls.
   C. washing the floors.
   D. changing the oil in the client's car.

5. Reports of a client's progress should include
   A. how much you like your job.
   B. what you think of the client's family.
   C. an analysis of the neighborhood.
   D. the client's level of daily activity.

6. Which of the following tasks is beyond the scope of practice of a home health aide?
   A. sterile dressing change
   B. catheter care
   C. personal care
   D. housecleaning

7. The case manager for a home health client is usually a
   A. physical therapist.
   B. physician.
   C. registered nurse.
   D. nursing assistant.

8. Arriving to work on time, every time, is an example of
   A. empathy.
   B. adaptability.
   C. honesty.
   D. dependability.

9. Storing and using materials efficiently in a client's home is an example of
   A. time management.
   B. time allotment.
   C. resource management.
   D. personal management.

10. Another term for a client care record is
    A. time/travel record.
    B. daily report.
    C. expense report.
    D. nurses' notes.

CHAPTER 26

OBJECTIVES

- Identify the basic nutrients and describe their functions.
- Identify food sources for the basic nutrients.
- Describe the MyPyramid food guidance system.
- Demonstrate the procedures for preparing and assisting patients with meals.
- Describe precautions to be taken when feeding a patient with swallowing problems.

- Explain how to measure and document food intake.
- Explain the importance of fluid balance.
- Demonstrate how to measure and record fluid intake.

- Describe alternative methods to meet food and fluid needs.
- Identify factors that influence dietary habits and preferences.
- Describe special diets and explain why they may be ordered.

Nutrition

Americans with Disabilities Act A federal law that requires a specific level of health care access for people who have a physical or mental impairment that substantially limits their ability to care for themselves.

anorexia Abnormal loss of appetite.

appetite The desire for food.

aspiration The breathing in or leaking of fluids (such as vomit) into the lung.

carbohydrate An organic chemical that is the body's primary source of energy.

congestive heart failure The heart's inability to pump effectively, which can result in the buildup of excess fluid in the lungs.

dehydration A decrease in the amount of water in body tissues occurring when fluid output exceeds fluid input. It can be dangerous when the body does not have the amount of fluid it needs to function.

edema An increase in fluid in body tissues that occurs when fluid input exceeds fluid output. It appears as swelling and can result in life-threatening complications.

emesis Vomit.

fat An organic compound that provides the body with stored energy and helps the body use certain vitamins.

gastrostomy tube A tube inserted surgically through the abdomen and into the stomach for feeding.

graduate A transparent container with a numerical scale marked on the side for the measurement of fluids.

intake A measure of all liquids a patient takes in.

intravenous (IV) nutrition therapy The continuous infusion of fluid and nutrients through a needle inserted into a vein.

minerals Inorganic chemicals that are essential to many body processes and functions.

nasogastric tube A tube inserted through the nose and into the stomach that can be used for feeding.

nothing by mouth (NPO) A doctor's order meaning that the patient cannot eat or drink anything by mouth. NPO stands for the Latin term *nil per os*, which means "nothing by mouth."

nutrient A chemical substance that enables the body to grow and heal itself.

nutrition The process of taking food and fluids into the body for growth, healing, and maintenance of body functions.

output A measure of any fluid a patient loses or that is removed.

proteins Organic (carbon-containing) chemicals that are present in every body cell. Proteins are responsible for the development and rebuilding of cells and tissues.

vitamins Important organic nutrients used by the body for a variety of body processes and functions.

Food

A well-balanced diet and good eating habits are important even to the healthiest of people. Proper diet and nutrition take on even more importance when a person is ill. **Nutrition** is the process of taking food and fluids into the body for growth, healing, and maintaining body functions.

Nutrients

The food we eat provides nourishment to the body. Foods contain chemical substances called **nutrients**, which enable the body to grow and to heal itself. The body needs many different nutrients to function properly. Nutrients are grouped into five categories: proteins, carbohydrates, fats, vitamins, and minerals. **See Figure 26-1.**

Proteins. One of the most important nutrients is protein. **Proteins** are *organic* (carbon-containing) chemicals that are present in every body cell. Without proteins, new cells could not develop. Existing cells could not rebuild themselves. Foods that are highest in protein come from animals. They include meat, fish, eggs, milk, cheese, and poultry. Protein is also found in cereals, grains, nuts, and dry beans and peas.

Carbohydrates. A **carbohydrate** is an organic chemical that provides energy to the body. Carbohydrates also provide the body with fiber. Fiber is important for bowel regularity. The fiber in carbohydrates is not digested. It provides bulk for bowel elimination. Foods that are high in carbohydrates include grains, legumes (beans, soybeans, peas, and lentils), potatoes, milk, fruits, vegetables, and sugar.

Fats. The body stores energy in the form of an organic compound called **fat**. When people eat more fats, carbohydrates, or proteins than their bodies need, the excess is stored as fat. However, fat is also a nutrient. It adds flavor to food and helps the body use certain vitamins. Butter, eggs, cheese, whole milk, nuts, and some meats are high in fat.

Vitamins. The body requires very small amounts of several organic substances called **vitamins**. Vitamins are used by the body for a variety of functions. They promote growth and boost the body's defenses against illness and disease.

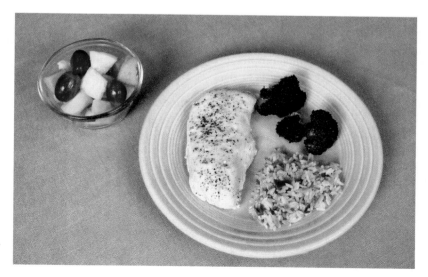

○ **Figure 26-1. To obtain all of the nutrients your body needs, it is important to eat a variety of healthful foods.**

Vital Skills READING

Paraphrasing

How can you tell if you really understand what you are reading? One way is to paraphrase the information you have read. When you *paraphrase* something, you say or write it in your own words.

Example:

You read: Many nutritionists and dietitians consider water to be the most important nutrient because it sustains life. Without water, a person could not live for more than about a week.

Possible paraphrase: Many experts say that water is the most important nutrient because people can't live without it for more than a week.

Reading, writing, and speaking are controlled separately in the human brain. By putting the information in your own words, you process it using more than one part of your brain. That gives you a better chance of remembering the information.

Practice

Read the paragraph below about carbohydrates. When you have finished, write a paraphrased version of the paragraph. You may also want to work with a partner to explain the contents of the paragraph in your own words. The more ways you find to paraphrase, the better you will remember the information.

There are two basic types of carbohydrates. *Simple* carbohydrates consist mostly of what we think of as sugars. Glucose, sucrose (table sugar), and fructose are examples of simple carbohydrates. They consist of one, two, or sometimes three units of sugar contained in single molecules. *Complex* carbohydrates have many more units of sugar—sometimes hundreds or thousands in a single molecule. These carbohydrates can be classified as high-fiber or low-fiber. Examples of high-fiber complex carbohydrates include broccoli and avocados. Examples of low-fiber complex carbohydrates include grains, potatoes, and rice.

Vitamins can be either fat soluble or water soluble. Fat-soluble vitamins are not easily dissolved in water, so they can be stored in the body. Vitamins A, D, E, and K are fat-soluble vitamins. Water-soluble vitamins, such as vitamins B and C, dissolve in water. The body cannot store more than small quantities of these vitamins, so people must include them in their nutritional plans. Vitamins are found in many foods, particularly in fruits and vegetables.

Minerals. Another class of nutrients includes inorganic chemicals (chemicals that do not contain carbon) called **minerals**. Minerals are essential to many body processes and functions. They help the body build bone and tissue, regulate the chemistry of body fluids, and maintain nerve and muscle functioning. Calcium, iodine, iron, phosphorus, potassium, and sodium are the most common minerals. Minerals are found in water and in foods such as leafy green vegetables and whole grains.

Food Groups

A balanced diet includes foods from the five different food groups plus oils, as established by the U.S. Department of Agriculture (USDA):

- Grains
- Vegetables
- Fruits
- Milk
- Meat and Beans
- (Oils—not a food group, but essential for good health)

The USDA's MyPyramid food guidance system provides nutritional guidelines for consumers and encourages them to make healthy food choices and to be active every day. The foods in each group provide varying amounts of nutrients. **See Figure 26-2.**

Grains. This group includes whole-grain cereals, breads, crackers, rice, and pasta. Consumers are advised to select whole grains for at least half of the grains they eat. This group encompasses one of the larger segments of the pyramid, so a larger portion of a person's diet should be whole grains. The primary nutrients in this group are carbohydrates, protein, vitamins, and minerals (iron, niacin, riboflavin, and thiamine).

Vegetables. Vegetables provide carbohydrates and vitamins (especially vitamins A and C). A variety of dark green, leafy vegetables, orange vegetables such as carrots and sweet potatoes, and dry beans and peas are recommended.

Fruits. Low in fat, fruits provide carbohydrates, vitamins A and C, potassium, and other minerals. The MyPyramid food guidance system emphasizes eating a variety of fresh, frozen, canned, and dried fruits.

Milk. Milk and milk products provide protein, carbohydrates, fat, calcium, and riboflavin. Low-fat or fat-free choices are best when choosing milk, yogurt, and other milk products. Calcium-fortified foods and beverages are recommended for people who cannot drink milk.

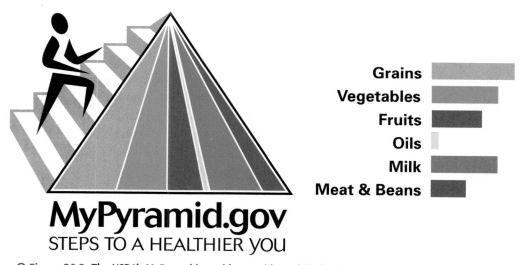

O **Figure 26-2.** The USDA's MyPyramid provides a guide to daily food choices.

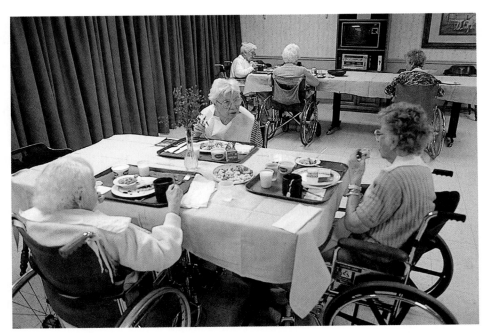

O **Figure 26-3.** Residents who are able to eat in the dining area can socialize during meals.

Meat and Beans. The body receives protein, fat, vitamins (primarily thiamine), and minerals (primarily iron) from this group. It includes nuts, dry beans, and peas in addition to beef, pork, poultry, and other meats and fish. Choosing low-fat or lean meats and poultry and eating more fish, beans, nuts, and seeds is recommended. Preparation of meats through grilling, broiling, and baking also minimizes the fat content.

Oils. Foods in this category include oil, butter, and fats. Most fat sources should be from fish, nuts, and vegetable oils. Butter, stick margarine, shortening, and lard should be limited.

A well-balanced diet includes servings from each food group in proportion to each individual person's daily nutritional needs. Individual nutritional needs are now calculated by a person's age, sex, and activity level. For example, young children may require more fat in their diet for their increased energy needs, whereas elderly people may need to restrict the amount of fat in their diet.

Serving Food

Residents who are able usually eat in a common dining area. **See Figure 26-3.** Some facilities group types of residents together in eating areas. For example, residents with Alzheimer's disease may eat together in a small group so that nursing assistants can pay close attention to them and make sure they eat while they socialize. Many facilities also have snack areas where residents can go to get fruit or juice during the day.

Some residents and patients must eat in bed because they are unable to get up and go to a dining area. Nursing assistants play various roles in assisting these patients, depending on their needs.

Procedure 26-1

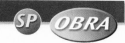

Preparing a Patient for a Meal

Equipment: urinal or bedpan • equipment for oral hygiene • wash basin • soap • washcloth • towel • robe • slippers

1. Identify the patient, check the ID bracelet, and call the patient by name.
2. Introduce yourself.
3. Explain the procedure to the patient.
4. Wash your hands.
5. Provide privacy.
6. Assist the patient as necessary with oral hygiene.
7. Ask the patient if the bedpan or urinal is needed. If the patient is able to walk to the bathroom, offer the robe and slippers. Assist if necessary.
8. Provide the patient with the wash basin, soap, and a washcloth and towel for hand-washing. Assist if necessary.
9. If the patient is able to sit in a chair for meals:
   a. Provide the robe and slippers.
   b. Help the patient to the chair.
   c. Place the overbed table in a comfortable position for eating (waist level is usually best). **See Figure 26-4.** Make sure it is clear of objects and the surface is clean. Go to Step 11.

○ Figure 26-4. Help the resident to a chair and position the overbed table for eating. Be sure the surface of the table is clear and clean.

10. If the patient is unable to get out of bed to eat:
    a. If instructed, make sure the bed rails on both sides of the bed are in the raised and locked position.
    b. Raise the head of the bed until the patient is in a sitting position.
    c. Move the overbed table to a comfortable position for eating. Make sure it is clear of objects and the surface is clean.
11. Make sure the patient can reach the signal light.
12. Unscreen the patient.
13. Wash your hands.

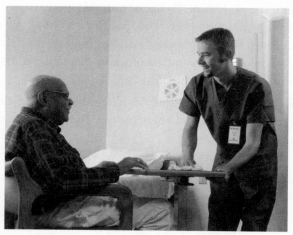

Patients with Disabilities

Most health care facilities have procedures and adaptive devices in place for patients who have disabilities. In fact, the **Americans with Disabilities Act** requires a specific level of health care access for people who have a physical or mental impairment that substantially limits their ability to care for themselves.

As a nursing assistant, you can help patients who have these disabilities get the nutrition they need. You can start by understanding and being sensitive to the special needs these patients have. For example, routine actions such as identifying yourself when you come into the patient's room and explaining what you plan to do become even more important if the patient is blind.

Procedure 26-2

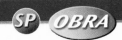

Serving a Meal in a Patient's Room

Equipment: food tray

1. Wash your hands.
2. Identify the patient, check the ID bracelet, and call the patient by name.
3. Introduce yourself.
4. Check to make sure the tray contains the correct diet for the patient. Be sure it includes all the items noted on the dietary card. Also be sure that it does not contain forbidden foods or condiments if the patient is on a restricted diet. For example, a tray for a patient on a sodium-restricted diet should not have salt packets.
5. Help the patient move to a sitting position in bed or in the chair.
6. Place the overbed table in a comfortable position for eating. Make sure it is clear of objects and the surface is clean.
7. Uncover food that is covered. Open all cartons, boxes, and containers. **See Figure 26-5.** If there is any food the patient cannot cut on his or her own, provide assistance.
8. Make sure the patient can reach the utensils, napkin, and all food items.
9. Ask if the patient needs any further help. If the patient does not need further assistance, leave the room.
10. When the patient is finished eating, return to the room and remove the tray. If ordered, measure and record the type of foods and liquids that were consumed and the quantity of each.
11. If any food or drink was spilled, clean it up now.
12. If appropriate, help the patient return to bed.
13. Assist with oral hygiene as needed.

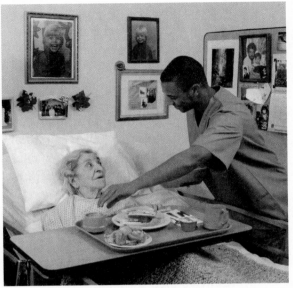

O **Figure 26-5. Prepare the tray for the patient by uncovering the food and opening all containers and cartons.**

14. Check to make sure the patient is comfortable and that the body is aligned properly.
15. Make sure the signal light is within the patient's reach.
16. Wash your hands.

SAFETY FIRST

Patients should not lie flat in the bed immediately after eating. Doing so can cause reflux, or the return of food back into the esophagus. Reflux can cause pain and, over a long period, can result in more serious disease.

Procedure 26-3

Serving a Meal to a Blind Patient

Equipment: food tray

1. Wash your hands.
2. Identify the patient, check the ID bracelet, and call the patient by name.
3. Introduce yourself.
4. Explain to the patient that you are going to feed him or her.
5. Help the patient move to a sitting position.
6. Place the overbed table in a comfortable position for you and the patient. Make sure it is clear of objects and the surface is clean.
7. Check to make sure the food tray is the correct diet for the patient. Be sure it contains all the items noted on the dietary card. Also be sure that it does not contain forbidden foods or condiments if the patient is on a restricted diet.
8. Place a napkin under the patient's chin.
9. Remove the covers from all food that is covered. Open all cartons, boxes, and containers. Place a straw in the cold beverage container. Prepare the food into small servings that will take up half a spoonful at most. Cut all food that is not bite-sized. Butter breads, season foods, and fix coffee or tea according to the patient's preferences and in accordance with any dietary restrictions. As you are doing these things, describe the food on the tray.
10. Ask the patient to imagine that the tray is a clock face. Use the numbers on a clock to describe the position of the food to the patient. For example, the bread is at 9 o'clock. **See Figure 26-6.**
11. If the patient can feed him- or herself, encourage the patient to do so. Tell the patient the position of the spoon. Guide the patient's hand to the spoon if necessary. Go to Step 16.
12. If the patient cannot feed him- or herself, follow Steps 13 through 15.

13. Feed the patient the food on the tray in a logical order (appetizer, then the main course, followed by coffee or tea and dessert). If the appetizer is soup or juice, you can alternate either of those with the main course since liquids may fill the patient up too fast. It is better for the patient to have at least some of each item on the tray. Fill the spoon half full with food. As you bring the spoon to the patient's mouth, tell the patient what it is. Warn the patient if the food is hot. Make sure it is not too hot to be served. (To test the heat of the food, let one drop fall onto your finger and feel the temperature before serving. Never touch food that is then going to be served to the patient.)
14. Place the tip of the spoon on one side of the patient's lower lip. Remove the spoon once the patient has taken the food off the spoon. Wait until the patient has finished chewing before offering something to drink. Do not rush the patient.

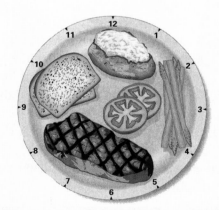

O **Figure 26-6.** When assisting blind patients who can feed themselves, describe the position of food on the plate as hours on a clock. The potato is at 12:00 in this drawing.

║SAFETY FIRST║

Never provide a straw with a hot beverage. Drinking a hot beverage through a straw can severely burn the mouth, tongue, and throat. For a blind patient, make sure that the edge of the cup of hot beverage is not hot enough to burn the patient's lips or fingers.

║SAFETY FIRST║

Patients should not lie flat in the bed immediately after eating. Doing so can cause reflux, or the return of food back into the esophagus. Reflux can cause pain and, over a long period, can result in more serious disease.

15. Offer the patient drinks between spoonfuls of solid food. To serve liquids, guide the straw (if a cold beverage) or the edge of the cup (if a hot beverage) to the patient's lips.
16. When the patient finishes, help him or her wipe the mouth with a clean napkin. Help the patient wash his or her hands.
17. Remove the tray and the overbed table. If ordered, measure and record the type of foods and liquids that were consumed and the quantity of each.

18. If any food or drink was spilled, clean it up now.
19. Check to make sure that the patient is comfortable and the body is aligned properly.
20. Make sure the signal light is within the patient's reach.
21. Wash your hands and report to the nurse.

Patients Who Need Assistance to Eat

Nursing assistants sometimes care for patients who are unable to feed themselves because of illness or injury. Some people are completely unable to feed themselves, while others need only some assistance. A variety of assistive devices are available to promote independent eating, such as specially designed implements, rounded plates with edges, plate guards, and spill-proof cups. **See Figure 26-7.**

○ **Figure 26-7.** Assistive devices that can be used by patients to eat independently.

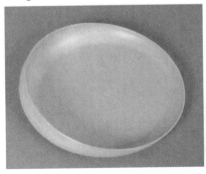
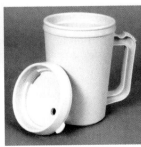
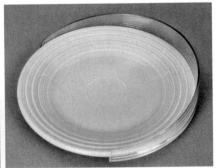

Communicating with Visually Impaired Patients

At some time in your career, you may need to work with patients who are *visually impaired* (partially or totally blind). Communication is the key to working with these patients effectively.

Remember that you must respond to each patient's needs on an individual basis. Identify barriers to communication and work to remove them. Here are a few communication tips for working with visually impaired patients:

- When you enter the patient's room, call the patient by name. Immediately identify yourself and explain why you are there.
- Always speak directly to the patient in a conversational manner. Do not raise your voice.
- Explain procedures carefully before you perform them. For some procedures, you may permit the patient to inspect or handle the equipment that will be used.
- Offer to read written diets or menu plans and other documents.

- Never leave the room without ensuring that the call button is within the patient's reach and that the patient knows where it is. Instruct new patients on how to use the call button.
- Do not assume that a particular patient can or cannot see well enough to complete a specific task. If you are not sure, ask the patient.

Practice

In teams of two, practice communicating with visually impaired patients. Take turns being the patient and the nursing assistant. A semi-transparent scarf may help you simulate partial blindness. The goals of this exercise are (1) to improve your communication skills and (2) to find out firsthand the special needs of visually impaired patients. As a nursing assistant, can you help meet these needs?

Still other patients are physically capable of feeding themselves but have been ordered not to for medical reasons, such as having a tendency to choke. It is important to provide support and encouragement to these patients and to ensure that their dignity is maintained.

Follow these precautions when feeding a patient with swallowing problems:
- Be gentle and patient.
- Avoid rushing the mealtime experience.
- Position the patient upright at all times.
- Allow more time to chew and swallow food.
- Feed the patient with a spoon to prevent injury.
- Fill the spoon only about half full of food.
- Provide sips of liquid after the patient swallows solid food.
- Reduce distractions and conversations while eating.
- Do not leave the patient alone while eating.
- Follow any additional recommendations from the doctor or speech pathologist.
- Stop any food or liquid that is accompanied by consistent coughing or throat clearing.
- Report any difficulties, such as choking or difficulty swallowing, to the registered nurse right away.

Procedure 26-4

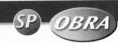

Feeding Patients Who Cannot Feed Themselves

Equipment: food tray

1. Wash your hands.
2. Identify the patient, check the ID bracelet, and call the patient by name.
3. Introduce yourself.
4. Explain to the patient that you are going to feed him or her.
5. Help the patient move to a sitting position or, if the patient cannot sit, position him or her on the side with the head slightly raised.
6. Place the overbed table in a comfortable position for you and the patient. Make sure it is clear of objects and the surface is clean.
7. Check to make sure the food tray is the correct diet for the patient. Be sure it contains all the items noted on the dietary card.
8. Place a napkin under the patient's chin.
9. Remove the covers from all food that is covered. Open all cartons, boxes, and containers. Place a straw in the cold beverage container. Prepare the food into small servings that will take up half a spoonful at most. Cut all food that is not bite-sized. Butter breads, season foods, and fix coffee or tea according to the patient's preferences and in accordance with any dietary restrictions.
10. Feed the patient the food on the tray in a logical order (appetizer, such as soup or juice, then the main course, followed by coffee or tea and dessert). Fill the spoon half full with food. Warn the patient if the food is hot. Make sure it is not too hot to be served.
11. Place the tip of the spoon in one side of the patient's mouth. Remove the spoon once the patient has taken the food off the spoon. Wait until the patient finishes chewing before offering something to drink. Do not rush the patient.
12. Offer the patient drinks between spoonfuls of solid food. To serve liquids, guide the straw (if a cold beverage) or the edge of the cup (if a hot beverage) to the patient's lips.

SAFETY FIRST

Never provide a straw with a hot beverage. Drinking a hot beverage through a straw can severely burn the mouth, tongue, and throat.

13. When the patient finishes, wipe the mouth with a clean napkin.
14. Remove the tray and the overbed table. If ordered, measure and record the type of foods and liquids that were consumed and the quantity of each.
15. If any food or drink was spilled, clean it up now.
16. Check to make sure the patient is comfortable and that the body is aligned properly.

SAFETY FIRST

Patients should not lie flat in the bed immediately after eating. Doing so can cause reflux, or the return of food back into the esophagus. Reflux can cause pain and, over a long period, can result in more serious disease.

17. Make sure the signal light is within the patient's reach.
18. Wash your hands.

Documenting Intake of Food

Some facilities may require that a patient's food intake be documented. Usually, the percentage of total food eaten is recorded after each meal. The doctor may also order a calorie count to determine a patient's food intake more accurately. The caregiver should record the portion of each food consumed. **See Figure 26-8.** The dietitian will then calculate the calories consumed and report the results to the doctor.

Fluid Balance in the Body

To maintain good health, the amount of fluid that enters the body must be equal to the amount of fluid that leaves the body. When fluid output exceeds fluid intake, dehydration can occur. **Dehydration** occurs when the body does not have as much fluid as it needs to function. It is a decrease (often sudden) in the amount of water in body tissues.

Dehydration is a condition that can be dangerous. Warning signs that may indicate a person is at risk for dehydration include:

- Dry mouth.
- Cracked lips.
- Sunken eyes.
- Dark urine.
- Confused or tired state.
- Consumption of less than 1500 mL of fluid per day.

Conversely, if fluid intake is greater than fluid output, tissues in the body retain the excess fluid. This condition is called **edema**. Excess fluid can build up in the lungs due to the heart's inability to pump effectively, a condition called **congestive heart failure**. Both edema and congestive heart failure can result in life-threatening complications. The first sign of excess fluid is often ankle edema, which causes the ankles to swell. **See Figure 26-9.**

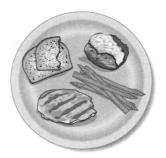

25% Food
Eaten

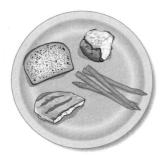

50% Food
Eaten

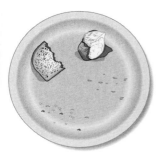

75% Food
Eaten

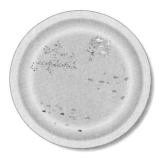

100% Food
Eaten

○ **Figure 26-8.** Document the food consumed by a patient at each meal, including an estimate of the percentage of food eaten.

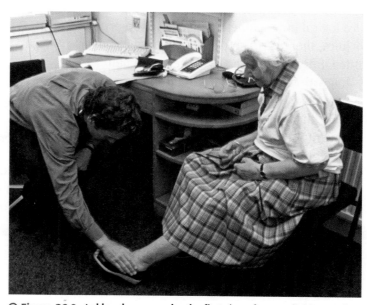

○ **Figure 26-9.** Ankle edema may be the first sign of excess fluid retention.

Adults need to take in 2000 to 2500 mL of fluids a day, depending on body weight. The minimum fluid intake for an adult is 1500 mL. Infants and children require a greater minimum daily fluid intake. Certain conditions, including extreme heat, sweating, fever, illness, and exercise, increase the body's need for fluids.

Special Orders for Fluid Intake

A doctor may specify the amount of fluid a patient can have during a 24-hour period. For example, the doctor may order "encourage fluids" (or "force fluids"), "restrict fluids," or "nothing by mouth (NPO)."

Encourage Fluids. This order is given for patients who need encouragement to take in more fluids. *Note:* The term "force fluids" is an older term for "encourage fluids." It is now being used less and less frequently, but you may see it on a doctor's order.

Restrict Fluids. This order is given for patients with conditions such as edema or kidney failure, whose fluid intake needs to be limited to a certain amount per day. It is important to measure fluids accurately when you are taking care of a patient on restricted fluids.

Nothing by Mouth. A **nothing by mouth (NPO)** order means that the patient is not allowed to eat or drink anything. NPO comes from the Latin *nil per os,* which means "nothing by mouth." A doctor may give an NPO order prior to surgery or diagnostic procedures, as a therapy to rest the gastrointestinal tract, or as a precaution when a nutritional problem is still unknown. An NPO order is usually posted both on the chart and above the bed.

Measuring Fluid Intake and Output

Measuring and recording fluid intake and output (I & O) are important aspects of patient care. For example, the health care team may examine intake and output to monitor a patient's kidney function or to evaluate the effects of treatments. In these situations, a record of intake and output is usually maintained near the patient's bed for convenience. **See Figure 26-10.** Information recorded there is transferred to the patient's record, usually at the end of each shift.

Resident Name _____
Room Number _____
Date _____

INTAKE		OUTPUT			
Time	Solution Amount	Time	Urine Amount	Time	Other Amount (Emesis, etc.)
Shift Total					
Shift Total					
Shift Total					
24-Hour Total					

○ **Figure 26-10. An example of an I & O sheet.**

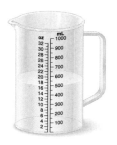

Figure 26-11. A graduate for measuring fluids. The fluid is at 500 mL (16.9 oz).

Fluid **intake** is a measure of all liquids the patient takes in. Fluids include water, ice chips, milk, coffee, tea, juices, soft drinks, and any other liquid a patient may drink. Soft foods such as ice cream, sherbet, hot cereals, pudding, gelatin, and popsicles are also measured. Fluid intake also includes fluids given intravenously or by feeding tube. Fluid **output** is a measure of any fluid a person loses or that is removed, such as urine, diarrhea, liquid draining from a wound, and **emesis** (vomit).

Fluids are generally measured using the metric system using either milliliters (mL) or cubic centimeters (cc). They are poured into a measuring container known as a **graduate**. **See Figure 26-11.** Graduates have a numerical scale marked on the side to measure the amount of liquid in the container.

Vital Skills MATH

Converting Liquid Measures

Tables that convert ounces to milliliters are available in most facilities. However, you should know how to do the math yourself as a backup measure. The following table shows some common factors for converting between U.S. (ounces, pints, etc.) and metric units.

To use the table, find the row in the table that converts to the units you need. Then multiply the first column by the conversion factor in the second column to obtain the measurement in the units listed in the third column.

Example: A patient has consumed one and a half pints of water today. How many liters did the patient drink?

pints × .047 = liters
1.5 pints × .047 = 0.705 liter

Practice

Use the conversion factors in Table 26-1 to answer the following questions.
1. Ms. G. drank 84 fluid ounces of water today. How many milliliters of water did she drink?
2. Mr. R. ate two 8-ounce helpings of sherbet and drank 38 ounces of water during your shift. How many cubic centimeters of fluid did he have?

Table 26-1.

Capacity (Liquid Measure)
Fluid ounces × 29.57 = cubic centimeters or milliliters
Pints × 0.47 = liters
Quarts × 0.95 = liters
Gallons × 3.8 = liters
Cubic centimeters or milliliters × 0.0338 = fluid ounces
Liters × 2.1 = pints
Liters × 1.06 = quarts
Liters × 0.26 = gallons

Procedure 26-5

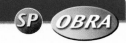

Measuring and Recording Fluid Intake

Equipment: intake and output record • graduate

1. Identify the patient, check the ID bracelet, and call the patient by name.
2. Introduce yourself.
3. Explain the procedure to the patient.
4. Pour the liquid that is left over from the patient's serving into the graduate.
5. Place the graduate on a level surface. At eye level, read the measurement of the amount of liquid.
6. Determine the full amount of the serving (usually listed on the I & O record).
7. Subtract the leftover amount from the full serving amount (for example, 300 mL full serving − 140 mL left = 160 mL consumed).
8. Note this amount.
9. Empty the graduate.
10. Repeat Steps 4 through 10 for all other leftover liquids. Make sure the graduate is empty before pouring another liquid into the container.
11. Add the amounts noted in Steps 8 and 10. This is the total intake.
12. Record the time and the amount as instructed.
13. Clean all the equipment and return it to its proper storage place.
14. Wash your hands.

Drinking Water

As a nursing assistant, one of your responsibilities is to provide patients with a fresh supply of drinking water. **See Figure 26-12.** Some patients may not be allowed drinking water at certain times. Other patients may be allowed only a limited amount per day. Still others may forget the importance of drinking water and may need to be reminded or offered water frequently.

Patients who are permitted to have drinking water should be provided with fresh water many times a day. Follow the rules of medical asepsis when serving drinking water.

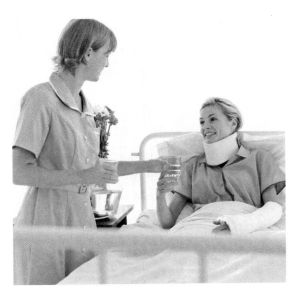

○ Figure 26-12. **Provide fresh drinking water frequently to patients who are permitted to have it.**

Alternative Methods to Meet Food and Fluid Needs

Some people are unable to eat or drink either by themselves or with assistance. These people may receive nutrition through feeding tubes or through intravenous nutrition therapy.

Tube Feedings

Several kinds of tubes are used to provide alternative nutrition. The **nasogastric tube** is inserted through the nose and goes through the esophagus to the stomach. **See Figure 26-13.** Nursing assistants must remember that the head of the bed must be elevated 30 degrees if a person has a nasogastric tube in place. Many patients find nasogastric tubes uncomfortable and prefer a **gastrostomy tube**, which is inserted through a small incision in the stomach area. **See Figure 26-14.**

Nursing assistants never prescribe or set up tube feedings, but they observe and care for patients with feeding tubes. They watch for signs of trouble, such as **aspiration**, which is the breathing or leaking of fluid into the lungs. In some states, the nursing assistant is also required to note the amount of feeding given and to observe the rate at which the feeding flows into the stomach.

Nursing assistants do not make decisions regarding tube feedings. It is important that any and all concerns be reported immediately to your supervisor.

- Report any unusual signs or symptoms to the nurse, including nausea, vomiting, diarrhea, or cramping.
- Keep the head of the bed up at least 30 degrees.
- Watch for signs of coughing or difficulty breathing and report to the nurse immediately.
- Observe for an enlarged abdomen.
- Provide frequent oral care.
- Observe for and report irritation, redness, or swelling of the nostril where a nasogastric tube is inserted.
- Observe for and report signs of redness or swelling at or near the site opening of a gastrostomy tube.

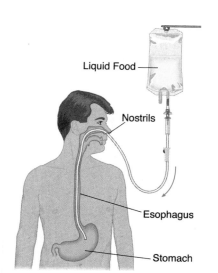

○ **Figure 26-13.** A nasogastric tube provides liquid nourishment through a tube that has been inserted through the nose and down the esophagus into the stomach.

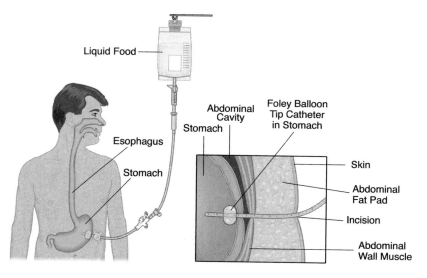

○ **Figure 26-14.** A gastrostomy tube provides a means of nourishment for long-term use.

Compare and Contrast

One way to approach writing a report is to compare and contrast sources of information. When you *compare* two or more sources, you look for how they are alike. When you *contrast*, you look for how they are different. By looking at several sources, you help make sure that your report will not be biased (one-sided). As you read each source, think about how the information agrees or does not agree with the information in other articles. Make notes as you do your research.

After you have read all of the sources, use your notes to create an impartial (not one-sided) report on the subject. Explain the points on which the sources you used agreed and disagreed, and draw your own conclusions.

Be sure to give credit to each source you use in your report.

Practice

Using your school or local library or the Internet, research gastrostomy tubes and nasogastric tubes. Find out how they are alike and how they are different. Do any of your sources disagree with one another? Write a report based on your research. Compare and contrast gastrostomy tubes and nasogastric tubes. Also compare and contrast your sources of information. Remember to give credit to any sources you use for your report.

Intravenous Nutrition Therapy

Another way to receive nutrition is through **intravenous (IV) nutrition therapy**. In this therapy, a specific fluid is ordered by a doctor when a patient cannot take nutrition by mouth. The fluid is *infused*, or taken into the patient's body, through an intravenous setup. A patient may also receive blood or medications through an IV line. Although nursing assistants are never responsible for IV therapy, patients in their care may have IV infusions. It is important to understand how to observe and assist these patients.

IV Setup. When a doctor has ordered an IV, a registered nurse starts and maintains the infusion. First, a needle connected to a small catheter is inserted into a vein. Then the catheter is attached to tubing leading to a container of the prescribed intravenous fluid. The flow of fluid is adjusted to the prescribed rate. Fluid drips from the container (a bag or bottle) into the drip chamber, and then into the patient. The clamp regulates the flow. **See Figure 26-15.**

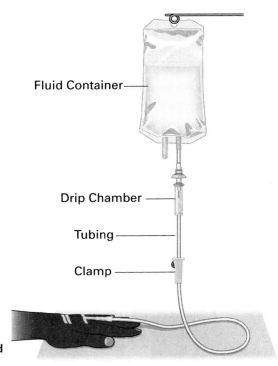

Fluid Container

Drip Chamber

Tubing

Clamp

○ **Figure 26-15. An IV setup. A catheter inserted into the patient's arm or hand is connected to the sterile IV fluid supply by flexible tubing.**

Special Care Requirements of Patients with an IV. When you assist patients who have an IV infusion:

- Never change the position of the clamp. If it moves, the flow rate of the fluid will change. If the fluid flows too quickly, it will cause the patient to receive too much fluid or, more importantly, medication. If it runs too slowly, it may cause insufficient supply of fluid or medication.
- Be careful not to move the catheter when changing a gown.
- When you help a patient walk, be careful to protect the IV solution container, tubing, and catheter. A rolling IV pole is useful.
- Encourage the patient to keep the arm with the infusion in a comfortable position. If the catheter becomes clogged, blocked, or bent, a new infusion must be started, which causes more discomfort.
- Never lower the IV solution container below the patient's heart. This would cause blood to back up in the tubing from the insertion site.

Notify the nurse or other supervisor immediately if you observe the following:

- The IV container is nearly empty.
- No fluid is dripping from the container to the drip chamber.
- Redness, swelling, pain, or leakage at the infusion site (where the catheter enters the patient's body).
- Blood in the tubing.
- Air bubbles in the tubing.

Procedure 26-6

Dressing a Patient Who Has an IV

Equipment: clean gown or clothing

1. Identify the patient and introduce yourself. Call the patient by name.
2. Provide privacy.
3. Explain the procedure to the patient.
4. Wash your hands.
5. Remove the gown or article of clothing from the arm without the IV.
6. Move the gown or item of clothing down the arm that has the IV. Slowly remove the arm and hand from the sleeve. *Never* disconnect the IV tubing to change the person's gown or garment.
7. Keep the sleeve gathered. Slide your hand along the tubing to the IV solution container (the bag or bottle).
8. Remove the container from the pole. Slide the sleeve over it. Hold the container above the patient's arm, and do not pull or tug on the tubing. **See Figure 26-16.**

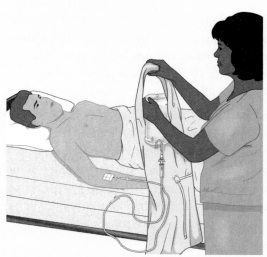

O **Figure 26-16. Remove the patient's gown over the IV setup without disconnecting the IV.**

9. Replace the container on the pole.
10. Gather the sleeve of the clean gown that will go on the arm with the IV. Remove the container from the pole, and slip the sleeve over the bottle. Hang the container back on the pole.
11. Slide the sleeve over the tubing, hand, arm, and IV site. Then slide the sleeve onto the patient's shoulder. **See Figure 26-17.**
12. Put the other side of the garment on the patient and fasten it.
13. Make sure the patient is comfortable.
14. Unscreen the patient, if appropriate, and remove the soiled garment.
15. Wash your hands.
16. Check the patient and the IV site.
17. Ask the nurse to check the IV flow rate.

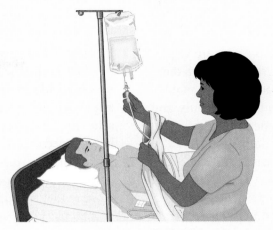

O **Figure 26-17.** To dress the patient in a clean gown, reverse the process. Slide the arm of the gown over the IV bag and tubing and then onto the patient's arm.

Dietary Preferences and Restrictions

People's eating habits and diets vary greatly. When they enter a hospital or long-term care facility, these differences may influence their appetite and willingness to eat the foods they are offered. This, in turn, may affect their general health or even their recovery rate.

Factors That Affect Diet

Many factors influence dietary habits and preferences. Some of the more important factors include age, financial situation, illness, and cultural, geographic, and religious personal choice differences.

Age. A person's age can affect dietary preferences significantly. For example, children's food preferences are generally quite limited when they are very young. Older adults may have less appetite than when they were young. **Appetite** is the desire for food. Elderly people have a tendency to lose their sense of taste and smell, so food may no longer be enjoyable. Their appetites may suffer as a result.

Culture. Culture also influences food preparation. Americans, for example, eat large quantities of processed foods. Some cultures eat more raw foods. Other cultures favor frying or smoking foods.

Geography. Eating habits are affected in various regions of the world by the ability to produce certain types of food. For example, rice grows well in the Far East. People in areas of the world that are surrounded by water typically consume greater quantities of fish.

Religion. Some religions have strict dietary rules. Not all members of a faith follow all of its dietary guidelines, but you should be sensitive to religious dietary rules and respect a patient's requests. Some religions require fasting or other dietary limitations at different times. Others restrict specific foods, such as certain meats.

Financial Situation. A person's income can also affect diet. People in lower socio-economic groups tend to have less income available for purchasing food. They may not be able to afford more expensive foods, such as meats. Sometimes people with low incomes are more susceptible to vitamin and mineral deficiencies.

Personal Choice. People also have strong personal preferences about food. These preferences may be based on taste, smell, appearance, and other factors. Some people avoid certain foods because of allergies, while others avoid foods that trigger adverse reactions. For example, people who suffer from migraine headaches may avoid foods that tend to trigger a headache, such as red wine, chocolate, or aged cheese.

Dental Health. People who wear dentures may wish to avoid certain foods to minimize problems with their dentures. This is particularly true of people whose dentures may be broken or ill-fitting. In some cases, people may need dentures but not be able to afford them. Absent or ill-fitting dentures are often responsible for poor eating habits in the elderly.

Illness. Many illnesses and diseases can make it difficult for a person to eat an adequate amount of nutrients. People who are ill sometimes have a poor appetite. **Anorexia** is the abnormal loss of appetite. Individuals who are depressed, anxious, or afraid may not have much of an appetite. Medication may also cause loss of appetite.

Patients who have no appetite still need to eat. Without food, the body cannot get the nutrients it needs to function. You can encourage patients suffering from a variety of illnesses to eat by suggesting that they:

- Eat foods higher in calories or protein first.
- Eat more frequent meals or snacks throughout the day.
- Allow time to rest before meals.

Special Diets

Doctors put patients on special diets for many reasons. Special diets can be prescribed to correct nutritional deficiencies, to remove or limit foods that worsen someone's health, or to increase or reduce a patient's weight. **See Figure 26-18.** Commonly prescribed special diets include:

- **Clear liquid diet**—clear liquids only, such as water, ginger ale, black coffee, apple juice, bouillon, tea, and gelatin without fruit.
- **Full liquid diet**—a transition diet between clear liquids and solid foods. It consists of all the liquids included in the clear liquid diet, plus nonclear liquids (such as milk) and nonsolid foods (such as ice cream, custard, fruit and vegetable juices, strained soups, and some cooked cereals).
- **Soft diet**—foods that are easy to digest and require no chewing: all liquids, as well as ground-up meat, pureed or mashed vegetables, strained cereals, puddings, and eggs. A special type of soft diet is the pureed diet, in which food is pureed in a blender until it reaches a smooth consistency.
- **Light diet**—excludes foods that are difficult to digest. Most foods are prepared by baking, broiling, or boiling. Fried foods, rich foods, and spicy foods are not allowed.
- **Bland diet**—foods that are not irritating to the stomach. Alcohol, caffeine, spicy or hot pepper foods, fried foods, and foods high in fat content are not allowed.

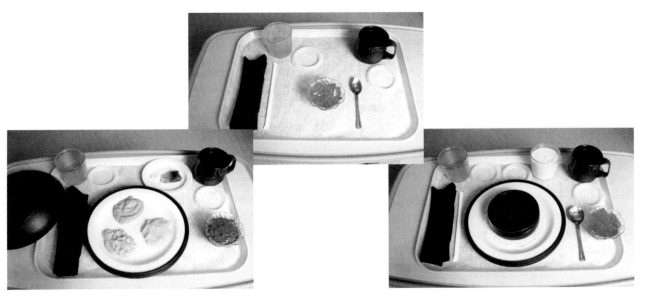

○ **Figure 26-18.** Special diets are ordered for patients based on their medical or therapeutic needs.

- **Calorie-restricted diet**—limits the caloric intake of the patient to a certain level (for example, 1000 calories per day). High-calorie foods, such as cake, cookies, and ice cream, are not allowed. Meats and breads are allowed in limited amounts.
- **High-fiber diet**—includes greater than normal amounts of fiber-containing foods, such as whole grains, fruits, and vegetables.
- **Low-fat/low-cholesterol diet**—excludes foods that are high in fat and cholesterol, such as whole milk, ice cream, butter, eggs, many meats, and fried foods.
- **Sodium-restricted diet**—sodium (salt) intake is monitored and restricted. There are different levels of sodium restrictions:
  - 2000–3000 mg per day—A minimal amount of salt is used for cooking, but no salt is added to already-cooked foods. High-salt foods such as pickles, olives, potato chips, and most luncheon meats are avoided.
  - 1000 mg per day—Food is prepared without salt and salt is not added at the table. Foods high in salt are avoided. Special low-salt versions of common foods, such as bread, are used instead of standard products.
  - 800 mg per day—No-salt substitutes are added to lower sodium intake further.
  - 500 mg per day—This is a rigid sodium-restricted diet. In addition to restrictions mentioned above, it limits consumption of milk, eggs, and meat.
  - 250 mg per day—This is the most extreme sodium-restricted diet. All efforts are made to keep sodium intake to a minimal level. For example, someone on this diet must avoid regular milk and use a low-sodium milk instead.
- **Diabetic diet**—A doctor usually determines the exact amount of various nutrients someone with diabetes needs. People with diabetes must eat their meals and between-meal snacks at specific intervals to maintain blood-sugar levels. The American Diabetes Association publishes exchange lists that group foods that have similar food values. Exchange lists are used by dietitians to plan and prepare meals for patients and residents. Diabetes is discussed further in Chapter 23.

Chapter Summary

- A well-balanced diet includes appropriate amounts of the following nutrients: proteins, carbohydrates, fats, vitamins, and minerals.

- The MyPyramid food guidance system provides individual guidelines for consumers based upon a person's age, sex, and activity level.

- The nursing assistant may be responsible for preparing patients for and assisting them with meals in a variety of situations.

- Nursing assistants are often required to document a patient's food intake.

- Fluid balance in the body is essential to maintain good health.

- Measuring and recording fluid intake and output is an important aspect of patient care.

- When people are unable to eat or drink, they may receive nutrition through nasogastric or gastrostomy tubes or through intravenous nutrition therapy.

- The nursing assistant should understand special diets in order to assist people with unique nutritional needs.

VOCABULARY REVIEW

Directions: Match the letter of each definition in the second column with the correct vocabulary term in the first column. Write your answers on a separate sheet of paper.

Vocabulary

1. anorexia
2. carbohydrate
3. congestive heart failure
4. dehydration
5. edema
6. emesis
7. fat
8. gastrostomy tube
9. intake
10. intravenous nutrition therapy
11. nasogastric tube
12. nutrient
13. nutrition
14. output
15. protein

Definitions

A. A measure of all liquids the patient takes in
B. The process of taking food and fluids into the body for growth, healing, and maintenance of body functions
C. The heart's inability to pump effectively, which can result in a buildup of excessive fluid in the lungs
D. An organic chemical that is responsible for the development and rebuilding of cells and tissues
E. A decrease in the amount of fluid the body needs to function
F. An organic chemical that is the body's primary source of energy
G. A chemical substance that enables the body to grow and heal itself
H. A tube inserted surgically through the abdomen and into the stomach for feeding
I. Loss of appetite
J. Increase in fluid in body tissues
K. A tube inserted through the nose and into the stomach
L. Vomit
M. Any fluid a person loses or that is removed from the body
N. An organic chemical that provides the body with stored energy
O. Continuous infusion of fluid and nutrients into a vein

Check Your Knowledge

Review Questions: Answer each of the following questions on a separate sheet of paper.

1. Which nutrient is an organic chemical present in every body cell?

2. Review the MyPyramid food guidance system and list at least four foods from each of the five food groups.

3. Name six warning signs for dehydration.

4. What medical condition may occur if fluid builds up in the lungs because the heart can't pump effectively?

5. Explain what is meant by NPO. Why might a patient be NPO?

6. Identify three alternative methods to provide fluid and nutrition to patients.

7. Name five factors that might influence a person's dietary preferences.

8. Why do patients who have no appetite still need to eat?

9. List three examples of foods that might be included on a full liquid diet.

10. What is the difference between a bland diet and a light diet?

True or False: Read each statement carefully. Then write *True* or *False* by the statement number on a separate sheet of paper.

1. Carbohydrates provide the body with energy.

2. Mealtime should be considered a time for eating only, keeping conversations and socializing to a minimum.

3. It is often the nursing assistant's responsibility to check the accuracy of each meal served.

4. When feeding patients who cannot feed themselves, position them on their side with the head of the bed flat.

5. While feeding a person who begins to cough or choke, offer large amounts of water to help the patient swallow the food given.

Think and Decide

Directions: Think about each of the following scenarios. Answer each question on a separate sheet of paper.

1. You are feeding Mrs. G., a long-term care resident with swallowing difficulties, when another nursing assistant asks you to help her change a patient's bed linens in a room up the hall. What action(s) should you take?

2. A 45-year-old hospital patient who is NPO following surgery has a dry mouth and dark urine. When you help him sit up on the side of the bed, you notice his IV is leaking. What should you do?

3. A patient had 900 mL of water in her water pitcher at 7:00 AM. It is now 3:00 PM and according to your facility, it is time to complete all documentation on this patient. There is still water left in the pitcher. What would you document?

4. Mr. N. is receiving nutrition through a nasogastric tube. When you check his condition, you observe that he is having difficulty breathing. What action should you take?

5. You are caring for a hospital patient who is recovering from abdominal surgery. She is receiving nutrition through an IV. While you are assisting her to walk in the hall, you observe blood in the IV tubing. What should you do?

6. A hospital patient is given a regular diet for breakfast. You remember that this patient is unable to chew solid foods due to a recent stroke. The family tells you not to worry, because they will watch the patient carefully. What should you do?

7. A long-term care resident with pneumonia is too tired to eat. What can you do to assist this patient in maintaining his daily nutritional requirements?

8. You arrive at the home of your client, Mrs. D., who has congestive heart failure. Her doctor has ordered a sodium-restricted diet of 500 mg per day. Mrs. D. has been preparing her own meals. While checking her vital signs, you observe that her blood pressure is 170/110 mm Hg and that her legs are swollen. What should you do?

CNA Certification Exam Prep

Directions: This practice test contains ten questions. Each question has four suggested answers. For each question, choose the ONE that best answers the question or completes the statement. Write your answers on a separate sheet of paper.

1. Examples of nutrients are
    A. proteins, fats, vegetables.
    B. carbohydrates, minerals, fruits.
    C. vitamins, proteins, minerals.
    D. vegetables, puddings, and minerals.

2. Vitamins A, D, E, and K are
    A. water soluble, so they cannot be stored in the body.
    B. fat soluble, so they can be stored in the body.
    C. water soluble, so they can easily be dissolved in water.
    D. fat soluble, so they can easily be dissolved in water.

3. Inorganic chemicals that are essential to many body processes and functions are
    A. carbohydrates.
    B. nutrients.
    C. proteins.
    D. minerals.

4. When assisting a blind patient to eat, if possible you should always try to
    A. feed the patient.
    B. serve only cold beverages to avoid burns.
    C. encourage the patient to feed himself or herself.
    D. provide a straw for all liquids.

5. When feeding a resident,
    A. alternate food and beverages.
    B. offer all the cold foods first.
    C. offer all the beverages first.
    D. fill the spoon to capacity.

6. Food intake is measured by
    A. counting the spoonfuls of food eaten.
    B. using percentages for solid foods.
    C. asking the resident.
    D. weighing the food left on the dishes.

7. Residents with Alzheimer's disease should be offered fluids at regular intervals to
    A. keep the bladder functioning.
    B. prevent dehydration.
    C. keep them from thinking of food.
    D. help them stay cool.

8. The breathing in or leaking of fluid into the lungs is
    A. dehydration.
    B. congestive heart failure.
    C. edema.
    D. aspiration.

9. When caring for a resident with a gastrostomy tube, you should
    A. make sure she lies flat while eating.
    B. offer her fluids by mouth frequently.
    C. observe for an enlarged abdomen.
    D. check her vital signs frequently.

10. A resident complains of nausea and vomits after eating only a third of her meal. You should
    A. encourage her to take a few more bites.
    B. leave the room immediately.
    C. return her tray to the cart.
    D. report the incident to the nurse.

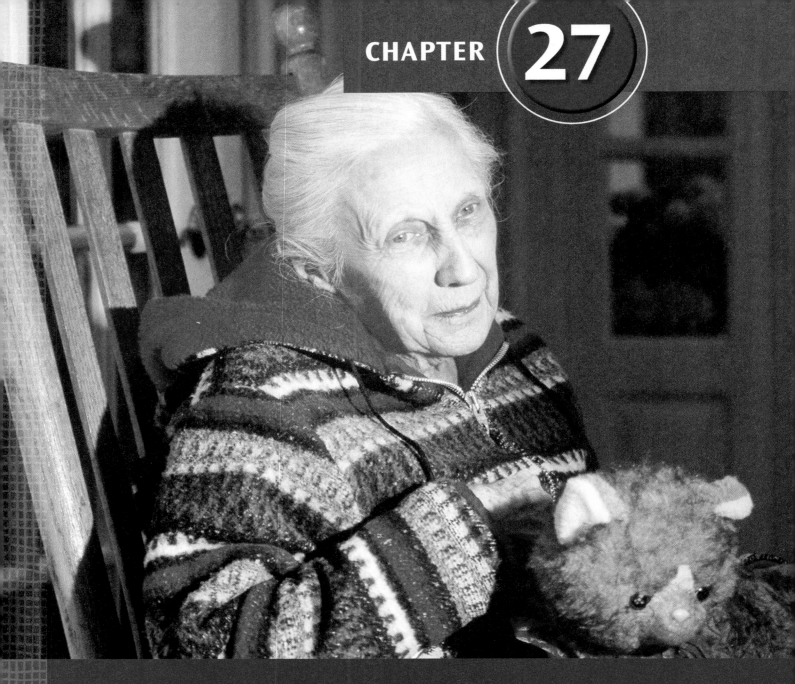

CHAPTER (27)

OBJECTIVES

- **Describe common coping and defense mechanisms and contrast effective and ineffective mechanisms.**
- **Identify causes or contributing factors of certain mental disorders and mental states.**
- **Describe observations and caregiving for patients with mental disorders.**

- **Describe ways a nursing assistant can help a patient with depression.**
- **Identify causes of dementia.**
- **Describe observations and caregiving for patients with dementia.**
- **Explain the difference between reality orientation therapy and validation therapy.**

- **Describe substance abuse and identify signs and symptoms to observe for.**
- **List ways that nursing assistants can help carry out a patient's treatment plan.**
- **Describe the developmental levels of mental retardation.**

Understanding Mental Health

VOCABULARY

agitation A state of extreme restlessness.

Alzheimer's disease A progressive, irreversible mental disorder accompanied by the gradual loss of intellectual and physical abilities.

anxiety A feeling of dread or discomfort that occurs without a specific reason.

assessment The process of observing for mental or psychological changes in patients.

confusion A mental state in which the patient is unaware of time, the environment, or the self.

delirium The acute, temporary mental state characterized by rambling or incoherent speech, a change in level of consciousness, confusion, extreme agitation and restlessness, or hallucinations; acute confusion.

delusion A false belief about oneself or others or about events.

dementia An irreversible, progressive loss in mental function, usually due to damage or disease of the brain; chronic confusion.

depression A mood disorder marked by extreme sadness and hopelessness.

disorientation A mental state in which the patient is confused and unaware of surroundings.

hallucination A false perception of reality that may include hearing voices or seeing objects or people that do not exist.

mental disorder A condition in which a person's thoughts interfere with normal daily functioning and a sense of well-being.

mental health A state of well-being of the mind and the emotions.

mental retardation A slowness or limitation of intellectual ability.

paranoia The false belief that others intend to do harm.

psychosis The general term for any severe disorder in which a person loses contact with reality.

reality orientation A technique for guiding disoriented patients back to reality. It is based on constant repetition of information.

schizophrenia A thought disorder that may include disorganized speech and behavior, irrational and illogical thoughts, social withdrawal, and an inability to make choices or decisions.

substance abuse Maladaptive behavior in which use of a chemical substance, such as alcohol, tobacco, or prescription or illegal drugs, has a negative impact on a person's life.

suicide The taking of one's own life.

sundowning Becoming upset, agitated, or disoriented in the late afternoon or evening.

validation therapy A communication technique that shows respect and maintains patients' dignity by acknowledging their reality.

Mental Health

Mental health is a state of well-being of the mind and the emotions. Physical and mental health are interrelated. A long physical illness can affect a patient's mental health. A patient with a mental disorder may become physically ill from lack of personal interest and care.

One of the hallmarks of good mental health is being able to adapt to change. Sometimes, however, we feel overwhelmed by change and then we experience stress. *Adaptive behavior* is the behavior we use to cope with stress. *Coping mechanisms* are conscious ways of handling stress. For example, some positive coping mechanisms are exercise, talking about our problems with friends, or just taking time out to relax. Sometimes people rely on negative coping mechanisms, such as overeating (or not eating enough), smoking, using drugs or alcohol, or arguing or fighting with others.

People also deal with stress by using *defense mechanisms*, which are unconscious ways of protecting the self from bad feelings, such as shame, anxiety, fear, or loss of self-esteem. Some defense mechanisms are:

- *Compensation:* Making up for feeling inadequate in one area by stressing strengths in others. For example, a patient who feels self-conscious about his paralysis constantly tells jokes to distract people from his physical condition.
- *Denial:* Blocking out or refusing to believe what is actually true, especially if it is frightening or unpleasant. A patient may refuse to believe that she has coronary artery disease, because her mother died of this disease.
- *Rationalization:* Justifying illogical behavior or poor performance by making excuses. A resident who is not reaching rehabilitation goals says that the goals are unrealistic.
- *Regression:* Returning to an earlier state or condition. A 7-year-old girl who is frightened about being in the hospital begins wetting the bed at night.
- *Projection:* Blaming others for one's own shortcomings. A patient in a drug-rehabilitation program blames his former employer for losing his job.

People with health problems may use coping and defense mechanisms as they struggle with fears about their changing condition and the loss of strength and abilities. Nursing assistants can help patients by learning to recognize coping and defense mechanisms and by providing emotional support and empathy.

Mental Disorders

Some patients you will care for suffer from a mental disorder. A **mental disorder** is a condition in which a person's thoughts interfere with normal daily functioning and a sense of well-being. People with mental disorders may have difficulty adjusting and handling situations and life events.

Set Aside Time to Read

Becoming a good reader takes practice—and that means reading, reading, and more reading. Good readers make reading a habit. They pack a novel in their purse when they know they are going to be waiting at the doctor's office. Or they pick up a newspaper on their way to work, to read at lunchtime. Reading is part of life for good readers.

Here are some tips for increasing your reading time:

• Set aside some time each day to read. Many people like to relax before going to sleep by reading. Keep a novel or magazine on your nightstand and read for half an hour before you turn out the light.

• Subscribe to a new magazine. Try something different—maybe a travel magazine, or a home improvement magazine.

Practice

How much do you currently read? Keep a journal of your reading time and then try to increase your current reading time by at least half an hour a day. Record how much time you spend reading.

Patients with mental disorders should be treated with understanding. Mental disorders are illnesses. Do not judge or blame patients for their mental problems. The way you interact with the patient—the words you use, your tone of voice, your body language—affects the patient's feelings.

Contributing Factors

Causes of mental disorders are complex and varied and are often unknown. However, stress from social and cultural pressure can contribute to mental disorder. Other contributing factors include:

• Ineffective coping mechanisms
• Substance abuse
• Brain damage or disease
• Aging
• Chemical imbalances in the body
• Genetic origins

Mental States

There are many categories of mental disorders. A diagnosis of a mental disorder may be complicated. Similar symptoms and behaviors can occur in many disorders. *Psychiatry* is the medical specialty that deals with the diagnosis and treatment of mental disorders. *Psychology* is the study of the mind and behavior. The word *psychological* refers to the study of the mind. Psychiatrists and psychologists try to classify a patient's specific mental disorder in order to determine the best treatment.

Mental health disorders range from mild to severe. Some change over time. Mental disorders are composed of a variety of altered mental states that affect a person's ability to think, learn, and remember. These conditions can range from mild to severe. Some are temporary, and others are permanent. When observing patients for changes, nursing assistants should be familiar with these altered states.

Confusion. In the mental state of **confusion**, the patient may be unaware of time, the environment, or the self. When confused, the patient may be unable to concentrate, may get lost, or may be unable to follow directions or ask for help. Confusion can be caused by a physical condition, such as dehydration, hypoglycemia, or a reaction to medication. It may be related to disease, an infection, or a high fever. People who have recently lost their sight or hearing can become confused. Injury or trauma to the head or brain is another cause of confusion. Confusion can also be a component of some mental disorders. Confusion is reversible if the underlying cause is resolved.

Disorientation. This condition is more severe than confusion. With **disorientation**, the patient is confused and unaware of surroundings. The patient is frequently unable to recognize people and places, or to remember events. Simple questions such as "Who are you?" or "What day of the week is it?" cannot be answered. Disorientation can result from physical problems such as blindness, deafness, or brain injury, or conditions such as hypotension, anemia, or uremia. Some medications cause disorientation. It may be temporary or long-lasting. Some people become disoriented when their environment changes, such as when moving from home to a long-term care facility. **See Figure 27-1.**

Reality orientation is a technique for guiding disoriented patients back to reality. It is based on constant repetition of information. Follow these reality orientation techniques:
- Repeat the patient's name often.
- Identify yourself each time you visit.
- Speak slowly, distinctly, and calmly.
- Use simple words the patient can understand.
- Repeat the day, date, and time often.
- Put a calendar and clocks in sight so the patient can easily refer to them. Make sure the print is big enough for the patient to read.
- Open shades or curtains during the day and close them at night, to help distinguish between night and day.
- Discuss familiar topics, people, places, and events.
- Give easy-to-understand instructions and repeat them as often as necessary.
- Ask simple questions and allow time for responses.

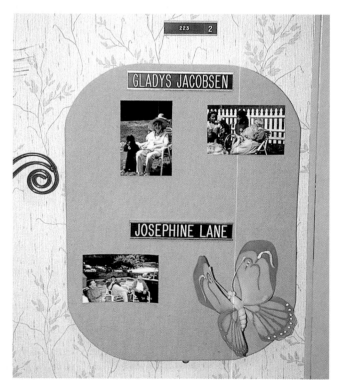

○ **Figure 27-1.** Residents who are disoriented may have trouble finding their own rooms. A few items on a memory board outside the room can sometimes help a resident remember where his or her room is located.

- Do not rush the patient.
- Maintain a daily routine. Give plenty of notice if the routine is going to change.

Delirium. The acute, temporary state of **delirium** is characterized by rambling or incoherent speech, a change in level of consciousness, confusion, extreme agitation and restlessness, or hallucinations. Delirium is usually caused by a physical condition, such as a high fever, traumatic injury, or sudden withdrawal from excessive alcohol intake. It is also known as *acute confusion*, because it begins suddenly and is usually reversible after treatment for the physical condition.

Anxiety. The feeling of dread or discomfort that occurs without a specific reason is called **anxiety.** Patients with anxiety often have rapid breathing, increased heart rate, and muscle tension. Anxiety can sometimes be relieved by talk therapy or medication. Some patients can control their anxiety by exercising strenuously or engaging in another activity, such as a craft, that distracts them from their thoughts.

Agitation. The state of extreme restlessness is called **agitation.** It is especially common in the elderly and patients with dementia. A patient may exhibit inappropriate and sometimes aggressive verbal and physical behaviors, such as cursing, spitting, screaming, hitting, biting, and fighting. Sometimes a warm bath or physical activity helps calm agitation. Intervention at the first sign of agitation can help prevent the behavior from becoming violent or requiring extreme measures to control the behavior.

When caring for a patient who is confused, disoriented, delirious, anxious, or agitated:
- Approach slowly so you do not startle the patient.
- Stay calm and maintain eye contact.
- Call the patient by name.
- Do not argue with or confront the patient.
- Minimize sensory stimulation, if possible. Remove the patient to a calmer environment.
- Speak in a slow, soft, calm voice.
- Protect yourself and the patient from harm.
- Ask about basic needs, such as the need to use the bathroom, or whether the patient is in pain.
- Identify and validate the patient's feelings by saying, "I see that you are upset" or "You have every right to be concerned."
- Do not restrain the patient unless ordered to do so by a physician or nurse.

When caring for patients with mental disorders, nursing assistants should also observe for the following behaviors:
- Emotional withdrawal
- Sleep disturbances
- Poor concentration
- Aggression
- Inappropriate sexual behavior
- Self-injurious behavior. This can include **suicide,** the taking of one's own life.
- Bizarre or deviant behavior. (*Deviant* means "abnormal.")

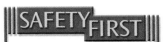

SAFETY FIRST

Nursing assistants who work with patients with some mental disorders are at risk of being injured if a patient becomes severely agitated or violent. Learn your facility's protocols for handling this type of crisis. Many employers offer or require training in crisis intervention.

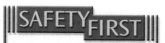

Depression

Depression is a mood disorder marked by extreme sadness and hopelessness. It appears in every age group, even in very young children. It is the most common mental disorder in elderly people. Symptoms of depression are fatigue, apathy, and physical disorders, such as headaches, backaches, joint pain, loss of appetite, and stomach problems.

Feeling depressed is not always a sign of illness. In some life situations, mild depression comes before an effort to change or accept a new situation. It is normal to be depressed during the natural grieving process, such as after the loss of a loved one. This is *situational depression*. It is not the mood disorder known as depression.

Depression can have physical and psychological causes. It can be caused by an imbalance in brain chemistry or the side effects of some medications. An older adult may become depressed over the loss of a spouse, friends or other family members, physical illness, body changes associated with aging, loss of purpose in life, and loneliness.

Depression becomes a mental disorder when it is long lasting and is accompanied by a nearly total inability to function. Symptoms can include:
- Losing interest in the world and surroundings
- The slowing down of movement and speech
- Withdrawal from other people
- Forgetfulness and difficulty concentrating
- Sleep disturbances
- Suicidal thoughts and attempts

During your career as a nursing assistant, you will have many opportunities to make a difference in patients' lives. This is especially true when you work with older adults who are depressed. They need to believe they have something to live for. Encourage patients to talk and then listen closely. Take the patient's concerns seriously. Do not make such comments as, "You're just having a bad day. Things will be better tomorrow." These comments can make the patient feel worse. Sometimes just being there and listening is enough to brighten a depressed patient's day.

When caring for a depressed patient:
- Be calm and consistent in the care you give.
- Encourage the patient to use support services and to attend therapy sessions.
- Emphasize the positive aspects of the patient's life.
- Be realistic, while still giving hope. Never give false hope.
- Do not pity the patient.
- Help the patient develop self-esteem and self-worth by encouraging involvement in social activities. Encourage interaction with other people.
- Prevent the patient from becoming exhausted.

- Provide care in frequent, short intervals, so you have contact with the patient often during the day.
- Stress the patient's value to society. **See Figure 27-2.**
- Observe for sudden mood swings.
- Report all complaints to the charge nurse so physical, emotional, and psychosocial problems can be addressed.
- Immediately report changes in behavior, increased use of alcohol, or threats of suicide. Do not ignore a patient who seems to be "getting his or her affairs in order," giving away favorite possessions, or getting a will written and witnessed.

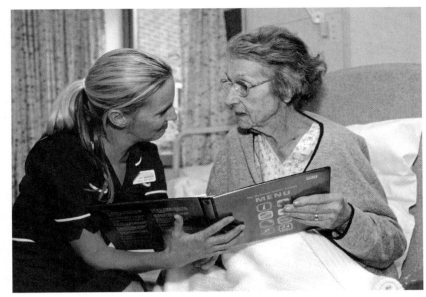

O **Figure 27-2.** Help the patient with depression feel valued by showing interest in what he or she has to say.

Schizophrenia and Psychosis

Schizophrenia is a thought disorder that may include disorganized speech and behavior, irrational and illogical thoughts, social withdrawal, and an inability to make choices or decisions. People with this mental disorder may demonstrate bizarre behaviors. They may present a *flat affect*, which means not showing any emotion. However, they are often in constant conflict with their emotions and thoughts, which makes coping more difficult. Schizophrenia typically begins in young adulthood and often lasts well into old age.

Psychosis is the general term for any severe disorder in which a person loses contact with reality. It is often experienced by patients with schizophrenia. However, psychosis can also be caused by side effects from some prescription drugs, substance abuse, or substance withdrawal.

These patients may have false perceptions of reality. A **delusion** is a false belief about oneself or others or about events. For example, someone with delusions may think that aliens are controlling his or her actions. A person may have a **hallucination**, such as hearing voices or seeing objects or people that do not exist. For instance, a patient may believe a deceased ancestor came to visit. Some patients experience **paranoia**, the false belief that others intend to do harm.

Nursing assistants can help by taking the following action:
- Make sure patients take medication regularly and on schedule. Report your observations about reactions to medications and therapy.
- Help patients with ADLs. They may not want to or understand why they should maintain personal hygiene. They may not wish to eat, sleep, or participate in activities. Encourage them to do what they can and help them with tasks they cannot perform.
- Keep patients involved in reality activities.

Vital Skills (WRITING)

Varying Sentence Length and Structure

What if every sentence in what you read had the same length and structure? It would be boring to read and you would lose interest fast. As you write, keep an ear out for variety. Are all your sentences the same length? Do they follow the same format? Read the paragraphs you write out loud. Do they sound monotonous? If so, you may need to vary the structure. For example, the two paragraphs below describe the same events. However, one uses a varied sentence structure. Does one sound better to your ear?

1. Mrs. Darcy was admitted on Friday. Mrs. Darcy had surgery in August. She had two stents put in. Mrs. Darcy may need another stent. Her doctor will decide on Monday. She may need a second surgery.

2. Mrs. Darcy was admitted on Friday. In August, she had surgery to place two stents. Her doctor thinks Mrs. Darcy may need another stent. He will decide on Monday whether she will need a second surgery.

The second paragraph has some variety to the sentence structure and doesn't sound as boring as the first.

Practice

Read the paragraph below and rewrite it to vary the sentence structure.

John came to work late today. He said he wasn't feeling well. He said he has food poisoning. He went out for lunch yesterday. He ate something bad at lunch. He says his symptoms are improving. He thinks he will feel better tomorrow.

- Actively listen. Patients may feel that nobody listens to them. Someone who is kind and listens is a rarity for these people. Your kindness may help them relax and feel more comfortable.
- Encourage family and friends to visit. Explain the value of these visits to the visitors.

If a patient having a psychotic episode expresses false perceptions to you, do not confront the patient. In severe situations, notify medical personnel. Some patients with psychosis harm themselves or others because their view of reality frightens or angers them in extreme ways. If you encounter patients with delusional thoughts, follow these guidelines:

- Do not confront patients or tell them they are wrong. The illness prevents them from understanding you, and they may believe that you will harm them. Confronting them might make them anxious or even angry. Talk about something that is realistic and may serve as a distraction.
- Be truthful and direct with the patient. Do not make promises to the patient unless you are able to keep them.
- Do not agree with or support any delusions the patient expresses.
- Try to reduce the patient's feelings of insecurity.

Dementias

Dementia is an irreversible, progressive loss in mental function, usually due to damage or disease of the brain. It is also called *chronic confusion*. Dementia can be the result of infections, injuries, Alzheimer's disease, AIDS, vascular disease, or long-term alcohol abuse. Some patients with dementia function independently, but others cannot perform the basic tasks of daily living. Some are aware of their environment, while others lose contact with reality. Specific symptoms include:

- Disorientation.
- Decreased ability to take care of one's needs.
- Impaired memory and judgment.
- Impaired attention span.
- Delusions.
- Incoherent or inappropriate speech.
- Personality change.

Assessment

Performing an **assessment** is the process of observing for mental or psychological changes in patients. An assessment provides the necessary information to plan for, implement, and evaluate care. Nurses are responsible for performing assessments. Most health care facilities have special *assessment tools*, or forms with checklists, to guide the nurse in gathering the assessment information. **See Figure 27-3.** Some checklists are brief, and some are lengthy and comprehensive. For

Mental Status Assessment

Patient's Name _____ Date _____

1. Behavior
- ❑ Cooperative
- ❑ Uncooperative
- ❑ Withdrawn
- ❑ Restless
- ❑ Hostile
- ❑ Aggressive
- ❑ Suspicious

2. Emotional State
- ❑ Depression
- ❑ Depressed mood
- ❑ Loss of interest
- ❑ Fatigue or loss of energy
- ❑ Decreased concentration
- ❑ Feelings of worthlessness
- ❑ Sleep disturbance

○ **Figure 27-3.** An example of an assessment tool that is used by the nurse to document the cognitive abilities of a patient.

example, a mental status assessment tool would include describing the patient's behavior, appearance, mobility, activities, body movement, emotional state, level of consciousness, memory, and judgment.

Nursing assistants often help the nurse with assessments. They care for patients for long periods of time throughout the day and night. This provides ample opportunity to notice changes in patients' behaviors or conditions. For example, they can observe patients for alertness, orientation, motor and sensory problems, fever, and seizures. Nursing assistants are not responsible for making decisions based on observations, so changes must be reported to the nurse as soon as possible.

Assessing change or identifying needs is difficult when caring for patients with dementia. They often have trouble communicating their concerns or problems. When caring for these patients, observe and report the following to the nurse:
- Changes in the level of consciousness, alertness, or behavior
- Changes in vital signs, appetite, or bowel or bladder function
- Changes in the ability to perform ADLs
- Increased weakness or pain
- Presence of seizures

Vital Skills (MATH)

Calculating Fluid Intake

You are a nursing assistant on the day shift, assigned to the Alzheimer wing in a long-term care facility. Frequent fluids are offered to the residents of this wing. The physician has written an order for Mr. Freiman to have at least 1000 cc of fluids during the day shift. Mr. Freiman consumed one container of grape juice, one of cranberry juice, 1 carton of milk, 1 cup of coffee, and half of his water. How much more than 1000 cc of fluids did he drink? (Juice containers hold 90 cc, the water pitcher holds 1000 cc, milk cartons hold 240 cc, and a coffee cup holds 240 cc.)

Add to find his total intake: 90 + 90 + 240 + 240 + 500 = 1160 cc

Subtract to find how much more than 1000 cc he drank: 1160 − 1000 = 160 cc

Practice

Another resident, Mrs. Gisela, is supposed to have 1200 cc of fluids during the day shift. By 1:30 PM, she has consumed two containers of orange juice, a carton of milk, a container of grape juice, and half of her water. How much more does she need to drink to equal 1200 cc?

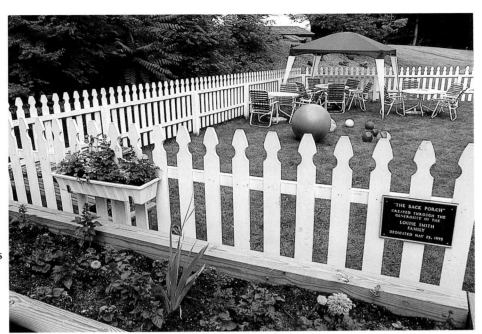

○ Figure 27-4. On nice days, a fenced area is used for residents with Alzheimer's disease during the sundowning period. In poor weather, the sundowning activity program is held in a recreation hall.

Alzheimer's Disease

The most common cause of dementia among the elderly is **Alzheimer's disease**. It is a progressive, irreversible mental disorder accompanied by the gradual loss of intellectual and physical abilities. The decline in intellectual functioning and judgment becomes severe. It affects the patient's ability to perform ADLs. The patient may experience mood changes, depression, and aggression. Alzheimer's disease also occurs in middle-aged people. The cause is unknown, but researchers believe that there is a genetic component in the development of the disease.

Patients with Alzheimer's disease behave in some characteristic ways. They may experience disorientation and memory loss. Disorientation can be so severe that patients forget their long-term spouses, may not recognize their own children, and may not know day from night.

Time of day can affect their behavior. In the late afternoon or evening, many patients with Alzheimer's disease become upset, agitated, or disoriented. This behavior is called **sundowning**. It is not known whether sundowning is caused by fatigue at the end of the day or by being upset by the change in lighting. **See Figure 27-4.**

Eventually, patients with Alzheimer's lose much of their physical functioning and become bedridden, or even comatose, and die. Alzheimer's disease is incurable. Therapies are being developed, however, that can slow the progression of the disease. Therapists also work with patients on maintaining speech, recapturing memories, and extending cognitive function as long as possible.

Alzheimer's patients progress through a series of stages at different rates. One patient may spend years with only minor symptoms and be able to lead a relatively normal life. Another patient's mental functioning may decline rapidly. The stages progress as follows:

- **Stage 1** Patients show slowing of reactions and understanding, and tend to be forgetful and indecisive. In this stage, patients are aware and concerned about these changes and may become depressed.
- **Stage 2** Patients tend to be disoriented and lose interest in surroundings. They may be moody and withdraw from social situations. Denial about the condition and blaming others are common. Patients have difficulty performing daily tasks.
- **Stage 3** Progression continues to poorer general functioning and more forgetfulness. Patients need more supervision because of wandering or inappropriate behaviors, such as urinating on public streets or screaming at strangers. Agitation is common. Some patients show unusual anger at this time. The anger may be a reflection of frustration and lack of understanding about what is happening. Patients begin to be unable to recognize family and friends. Speech may be affected, so needs can no longer be communicated. Patients may become restless, especially at night, and may have bowel and bladder incontinence.
- **Stage 4** The complete decline of mental functioning takes place. Patients must be confined or totally supervised, because they may wander and become lost or may harm themselves or others. They do not recognize family members. They may also lose control of most physical functioning, including the ability to walk, sit, eat, and control their bowels. Falls are common and seizures may occur. Sleep disturbances occur frequently. Although there is no timetable for how long a patient may remain in Stage 4, Alzheimer's disease eventually leads to coma and death.

Care of Patients with Dementia

Dementia is a difficult and frustrating disease for the patient and the family. During the course of the disease, basic communication skills break down and personality changes occur. Patients sometimes remember events from long ago but cannot remember something that happened minutes ago. This is called *short-term memory loss*, and can result in the patient asking the same question over and over again.

The patient begins acting in ways that are inconsistent with prior behavior. For example, a previously calm, even-tempered person may experience bursts of tears or fits of anger. Family members may feel that the patient has become a different person, someone they no longer know. Caring for a patient with dementia requires a great deal of patience. The psychological, emotional, physical, and social strains on the family can be enormous.

Contribute to the well-being of patients and their families by providing support and understanding. Be a good listener. When appropriate, encourage the family to talk about their experiences. Having someone to talk to about what they are going through can be extremely beneficial to family members.

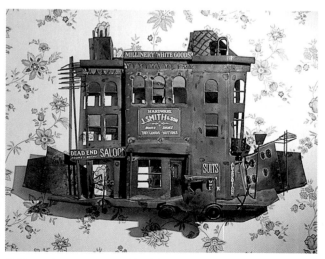

○ **Figure 27-5.** Patients with Alzheimer's disease often have problems with depth perception. Three-dimensional art may help them focus on and enjoy a piece of artwork.

Validation Therapy

Patients with Alzheimer's disease or dementia may be confused about events in their lives. They may not know where they are or what year it is. Caring for these patients can be challenging, because the patient may insist that some events are happening, even though it is clear to you that what they're describing can't be true. For example, Mr. Jackson has Alzheimer's disease and has been on the unit for several years. One day he insists that he needs to get ready for school, even though you know that he hasn't gone to school for more than 40 years.

Validation therapy is a way to communicate with patients with cognitive impairment who are confused about events. It shows them respect by validating their beliefs but redirects them towards reality. In this type of communication, you acknowledge that the person believes these events to be true. You may ask him (or her) to describe his beliefs further so that you can validate his concerns and relieve his anxiety. While you are acknowledging his feelings, however, you do not reinforce the belief itself.

For example, in the case of Mr. Jackson, you might say, "I understand that you want to get ready for school, but I need you to get ready to go to breakfast. Do you think you might want to get something to eat?" You would not say, "OK, Mr. Jackson, let's get you up and dressed so you can eat before you catch the school bus." Your communication with the patient should always be honest and not deceptive.

By responding in this way, you show that you respect what Mr. Jackson is feeling, but you help orient him to reality.

Practice

Mr. Benson is a patient with Alzheimer's disease. He is insisting that he needs to get into his car and pick up his daughter from school. He is agitated and is refusing to come to the dining room for lunch. You are aware that Mr. Benson has only one daughter who is grown and does not live nearby. You are also aware that Mr. Benson does not have a car and has not driven in at least five years. How should you handle this situation?

Occupational therapists may devise therapeutic programs for patients in the early stages of dementia. These programs encourage intellectual and social activity and may help patients remain calm. Some patients have shown improvement with these structured daily programs. A program might include working with words and numbers as mental exercise. This may include such simple activities as having patients repeat the day and date at certain intervals. It might also include complex activities such as working math or crossword puzzles. **See Figure 27-5.**

Abuse

Sometimes patients with dementia suffer abuse at the hands of their caregivers. These patients may not realize or remember what happened. If you see such behavior, immediately tell the nurse in charge. If no one in the facility will try to stop the abuse, call your state's abuse prevention hotline. Your first duty is the care and safety of your patients.

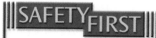

Patients with dementia, or any patients who may become confused or disoriented, should always wear identification in case they wander away. Keep a recent picture to use for identification as well.

Nursing assistants can encourage patients in Stages 1 and 2 of Alzheimer's disease to participate in activities such as *reminiscing*, or remembering and talking about past events in their lives. Reality orientation techniques may also be used. Patients who are in Stages 3 and 4, however, cannot be helped by these therapies. Trying to reorient the patient may increase agitation. For example, telling such a person that his or her mother has died can cause unnecessary pain and torment.

Patients in these later stages are living in their own reality. **Validation therapy** is a communication technique that shows respect and maintains patients' dignity by acknowledging their reality. It is a calm way to redirect agitated patients back to the present time and situation. First, ask about their belief. Then respond about what is upsetting them to *validate* (affirm or support) their concerns and relieve their anxiety. For example, an elderly patient becomes agitated because she cannot find the dog she had as a child. Her reality, or belief, is that she is a child and that her dog is lost. You can acknowledge that she wants to find the dog and then ask her to tell you about him. This distracts the patient from worrying about the dog but acknowledges her loving feelings for him.

When providing daily care to patients with dementia, follow these guidelines:

- Avoid sudden changes in environment and schedule. Moving even a chair or a picture may cause disorientation. Having meals or baths at the same time every day reassures patients.
- Keep environmental stimulation to a minimum. The environment should be quiet and calm.
- Help patients who are disoriented or have short-term memory loss by *cuing*, or prompting them about what to do next. For example, if the patient forgets that he or she is eating, continually prompt the patient to take a bite or a drink and to swallow.
- Distinguish day from night. Change the patient's clothes at regular times, turn lights on and off, open and close shades or curtains, and follow familiar daytime and nighttime routines to help the patient maintain a regular sleeping and waking schedule.
- Comfort by touch whenever appropriate. Alzheimer's patients may respond well to a comforting pat or touch on the hand or shoulder. Such gentle expressions may help the disoriented patient remain calm and focus on reality.
- Practice safety measures. Constantly supervise patients with dementia. **See Figure 27-6.** They tend to wander, may not be able to distinguish hot from cold, may drop or throw things, are often unsteady on their feet, and may eat poisons, medicine, or cleaners. Their safety must be carefully guarded. To allow patients some freedom of movement, secure an area where they can move about but always be observed. In a home care situation, control the exits from an apartment, a house, or a fenced yard. Remove all potential hazards.

- Maintain adequate nutrition. Patients may not be able to communicate hunger or thirst or may not be aware of these needs. Some facilities record intake and output of patients with dementia.
- Promote and assist with personal hygiene. Patients become incontinent and are not able to bathe, comb their hair, brush their teeth, or dress properly. You can help maintain patients' dignity by making sure their daily hygiene needs are met. Patients who are neatly dressed and groomed are likely to be treated better by other people with whom they come into contact.

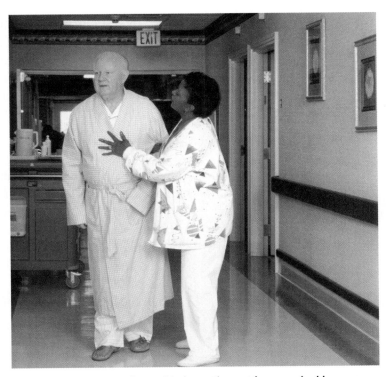

○ **Figure 27-6.** Some patients with dementia must be supervised because they may wander away or injure themselves.

Substance-Related Disorders

Substance abuse is maladaptive behavior in which use of a chemical substance, such as alcohol, tobacco, or prescription or illegal drugs, has a negative impact on a person's life. A number of chronic diseases, including heart disease, stroke, diabetes, liver disease, and mental disorders, result from substance abuse. Social problems can occur as well, such as problems with relationships, loss of employment, and financial ruin. Some people lose the ability to properly care for themselves or others who are dependent on them.

The overwhelming need to repeatedly use or consume a chemical substance is called *psychological dependence*. Some people are able to hide their dependency for years. Others show obvious signs of *intoxication*, the altered mental state due to the ingestion of a substance.

As a nursing assistant, you will probably encounter people who are suffering from drug and alcohol dependence as part of your work. Signs and symptoms vary, depending on the type of substance used, but may include:
- Changes in eating or sleeping habits and physical appearance
- Being defensive, angry, or withdrawn
- Erratic behavior and mood swings
- Unsteady gait
- Hand tremors
- Unexplained injuries
- Forgetfulness or lack of concentration
- Distorted or false perceptions, including psychosis

There are a number of treatments for drug and alcohol dependency. Most involve complete abstinence (the practice of staying completely away from the substance). Nursing assistants who work in a drug or alcohol treatment facility help residents maintain their sobriety. Understanding of the illness and patience are important traits for caregivers in this field.

Treatment Planning

Mental health and substance-abuse disorders can affect a patient's physical, emotional, mental, and social functioning. Treatment is based on the patient's ability to cope with the illness. An interdisciplinary team may include mental health nurses, mental health aides, counselors, psychiatrists, psychologists, social workers, medical physicians, pharmacists, occupational therapists, and nursing assistants. They are often all involved in the planning and implementation of a patient's care and treatment.

Within the individualized treatment plan, nursing assistants may have a significant role in carrying out a portion of the plan, including these tasks:
- Assistance with ADLs
- Participation in one-on-one activities, such as playing card games or watching television with the patient
- Participation in group activities, such as basketball, table tennis, or other sports
- Accompanying patients on field trips, or to appointments and examinations
- Maintaining patient safety as outlined in the treatment plan
- Observing and reporting significant changes in the patient's signs and symptoms
- Utilizing appropriate communication techniques

Mental Retardation

Mental retardation is a slowness or limitation of intellectual ability. It can result from a genetic disorder, birth trauma, or from a childhood disease or injury.

People with mental retardation vary greatly in their level of development. Some function at a very high level of independence, holding jobs, having families, driving cars, and participating in the normal social life of their communities. Others live at home and get help from their family. Some live in group homes. Some people live in long-term care facilities, because they need complete assistance with ADLs.

The level of severity is sometimes determined by intelligence quotient (IQ) tests. **Table 27-1** shows the developmental levels of mental retardation and the abilities normally seen with each level.

Elderly people with mental retardation often have the effects of aging combined with the disabilities of their condition. Nursing assistants who work with such residents need to understand the effects of mental retardation and aging.

These residents usually require repetition of actions or words before they understand what is wanted. They may act out and scream for no apparent reason. The nursing assistant can help by being calm, touching gently, and talking softly. Caring for these residents can be rewarding. You are helping someone live as comfortably as possible. Often, you receive in return unconditional love and acceptance.

○ **Table 27-1. Developmental Levels of Mental Retardation**

Developmental Level	Abilities
Mild	• Usually able to live independently • May be able to maintain a job • Assistance is minimal • Adequate social skills
Moderate	• Needs supervision with living skills but can perform some ADLs independently • Some difficulty with communicating • Low social skills
Severe	• Needs complete supervision and assistance for ADLs and living skills • Very little ability for verbal communication
Profound	• Requires continuous supervision • Almost no speech • May also have problems with mobility

Chapter Summary

- People use coping and defense mechanisms to deal with stress.

- Causes and contributing factors of mental disorders include social and cultural pressures, ineffective coping mechanisms, substance abuse, brain damage or disease, aging, chemical imbalances in the body, and genetic origins.

- Caring for patients with mental disorders includes helping with ADLs, providing safety, providing emotional support, and observing for changes.

- Depression is the most common mental disorder in elderly people.

- Dementia can be caused by infections, injuries, Alzheimer's disease, AIDS, vascular disease, or long-term alcohol abuse.

- Patients with Alzheimer's disease have symptoms of dementia but seem to have other, distinct characteristics as well.

- Caring for patients with dementia includes helping with ADLs, providing safety, providing emotional support, and observing for changes.

- Reality orientation therapy and validation therapy are used to help patients with disorientation and dementia.

- Substance abuse involves being psychologically dependent on chemical substances.

- Nursing assistants have a significant role in carrying out a portion of the patient's individualized treatment plan.

- Developmental levels of mental retardation vary greatly.

VOCABULARY REVIEW

Directions: Match the letter of each definition in the second column with the correct vocabulary term in the first column. Write your answers on a separate sheet of paper.

Vocabulary
1. agitation
2. anxiety
3. confusion
4. delusion
5. depression
6. hallucination
7. psychosis
8. schizophrenia
9. sundowning

Definitions
A. The general term for any severe disorder in which a person loses contact with reality
B. A thought disorder that may include disorganized speech and behavior, irrational and illogical thoughts, social withdrawal, and an inability to make choices or decisions
C. A false perception of reality that may include hearing voices or seeing objects or people that do not exist
D. A state of extreme restlessness
E. A mental state in which the patient is unaware of time, the environment, or the self
F. Becoming upset, agitated, or disoriented in the late afternoon or evening
G. A feeling of dread or discomfort that occurs without a specific reason
H. A false belief about oneself or others or about events
I. A mood disorder marked by extreme sadness and hopelessness

Check Your Knowledge

Review Questions: Answer each of the following questions on a separate sheet of paper.

1. What is a mental disorder?

2. List three behaviors or activities that might indicate that a patient is planning to commit suicide.

3. List three possible causes of psychosis.

4. What is the purpose of an assessment?

5. What symptoms would you expect to see in a patient with Alzheimer's disease who has progressed to Stage 3?

6. What is cuing?

7. Why is it important to maintain adequate nutrition for patients with dementia?

8. List four signs or symptoms of substance abuse.

9. Who may be involved in the interdisciplinary team when planning and implementing care and treatment for individual mental health patients?

10. What are the abilities of someone with moderate mental retardation?

True or False: Read each statement carefully. Then write *True* or *False* by the statement number on a separate sheet of paper.

1. People with mental disorders should do as much for themselves as they are able to handle.

2. Alzheimer's disease can be cured.

3. Sundowning is a normal reaction to darkness.

4. Always make sure you remove potential hazards when caring for a patient with Alzheimer's disease.

5. Group homes provide a supportive community setting for some people with mental retardation.

Think and Decide

Directions: Think about each of the following scenarios. Answer each question on a separate sheet of paper.

1. Mr. G. is a long-term care resident who has just recently been admitted with Stage 4 Alzheimer's disease. Mr. G.'s daughter is visiting him one afternoon and is upset when he doesn't remember who she is. How can the nursing assistant help the daughter?

2. Mrs. D. also has Stage 4 Alzheimer's disease. She rarely communicates her needs and is incontinent of bowel and bladder. What is the nursing assistant's role in caring for Mrs. D.?

3. You are working in a long-term care facility with elderly residents who suffer from depression, anxiety, confusion, dementia, psychosis, and disorientation. You are feeling particularly sad today, and you don't really feel like being at work. How does your mental well-being affect the residents you care for? What can you do to improve your mental health?

4. You are assisting Lydia, an 89-year-old resident who has dementia, to the commode. You observe that her weakness seems to have increased from yesterday. Lydia is also complaining of pain in her back. You remember also that she did not eat breakfast this morning because, she said, "I don't feel well." What should you do? Why?

5. A patient in the psychiatric facility where you are working is seeing mice crawling up and down the walls of his room. How should you communicate with this patient?

6. Jim, a long-term care resident, is sitting by the window when you come into the room. He refuses to make eye contact. He states that he hasn't slept and he has a headache. You try to talk to Jim, but he withdraws. You tell him to put on his call light if he needs anything. You leave the room knowing Jim is not all right. You need to report your suspicions to the nurse. Based on the information Jim has presented, what are you going to tell the nurse?

7. B.C. is a new resident at the long-term care facility where you work. She formed an immediate attachment to you and tells her visitors and other residents that you are her daughter, even though you are not. What is this perception of reality called? How can you best help B.C.?

8. Z.R. is a new patient at the alcohol treatment facility where you work. You have been asked to help keep Z.R.'s mind occupied using group or one-on-one activities. When you approach him with ideas for activities, he tells you he hates playing cards and that watching television makes him want a drink. What other activities might you try?

CNA Certification Exam Prep

Directions: This practice test contains ten questions. Each question has four suggested answers. For each question, choose the ONE that best answers the question or completes the statement. Write your answers on a separate sheet of paper.

1. Reality orientation is suggested for a confused patient. Which of the following might be part of his care plan?
   A. doubling his daily exercise
   B. changing his daily routines
   C. confronting inaccurate statements
   D. discussing familiar people and places

2. Mental health is
   A. well-being of the mind and emotions.
   B. a state of physical illness.
   C. a state of physical well-being.
   D. a state of chronic illness.

3. Which of the following is a sign of depression?
   A. withdrawal
   B. excitement
   C. insomnia
   D. good concentration

4. Which of the following can a nursing assistant do to help ensure the safety of a confused patient?
   A. shout to get his attention
   B. approach him from behind
   C. keep instructions simple
   D. ignore the patient

5. When talking to a person with delusions, it is best to
   A. challenge the person's thinking.
   B. ignore the person.
   C. avoid confrontations.
   D. call emergency personnel.

6. A defense mechanism in which a person blames other people for his own mistakes is
   A. projection.
   B. rationalization.
   C. regression.
   D. compensation.

7. The study of the mind and behavior is known as
   A. psychiatry.
   B. psychology.
   C. neurology.
   D. nephrology.

8. Another term for dementia is
   A. acute confusion.
   B. acute delusion.
   C. chronic confusion.
   D. chronic delusion.

9. An Alzheimer's patient is forgetful and is sometimes slow to understand, but is still well-oriented. At what stage is she?
   A. Stage 1
   B. Stage 2
   C. Stage 3
   D. Stage 4

10. A patient who remembers events from the past but cannot remember something that happened minutes ago is experiencing
    A. long-term paranoia.
    B. short-term paranoia.
    C. long-term memory loss.
    D. short-term memory loss.

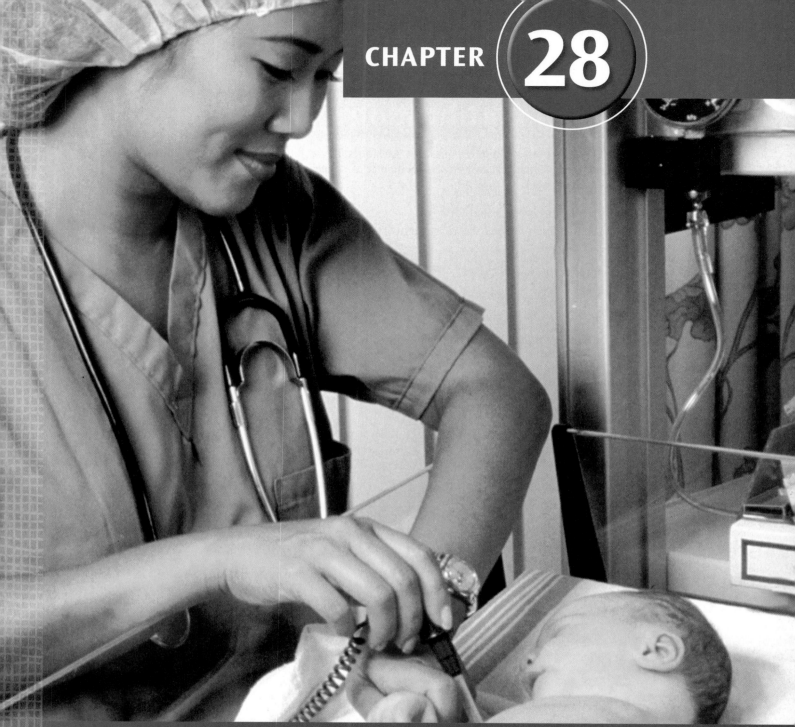

CHAPTER 28

OBJECTIVES

- Identify expanded roles available to nursing assistants after special training.
- Describe how a trained nursing assistant may safely assist patients with medications.
- Describe the trimesters of pregnancy, tests performed during the prenatal period, and reportable observations of patients in the prenatal period.
- Describe the signs of impending labor and the stages of labor.
- Describe how to care for the postpartum patient in a hospital and home setting.
- Demonstrate how to help a new mother breastfeed.
- Demonstrate how to bottle-feed and burp an infant.
- Demonstrate how to change an infant's diaper and provide care for the umbilical cord and a circumcision.
- Demonstrate how to weigh a newborn.

Nursing Assistant Specialties

VOCABULARY

breastfeeding The natural feeding of the mother's milk to an infant.

cesarean section (c-section) The delivery of a fetus by a surgical incision into the uterus through the abdomen.

circumcision The surgical removal of the foreskin on a boy's penis.

colostrum A thick, yellow fluid secreted from the mother's breast for the first few days after delivery that supplies babies with important antibodies.

episiotomy A small incision of the perineum made during delivery to avoid tearing of the tissue and to ease the baby's passage.

formula A milk mixture enhanced with extra nutrients to make it as close in content to breast milk as possible.

labor The process that begins with uterine contractions and ends with delivery of the baby.

letdown reflex The automatic release of breast milk in response to the presence of milk in the breasts.

lochia The normal discharge from the uterus after childbirth.

placenta The vascular organ lining the walls of the uterus from which the fetus derives nutrition and oxygen.

postpartum care The medical and supportive care given to a mother after childbirth.

prenatal care The medical care and monitoring a woman receives during her pregnancy to ensure optimum health for her and the developing baby.

rooting reflex The natural response that causes a baby to look for something to suck when the cheek is touched.

umbilical cord The structure that connects the fetus to the placenta during pregnancy.

Expanded Roles of Nursing Assistants

The nursing assistant's role may differ from state to state and facility to facility, depending on specific regulations. To ensure that safe and effective care is delivered, specialty training courses in a variety of topics may be provided to nursing assistants. These courses may include training in assisting a patient with medications, care of a woman during pregnancy and labor, or during and after childbirth, care of the newborn infant, expanded care of the geriatric patient, assisting the patient in surgery, drawing blood for testing (*phlebotomy*), and expanded care of the patient during rehabilitation.

Some training facilities issue a certificate to verify the additional specialty training that a nursing assistant completes. In all cases, however, nursing assistants always work under the direction and supervision of a licensed nurse.

This chapter presents information about three areas of specialty training:

- Assisting patients with taking self-administered, prescribed medications at home or in residential care facilities
- Care of women during pregnancy, labor and delivery, and the period following childbirth
- Care of the newborn

Assistance with Medications

Some states permit nursing assistants to help patients with prescribed, routine, nonnarcotic medications. Health care facilities and state agencies must identify specific, legal criteria before this practice can occur. This added role and responsibility depends on:

- State laws and facility policy and procedures.
- Additional training received by the nursing assistant.
- Appropriate delegation and supervision by a licensed nurse.

After training, the nursing assistant may receive a certificate. In some areas, the trained nursing assistant is called a *certified medication assistant*. Some states prefer not to use this title, because it may imply that the role is regulated by a governmental agency.

Assistance with medications is defined by state laws and regulations and varies greatly, not only from state to state, but also from setting to setting. It may be handled differently, for example, in home care and adult day care settings. The nursing assistant's role may involve assisting patients who cannot independently self-administer their own medications. It may apply only to clients in the home setting or only to residents of assisted-living facilities who need assistance. It could also include:

- A simple verbal reminder to a patient to take medications on time.
- Breaking a scored tablet if only half of a tablet is prescribed.
- Checking the drug label before the patient takes the medication, to ensure accuracy. **See Figure 28-1.**
- Crushing a tablet and assisting a patient with swallowing the pill in soft food.
- Helping a patient open medication containers.
- Providing and assisting with fluids in which to take oral medications.
- Assisting a patient with
  – Administration of oral medications

HealthTrust
Pharmacy (888) 555-1212

Rx: 7433149 Michaels, Russell
Dr. Saymore, Leona SAM 12-Apr-07
90 TAB Apo-Hydralazine 50mg
Hydralazine HCl 50mg
DIN: 00441635 APX Refills: 0
TAKE 1 TABLET DAILY EVERY
MORNING WITH ORANGE JUICE
KEEP OUT OF REACH OF CHILDREN

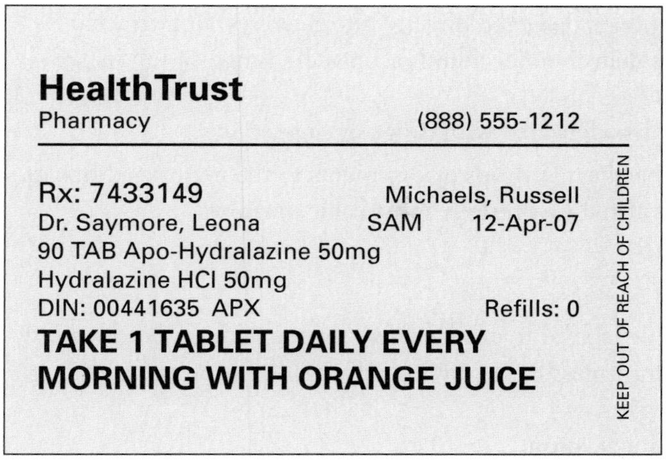

Figure 28-1. Read all of the information on the medication label before assisting the patient with the medication.

  – Instilling eye, ear, or nose drops
  – Application of topical medications
  – Administering medications through a gastric tube
  – Insertion of suppositories
- Ensuring that a patient takes the right drug, at the right time, in the right amount, using the right route.
- Documenting and reporting problems and concerns.
- Assisting with proper storage of patient medications.

Before you attempt to help patients or residents in any of these ways, it is important to find out what the laws are in your state, take the required educational program, and pass the exam.

SAFETY FIRST

A patient could become very ill or die if taking the wrong medication or taking it incorrectly. Before the patient actually takes the medication, check the following:
- Right person
- Right medication
- Right dose
- Right route
- Right time

Document all of the above according to facility policy.

Ensuring Safety

When agencies and facilities train nursing assistants to help patients with medications, they have certain requirements to ensure patient safety. They clarify the nursing assistant's role in order to prevent errors. They ensure that there is no opportunity for judgment or decision making by a person who is not qualified to do so. This includes the calculation of dosages, which is beyond the scope of practice for the nursing assistant.

Medication Routes

A medication route describes how the medication should be taken, as prescribed by the health care provider. The oral route, by mouth, is the most frequently prescribed. Oral medications come in liquid form, sprays, lozenges, tablets, and capsules. *Sublingual* medications are given under the tongue. *Buccal* medications are given in the cheek. Sublingual and buccal medications are to be dissolved in the mouth before swallowing.

Most oral medications are given with water or juice. Always check the instructions to determine if specific liquids should be avoided with certain medications. Some pills or tablets may need to be cut in half or crushed and mixed with food.

Some medications do not work effectively if taken by mouth. Some patients cannot take medications by mouth. Other common routes are:
- **Topical route.** Medication is applied directly on the skin surface, in creams, lotions, powders, sprays, or patches.
- **Gastrostomy route.** Medication is administered directly into the stomach through a tube that is surgically inserted.

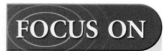

PRN Medications

Health care providers may order medications to be taken on a *PRN*, or as-needed, basis. Pain, anti-nausea, and asthma medications are sometimes prescribed in this way. Written instructions specify when and why the patient should take the medication. The nursing assistant may not decide when or whether to give a medication on a PRN order—this is the responsibility of the nurse.

- **Inhaled route.** Medication is delivered directly into the respiratory tract. Inhalers and nebulizers deliver either liquid or powdered medication in pre-mixed doses.
- **Nasal route.** Medication is delivered with drops or nose sprays.

Medication may also be given as drops or ointments to the eye or as drops in the ear. It may be given vaginally or rectally for specific purposes.

Medication Labels

All medications must be labeled to ensure safety for the patient. Do not assist a patient with medications unless the following information is on the label:
- Patient's full name
- Expiration date of the medication
- Name of the medication
- Amount (dose) of medication to take and the medication route
- How often the medication is to be taken
- Prescriber's name
- Pharmacy's name, address, and phone number

Medication Administration Records

Although medication administration records may look different in different facilities, all include the date, time, route, and signature of the person who assisted the patient. **See Figure 28-2.** Accurate and complete documentation of the medication given to a patient ensures patient safety. Document every medication the patient takes, including those taken without assistance. Also, ask the patient about known allergies and make sure that these are documented on the medication record.

MEDICATION ADMINISTRATION RECORD

DATE: _3/10/07_

RESIDENT NAME: _O'Brien, Charles_   APT#: _463_

PHARMACY: _Hometown_   DRUG ALLERGIES: _None_

MEDICATION	ROUTE	DOSE	TIME	SIGNATURE
Celebrex	oral	200 mg	0800	D. Vogel
Lanoxin	oral	0.125 mg	0200/0800/ 1400/2000	
Lorazepam	oral	0.5 mg	0200/0800/ 1400/2000	
Trazodone	oral	50 mg	0800/2000	

○ **Figure 28-2.** Medication records should include the patient's name, the date, the name of the medication, and the time, amount, route, and who gave it.

Vital Skills READING

Be a Critical Reader

Just because something is in print doesn't mean it is true. As a good reader, you should evaluate what you read and ask yourself questions about the material. For example, you might ask, is this likely? Is the author not telling me something important because it doesn't support his point of view? Is this information current? Has it been validated by other sources?

It is especially important to read critically when you're reading material on the Internet. Anyone can post a Web page on any topic, so carefully consider the source. Search for information that comes from a respected organization.

Practice

The editorial pages of newspapers contain opinion columns. Choose an editorial and evaluate it critically. Do you think the writer left out any important information?

Medication Storage

Any medication, whether prescription or over-the-counter, has the potential to do harm if handled improperly. Medications stored in health care or residential facilities should always be locked up to ensure safety. Medications stored in a patient's home should be placed out of reach of children and people who are cognitively impaired.

Follow the manufacturer's instructions for refrigeration, specific temperature limit requirements, and exposure to light. These can affect the chemical structure and effectiveness of some medications.

Pregnancy, Labor, and Postpartum Care

In some areas, nursing assistants must get special training to care for women during pregnancy and labor and delivery, and during the period after childbirth.

Prenatal Care

When a woman becomes pregnant, many physical and psychological changes begin to occur. **Prenatal care** is the medical care and monitoring a woman receives during her pregnancy to ensure optimum health for her and the developing baby.

An average pregnancy lasts for 40 weeks. To help calculate and monitor the expected changes that occur during a pregnancy, it is divided into 3 trimesters.

The First Trimester. This is the first 12 weeks of pregnancy, beginning with conception. As soon as possible after she suspects she is pregnant, a woman should go to a health care provider or a lab for a serum (blood) test or a urine test to confirm pregnancy. Other tests given during this period are:
- Prenatal panel, including blood tests, blood typing, rubella (measles) screening, hepatitis panel, and urinalysis
- For women 35 and older, blood tests for genetic disorders in the fetus

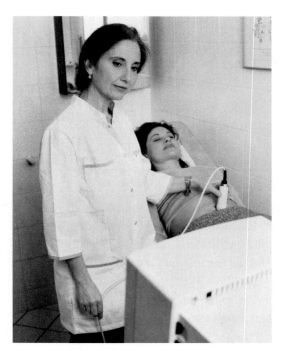

○ **Figure 28-3.** An ultrasound test is done early in the second trimester to determine the age and health of the fetus and its position in the uterus.

• For at-risk women, tests for gestational (during pregnancy) diabetes

The Second Trimester. This period is from week 13 through week 27. Screening tests are given to determine how mother and baby are doing. The first ultrasound test is performed early in the trimester. In this test, sound waves create an image of the fetus. It is performed to determine age and health of the fetus and its position in the uterus. A second ultrasound is done late in this trimester or early in the third. **See Figure 28-3.** Screening tests for hepatitis B, sexually transmitted infections, and diabetes are also performed. The test for diabetes is called a *glucose tolerance test.* It measures the glucose level in the blood. Tests for fetal genetic disorders and a pelvic examination may also be performed.

The Third Trimester. This period is from week 28 through week 40. Visits to the health care provider will become more frequent from about week 32. From this time, the goal of care is to ensure optimum health for the mother and fetus, to treat possible complications, and to make sure the fetus is growing and developing properly. Tests include cervical examination of the woman to check for signs of early labor and ultrasound. Fetal monitoring is performed if there are reasons to suspect problems with the mother or fetus.

Trained nursing assistants may be involved with prenatal care at a clinic or hospital, or in the home. They encourage good nutrition and health habits, and regular prenatal examinations. They observe and report the following signs and symptoms that could indicate serious problems for the mother or baby:

- Continuous vomiting
- Elevated temperature
- Severe or continuous pain
- Burning when urinating
- Dizziness and blurred vision
- Persistent headache
- Decreased or absent fetal movements
- Leaking of fluid or blood from the vagina
- Frequent uterine contractions (4 every 20 minutes)

Labor and Delivery

Labor is the process that begins with uterine contractions and ends with delivery of the baby. The nursing assistant provides supportive care to the woman in labor. Care may include measuring and recording vital signs, and observing for signs and symptoms of problems. The facility where you work may provide additional training to perform specialized tasks during labor and delivery. Signs of impending labor include:

- *Lightening,* or the lowering of the baby's head into the pelvis.
- Regular and predictable uterine contractions. They usually begin in the lower back and move around to the front of the lower abdomen. They increase in intensity, duration, and frequency.
- Dilation (expanding) of the cervix.
- Bloody vaginal discharge after the mucous plug is expelled from the cervix.
- The rupture of amniotic membranes. This can be a sudden gush of clear fluid from the woman's vagina or a slow, steady stream.

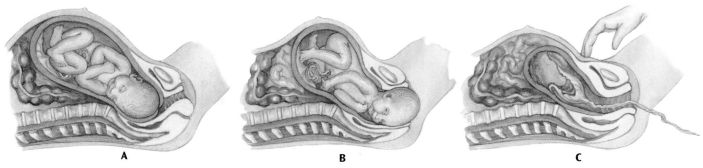

○ **Figure 28-4.** (A) During the first stage of labor, the cervix dilates. (B) The baby's head crowns at the opening of the birth canal at the beginning of the expulsion stage. (C) The mother delivers the placenta during the third stage.

Labor is divided into three stages to best measure the progression of the birth process.

- *Dilation stage.* This stage begins with true, regular uterine contractions and ends with complete dilation, which is the stretching and widening of the cervix.
- *Expulsion stage.* From complete dilation, this stage continues through the birth.
- *Placental stage.* This stage follows the birth through the delivery of the placenta and all its contents. The **placenta** is the vascular organ lining the walls of the uterus from which the fetus derives nutrition and oxygen. **See Figure 28-4.**

Pain Relief. Anesthesia can be given to the mother to ease the discomfort and pain of labor. A systemic analgesic can be injected into a vein or muscle. It affects the entire nervous system of the mother as well as the baby. An epidural block or a spinal block can be injected into the space around the spinal cord in the mother's lower back. This numbs only the lower half of the body. A pudendal block is local anesthesia delivered to the perineal area.

Cesarean Section. A **cesarean section** (**c-section**) is the delivery of the fetus by a surgical incision into the uterus through the abdomen. The health care professional may decide to perform a cesarean section because:

- Labor is not progressing normally.
- The fetus is too large to be delivered vaginally.
- The fetus has other health problems.
- The mother is HIV-positive or has active genital herpes or other health problems that create a risk to her or the fetus.
- There are problems with the placenta.

Postpartum Care

The medical and supportive care given to a mother after childbirth is called **postpartum care**. The postpartum period lasts for the mother's entire stay in the hospital as well as the time it takes to recuperate at home, usually around 6 weeks. Women who have had a normal vaginal delivery usually stay in the hospital from 1 to 3 days. Women who have had a cesarean delivery stay 4 or 5 days.

During the first 24 hours after childbirth, the mother receives the same type of care that a postoperative patient receives. Her vital signs are measured every 15 minutes for the first hour, and every hour thereafter. If she has had an epidural or spinal block, she is positioned flat on her back until the anesthesia wears off. Women who have had a cesarean section are treated as surgical patients.

After the mother is settled in her room, you may be asked to check her perineum and assist with elimination needs and perineal care. Perineal care is performed every few hours.

Encourage her to urinate as soon as she can after birth. You may need to measure the first void and defecation. Provide her with a bedpan or help her walk to the bathroom. After defecating or voiding, the mother should fill a squeezable bottle with warm water. Instruct her to spray the water over her perineal area to clean herself. If she is unable to urinate, immediately report to the nurse.

Check the perineum for color and for **lochia**, the normal discharge from the uterus after childbirth. At first, it is thick and red. It will decrease and become lighter in color. Report signs of tenderness or infection, swelling, and unusual odor.

The mother will need to use sanitary pads for some time after delivery. Place a disposable bed pad under her buttocks and help her put on a sanitary napkin. Show her how to remove the soiled sanitary napkin and replace it with a fresh one. Always lift the sanitary napkin away from the body from front to back. Show her where to discard used sanitary napkins. Tell her to wash her hands before applying a fresh napkin and not to touch the inside of the pad.

Check the episiotomy, if she had one. An **episiotomy** is a small incision of the perineum made during delivery to avoid tearing of the tissue and to ease the baby's passage. This cut is sutured (sewn) after delivery. Sitting down and getting up will be quite painful. Suggest that she squeeze her buttocks together and hold them in this position while sitting down or getting up to reduce pressure on the incision.

Vital Skills   COMMUNICATION

Working in a Team

Being a good nursing assistant means working well in a team. A *team* is a group of people who work together toward a common goal. The only way to accomplish the goal is if the team members work together. Teamwork can be challenging because team members may have different ideas about how to meet the goals.

Follow these tips for effective teamwork:

• *Set the goals of the team.* Work with your team members to establish the goals and commit them to paper so they are clear to everyone.

• *Plan your approach.* How will your team meet their goals? Assign tasks to each team member.

• *Keep the team goals in mind.* There may be times when you need to compromise. Do not take things personally as you work toward your goals.

Practice

With four or five classmates, create a team to meet a goal of your choosing. Brainstorm to come up with a goal. Choose a goal that can be met in two or three meetings. Meet with your team and work on your goal. Keep these questions in mind:

1. How can your team avoid conflict?
2. Should the team assign a leader?
3. What will your team do if someone doesn't fully participate?
4. What can you do individually to help your team be effective?

If she has pain in the perineal area, she can use specially medicated cleansing pads. Remind her to wipe from front to back. Placing an ice pack in the perineal area will provide relief for pain and swelling.

After the first few postpartum hours, most mothers are able to get out of bed with assistance and care for personal needs. Ask the mother to call you the first couple of times she wants to walk to the bathroom. Observe her walking to make sure she is strong enough to walk on her own. **See Figure 28-5.**

The new mother is allowed to shower as soon as she feels ready. Assist her to the shower and help her undress. Stay nearby in case she feels dizzy. She may also need help getting out of the shower, getting dressed, and walking back to bed.

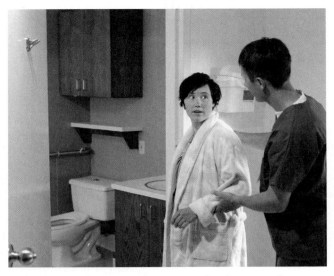

○ **Figure 28-5.** The new mother may need assistance getting to the bathroom and shower in the first hours after childbirth.

Breastfeeding

Breastfeeding is the feeding of the mother's milk to an infant. It is also called *nursing*. Both mother and baby have natural physical responses to promote nursing. Breastfed babies are put on the breast immediately after birth. At first the baby receives only colostrum. **Colostrum** is a thick yellow fluid secreted from the breast for the first few days after delivery. It supplies babies with important antibodies from the mother. Several days later, the mother's breast milk comes in. Breast milk provides infants with all the necessary nutrients to thrive and enzymes and antibodies that help prevent infection.

Breastfeeding is not always easy or automatic. One of your responsibilities may be to help and encourage the mother. Learning about the process will help you help her. The mother must drink plenty of liquids and eat nutritionally balanced meals to produce an adequate milk supply. A nursing mother needs 500 extra calories per day.

The **letdown reflex** is the automatic release of breast milk in response to the presence of milk in the breasts. However, the reflex takes conditioning. When a mother is learning to breastfeed, she should feed her baby in a relaxing environment. The letdown reflex can be upset by anxiety, fear, distraction, and fatigue. The **rooting reflex** is the natural response that causes a baby to look for something to suck when the cheek is touched. The baby must suck from the breast to stimulate milk production.

The baby is fed on demand so that the baby gets enough to eat and to establish the milk supply. Newborns may nurse up to 10 times a day for the first couple of weeks. Mother and baby then establish a nursing routine, usually every 3 to 4 hours.

When assisting a mother to breastfeed, wash your hands and help her wash hers. Offer her a beverage and provide privacy. Then follow these guidelines:

• Assist her into a comfortable position, such as sitting in a chair or lying on her side. She can support the baby with one arm and support her breast with the other hand.

• She should grasp her breast with thumb and forefinger just above the areola. Instruct her to brush the baby's cheek closest to the breast with the nipple. The

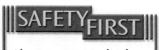

SAFETY FIRST

Always use standard precautions when caring for mother and baby in the hospital and the home.

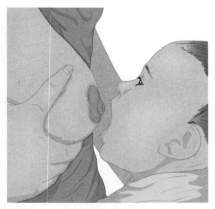

○ **Figure 28-6.** Instruct the mother to guide the nipple into the baby's mouth.

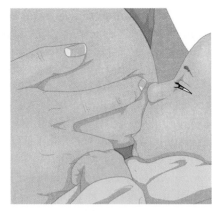

○ **Figure 28-7.** Using a finger to hold the breast away from the baby's nose.

baby will turn toward the nipple with its mouth open. She gently places her nipple and areola into the baby's mouth so the baby can latch on. **See Figure 28-6.** If this is temporarily painful for the mother, encourage her to relax. Instruct the mother to hold her breast away from the baby's nose so the baby can breathe properly. **See Figure 28-7.**

- The baby should nurse on the first breast for no more than 10 minutes. Teach the mother to break the baby's suction by placing her forefinger between the areola and the baby's mouth.
- Encourage her to burp the baby after feeding at the first breast. Burping releases the air from the baby's stomach. Then have her nurse the baby on the other breast until the baby falls asleep or loses interest. Burp the baby again.

Helping a New Mother at Home

Nursing assistants often work in the home caring for new mothers and their babies. The mother will tell you what she wants you to do while you are in the home. Some mothers want to take care of the baby and have you do household tasks. Others are happy to have a helping hand with the newborn. You may be asked to take care of the baby at certain times of the day so the mother can sleep or spend time with her older children.

She needs time to get to know and love her baby. She also needs time to sleep, eat nutritional meals, drink plenty of liquids—especially if she is breastfeeding—and take care of her physical and emotional needs. Your job is to guide, nurture, and help her heal.

Newborn Care

Nursing assistants often care for newborns in hospital nurseries. The nursing assistant helps the nursing staff feed, burp, diaper, clean, and observe infants.

Bottle-Feeding an Infant

Bottle-fed babies receive sugar water for the first day or two after birth, and then formula. **Formula** is a milk mixture enhanced with extra nutrients to make it as close in content to breast milk as possible. Formula provides the necessary nutrients for a baby to thrive, but it does not contain the enzymes and antibodies of mother's milk.

Formula can be given at room temperature or warmed. To warm the bottle, place it in a pan of warm water or a bottle warmer just before feeding. Put a few drops on your wrist to make sure the formula is warm, not hot. Do not use a microwave for warming formula, because it may heat unevenly.

Make feeding time peaceful. Sit in a comfortable chair and support the infant's head and shoulders in your arm. Place a bib under the baby's chin. Gently touch the cheek. The rooting reflex will make the baby turn its head and get ready to suck. Tilt the bottle and place the nipple in the infant's mouth. Keep the bottle upright so the nipple and neck remain filled with formula. Speak quietly to get the baby to focus on your face as you offer the bottle. **See Figure 28-8.** Let the infant drink at its own pace.

About halfway through the feeding, burp the baby. Continue feeding until the infant either finishes the bottle or stops sucking. Clean the baby's face and neck. Discard extra formula and disposable feeding supplies. Record the time and amount of the feeding.

Changing a Diaper

An average baby urinates at least 6 to 10 times in 24 hours. Breastfed babies usually have a bowel movement after every feeding. Bottle-fed babies have a bowel movement 2 to 4 times a day. A newborn's diaper is changed after every feeding, and more often if the baby seems uncomfortable. A typical newborn is changed 7 to 10 times a day.

The first feces after birth, passed within 24 hours, are called *meconium*. Meconium is black and tarry. Stools then become greenish-brown and very loose. After about a week, the infant's stools develop a regular color and consistency. Breastfed babies have yellow stools. Bottle-fed babies have brown stools.

Hospitals have changing tables or changing stations where all newborns are changed. The table is covered with a disposable pad that is discarded after each diaper change. When caring for a baby in the home, set up a changing table with all your supplies. Never leave a baby alone on a changing table. Have your supplies organized and within reach. If no changing table is available, use a waterproof pad in the crib.

Place the changing pad under the baby. Put on your gloves. Loosen the soiled diaper. Bring the front piece down between the legs. Use the front of the diaper to wipe feces off the baby's genitals and buttocks. Wipe from front to back. Hold the baby's ankles and gently lift the buttocks. Place the soiled diaper in a disposable bag or diaper pail.

Use a wet washcloth, disposable wipe, or a cotton ball dipped in water to clean the baby's perineal area. Wipe from front to back with a clean cotton ball, cloth, or wipe for each swab until the baby is clean. Be sure to pat skin dry. Open the clean diaper and place it under the baby's buttocks. Note any sign of irritation, such as diaper rash. Apply creams or ointments if necessary.

Pull the loose part of the diaper up between the legs and adjust so it fits snugly. Arrange a cloth diaper with the extra fold in the front for boys and in the back for girls. Gently point a boy's penis downward, so urine does not spray up out of the diaper. Fasten the diaper using the adhesive strips, diaper pins, or

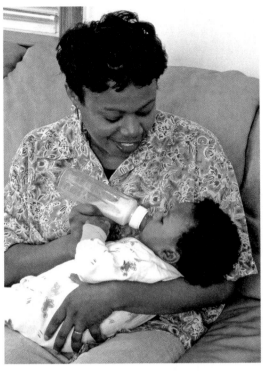

○ **Figure 28-8.** An infant's feeding time offers a chance to provide comfort and security.

Mixing Formula for Bottle Feeding

An infant is usually fed every three to four hours. Formula comes either pre-mixed or concentrated. Prepare the concentrated formula as follows: Mix one 8-oz can of concentrate with 8 oz of water. The infant will be bottle-fed every 4 hours. At each feeding, the infant will be offered 4 oz of formula.

Practice

Using the information provided, answer the following questions.
1. How many ounces of formula can you make from 1 can of concentrate?
2. How many 4-oz bottles of formula can be prepared from 1 can of concentrate?

SAFETY FIRST

If the baby does not drink all of the formula, discard what remains in the bottle. If left to sit, bacteria could grow. Do not refrigerate remaining formula. If the baby has a cold or other illness, microorganisms could remain on the nipple and re-infect the baby if used again. Use a clean bottle and nipple for each feeding.

diaper cover. Fasten diaper pins so they point away from the abdomen. **See Figure 28-9.** Report and record the following: the time of diaper change, the amount and color of urine or feces, ointments or creams used, and the condition of the skin.

Umbilical Cord Care

The **umbilical cord** connects the fetus to the placenta during pregnancy. It carries blood, oxygen, and nutrients to the fetus, and carries wastes away from the fetus. After birth, the umbilical cord is clamped and cut. The stump that remains on the baby turns black and falls off between 10 and 14 days after birth. The baby can be given a sponge bath but should not have a tub bath until it falls off. Keep it clean and dry, because it is a site for potential infection. Do not get the navel wet until the stump falls off. Tell the nurse or mother if the site oozes drainage, has an odor, or turns red.

Provide cord care each time you diaper a newborn. After you have cleaned the perineal area, place the clean diaper under the buttocks. Dip a cotton ball in alcohol or use an alcohol wipe to wipe the base of the umbilical stump. See **Figure 28-10.** Fold down the front of the diaper below the navel so it does not irritate the stump. Report umbilical cord care and the condition of the stump.

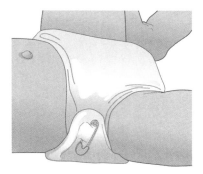

○ **Figure 28-9.** For safety, diaper pins are always pointed away from the abdomen.

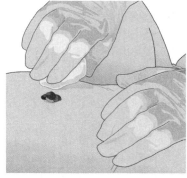

○ **Figure 28-10.** Gently wipe around the base of the umbilical stump.

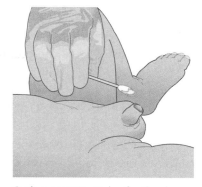

○ **Figure 28-11.** Caring for the circumcision site.

Care After Circumcision

Circumcision is the surgical removal of the foreskin on a boy's penis. It is usually performed in the hospital. Circumcisions usually heal in 2 to 3 days.

Care for the circumcision area while changing the baby's diaper. After you have cleaned the perineal area, place the clean diaper under the baby's buttocks. Put a generous amount of petroleum jelly on a gauze pad or cotton swab. Gently apply it to the penis. **See Figure 28-11.** A small amount of blood on the incision site or diaper is normal. Make sure the diaper is loose in that area. Wash your hands. Report and record circumcision care, including odor, drainage, or bleeding, and the condition of the skin.

Weighing a Newborn

The average baby weighs a little over 7 pounds at birth. Most babies lose about 1 ounce per day for the first couple of days. Then they gain about 1 ounce per day for the next 3 months.

The nurse may ask you to weigh a newborn. First, remove the baby's clothing, including the diaper. Clean the perineal area, if necessary. Wrap the baby in a blanket to keep it warm until you place it on the scale. Place the disposable pad on the scale and level the scale to zero. Place the baby on its back on the scale. Most infant scales have beveled sides to prevent the baby from falling. Some scales have a safety belt, which you should fasten. Keep one hand over the baby to keep it from falling.

Move the pointer of the pound calculation until it is almost level. Adjust the ounces calculation until the scale is level. Slide the pointers back to zero with one hand. Hold onto the baby with the other. Lift the baby from the scale and wrap it in the blanket. Remove the pad and discard it. Diaper and dress the baby. Return the baby to the bassinet or crib. Wash your hands. Record the time, date, and weight on the baby's chart.

Vital Skills — WRITING

Taking Notes

Being a good student means taking good notes. With good notes, it's easier to study later. Before class, review your notes from the last class and complete assigned readings. Then you're ready to build on the information you already have. Use one notebook for note-taking and bring it to class every time.

Focus on what the instructor says. Listen for cues that indicate that a particular point is important and worth writing down. For example, the instructor might start a sentence with, "It's important to remember that . . . ."

As you take notes, use abbreviations, and leave out small words such as *the* or *at*. After class, rewrite your notes. Add words you left out, and edit so that your sentences are complete. Rewriting is a good way for you to reinforce the information and see what you might need to spend extra time studying.

Practice

Tune in to a radio or television news talk show. Practice taking notes on what the speakers are saying.

Chapter Summary

- Nursing assistants may choose to complete additional training to expand their roles.

- Nursing assistants may assume a wide variety of roles when assisting with patient medications as delegated by a licensed nurse.

- Pregnancy is divided into trimesters to help women calculate and monitor the expected changes that occur during pregnancy. Certain tests are performed during this period, and certain signs and symptoms must be reported.

- There are certain signs of impending labor and stages of labor.

- Caring for a postpartum patient involves personal care and helping the patient meet her needs through emotional support and encouragement. Helping in the home may involve assistance with housekeeping, the baby, and the family.

- The nursing assistant can support and encourage a new mother to breastfeed her baby.

- Newborn care includes bottle-feeding and burping the infant, changing the diaper, caring for the umbilical cord and circumcision, and weighing the infant.

VOCABULARY REVIEW

Directions: Match the letter of each definition in the second column with the correct vocabulary term in the first column. Write your answers on a separate sheet of paper.

Vocabulary

1. cesarean section
2. circumcision
3. colostrum
4. episiotomy
5. letdown reflex
6. lochia
7. placenta
8. postpartum care
9. prenatal care
10. rooting reflex

Definitions

A. The medical and supportive care given to a mother after childbirth
B. A small incision of the perineum made during delivery to avoid tearing of the tissue and to ease the baby's passage
C. The natural response that causes a baby to look for something to suck when the cheek is touched
D. The surgical removal of the foreskin on a boy's penis
E. The delivery of a fetus by a surgical incision into the uterus through the abdomen
F. The vascular organ lining the walls of the uterus from which the fetus derives nutrition and oxygen
G. The automatic release of breast milk in response to the presence of milk in the breasts
H. A thick, yellow fluid secreted from the mother's breast for the first few days after delivery that supplies babies with important antibodies
I. The medical care and monitoring a woman receives during her pregnancy to ensure optimum health for her and the developing baby
J. The normal discharge from the uterus after childbirth

Check Your Knowledge

Review Questions: Answer each of the following questions on a separate sheet of paper.

1. List five topics of care in which a nursing assistant may obtain additional training for expanded roles within the scope of practice.

2. Why is it important to follow manufacturer's instructions for medication storage?

3. When is the first ultrasound done in a normal pregnancy?

4. How can a new mother clean her perineal area after defecating or voiding?

5. How soon can a new mother shower after a normal childbirth?

6. What is formula?

7. Why should babies be burped after feeding?

8. How many times does the average baby urinate in 24 hours?

9. What is the first feces that the new infant passes and what does it look like?

10. What is the average weight of a baby at birth?

True or False: Read each statement carefully. Then write *True* or *False* by the statement number on a separate sheet of paper.

1. The topical route for medication administration is the eye.

2. Fluid or blood leaking from a pregnant woman's vagina should be reported.

3. An infant may have a tub bath after the umbilical stump falls off.

4. Circumcisions normally take about 14 days to heal.

5. A baby loses weight in the first days after birth.

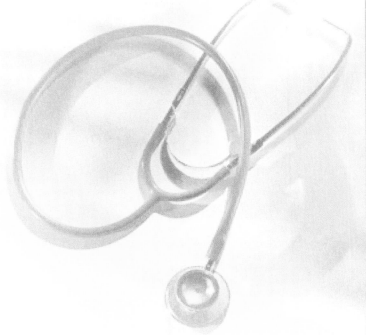

Think and Decide

Directions: Think about each of the following scenarios. Answer each question on a separate sheet of paper.

1. You have been trained to assist the residents with their medications in the long-term care facility where you work. Mrs. G.'s husband brings a medication for you to give her before bedtime. He tells you it is a laxative. The medication is not in its original container. What should you do? Why?

2. Mrs. C. is a new mother who is at home with her newborn infant. She is a single mother with no one to help her. You are assigned to help in her home. Mrs. C. wants to do everything for her baby and asks you to help with light housekeeping duties and to plan meals. Is this appropriate? What should you tell her?

3. You are assisting in the home of the young Ramirez family. They have a baby who is 5 days old. Elena, the mother, asks you to go upstairs and check on the baby. When you see the baby, you notice a rash on his chest. He has also vomited. What should you do?

4. You are assisting in the home of the Greene family. Mrs. Greene asks you why you are not warming her baby's bottle in the microwave. What should you tell Mrs. Greene?

5. Mrs. H. has had her newborn baby home for one week. She asks if you would give her baby a tub bath. What should you do?

6. Mrs. V. is a long-term care resident in your care during the evening shift. She had surgery recently and is in pain. When you enter the room, Mr. V. angrily demands that you give Mrs. V. her morphine pill. He claims he has asked the nurse three times, but the medicine still hasn't been administered. You have received training to assist with nonnarcotic medications. What should you do?

7. You are assisting in the home of Mrs. C., a new mother who has decided to breastfeed her baby. She is careful to eat nutritionally balanced meals and to drink plenty of fluids. However, you notice that the portions of food she prepares for herself are very small. When you ask her about the portions, she explains that now that she has had the baby, she wants to lose all the extra weight she gained during pregnancy. What should you tell Mrs. C.?

CNA Certification Exam Prep

Directions: This practice test contains ten questions. Each question has four suggested answers. For each question, choose the ONE that best answers the question or completes the statement. Write your answers on a separate sheet of paper.

1. Expanded roles of the nursing assistant include
   A. diagnosing illness.
   B. filling prescriptions.
   C. caring for newborn infants.
   D. creating patient care plans.

2. Medication that is applied as a cream or lotion is given by the
   A. oral route.
   B. inhaled route.
   C. ear route.
   D. topical route.

3. Which of the following tests is done within the first 12 weeks of pregnancy?
   A. prenatal panel
   B. ultrasound
   C. diabetes screen
   D. fetal monitoring

4. The period of pregnancy from week 28 through week 40 is the
   A. first trimester.
   B. second trimester.
   C. third trimester.
   D. fourth trimester.

5. The lowering of the baby's head into the mother's pelvis during labor is known as
   A. dilation.
   B. lightening.
   C. crowning.
   D. contracting.

6. The type of pain relief during the birth process that is injected into a vein or muscle is a(n)
   A. systemic analgesic.
   B. epidural block.
   C. spinal block.
   D. local analgesic.

7. The period of postpartum care usually lasts about
   A. 2 weeks.
   B. 4 weeks.
   C. 6 weeks.
   D. 8 weeks.

8. For the first few days after birth, bottle-fed babies receive
   A. formula.
   B. sugar water.
   C. colostrum.
   D. goat's milk.

9. Formula contains
   A. nutrients.
   B. colostrum.
   C. antibodies.
   D. enzymes.

10. After the first couple of days, how much weight do most babies gain per day for the first three months?
    A. 1 ounce
    B. 2 ounces
    C. 4 ounces
    D. 8 ounces

CHAPTER 29

OBJECTIVES

- Explain the stages of grief and the effect they may have on the terminally ill patient.
- Identify rights of the dying patient.

- Describe care options for terminally ill patients.
- Identify and meet the physical needs of terminally ill patients.

- Discuss the psychological needs of terminally ill patients and their families.
- Discuss ways to help the patient's family.

Caring for the Terminally Ill

hospice A facility or program that provides physical and emotional care and support for terminally ill patients and their families.

oral swab A small sponge on a stick used to moisten a patient's mouth to prevent painful cracking.

patient-controlled anesthesia (PCA) A pumping device that delivers a small dose of pain medication intravenously when the patient pushes a button.

quality of life The ability to enjoy the activities of life or to be satisfied with everyday living.

sacraments Rites or rituals, held to be sacred, to confer grace on an individual.

terminal illness An illness that is not curable and from which the person will eventually die.

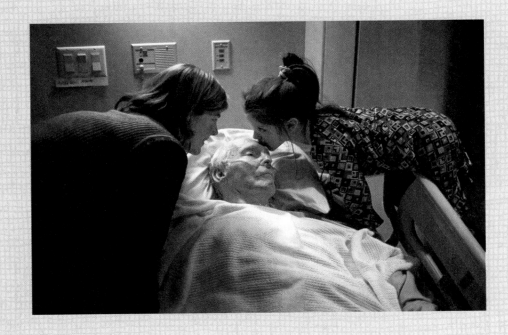

The Terminally Ill Patient

At various times in our lives, we must all deal with death and dying—our own or someone else's. Some deaths are sudden, and others are expected, but all have an impact on the dying person, as well as the family and caregivers.

A **terminal illness** is one that is not curable and from which the person will eventually die. As a nursing assistant, you may care for people who are terminally ill. When you care for such a person, you will help meet his or her physical, psychological, social, and spiritual needs. It is important for you to understand the dying process so that you can approach the dying person with caring, compassion, kindness, and respect.

You may be nervous or anxious the first few times you care for someone who is terminally ill. Many new nursing assistants worry about saying or doing the wrong thing. Working with someone who is dying may bring back painful memories of a loss of your own, too. You may find that your own fears about death and dying surface. Discuss any of these concerns with your supervisor. These are normal feelings and reactions, and with time and experience, you will find yourself less unsettled.

The Stages of Grief in Dying Patients

Dr. Elisabeth Kübler-Ross described the five stages of grief that people with terminal illnesses often experience. They are denial, anger, bargaining, depression, and acceptance. Not all people go through all of the stages before death. Let's look at the different stages. By understanding them, you will better understand the person and will be better able to help.

First Stage: Denial. The patient refuses to believe he or she is dying. This stage can last a few hours, days, or months. Some people are still in denial when they die.

Second Stage: Anger. The second stage includes anger and rage. The patient blames others and finds fault with loved ones—the very people he or she may need the most. Do not take the person's anger personally.

Third Stage: Bargaining. Often the patient attempts to "bargain" for more time. The patient makes promises to change or do specific things in exchange for more time. Bargaining is usually very private, so you may not see or experience this stage with the dying person.

Fourth Stage: Depression. The person may say little, cry, and seem sad. He or she may focus on losses and the loss of things to come.

Fifth Stage: Acceptance. The person is calm and at peace. This does not mean the end of life is near. It simply means the person has no more unfinished business. **See Figure 29-1.**

In all stages, maintain a positive, compassionate attitude toward the patient and the care you are providing. However, do not tell the patient not to worry and that everything will be okay. Such statements are clichés that can block communication and make patients feel that their fears do not matter to you. Giving false hope does not help the patient go through the emotional processes leading to acceptance of his or her condition.

Rights of the Dying Patient

People who have terminal illnesses have rights that are protected by federal and state laws. They have the right to:

- Be treated courteously and respectfully as a living human until they die.
- Have competent, compassionate care from caring people until they die.
- Participate in decisions concerning their care.
- Obtain relief from pain.
- Have their questions answered honestly.
- Have loved ones supported emotionally by the health care team.
- Die peacefully in a dignified manner.
- Not be alone when they die.

Nursing assistants can help with many of these items. For example, they can treat patients courteously and respectfully and provide competent, compassionate care. They can provide emotional support to the patient's family and friends. Other items are beyond the nursing assistant's scope of practice. For example, if a patient requests pain relief or an honest answer to a medical question, the nursing assistant should forward the requests to the nurse.

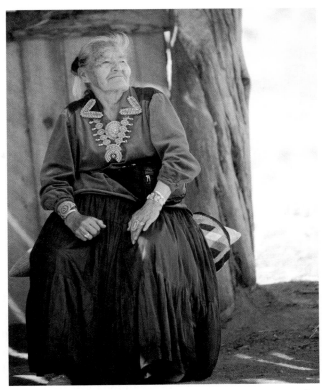

O **Figure 29-1.** Patients in the fifth stage of grief have accepted that death is near and have come to terms with it.

Some people make their end-of-life wishes known in advance through an advance directive or living will. They may have also appointed someone to act on their behalf if they cannot do so in a durable power of attorney. These documents give the patient and the patient's family specific rights. Many terminal patients also have DNR (do not resuscitate) orders. CPR is not performed on these patients if their breathing or heart stops. See Chapter 4 for a discussion of the patient's rights in these cases.

Care Options for Terminally Ill Patients

People with terminal illnesses usually have several options for receiving care. In some cases, the person may stay at home with part-time or full-time care. This care is often provided by nursing assistants, under the direction of an RN. Some patients require hospital care, and others may need the services available in a long-term care facility. The patient, family, and doctor generally weigh the patient's needs against the type of services provided by the different types of facilities before deciding how and where to care for the patient.

As you may recall from Chapter 2, **hospice** is a facility or program that provides physical and emotional care and support for terminally ill patients and their families. It can refer to either a type of care or a place where the care is provided. Hospice programs provide supportive, comfortable care for terminally ill people who are expected to die within 6 months.

Extraordinary medical care aimed at prolonging life is not the purpose of hospice care. People who choose hospice care usually do not want their illnesses prolonged by breathing machines or other artificial medical measures. They prefer to remain as pain-free as possible and to let death come as naturally as possible. Comfort measures, good skin care, and turning and repositioning are the main goals of hospice care. **See Figure 29-2.**

Another major goal of hospice organizations is to maintain or improve the quality of life of terminally ill patients. **Quality of life** is the ability to enjoy the activities of life or to be satisfied with everyday living. For terminally ill patients, maintaining quality of life is a challenging, yet important, aspect of care. As the patient's health declines, caregivers may try to find activities or pastimes that are within the patient's ability to stimulate interest and satisfaction.

Physical Care

Regardless of the setting, most terminally ill patients require physical care. Follow the care plan to determine the routine needs of the patient. The care plan should consist of group decisions made by the nursing staff, family members, the patient, and anyone else the patient wishes to include.

Check frequently to be sure the patient is comfortable. Help him or her move to the most comfortable position possible for breathing and avoiding pain. Patients with breathing difficulties are usually more comfortable in the semi-Fowler's position. To avoid pressure ulcers and other skin problems, patients' positions should be changed a minimum of every 2 hours. Keeping the patient in good body alignment can also promote comfort.

Terminally ill patients have the same personal hygiene needs as other patients. If anything, their needs are greater than that of other patients. Cleanliness, for example, can increase the patient's self-esteem and quality of life. The nursing assistant takes care of these needs on an ongoing basis.

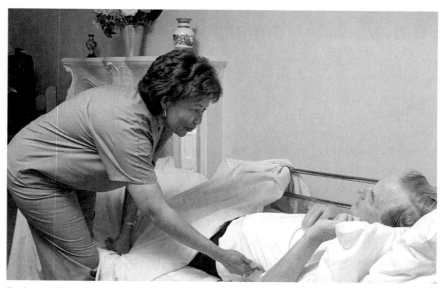

O **Figure 29-2.** The patient's comfort and quality of life are the main goals of hospice care.

Subtraction with Months

Many hospice programs accept only patients who are expected to die within 6 months. This is a guideline, not an absolute. In other words, if a patient lives for 7 months, he or she will not be thrown out of the hospice program after 6 months.

Suppose your patient entered a hospice program in February. The patient died in August of the same year. Did the patient die within the 6-month guideline?

Let's think this through.

1. There are 12 months in a year. They can be numbered 1 through 12, beginning with January.
2. February is the second month.
3. August is the eight month.

4. To find the difference between the second and the eight month, you subtract.

$$
\begin{array}{r}
8 \text{ (August)} \\
- \ 2 \text{ (February)} \\
\hline
6 \ \text{months difference}
\end{array}
$$

The patient died within the 6-month guideline.

> **Practice**
>
> 1. If a patient enters a hospice program in March and dies in December, how long was the patient in the hospice program?
> 2. If a patient enters a hospice program in August and dies in November, how long was the patient in the hospice program?

Nutritional Needs

Patients who are nearing death often have decreased appetites. Sometimes, the patient's chart has specific dietary instructions. However, if you have no specific instructions and the patient has no appetite or seems uninterested in food, try offering liquid or semi-liquid nutrition. This may be more appealing, since it is easier to swallow.

For a terminally ill patient, a balanced diet should not be the prime consideration. Trying favorite foods and small, frequent feedings may appeal to patients. Also, whenever possible, ask patients what they would like to eat. The staff should attempt to provide such foods, or the family can be asked to bring in favorite foods. Do not force patients to eat or drink, however.

Elimination Needs

Some terminally ill patients lose bowel and/or bladder control in the later stages of the illness. It is important to keep these patients' skin clean and their bed linens fresh. Clean the patient's perineal area as often as necessary. Since soap may be too drying, ask your supervisor about using a special cleanser or moisturizing soap to keep the skin soft. Change bed linens whenever they become soiled or moist. Remember that your primary responsibility is to make sure the patient is comfortable.

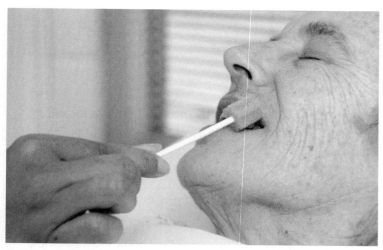
○ **Figure 29-3.** Using an oral swab to moisten the patient's lips helps avoid uncomfortable cracking of the lips.

Care of the Mouth and Nose

Patients with a terminal illness often have special oral hygiene needs. Some patients develop painful sores in the mouth and others have bleeding gums. If a patient is bleeding from the mouth, gently wipe the area with a damp washcloth. Patients approaching death often have a dry mouth and lips and require more frequent oral hygiene. Offer the patient drinking water as often as permitted. Use an **oral swab** (a small sponge on a stick) to swab the lips with a lubricant to provide lasting moisture and to prevent cracking. **See Figure 29-3.**

Some patients secrete excess mucus or other fluids in the mouth. This interferes with swallowing and may cause choking. Inform your nursing supervisor if you see this happening. The nurse can remove excess secretions by suction.

Patients with oxygen or other tubes in the nose may experience irritation and crusting of the nostrils. The nose area should be cleaned gently. The nurse may recommend applying a lubricant.

Vision and Hearing

The patient's vision, hearing, and speech may be affected as a terminal illness progresses. Vision may become blurred and eventually fail. If a patient has failing vision, it is especially important to explain what you are going to do before you do it. Good eye care is also important. Secretions may form in the corners of the eyes. Wipe them gently with a cool washcloth. Wash your hands afterward.

Hearing is the last function lost in many dying patients. Many people hear up to the moment of death. Encourage the family to talk to their loved ones. They may not seem to be awake, but they may be able to hear. Also, provide reassurance and explanations about care even if the patient seems unresponsive. Offer words of comfort.

Psychological Needs

All dying patients have psychological needs, whether expressed or unexpressed. Some of their needs will be met by family, friends, clergy, or a counselor. You may have the opportunity to meet some of the patient's emotional needs. Some patients want to talk about their fears and concerns, and by being a good listener, you give them opportunities to express feelings and worries. Patients often feel less afraid and alone when they have someone to talk to. Besides listening, your touch may comfort many patients. Giving a gentle back rub may comfort some patients. Playing soft music while simply holding the person's hand may be calming.

Reminiscing Therapy

Caring for terminally ill patients can be difficult. It might be hard to feel that you are making a difference as their life comes to an end. One way to communicate with terminally ill patients is through reminiscing therapy.

Listen and talk with the person about his or her past experiences, activities, and memories. Use photographs or other objects to prompt the person to recall memories.

Reminiscing is a way for people to make sense of their lives and to reflect on what they have accomplished. By listening and talking about the past, nursing assistants can provide a source of comfort to terminally ill patients.

Practice

With a partner, practice reminiscing therapy. Take turns playing the role of patient and nursing assistant. How would you react if the patient told you something you found disagreeable?

Emotional and Social Needs

When caring for a terminally ill patient, your primary responsibility is to do what you can to make the patient comfortable. Often, you will also have the opportunity to meet some of the patient's emotional needs.

Patients without support systems such as friends and family may be especially susceptible to depression. Their social needs—to be part of a group or family, to talk to other people—may not be met without assistance from the health care team.

Spiritual and Cultural Needs

People differ in their spiritual beliefs and practices. Some belong to organized religions and attend worship services regularly. Some people are spiritual, but do not participate in an organized religion. Still others do not believe in a spiritual being. Whatever the person's beliefs, your role is to listen if they want to discuss spiritual issues. Listen without judging the person's beliefs, however different they may be from your own.

Most facilities also have counselors on staff who listen to the patient and provide support. If a patient has a religious affiliation, your supervisor may call the patient's priest, minister, or rabbi. **See Figure 29-4.**

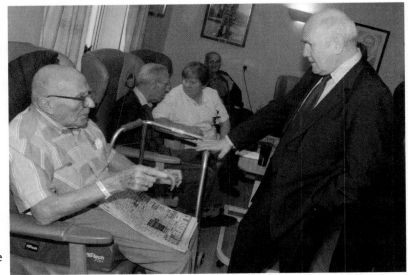

○ **Figure 29-4.** Sometimes a spiritual leader from the patient's religious organization can help ease a patient's fears.

Sometimes people who are facing their own deaths feel a greater need for spiritual faith. In some religions, special sacraments are administered to people who are sick or dying. **Sacraments** are rites or rituals, held to be sacred, that confer grace on an individual. Some people want to spend more time in prayer, sometimes with a member of the clergy. Unless doctors' orders prohibit, patients should have privacy during visits from the clergy. If the patient expresses a desire to speak with clergy but is not attached to a specific church, speak to your supervisor about arranging a visit from a staff chaplain or local clergy. Many clergy are "on call" and rotate times they are available to come to the hospital or nursing facility.

Helping the Patient's Family

You may also have the opportunity to help the patient's family cope with the situation. Whether dealing with the patient's needs or the family's needs, your role is to be helpful and cooperative. Everyone involved is going through a difficult emotional experience. Different family members have different feelings and reactions. Many family members want to spend as much time as possible with the patient. Whenever possible, leave the patient alone with his or her family. Private time is important. Do whatever you can to make this private time possible. Respect the person's need for privacy.

Vital Skills — WRITING

Avoiding Common Writing Mistakes

All writers make common mistakes at one time or another. With practice, you can avoid some of these common errors, or learn how to spot them in your own writing and make corrections. Two common writing errors are:

- Subjects and verbs that don't agree
  Incorrect: The children she saw on the playground is in the waiting room.

  The subject is *children* (plural) and the verb is *is* (singular).
  Correct: The children she saw on the playground are in the waiting room.
- Misplaced apostrophes; for example, *it's* is a contraction that stands for "it is" or "it has." *Its* is a possessive pronoun meaning "belonging to it."

Incorrect: Dr. Drake said the wound would heal on it's own.
Correct: Dr. Drake said the wound would heal on its own.

Practice

Correct the sentences below. There may be more than one error in a sentence.

1. The children in the fourth-floor play area is ready for lunch.
2. Its not clear whether she understood that her prescription had expired.
3. The patient in room 416 are reading to his grandchildren.
4. She said the cat scratched her when she picked up one of it's kittens.

Guidelines for helping the patient's family include:

- Allow the family as much private time with the patient as treatment permits.
- Be sensitive to the family's emotions. Do not judge words or behavior.
- Ask if the family has any special requests or needs.
- Be supportive and understanding. Be a good listener when family members want to talk.
- Tell the family where to find food, a telephone, a lounge, and whatever else they need.
- If family members stay at the facility overnight, help them find a place to rest. In the hospital setting, a cot usually can be brought into the patient's room.
- If permitted, allow the family to participate in some of the patient's basic care (for example, bathing, grooming, or feeding) if the family requests. **See Figure 29-5.**

In some cultures, family members are very involved with the care of the dying person. Include them in the patient's care when possible. Assist them whenever you can. Ask family members what they want you to do. This is a very emotional time. Be respectful of their wishes.

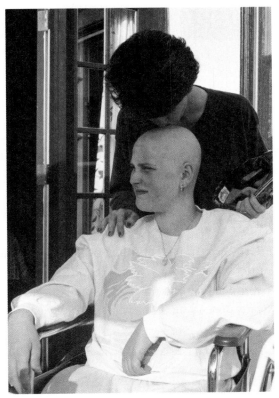

○ **Figure 29-5.** Allow the family to help with the patient's care. In many cultures, giving care to a dying family member is an act of love and respect.

Vital Skills   READING

Vary Your Reading Rate

A good reader varies reading speed. When scanning a reference book in the library, you'll probably read at a different rate than you would a novel. Just as you don't want to speed-read a poem, you might not read every single word of the manual that came with your new MP3 player.

As you become a better reader, you'll learn to adjust your reading rate and the transition will become natural to you. These factors might influence your reading rate:

- *The difficulty of the reading material.* Sometimes a difficult paragraph can take as long to read as an entire page. If there are words that are new to you or you don't understand a passage, slow down and re-read.

- *The purpose for reading.* If you are studying for a test, you'll take your time with the reading material to make sure you understand each concept before you move on. If you're reading a novel, however, you may read more quickly.

Practice

Gather four or five different kinds of reading material: a magazine article, junk mail, a novel, a textbook, a recipe, a poem, and the phone book. Read from each and think about your reading rate. Can you feel yourself speed up or slow down depending on the material?

Chapter Summary

- Terminal illness is an illness without hope of recovery, from which the patient is expected to die.
- Your own feelings about working with the terminally ill are important and can be discussed with a supervisor.
- Terminally ill patients often experience five stages of grief before dying.
- Terminally ill patients have several options for health care, depending on their individual needs.

- Terminally ill patients have the same physical needs as all other patients and should receive the same quality of care as any other patient.
- Psychological needs include emotional, social, and spiritual needs. Paying attention to these needs can help comfort the patient.
- The family of terminally ill patients also needs care and attention.

VOCABULARY REVIEW

Directions: Match the letter of each definition in the second column with the correct vocabulary term in the first column. Write your answers on a separate sheet of paper.

Vocabulary

1. hospice
2. oral swab
3. patient-controlled anesthesia
4. quality of life
5. sacraments
6. terminal illness

Definitions

A. A pumping device that delivers pain medication when a patient pushes a button
B. An illness that is not curable and from which the person will eventually die
C. Rites or rituals, held to be sacred, to confer grace on an individual
D. A small sponge on a stick used to moisten a patient's mouth to prevent painful cracking
E. The ability to enjoy the activities of life or to be satisfied with everyday living
F. A facility or program that provides physical and emotional care and support for terminally ill patients and their families

Check Your Knowledge

Review Questions: Answer each of the following questions on a separate sheet of paper.

1. What should you do if you are assigned to care for a terminally ill patient and you are nervous or uneasy about it?

2. What are the five stages of grief associated with dying?

3. Name three care options for terminally ill patients.

4. What is hospice?

5. Explain the importance of quality of life for a terminally ill patient.

6. Who is involved in the decisions reflected in a terminally ill patient's care plan?

7. What special mouth care needs might terminally ill patients have?

8. What can you do to make a patient with dry, cracked lips more comfortable?

9. In general, how might you meet the psychological needs of a terminally ill patient?

10. How can you help the family of a terminally ill patient?

True or False: Read each statement carefully. Then write *True* or *False* by the statement number on a separate sheet of paper.

1. Upon learning they have a terminal illness, most people respond in the same way.

2. The patient's family should be allowed to spend as much time as medically permissible with the patient.

3. Patients who have a need to talk about their fears should always be referred to a counselor.

4. Patients who are not members of a religious organization do not have spiritual needs.

5. The nursing assistant's primary responsibility when caring for a terminally ill patient is to reassure the patient that everything will be okay.

Think and Decide

Directions: Think about each of the following scenarios. Answer each question on a separate sheet of paper.

1. E.M. has a terminal illness. She has been crying often. You ask her what the matter is and she turns away from you. She says she just wants to be left alone. Which stage of the grieving process might E.M. be in? What might you do for her?

2. Mr. H. has just been notified by his doctor that he has terminal stomach cancer and has less than 6 months to live. He has made a choice to seek no further treatment. He wishes to stay in his own home until death. What type of care will be given to Mr. H.? What health care organization may help care for him?

3. Mr. D. has amyotrophic lateral sclerosis (Lou Gehrig's disease). As this terminal illness progresses, he has had more and more trouble controlling muscle movements. His doctor has finally told him that he can no longer safely live alone. Mr. D. is horrified by the thought of living and dying in a long-term care facility, and he has no family to help. What other option does Mr. D. have?

4. Mrs. U. has a nonoperable cancer that has not responded to radiation or chemotherapy, and the doctors give her only a month to live. She is excited this morning when you arrive to help with her personal care. She says she knows now that she will live until her grandson graduates from college, two years from now. "You see," she says, "I've promised to help organize a charity bazaar here at the facility every year so that I can live a few more years." What stage of grief is Mrs. U. experiencing? How should you answer?

5. P.J. is a terminally ill patient in a long-term care facility who seems to grow weaker every day. Today she has refused both lunch and dinner, saying that she is not hungry. What might you do for her?

6. Mr. N. had a massive stroke a few days ago and has been unconscious since then. He is not expected to live. Mr. N.'s family is here to visit. They are talking softly about how awful it is to see him like this and what a shame it is that he is dying. What, if anything, might you do for Mr. N.?

CNA Certification Exam Prep

Directions: This practice test contains ten questions. Each question has four suggested answers. For each question, choose the ONE that best answers the question or completes the statement. Write your answers on a separate sheet of paper.

1. An illness that cannot be cured and from which the patient will eventually die is a(n)
   A. chronic illness.
   B. acute illness.
   C. terminal illness.
   D. transient illness.

2. The stage of grief in which a person finds fault with everything and blames others is
   A. the first stage: denial.
   B. the second stage: anger.
   C. the third stage: bargaining.
   D. the fourth stage: depression.

3. A dying patient has the right to
   A. be cured of the terminal illness.
   B. be treated for free until death.
   C. threaten his or her caregivers.
   D. obtain relief from pain.

4. If a patient has a DNR order,
   A. CPR is not performed on the patient if breathing or the heart stops.
   B. the patient may not be given anything by mouth.
   C. relatives can make decisions for the patient if he or she cannot.
   D. an appointed person can act on the patient's behalf.

5. One of the main goals of hospice care is to
   A. attempt to cure the patient.
   B. perform transplant surgery.
   C. maintain or improve quality of life.
   D. rehabilitate the patient.

6. If you notice a terminally ill patient having trouble swallowing, you should
   A. offer the patient water frequently.
   B. inform your supervisor immediately.
   C. suction the patient's mouth.
   D. not feed the patient.

7. A dying patient who is in denial
   A. tries to bargain for more time.
   B. focuses on losses.
   C. finds fault with everyone.
   D. refuses to believe he or she is dying.

8. Hospice organizations generally care for patients who are expected to die within
   A. 6 months.
   B. 1 year.
   C. 5 years.
   D. 10 years.

9. A device that allows a patient to obtain small amounts of pain medication on demand is called
   A. patient-controlled anesthesia.
   B. self-ordered medication.
   C. over-the-counter medication.
   D. terminal anesthesia.

10. The ability to enjoy the activities of life is called the
    A. life span.
    B. quality of life.
    C. quantity of life.
    D. life goals.

CHAPTER 30

OBJECTIVES

- List the typical signs of approaching death.

- List the four indications of death.

- Demonstrate typical post-mortem care.

Death and Postmortem Care

death rattle A gurgle or rattle caused by accumulating mucus at the back of the throat of a dying patient.

expires Dies.

morgue A place where bodies are kept until burial arrangements have been made.

mottled Having an irregular pattern of patches or spots of different colors.

no-code orders Another term for DNR (do not resuscitate) orders.

organ donor A person who has agreed to donate tissue or organs to others when he or she dies.

postmortem care Care after death.

resuscitation Lifesaving measures on a person whose breathing and/or heart has stopped.

rigor mortis The stiffening of a body 2 to 4 hours after death.

shroud A cloth used to wrap a person's body for burial.

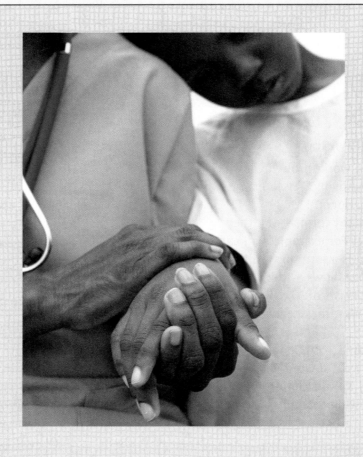

Grieving with the Person Who Is Dying

When they learn that death is near, people at various ages usually have different attitudes. However, almost everyone has some fears or concerns about death. They may be afraid of the unknown, or of being alone.

As you provide care for dying patients, your role is to listen and accept the emotions they are experiencing. You may encourage them to talk about their feelings, or you may need to understand their nonverbal communications. Each person's ideas about what happens when we die are different. Do not judge patients' ideas. You cannot help them achieve acceptance. You can, however, provide the emotional support that will help them move toward death in the way that is most comforting for them. Your own acceptance of death as a natural part of life can provide you with strength to help meet patients' needs.

Signs of Approaching Death

Sometimes death comes gradually. In other situations, death may occur more rapidly. A patient may have been terminally ill for a long time, or may die after a surgical procedure or medical emergency. As you provide care for a dying patient, you will need to observe the physical signs of approaching death. In a home care situation, you give the client the same kind of care as always.

There are five basic signs of approaching death. They are: decreased circulation, decreased respiration, loss of muscle control, decreased organ function, and changes in mental state. As you watch for these signs of impending death, notice any changes in the patient's condition. Report these changes to your supervisor. Notify the family as instructed.

Vital Skills — WRITING

Creative Writing: Poetry

Writing can help you work through your feelings about death and dying. Try to express your feelings by writing a poem.

Poems can take many forms—and they don't have to rhyme! For example, you can try writing haiku. *Haiku* is a form of traditional Japanese poetry that follows a specific format. It has 3 lines and consists of 17 syllables. The first line has 5 syllables, the second has 7, and the third has 5.

You can also try an acrostic poem. In this type of poetry, you write a word vertically. Each letter of the word is the first letter in a line of the poem. The following example is an acrostic poem about a hospital.

Healing
Open
Safe
Patients
Illness
Touching
All
Lives

Practice

Write a haiku or acrostic poem about death and dying. You may want to share your poem with classmates.

Decreased Circulation

As the heart begins to fail, blood circulation slows. Body temperature rises. The pulse may be rapid or weak or both; it also becomes irregular. Blood pressure falls.

As a result, the hands and feet may become cold, and the face pales. The patient's skin may feel cold, even though the patient may perspire heavily. The extremities (arms and hands, legs and feet) may become **mottled** (an irregular pattern of patches or spots of skin that have different colors). The skin changes to ashen and then to a blue color. As circulation to the brain decreases, less blood reaches the brain, and the sense of pain is diminished.

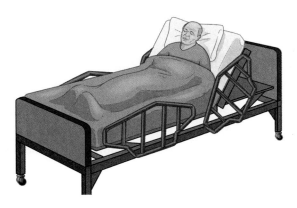

O **Figure 30-1.** When breathing becomes difficult, some patients find relief in the semi-Fowler's position.

Decreased Respiration

Breathing may become more difficult. Fluids that gather in the throat and bronchial tubes may result in a **death rattle**—a gurgle or rattle caused by accumulating mucus at the back of the throat of a dying patient. Avoid positioning the patient flat or prone. Remember that patients who have difficulty breathing are often helped by the semi-Fowler's position. **See Figure 30-1.**

As the respiratory system fails, Cheyne-Stokes respirations may be observed. (See Chapter 7 for more information about Cheyne-Stokes respirations.) Immediately before death, the pulse is almost gone and respiration stops.

If the patient is on oxygen, observe for signs of dry nostrils. You might be asked to clean the nostrils with a lubricant. Also keep the lips moist. A lip balm may help.

Loss of Muscle Control

The dying patient loses voluntary and involuntary muscle control. The jaw may drop, the eyes may fail to close or stare into space, and the mouth may hang open. The patient may no longer be able to speak or control swallowing saliva. He or she may also lose or partially lose sensation in the extremities.

The nursing assistant can help by maintaining oral and personal hygiene. Patients lose control of elimination and need to be kept clean, dry, and comfortable. Be observant and change the bedding as required.

Decreased Organ Function

As the patient nears death, other vital organs besides the heart and lungs begin to shut down. Peristalsis decreases, and digestion ceases. The kidneys begin to fail, resulting in decreased urine production and extreme swelling. Toxins are no longer being removed efficiently from the patient's body, because of the combination of decreased blood circulation and kidney failure.

Changes in Mental State

Some patients become confused or disoriented as they near death. Other people are alert up to the moment of death. Some people's conditions even seem to improve just before death. Keep the room as pleasant as possible by removing unneeded equipment and arranging mementos so the patient can easily see them.

FOCUS ON

Understanding Reactions

Nursing assistants often have close contact with the friends and family of a dying patient. Reactions of friends and family vary considerably. Some may openly grieve for their loved one, while others may be reserved in expressing their feelings. Nursing assistants can be friendly, available for communication, efficient, and kind in their caregiving, and not make judgments about the reactions of family members. Customs and relationships are unique to each family and should be respected.

Calculating Frequency of Respirations

Cheyne-Stokes respirations are alternating deep breaths with very shallow breaths and even an absence of a breath (apnea) for a period of 10 to 20 seconds.

You are checking a patient's vitals and notice Cheyne-Stokes respirations. You record a total of 6 respirations and 3 episodes of apnea. Each apneic episode lasted 10 seconds. Calculate the frequency of breaths during the periods in which the patient was breathing.

1. You checked the respirations for 1 minute, which is 60 seconds.
2. There were 3 episodes of apnea, each lasting 30 seconds, so the patient was apneic for 3 × 10 = 30 seconds.
3. Therefore, the patient was breathing for 60 − 30 = 30 seconds.
4. You counted a total of 6 respirations. You now know that those respirations occurred during 30 seconds. Divide 30 seconds by 6 breaths to find the frequency of breaths: 30 ÷ 6 = 5 breaths.

Practice

During a one-minute period, you count 7 respirations. The patient had two episodes of apnea, one lasting 15 seconds and the other 10 seconds. What is the frequency of breaths while the patient was breathing?

Avoid glaring light, but do not darken the room, because this may frighten the patient. Remember that hearing is the last remaining sense, so talk to the person and explain what you are doing. Be aware of your comments, because the patient may be able to hear you even if he or she cannot see or speak.

Signs of Death

The physician or, in some cases, the head nurse is responsible for certifying death and notifying the family. After a patient **expires**, or dies, the following signs are observed:

1. There is no pulse.
2. There is no respiration.
3. There is no blood pressure.
4. The patient's eyes are fixed and dilated.

When the patient has stopped breathing or lacks a pulse, the nurse will follow the patient's care plan. If there is no DNR (do not resuscitate) order, the nurse may initiate **resuscitation** (lifesaving measures). Terminally ill patients, however, often have DNR orders. You may also hear these orders called **no-code orders**. In these cases, no attempt is made at resuscitation. If the patient is an **organ donor** (a person who has agreed to donate tissue or organs to others when he or she dies), arrangements for the donation are made when the patient dies.

Remember as you work with patients who are dying or deceased that confidentiality is still in force. Health care workers have a duty to hold the patient's information confidential at all times, even at death.

Postmortem Care

The goal of **postmortem care** (care after death) is to maintain the body's hygiene and appearance. Do not begin to assist the nurse with postmortem care until you are instructed to do so.

You may be asked to elevate the head and gently straighten the limbs. The body may release fluids such as urine or feces. Blood may be released from the nose. Carefully cleanse the body with warm water, and wipe off discharges. **See Figure 30-2.** Be sure to follow standard precautions. After 2 to 4 hours, the body starts to become stiff, a condition called **rigor mortis**.

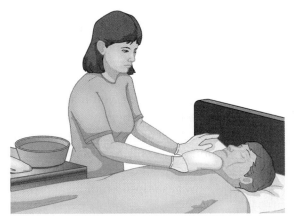

○ **Figure 30-2.** Gently cleanse the body with warm water.

Sometimes, family and friends stay close by during the physician's examination of the body. They may wish to see the body before it is removed to a **morgue** (a place where bodies are kept until burial arrangements have been made) or a funeral home. If the family is not present when the patient dies, they are notified of the death, usually by the nurse or physician. Long-term care facilities have procedures for family notification and for postmortem care. In a home care situation, notify your supervisor or the family, as instructed, and wait until the doctor or medical supervisor arrives.

If the family wishes to view the body, it will remain in the room until they arrive. In preparation, straighten the room and remove all extra equipment. Gather the patient's personal possessions and check them against an inventory list before releasing them to the family. Follow your facility's procedure.

Postmortem care is provided in the facility or in a funeral home. If you are providing postmortem care, the process will be similar to the steps described in Procedure 30-1.

Vital Skills (READING)

Reading Circle

A reading circle is a group of people who read a book and then meet to discuss it. Starting your own reading circle is a great way to gain practice as a reader and to get into the habit of reading. It can help you deal with issues that upset you or that you have questions about, such as death and dying.

Talking with members of your reading circle can help you see what you might be missing when you read. Others might pick up things from the book that you missed, and vice versa. Each member brings a unique perspective to the group. Hearing what other people think about a book—and sharing your thoughts—can help you better understand your feelings.

Participating in a reading circle can also be an enjoyable social experience. Many reading circles get together once a week to share books, food, ideas, and maybe some laughs.

Practice

With three or four classmates, set up a reading circle and choose a text to read. For your first reading selection, choose a book that relates to death and dying. Allow two weeks to read the book and then meet to discuss it. Below are some questions to get your discussion started:
- Who was your favorite character?
- Which character did you identify with most?
- Did this book change your thoughts about dying?

Vital Skills COMMUNICATION

Teaching Others

As a nursing assistant, you may be called on to teach a skill to others or to train a new employee. Effective teaching is not something that comes naturally to everyone, but you can learn to be an effective teacher with some practice. Keep these tips in mind when you teach.

- *Know what you are teaching.* If you aren't sure how to do something, it will be difficult for you to teach someone else to do it. Stick to teaching things you know about.
- *Be clear.* Outline the steps or objectives that you want to convey and stick to the outline.
- *Ask for feedback.* Ask the people you teach if they have any questions.

- *Be patient.* Remember that everyone learns at a different rate. Things that may seem easy to you might take others a bit longer to grasp.
- *Ask for suggestions.* Use constructive criticism to learn how to become a better teacher.

Practice

In groups of three or four, take turns being the teacher. Teach your classmates a skill of your choosing, being mindful of the tips given. Be sure to ask for their feedback so you can work on becoming a better teacher.

Procedure 30-1

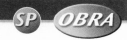

Providing Postmortem Care

Equipment: postmortem kit • washcloth and towels • warm water • disposable gloves • tape and dressings

1. Wash your hands.
2. Provide privacy. Work quietly.
3. Raise the bed to the highest comfortable level for working and make sure the bed is flat.
4. Put on gloves.
5. Position the body on its back.
6. Elevate the head and shoulders on a pillow.
7. Close the eyes by gently pulling the upper eyelid down over the eyeball. Put a moistened gauze pad on each eyelid if the eyes are being donated to an eye bank.
8. Replace dentures or artificial eyes, unless otherwise instructed.
9. Close the mouth.
10. If instructed, remove drainage bags, bottles, and containers. After checking with the nurse, remove tubes or catheters. The policy

on removal of these items varies, so make sure you have permission.
11. Remove and list jewelry except engagement and wedding rings (check the facility's procedure).
12. Bathe and dry soiled areas as needed.
13. Place a bed protector under the buttocks and put on clean dressings.
14. Groom hair.
15. Fill out the identification tags and attach one to the right ankle or right big toe.
16. Cover the body up to the shoulders if the family will view it.
17. Gather all possessions in a labeled bag.
18. Remove all equipment and supplies except the **shroud** (cloth used to wrap the body for burial) or disposable sheet and tags.
19. Remove gloves and wash your hands.

20. Make sure the room is neat and softly lit.
21. Provide privacy while the body is viewed. Allow the family as much time as needed. Give the family the person's possessions.
22. Get a stretcher.
23. Put on gloves.
24. Follow the procedures of the facility. Some facilities use a disposable sheet to cover the entire body. Others place the body on the shroud. If a shroud is used, follow Steps 25 through 29. If a disposable sheet is used, cover the body with the disposable sheet and skip to Step 30.
25. Place the body on the shroud. **See Figure 30-3.**
26. Bring the top down over the head. **See Figure 30-4.**
27. Fold the bottom up over the feet. **See Figure 30-5.**
28. Fold the sides over the body and secure the shroud. **See Figure 30-6.**

29. Apply an identification tag to the shroud.
30. With assistance from other workers, move the body to the stretcher.
31. If a funeral home or mortuary will pick up the body, wait until the family leaves. Then shut the patient's door and await arrival of personnel from the funeral home or mortuary.
32. If the body is to be transported to the morgue, transport it discreetly, making sure the doors to other patient rooms along the hallway are closed.
33. Return the stretcher to its proper location.
34. Remove all linens and supplies from the patient's room and place them in the soiled utility area.
35. Remove the gloves and wash your hands.
36. Report to the nurse the time the body was transported and what was done with the patient's personal belongings.

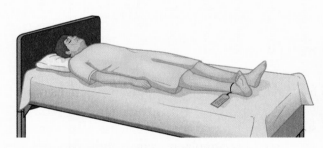

○ **Figure 30-3. Position the body on the shroud.**

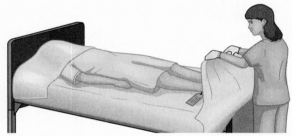

○ **Figure 30-5. Fold the shroud up over the person's feet.**

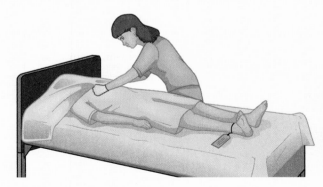

○ **Figure 30-4. Cover the head.**

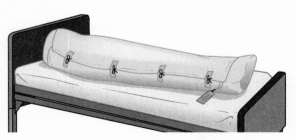

○ **Figure 30-6. Fold the sides over the body and secure the shroud.**

Chapter Summary

- Signs of approaching death include decreased circulation, decreased respiration, loss of muscle control, decreased organ function, and changes in mental state.

- Signs of death include lack of pulse, respiration, and blood pressure, and fixed, dilated eyes.

- When a patient dies, health care workers follow any advance directives, DNR/no-code orders, and organ donation instructions listed in the patient's medical record.

- Postmortem care maintains the body's appearance and prepares it for transport to the morgue or funeral home.

- Health care workers should be sensitive to family needs and emotions when a patient nears death and dies.

VOCABULARY REVIEW

Directions: Match the letter of each definition in the second column with the correct vocabulary term in the first column. Write your answers on a separate sheet of paper.

Vocabulary

1. death rattle
2. expires
3. morgue
4. mottled
5. no-code orders
6. organ donor
7. postmortem care
8. resuscitation
9. rigor mortis
10. shroud

Definitions

A. Dies
B. A place where bodies are kept until burial arrangements have been made
C. A cloth used to wrap a person's body for burial
D. A person who has agreed to donate tissue or organs to others when he or she dies
E. Lifesaving measures
F. A gurgle or rattle caused by accumulating mucus at the back of the throat of a dying person
G. Another term for DNR orders
H. The stiffening of a body 2 to 4 hours after death
I. Care after death
J. Having an irregular pattern of patches or spots of different colors

Check Your Knowledge

Review Questions: Answer each of the following questions on a separate sheet of paper.

1. What is your role when caring for a patient who is near death?

2. What should you do if you notice signs of approaching death?

3. What may happen to the skin of a person who is near death?

4. What is a death rattle?

5. How can you tell if the kidneys have begun to fail?

6. Name the four signs of death.

7. What is the name of the condition that occurs 2 to 4 hours after death, when the body begins to stiffen?

8. Where are bodies kept until burial arrangements can be made?

9. What should you do when providing postmortem care if a patient's eyes are being donated to an eye bank?

10. Briefly describe how to wrap a body in a shroud.

True or False: Read each statement carefully. Then write *True* or *False* by the statement number on a separate sheet of paper.

1. A person who is near death is always unconscious.

2. As blood circulation slows down in the dying patient, the patient's body temperature increases.

3. As a person's respiratory system fails, Cheyne-Stokes respirations may be observed.

4. You should keep the room of a dying patient as dark as possible.

5. If a patient dies without family present, it is the nursing assistant's duty to inform the family.

Think and Decide

Directions: Think about each of the following scenarios. Answer each question on a separate sheet of paper.

1. J.T. has terminal lung cancer. He has a living will and has named his son as power of attorney of durable health care. J.T. has specified that he be a DNR and his son agrees. What will the health care staff do when J.T. dies?

2. S.D. is a dying patient in your care. Her family has asked to be involved in S.D.'s care as she nears death. Why is this important? What should you do?

3. Mr. Young is a terminally ill patient in your care at a long-term care facility. When you enter his room this morning, you think that his breathing seems different. You listen carefully and hear a gurgling sound as he breathes. His skin seems cold, and his arms are mottled. What should you do?

4. You are working in an acute care unit at the hospital. A patient is brought in from the Emergency Department after having been involved in a serious motor vehicle accident. He had been riding a motorcycle without wearing a helmet, and he has severe head injuries. His condition worsens, and it becomes apparent that he is approaching death. His family is present; they keep asking again and again, "Why? Why did this happen to him?" What should you do?

5. A.K. is a terminally ill patient in your care. A.K.'s family has been notified that she has only a few days left, and they have been staying close to her. A family member approaches you in the hall and asks if there is anything you can do about the oxygen A.K. is receiving. He says the oxygen tube in her nose is making her nostrils dry and painful. What should you do?

6. You are caring for a hospital patient who was brought in unconscious and without identification. The patient is near death, but without knowing who he is, health care workers cannot notify his family. When he dies a few hours later, what procedures should be followed?

7. Mrs. B. is a terminally ill patient in your care at a long-term care facility. At 3:00 AM, she calls you into her room, which has been darkened to help her sleep. She says she is frightened. She explains that she "has a feeling" that she is near death. What can you do for Mrs. B.?

CNA Certification Exam Prep

Directions: This practice test contains ten questions. Each question has four suggested answers. For each question, choose the ONE that best answers the question or completes the statement. Write your answers on a separate sheet of paper.

1. One of the signs of approaching death is
   A. decreased circulation.
   B. increased respiratory rate.
   C. increased urinary output.
   D. lower body temperature.

2. Care given to a person after death is called
   A. antebellum care.
   B. antemortem care.
   C. postmortem care.
   D. postoperative care.

3. When a person begins losing muscle control,
   A. the mouth may hang open.
   B. the hair may begin to fall out.
   C. the muscles contract violently.
   D. dementia sets in.

4. A dying patient's urine output has decreased markedly in the last 12 hours. Which organ(s) may be shutting down?
   A. pancreas
   B. kidneys
   C. lungs
   D. liver

5. Where on an expired patient should you put the identification tag?
   A. on the right wrist or right forefinger
   B. on the left wrist or left forefinger
   C. on the left ankle or left big toe
   D. on the right ankle or right big toe

6. What can be used instead of a shroud?
   A. disposable sheet
   B. pillowcase
   C. bed protector
   D. warm blanket

7. Which of the following is a sign of death?
   A. Cheyne-Stokes respiration
   B. profuse sweating
   C. decreased heart rate
   D. no blood pressure

8. Do not resuscitate a patient with a(n)
   A. out-of-state license.
   B. PRN order for pain medication.
   C. no-code order.
   D. organ donation card.

9. Rigor mortis occurs
   A. 1 to 2 hours before death.
   B. 2 to 4 hours after death.
   C. 6 to 8 hours after death.
   D. 10 to 12 hours after death.

10. If a funeral home is to pick up a deceased patient from a long-term care facility, the nursing assistant should
    A. stay with the body until the funeral home personnel arrive.
    B. close the patient's door and leave the body alone.
    C. transport the body promptly to the facility entry.
    D. transport the body to the morgue for temporary storage.

Glossary

A

abandonment. Ending help or support without providing notice or getting the client's consent; leaving without notice. (Ch. 25)

abbreviation. A shortened form of a word or phrase. (Ch. 12)

ABC Class fire extinguisher. An extinguisher used for all types of fires. (Ch. 6)

abdominal distension. Abnormal swelling of the abdomen. (Ch. 19)

abuse. The willful mistreatment of someone. (Ch. 4)

acquired immunodeficiency syndrome (AIDS). A syndrome caused by the human immunodeficiency virus that attacks the immune system and affects the body's ability to fight other diseases. (Ch. 23)

acronym. An abbreviation made up of the first letters of each word in a phrase. (Ch. 12)

active listening. A listening technique that consists of restatement, reflection, and clarification. (Ch. 13)

activities of daily living (ADLs). The physical tasks necessary to maintain oneself. They include eating, self-care, grooming, dressing, and mobility. (Ch. 5)

ADLs (activities of daily living). The physical tasks necessary to maintain oneself. They include eating, self-care, grooming, dressing, and mobility. (Ch. 5)

admission. The official entry of a person into a health care facility. (Ch. 15)

admissions checklist. A standard form a health care facility uses for initial impressions and a baseline assessment of a new patient. (Ch. 15)

adult day-care center. A facility that provides care for adult (usually elderly) clients during the day. (Ch. 2)

advance directive. A legal document that specifies how medical decisions should be made in the future if a person becomes unable to make them. (Ch. 4)

AED (automated external defibrillator). An automatic, portable device that is used to deliver an electric shock to someone in cardiac arrest. (Ch. 17)

aerosol therapy. Moisture and/or medication inhaled into the lungs. (Ch. 6)

agitation. A state of extreme restlessness. (Ch. 27)

AIDS (acquired immunodeficiency syndrome). A syndrome caused by the human immunodeficiency virus that attacks the immune system and affects the body's ability to fight other diseases. (Ch. 23)

All Class fire extinguisher. An extinguisher used for all types of fires. (Ch. 6)

alveoli. Tiny air sacs in the lungs. (Ch. 9)

Alzheimer's disease. A degenerative disorder of the brain that affects thinking, memory, judgment, and speech. (Ch. 9) A progressive, irreversible mental disorder accompanied by the gradual loss of intellectual and physical abilities. (Ch. 27)

ambulate. Walk or move around freely without being restricted to a bed or wheelchair. (Ch. 24)

ambulatory. Able to walk with or without the help of a walking aid. (Ch. 6)

ambulatory surgery. Surgery that does not require a hospital stay. (Ch. 20)

Americans with Disabilities Act. A federal law that requires a specific level of health care access for people who have a physical or mental impairment that substantially limits their ability to care for themselves. (Ch. 26)

anal incontinence. The inability to control the passing of feces or gas. (Ch. 19)

anatomical plane. An imaginary flat surface that separates two sections of the body or of an organ. (Ch. 9)

anatomical position. The position of the body used in anatomical descriptions: standing upright, facing forward, arms at the side, palms facing forward, feet slightly apart. (Ch. 9)

anatomy. The basic structures of the human body. (Ch. 10)

anesthesia. The loss of sensation or the ability to feel pain. (Ch. 20)

anesthetic. A drug or an agent given to patients to produce a loss of sensation. (Ch. 20)

angina pectoris. Severe pain or pressure in the chest caused by reduced blood flow and an inadequate oxygen supply to the heart muscle. (Ch. 23)

anorexia. Abnormal loss of appetite. (Ch. 26)

antibodies. Specialized proteins that fight disease. (Ch. 10)

antiembolic stockings. Stockings made of elastic fabric that provide support, promote blood flow, and prevent the formation of blood clots. (Ch. 18)

antisepsis. Using chemicals to kill pathogens or to stop their growth. (Ch. 11)

anxiety. A feeling of dread or discomfort that occurs without a specific reason. (Ch. 27)

aphasia. The inability or impaired ability to communicate through speech, writing, or signs. (Ch. 23)

apical pulse. The pulse felt over the apex of the heart. The apex is the tip of the heart. It is located just below the left nipple. (Ch. 7)

apical-radial pulse. Measurement of the apical and radial pulse at the same time. (Ch. 7)

apnea. The lack of respirations. (Ch. 7)

appetite. The desire for food. (Ch. 26)

application form. A questionnaire filled out by a job applicant that summarizes the person's qualifications. (Ch. 3)

aquamatic pad. An electric heating pad containing tubes filled with circulating water. (Ch. 18)

artery. A blood vessel that carries blood away from the heart. (Ch. 10)

asepsis. The condition of being free of pathogens. (Ch. 11)

aspiration. The breathing in or leaking of fluids (such as vomit) into the lung. (Ch. 26)

assault. The attempt or threat to touch another person's body without the person's consent. (Ch. 4)

assessment. The process of observing for mental or psychological changes in patients. (Ch. 27)

assisted-living facility. A residential complex, usually for the elderly or people with disabilities, where residents live in their own units but where health care services are provided as necessary. (Ch. 2)

asthma. A respiratory disease caused by narrowing and inflammation of the airways in response to triggers. (Ch. 23)

atelectasis. The collapse of a lung or part of a lung; one of the possible complications of surgery. (Ch. 20)

atherosclerosis. A condition in which fat deposits build up on the inner walls of blood vessels. (Ch. 23)

atria. The two upper chambers of the heart. (Ch. 9)

atrophic skin. Skin that has become thinner, fragile, and less elastic due to aging. (Ch. 22)

autoclave. A pressurized steam sterilizer. (Ch. 11)

automated external defibrillator (AED). An automatic, portable device that is used to deliver an electric shock to someone in cardiac arrest. (Ch. 17)

autonomy. Independence and the freedom to make one's own decisions about health care and other life issues. (Ch. 24)

B

basic life support. The series of actions taken to maintain life in an emergency. (Ch. 17)

bath blanket. A lightweight blanket used to provide warmth and privacy when changing the bed while the patient is in it and when the patient is bathing or using the bedpan. (Ch. 14)

battery. Touching another person's body without the person's consent. (Ch. 4)

bed cradle. A device or frame placed on the bed at the resident's feet to keep pressure from the top linens off the feet. (Ch. 24)

bed pad. An absorbent pad placed between the bottom sheet and the patient to protect the linen from becoming wet or soiled. (Ch. 14)

bedpan. A plastic container used by patients who are bedridden to urinate or defecate. (Ch. 19)

bed rest. Confined to bed by a doctor's order. (Ch. 24)

bedridden. Confined to bed. (Ch. 16)

bioethics. The study of the ethical questions and problems associated with medical research and delivery of health care. (Ch. 2)

bloodborne pathogen. A disease-causing organism found in blood or other body fluids. (Ch. 11)

blood pressure. A measure of the force of the blood flow against artery walls. (Ch. 7)

body alignment. The proper positioning of the head, back, and limbs in a straight line. (Ch. 16)

body fluids. The body's secretions: sputum, semen, mucus, vaginal excretions, urine, feces, blood, saliva, tears, vomit, sweat, cerebrospinal fluid, amniotic fluid, breast milk, and excretions from wounds. (Ch. 11)

body language. All of the mannerisms and gestures used in communication. (Ch. 13)

body mechanics. The positions and movements that help the body maintain proper posture and prevent injury. (Ch. 16)

body support. A brace that supports the back when worn properly to perform lifting, moving, or transferring tasks. (Ch. 16)

body temperature. An indicator of the amount of heat in the body. The body temperature equals the amount of heat produced by the body less the amount of heat lost by the body. (Ch. 7)

bradycardia. A slow heart rate; fewer than 60 pulse beats per minute. (Ch. 7)

bradypnea. Slow breathing; fewer than 12 breaths per minute. (Ch. 7)

brainstem. The portion of the brain that houses the control centers for the body's involuntary activities, such as respiration and heartbeat. (Ch. 9)

breastfeeding. The natural feeding of the mother's milk to an infant. (Ch. 28)

C

call signal. A one-way communication device that must be kept within the patient's easy reach. The signal goes off at a main terminal. (Ch. 13)

cancer. A malignant (harmful), uncontrolled growth of abnormal cells. Cancer generally invades healthy tissue and stops normal body functioning. (Ch. 23)

capillary. Small blood vessel that connects the ends of arterioles with venules. (Ch. 10)

carbohydrate. An organic chemical that is the body's primary source of energy. (Ch. 26)

cardiac arrest. The condition that occurs when the heart and breathing suddenly stop. (Ch. 17)

cardiopulmonary resuscitation (CPR). A form of basic life support that includes activation of EMS and procedures that support both breathing and circulation. (Ch. 17)

career portfolio. A collection of educational and professional achievements. (Ch. 3)

caregiver. A person who provides direct care for someone who is in need. (Ch. 1)

case manager. The supervising nurse in a home health care agency who plans and oversees the care of the client and provides assignments to the home health aide. (Ch. 25)

catheter. A tube used to drain fluid into or out of the body. (Ch. 19)

cavity. A space within the body. (Ch. 9)

CDC (Centers for Disease Control and Prevention). A division of the U.S. Department of Health and Human Services (HHS) that works to protect the public health. (Ch. 11)

cell. The simplest living unit of the body structure. (Ch. 9)

Centers for Disease Control and Prevention (CDC). A division of the U.S. Department of Health and Human Services (HHS) that works to protect the public health. (Ch. 11)

cerebellum. The part of the brain that coordinates activities of the muscles and helps maintain balance. (Ch. 9)

cerebrovascular accident (CVA). A sudden interruption in the blood supply to the brain; a stroke. (Ch. 23)

cerebrum. The largest section of the brain. It is responsible for intelligence and thought. (Ch. 9)

cesarean section (c-section). The delivery of a fetus by a surgical incision into the uterus through the abdomen. (Ch. 28)

chain of command. A "ladder" of responsibility that defines who can assign tasks to whom in an organization. (Ch. 1)

chain of infection. The series of six conditions that together produce infection. (Ch. 11)

charge nurse. A nurse who supervises other nurses or who is in charge of a department. (Ch. 1)

charting. The process of writing down the observations you make and the treatments and procedures you perform. (Ch. 13)

chemical restraints. Medications given to decrease activity and control behavior. (Ch. 6)

chemotherapy. A therapy that uses drugs to destroy or slow the growth of cancer cells. (Ch. 23)

Cheyne-Stokes breathing. A pattern of breathing in which a series of very deep breaths is followed by very short, shallow breaths. (Ch. 7)

CHF (congestive heart failure). The heart's inability to pump effectively, which can result in a buildup of excess fluid in the lungs. (Ch. 23, Ch. 26)

chronic. Lasting a long time (as of an illness or condition). (Ch. 23)

chronic bronchitis. Inflammation in the lungs, with increased mucus production and a chronic productive cough that is present for at least three months in two successive years. (Ch. 23)

chronic obstructive pulmonary disease (COPD). A group of chronic, progressive lung diseases characterized by airway obstruction and a loss of elasticity of the lungs. (Ch. 23)

circumcision. The surgical removal of the foreskin on a boy's penis. (Ch. 28)

Class A fire extinguisher. An extinguisher used for fires involving combustibles. (Ch. 6)

Class B fire extinguisher. An extinguisher used for fires involving grease. (Ch. 6)

Class C fire extinguisher. An extinguisher for electrical fires and flammable gases. (Ch. 6)

client. A person receiving service from a health care provider. (Ch. 2)

client care record. A record of all the care given to a home health care client. (Ch. 25)

clinic. A facility for the diagnosis and treatment of outpatients. (Ch. 2)

closed bed. A bed in a health care facility that is not currently in use. (Ch. 14)

coercion. An attempt to force someone to do something against his or her will. (Ch. 4)

cold compress. A cold folded and moistened cloth or towel that is placed over a small area of the body for cold moist therapy. (Ch. 18)

cold pack. A dry cold treatment that is applied or wrapped around an area of the body. (Ch. 18)

colostomy. An artificial opening from the colon (large intestine) to the abdominal wall. (Ch. 19)

colostrum. A thick, yellow fluid secreted from the mother's breast for the first few days after delivery that supplies babies with important antibodies. (Ch. 28)

combining form. A word part plus a vowel to make the word easier to pronounce. (Ch. 12)

communication. The exchange of information. (Ch. 13)

condom catheter. An external drainage catheter with a rubber sheath that is placed over the penis and attached to a drainage bag to assist urination. (Ch. 19)

confidentiality. Keeping information about a patient private. (Ch. 4)

confusion. A mental state in which the patient is unaware of time, the environment, or the self. (Ch. 27)

congestive heart failure (CHF). The heart's inability to pump effectively, which can result in a buildup of excess fluid in the lungs. (Ch. 23, Ch. 26)

conscientiousness. Being careful, thorough, and accurate when you complete assignments. (Ch. 1)

constipation. Difficulty in fecal elimination. (Ch. 19)

constrict. To narrow. (Ch. 10)

continuing education. Programs for adult learners at high schools, colleges, and universities. (Ch. 3)

continuum of care. A system that provides health care for people throughout their life span. (Ch. 2)

COPD (chronic obstructive pulmonary disease). A group of chronic, progressive lung diseases characterized by airway obstruction and a loss of elasticity of the lungs. (Ch. 23)

cover letter. A short letter that introduces you to an employer. It explains why you are sending your résumé and why you are the right person for the job. (Ch. 3)

CPR (cardiopulmonary resuscitation). A form of basic life support that includes activation of EMS and procedures that support both breathing and circulation. (Ch. 17)

croupette. A small portable oxygen device that resembles a tent, used for infants and young children. (Ch. 6)

culture. The accumulation of customs, values, and beliefs shared by a people. (Ch. 5)

CVA (cerebrovascular accident). A sudden interruption in the blood supply to the brain; a stroke. (Ch. 23)

cyanosis. A bluish discoloration or darkening of the skin, eyelids, lips, or fingernails caused by insufficient oxygen in the blood. (Ch. 18)

D

dandruff. White flakes on the hair and scalp accompanied by itching. (Ch. 22)

dangle. To sit up and allow the legs to hang loosely over the side of the bed for a short while. (Ch. 16)

data. Information entered and stored in a computer. (Ch. 13)

death rattle. A gurgle or rattle caused by accumulating mucus at the back of the throat of a dying patient. (Ch. 30)

decubitus ulcer. An area of the skin that has broken down because of constant pressure or friction. Also called *bedsore, pressure sore,* or *pressure ulcer.* (Ch. 22)

defecation. The passing of feces from the body. (Ch. 19)

defense mechanisms. Unconscious ways of protecting the self from bad feelings, such as shame, anxiety, fear, or loss of self-esteem. (Ch. 5)

defibrillation. The delivery of an electric shock to a patient's chest to re-establish the heart rhythm. (Ch. 17)

dehydration. A decrease in the amount of water in body tissues occurring when fluid output exceeds fluid input. It can be dangerous when the body does not have the amount of fluid it needs to function. (Ch. 26)

delegation. The process of assigning tasks to other trained or qualified people. (Ch. 1)

delirium. The acute, temporary mental state characterized by rambling or incoherent speech, a change in level of consciousness, confusion, extreme agitation and restlessness, or hallucinations; acute confusion. (Ch. 27)

delusion. A false belief about oneself or others or about events. (Ch. 27)

dementia. An irreversible, progressive loss in mental function, usually due to damage or disease of the brain; chronic confusion. (Ch. 27)

dentifrice. An oral cleaning agent, such as a paste, gel, powder, or liquid. (Ch. 22)

dentures. False teeth. (Ch. 22)

depression. A mood disorder marked by extreme sadness and hopelessness. (Ch. 27)

dermatitis. An irritation or inflammation usually seen as an itchy, red rash. (Ch. 22)

dermis. The inner layer of the skin. (Ch. 9)

development. The process of acquiring motor (movement) skills, language skills, social skills, and cognitive (learning) skills. (Ch. 8)

developmental tasks. The set of tasks that must be accomplished to complete a stage of development. (Ch. 8)

diabetes mellitus. A disease of the pancreas caused by destruction or damage to the islet cells. (Ch. 9)

diarrhea. The passage of frequent watery stools. (Ch. 19)

diastole. The period during which the heart muscle relaxes; the heart is at rest. (Ch. 7)

diastolic pressure. A measure of the pressure in the arteries between beats, when the heart is at rest. (Ch. 7)

digestion. The process of breaking down foods into usable nutrients, absorbing nutrients, and excreting waste products. (Ch. 10)

dilate. To expand. (Ch. 10)

directional terms. Words used to describe a body location or direction. (Ch. 9)

disability. An impairment of function. (Ch. 21)

disaster. A sudden event that injures many people and causes major damage. (Ch. 6)

discharge. A patient's authorized release from a health care facility. (Ch. 15)

discharge instructions. Written documents that outline the information the patient needs about ongoing care. (Ch. 15)

discharge interview. A meeting of the patient, family members, caregivers, and other interested parties with the nurse to learn how to continue the healing process and provide patient care. (Ch. 15)

discharge plan. A plan that outlines ongoing patient care following discharge. (Ch. 15)

discrimination. Treating a patient unfairly because of race, religion, sex, ethnic origin, age, or physical disability. (Ch. 4)

disinfection. A cleaning process that uses strong chemicals to kill most pathogens. (Ch. 11)

disorientation. A mental state in which the patient is confused and unaware of surroundings. (Ch. 27)

domestic violence. The act of physically injuring, or causing to be injured, a family member or someone else who lives in the home. (Ch. 25)

do not resuscitate (DNR) form. A medical treatment order that tells health care providers not to use cardiopulmonary resuscitation (CPR) on a person if the person's heart or breathing stops. (Ch. 4)

dorsal. The back of the body. (Ch. 9)

dorsal recumbent position. The patient is positioned lying flat on the back with the legs close together, the knees flexed, and the soles of the feet flat on the mattress. (Ch. 16)

draping. Covering part or all of a patient's body with a sheet, blanket, or other material. (Ch. 16)

draw sheet. A small sheet placed over the middle of the bottom sheet to help lift and move a person up in bed. (Ch. 14)

dyspnea. Difficult, labored, or painful breathing. (Ch. 7)

E

edema. An increase in fluid in body tissues that occurs when fluid input exceeds fluid output. It appears as swelling and can result in life-threatening complications. (Ch. 26)

ejaculation. The expelling of semen from the body. (Ch. 8)

elastic bandage. A long strip of stretchy material that provides support and protection to extremities and joints. (Ch. 18)

elderly. A broad term that describes people in the later years of their lives. (Ch. 24)

elimination. The excretion or removal of waste from the body. (Ch. 19)

embolism. An obstruction in a blood vessel caused by an embolus. (Ch. 20)

embolus. A blood clot or other matter that has broken away and travels through the bloodstream. (Ch. 20)

emergency. An event calling for immediate action. (Ch. 6, Ch. 17)

emergency medical services (EMS). A community network of equipment, facilities, and specially trained personnel set up to provide treatment and care during emergencies. (Ch. 17)

emesis. Vomit. (Ch. 26)

emotional well-being. A state of feeling contented and happy. (Ch. 5)

empathy. Being able to understand or imagine how it would feel to be in someone else's situation. (Ch. 1)

emphysema. A condition in which the air spaces in the lungs become enlarged and overinflated, resulting in the loss of elasticity. (Ch. 23)

EMS (emergency medical services). A community network of equipment, facilities, and specially trained personnel set up to provide treatment and care during emergencies. (Ch. 17)

enema. A liquid solution placed into the rectum to loosen stools and to remove feces. (Ch. 19)

entrepreneur. A person who plans, organizes, and then runs a business. (Ch. 3)

epidermis. The outer layer of the skin. (Ch. 9)

epilepsy. A disease in which a person has recurrent seizures. (Ch. 17)

episiotomy. A small incision of the perineum made during delivery to avoid tearing of the tissue and to ease the baby's passage. (Ch. 28)

esteem needs. Those needs that must be met to have a feeling of self-worth. (Ch. 5)

ethical standards. The set of rules for proper personal and professional conduct. (Ch. 4)

excoriations. Surface skin problems, such as scratches or scrapes. (Ch. 22)

expires. Dies. (Ch. 30)

exploitation. Taking advantage of someone financially, physically, or in any other manner. (Ch. 4)

external bleeding. Loss of blood on the outer surface of the body. (Ch. 17)

F

face mask. An oxygen delivery device that covers the nose and mouth. (Ch. 6)

fanfold. Turn back (bed linens) in an accordion fashion. (Ch. 14)

fat. An organic compound that provides the body with stored energy and helps the body use certain vitamins. (Ch. 26)

FBAO (foreign body airway obstruction). The prevention of air from entering the lungs caused by a foreign object caught in the throat. (Ch. 17)

fecal impaction. A collection of hardened feces in the intestines. (Ch. 19)

fecal occult blood test (FOBT). A test used to detect the presence of hidden (occult) blood in the stool. (Ch. 19)

feces. The waste material from the large intestine, or bowel. (Ch. 19)

feedback. The response to a communication message. (Ch. 13)

fire blanket. A blanket made of strong material that does not burn easily. Used to smother small fires and sometimes to transport patients. (Ch. 6)

first aid. The first care given to an injured or ill person in an emergency before medical help arrives. (Ch. 17)

flatulence. The excessive creation and buildup of gas in the stomach and intestines. (Ch. 19)

flow sheet. A chart in the medical record used to record different types of data. (Ch. 13)

FOBT (fecal occult blood test). A test used to detect the presence of hidden (occult) blood in the stool. (Ch. 19)

foot board. A device placed at the foot of a resident's mattress to prevent the plantar flexion that leads to foot drop. (Ch. 24)

foot drop. A condition in which the foot falls down, or droops, at the ankle. (Ch. 24)

foreign body airway obstruction (FBAO). The prevention of air from entering the lungs caused by a foreign object caught in the throat. (Ch. 17)

formula. A milk mixture enhanced with extra nutrients to make it as close in content to breast milk as possible. (Ch. 28)

Fowler's position. A semisitting position with the head of the bed raised between a 45° and 60° angle and the knees slightly flexed. (Ch. 16)

fracture. A broken bone. (Ch. 21)

fracture pan. A type of bedpan used by patients who are unable to raise their hips high enough to sit on a regular bedpan. (Ch. 19)

friction. A force caused by the rubbing of one surface against another. (Ch. 16)

G

gangrene. The death of tissue, usually caused by poor blood circulation. (Ch. 23)

gas exchange. The process of moving oxygen into the blood and removing carbon dioxide from the blood. (Ch. 10)

gastrostomy tube. A tube inserted surgically through the abdomen and into the stomach for feeding. (Ch. 26)

generalized seizure. Convulsions that involve all or part of the body and are characterized by a loss of consciousness. (Ch. 17)

geriatrics. A health care specialty that meets the health care needs of elderly people. (Ch. 24)

glands. Organs that create chemicals needed for proper body functioning. (Ch. 10)

graduate. A transparent container with a numerical scale marked on the side for the measurement of fluids. (Ch. 26)

graphic chart. A chart in the medical record used to record observations and measurements. (Ch. 13)

grievance. A formal complaint. (Ch. 4)

grooming. Making the appearance neat. (Ch. 22)

group home. A small facility that serves as a residence for several people with long-term physical or mental disabilities. (Ch. 2)

growth. The process of changing physically in ways that can be measured. (Ch. 8)

H

halitosis. Bad breath. (Ch. 22)

hallucination. A false perception of reality that may include hearing voices or seeing objects or people that do not exist. (Ch. 27)

hand rail. A rail that is placed along a hallway, in a bathroom, or in a stairway to steady ambulatory patients and prevent falls. (Ch. 6)

harassment. Troubling, tormenting, offending, or worrying a person by one's behavior or speech. (Ch. 4)

hazardous material. Any agent that has the potential to cause harm. (Ch. 6)

head nurse. The nurse who supervises the nurses and nursing assistants on each shift. (Ch. 1)

health. A state of complete physical, mental, emotional, and social well-being. (Ch. 5)

health care proxy. A legal document appointing someone, often a friend or family member, to make health care decisions on your behalf. (Ch. 4)

health care team. Everyone involved in making and carrying out health care decisions. The patient is the center of the health care team. (Ch. 1)

Health Insurance Portability and Accountability Act (HIPAA). A federal regulation protecting the security of medical records and patients' privacy. (Ch. 2)

heat exhaustion. A condition caused by prolonged exposure to heat over hours to days that results in a slightly elevated body temperature and signs of dehydration. (Ch. 17)

heat stroke. A severe and possibly fatal condition caused by exposure to extreme heat and characterized by confusion and high fever. (Ch. 17)

Heimlich maneuver. A first-aid procedure for dislodging an item that is causing a person to choke. (Ch. 17)

hemiparesis. Paralysis or numbness on only one side of the body. (Ch. 22)

hemoglobin. An iron-containing protein in red blood cells that carries oxygen and gives blood its red color. (Ch. 10)

hemorrhage. The sudden and extreme loss of blood. (Ch. 17)

hemorrhoids. Distended veins surrounding the rectum. (Ch. 19)

hemostasis. The prevention of blood loss. (Ch. 10)

hepatitis. An inflammatory disease of the liver caused by a virus. (Ch. 9)

HIPAA (Health Insurance Portability and Accountability Act). A federal regulation protecting the security of medical records and patients' privacy. (Ch. 2)

HIV (human immunodeficiency virus). A virus that is transmitted through blood and body fluid contact and causes AIDS. (Ch. 23)

home health aide. A person who provides basic personal care and health-related services for a client in the client's home. (Ch. 2, Ch. 25)

homeostasis. The body's state of good health and stability in the face of constant change. (Ch. 9)

horizontal recumbent position. The patient is positioned lying flat on the back with the legs close together. (Ch. 16)

hormone. Chemical substance that regulates and controls the activities of cells. (Ch. 10)

hospice. A facility or a program that provides physical and emotional care and support for terminally ill patients and their families. (Ch. 2, Ch. 29)

hospital. A facility that provides medical or surgical care to sick or injured people who stay overnight or longer. Many hospitals also provide outpatient services. (Ch. 2)

host. A person who harbors pathogens. (Ch. 11)

human immunodeficiency virus (HIV). A virus that is transmitted through blood and body fluid contact and causes AIDS. (Ch. 23)

hygiene. A condition of cleanliness and health. (Ch. 1, Ch. 22)

hyperglycemia. A condition that occurs when the blood glucose level is abnormally high. (Ch. 23)

hypertension. Abnormally high blood pressure. (Ch. 7)

hyperthermia. A dangerous condition in which body temperature is elevated above the normal range. (Ch. 17)

hypoglycemia. A condition that occurs when the blood glucose level is abnormally low. (Ch. 23)

hypotension. Abnormally low blood pressure. (Ch. 7)

hypothermia. A condition in which the core body temperature drops below 95° F (35° C) caused by prolonged exposure to the cold. (Ch. 17)

I

identity. An individual's uniqueness and sense of self. (Ch. 8)

ileostomy. An artificial opening between the small intestine and the abdominal wall. (Ch. 19)

illness. Sickness, disease, or an ailment. (Ch. 5)

immobilize. To restrict movement. (Ch. 21)

immunity. The body's resistance to a particular disease. (Ch. 11)

immunization. The process of providing protection against specific communicable diseases. (Ch. 8)

incentive spirometer. A device used to promote and measure maximum effort of deep breathing to prevent atelectasis. (Ch. 20)

incident. An accident, error, or unusual event. (Ch. 6)

incident report. A form used to report accidents, errors, or unusual events. (Ch. 6)

indwelling catheter. A catheter that is left in the bladder over a period of time to continuously drain urine. (Ch. 19)

infection. A disease caused by a group of pathogenic microorganisms that invade and multiply within the body. (Ch. 11)

infectious diseases. Diseases that are transmitted from one person to another through the chain of infection. (Ch. 11)

inflammatory response. The body's built-in defense mechanism. (Ch. 11)

informed consent. A patient's understanding and agreement to an action or procedure that has been explained. (Ch. 4)

insulin. A hormone produced by the pancreas that the body uses to convert glucose into energy. (Ch. 23)

intake. A measure of all liquids a patient takes in. (Ch. 26)

intentional tort. Causing harm or injury to a person or property on purpose. (Ch. 4)

intercom. A two-way device in a patient's room that permits patients to talk and to listen to a health care worker at a main terminal. (Ch. 13)

intermittent pneumatic compression device. A device that is wrapped around the legs and connected to a pump that inflates and deflates to promote circulation and help prevent blood clots. (Ch. 20)

internal bleeding. Loss of blood inside the body or under the skin from an organ, blood vessels, or other internal tissues. (Ch. 17)

intravenous (IV) nutrition therapy. The continuous infusion of fluid and nutrients through a needle inserted into a vein. (Ch. 26)

invasion of privacy. A violation of law that occurs when a patient is not protected from unwanted visitors or from unwanted release of confidential information. (Ch. 4)

islet cells. Cells that produce and secrete the hormone insulin in the pancreas. (Ch. 9)

isolation precautions. Guidelines to follow to prevent the spread of infectious diseases. (Ch. 11)

J

JCAHO (Joint Commission on Accreditation of Healthcare Organizations). An independent, not-for-profit organization that sets the standards by which health care quality is measured. (Ch. 2)

job interview. A formal meeting between a job candidate and an employer. (Ch. 3)

job shadowing. Following another employee on the job to learn the routine. (Ch. 3)

Joint Commission on Accreditation of Healthcare Organizations (JCAHO). An independent, not-for-profit organization that sets the standards by which health care quality is measured. (Ch. 2)

K

kidney dialysis. A process in which a machine is attached to a patient's circulatory system, by a catheter or some other device, to remove waste products from the blood. (Ch. 23)

kidney (renal) failure. A chronic condition that involves gradual, progressive, and irreversible damage to the kidneys. (Ch. 23)

knee-chest. The patient lies face down with knees flexed at a 90° angle and the chest touching the bed or table. (Ch. 16)

L

labor. The process that begins with uterine contractions and ends with delivery of the baby. (Ch. 28)

lateral. The patient is lying on his or her side. (Ch. 16)

legal rights. The rights of all people under the law. (Ch. 4)

lesion. A break in the skin or mucous membranes. (Ch. 22)

letdown reflex. The automatic release of breast milk in response to the presence of milk in the breasts. (Ch. 28)

liability. Legal responsibility for what someone does or fails to do. (Ch. 4)

licensed practical nurse (LPN). A nurse who has completed a one- to two-year training program and has passed a state licensing exam. LPNs work under the supervision of an RN, a doctor, or a dentist. (Ch. 1)

licensed vocational nurse (LVN). A nurse who has completed a practical nursing program taught either in public vocational high schools or other state-approved programs. LVNs work under the supervision of an RN, a doctor, or a dentist. (Ch. 1)

living will. A legal document stating how a person wishes to be treated in the event of serious or catastrophic illness. (Ch. 4)

lochia. The normal discharge from the uterus after childbirth. (Ch. 28)

log-in. The unique ID a person uses to access a secure computer system. (Ch. 13)

logrolling. A method for turning the patient onto the side in one movement to keep the spine aligned. (Ch. 16)

long-term care facility. A residential facility that provides care for people with chronic disorders or disabilities who need assistance with daily care. (Ch. 2)

M

malpractice. The act or conduct of a trained health care provider that does not meet established standards or that goes beyond the provider's skill or scope of practice and results in harm. (Ch. 4)

material safety data sheet (MSDS). A document that provides information about the potential hazards associated with a particular substance. (Ch. 6)

mechanical lift. A lifting device that assists in raising, lowering, and transferring patients. (Ch. 16)

Medicaid. Federal and state health care funding for people who meet certain guidelines. (Ch. 2)

medical asepsis. The practice of minimizing or reducing the spread of pathogens. (Ch. 11)

medical record. A written or computerized record documenting a patient's care, condition, treatment, and response to treatment. (Ch. 13)

medical terminology. The specialized language used by the health care professions. (Ch. 12)

Medicare. Federal health care funding for people over age 65 and for people under 65 with certain disabilities. (Ch. 2)

medium. The way or means in which information is sent or received. (Ch. 13)

menarche. The first menstrual period and the beginning of puberty in girls. (Ch. 8)

menopause. The natural stopping of menstruation that marks the end of the childbearing stage. (Ch. 8)

menstruation. The cyclic process of the blood and tissue lining the uterus being discharged through the vagina. (Ch. 10)

mental disorder. A condition in which a person's thoughts interfere with normal daily functioning and a sense of well-being. (Ch. 27)

mental health. A state of well-being of the mind and the emotions. (Ch. 27)

mental retardation. A slowness or limitation of intellectual ability. (Ch. 27)

message. The information a sender wants to convey. (Ch. 13)

microorganism. A living plant or animal that is too small to be seen without magnification. (Ch. 11)

minerals. Inorganic chemicals that are essential to many body processes and functions. (Ch. 26)

mitered corner. A corner of bed linens that is angled and tucked to lie flat against the mattress. (Ch. 14)

morgue. A place where bodies are kept until burial arrangements have been made. (Ch. 30)

mottled. Having an irregular pattern of patches or spots of different colors. (Ch. 30)

MS (multiple sclerosis). A progressive disease of the nervous system that affects how nerve impulses are sent to and from the brain. (Ch. 23)

MSDS (material safety data sheet). A document that provides information about the potential hazards associated with a particular substance. (Ch. 6)

multiple sclerosis (MS). A progressive disease of the nervous system that affects how nerve impulses are sent to and from the brain. (Ch. 23)

muscle atrophy. A condition in which the muscles decrease in size and waste away from lack of use. (Ch. 24)

muscle contracture. Deep, painful tightening and shortening of the muscles that cannot easily be relieved. (Ch. 24)

myocardial infarction. An event in which the blood supply to the myocardium—the heart muscle—is reduced or completely stopped. Also called *heart attack.* (Ch. 9)

N

nasal cannula. An oxygen delivery device made of plastic tubing with two prongs that are inserted into the nostrils. (Ch. 6)

nasal catheter. An oxygen delivery device made of a small plastic or rubber tube that is inserted into a patient's nose. (Ch. 6)

nasogastric tube. A tube inserted through the nose and into the stomach that can be used for feeding. (Ch. 26)

need. Anything that is necessary to maintain life and well-being. (Ch. 5)

negligence. The failure of a trained health care provider to perform in a reasonable, careful manner and according to established standards, which results in unintentionally causing harm. (Ch. 4)

neonate. A newborn baby in the first 4 weeks after birth. (Ch. 8)

networking. Communicating with people you know to share information. (Ch. 3)

no-code orders. Another term for DNR (do not resuscitate) orders. (Ch. 30)

noninfectious disease. A disease that cannot be transmitted from one person to another. (Ch. 11)

nonpathogen. A microorganism that does not cause disease or infection. (Ch. 11)

nonverbal communication. All forms of communication except words. (Ch. 13)

nosocomial infection. An infection that a patient acquires while in a health care facility. (Ch. 11)

nothing by mouth (NPO). A doctor's order meaning that the patient cannot eat or drink anything by mouth. NPO stands for the Latin term *nil per os*, which means "nothing by mouth." (Ch. 26)

NPO (nothing by mouth). A doctor's order meaning that the patient cannot eat or drink anything by mouth. NPO stands for the Latin term *nil per os*, which means "nothing by mouth." (Ch. 26)

nurses' notes. Nurses' written documentation about a patient's condition. (Ch. 13)

nursing assistant. A person who is trained and state-approved to give basic personal care to patients in a health care facility, especially one that provides long-term care. (Ch. 1)

nursing care plan. A document that details the care required for a patient. Nursing care plans are developed by the health care team and coordinated by a nurse. (Ch. 13)

nutrient. A chemical substance that enables the body to grow and heal itself. (Ch. 26)

nutrition. The process of taking food and fluids into the body for growth, healing, and maintenance of body functions. (Ch. 26)

O

objective information. Information you collect about a patient using your senses. (Ch. 13)

objectivity. The ability to see and accept facts or conditions as they are, without a personal interpretation or bias. (Ch. 1)

OBRA (Omnibus Budget Reconciliation Act of 1987). A congressional act that established the minimum federal requirements for nursing assistants working in long-term care facilities. (Ch. 1) Federal regulation that protects residents in long-term care facilities and ensures their quality of care. (Ch. 2)

observation. Something that you can see, hear, smell, or touch that provides information about a patient, such as a physical change or a change in behavior. (Ch. 13)

Occupational Safety and Health Administration (OSHA). The federal government agency that protects the health and safety of employees. (Ch. 2)

occupied bed. A bed that is made while the patient or resident is in it. (Ch. 14)

ombudsman. A person who supports the health, welfare, safety, and rights of residents in long-term care facilities. (Ch. 4)

Omnibus Budget Reconciliation Act (OBRA). A congressional act that established the minimum federal requirements for nursing assistants working in long-term care facilities. (Ch. 1) Federal regulation that protects residents in long-term care facilities and ensures their quality of care. (Ch. 2)

open bed. A bed that is used by a resident who gets up during the day. (Ch. 14)

oral hygiene. The practices that clean and maintain the mouth, teeth, and dentures. (Ch. 22)

oral swab. A disposable, soft foam swab used for oral care. Some contain a dentifrice. (Ch. 22) A small sponge on a stick used to moisten a patient's mouth to prevent painful cracking. (Ch. 29)

organ. Any major body structure made up of two or more tissues working together that performs a specific function. (Ch. 9)

organ donation form. A legal document that states a person's wish to donate all or some organs and tissues to people who need them or to train health care workers. (Ch. 4)

organ donor. A person who has agreed to donate tissue or organs to others when he or she dies. (Ch. 30)

orientation. A program that explains an employer's policies, procedures, and benefits to a new employee. (Ch. 3)

orthostatic hypotension. A drop in blood pressure when a change in position occurs. (Ch. 16)

orthotic device. A device applied to the body to immobilize a bone, joint, or muscles in order to restore or improve function, or prevent deformity of the body part. (Ch. 21)

OSHA (Occupational Safety and Health Administration). The federal government agency that protects the health and safety of employees. (Ch. 2)

osteoporosis. Loss of bone density, causing bones to become brittle and break more easily. (Ch. 24)

ostomy. The surgical creation of an artificial opening in the body. (Ch. 19)

output. A measure of any fluid a patient loses or that is removed. (Ch. 26)

oxygen. A colorless, odorless, tasteless gas that is essential for life. (Ch. 6)

oxygen tent. A plastic covering on a frame that is placed over a patient's upper body. It delivers a higher percentage of oxygen than is available in air. (Ch. 6)

P

paranoia. The false belief that others intend to do harm. (Ch. 27)

paresis. Partial paralysis. (Ch. 22)

Parkinson's disease. A progressive disease that affects the part of the brain that handles muscular control and function. (Ch. 23)

partial seizure. A seizure in which the patient remains conscious and appears to stare blankly. (Ch. 17)

P.A.S.S. The sequence of critical steps when using a fire extinguisher. (Ch. 6)

password. A secret code made up of letters, numbers, and/or symbols, used to access a secure computer system. (Ch. 13)

pathogen. A microorganism that causes disease or infection. (Ch. 11)

patient. A person receiving health care services in a health care provider's office, a clinic, or a hospital. (Ch. 2)

patient-controlled anesthesia (PCA). A pumping device that delivers a small dose of pain medication intravenously when the patient pushes a button. (Ch. 29)

Patient's Bill of Rights. The guidelines that health care staff must follow to ensure that patients are protected in the hospital. (Ch. 4)

PCA (patient-controlled anesthesia). A pumping device that delivers a small dose of pain medication intravenously when the patient pushes a button. (Ch. 29)

pedal pulse. The pulse measured over the dorsalis pedis artery on the top of the foot. (Ch. 7)

pediculosis. A parasitic infestation of head lice. (Ch. 22)

perineal care. The care given to the genital and rectal areas. (Ch. 22)

perineum. The genital and rectal areas. (Ch. 22)

periodontal disease. Disease that affects the supporting structures of the teeth and gums, and can lead to decay and eventually loss of teeth. (Ch. 22)

peristalsis. Involuntary muscular, rhythmic contraction that propels contents through an organ. (Ch. 10)

personal data sheet. A document containing the personal information likely to be needed when applying for a job. (Ch. 3)

personality. The accumulation of individual traits that distinguish someone. (Ch. 8)

personal protective equipment (PPE). Special clothing or gear worn to protect against different types of hazards. (Ch. 6)

phlebitis. An inflammation of the veins. (Ch. 18)

physical needs. The basic human needs for oxygen, food, water, sleep, elimination, and shelter. (Ch. 5)

physical restraints. Protective devices that limit movement and keep patients from harming themselves or others. (Ch. 6)

physiology. The functions of systems in the human body. (Ch. 10)

placenta. The vascular organ lining the walls of the uterus from which the fetus derives nutrition and oxygen. (Ch. 28)

plantar flexion. Bending of the foot downward. (Ch. 24)

plasma. The liquid part of the blood that carries blood cells, nutrients, antibodies, chemicals, gases, and waste products within the body. (Ch. 10)

platelets. Irregular, disc-shaped solids in the blood that play a critical role in hemostasis. (Ch. 10)

poison. Any substance that is toxic to humans and can change the function of body organs and adversely affect the patient's health. (Ch. 17)

postmortem care. Care after death. (Ch. 30)

postoperatively. The period of time after surgery. (Ch. 18)

postoperative period. The time after surgery that begins when the patient is transported from the operating room to the recovery room. (Ch. 20)

postpartum care. The medical and supportive care given to a mother after childbirth. (Ch. 28)

PPE (personal protective equipment). Special clothing or gear worn to protect against different types of hazards. (Ch. 6)

prefix. A word part that comes before a root word or a combining form and modifies its meaning. (Ch. 12)

prehypertension. Blood pressure that is slightly higher than normal. (Ch. 7)

prenatal care. The medical care and monitoring a woman receives during her pregnancy to ensure optimum health for her and the developing baby. (Ch. 28)

preoperative period. The time when the patient is admitted to the hospital until the patient goes to surgery. (Ch. 20)

pressure sore. An area on the skin that is broken down. Also called *bedsore*, *decubitus ulcer*, or *pressure ulcer*. (Ch. 16, Ch. 22)

primary caregiver. The person who is mainly responsible for meeting a child's basic needs. (Ch. 8)

privacy. Freedom from intrusion of any kind. (Ch. 4)

procedures. Established methods of doing patient care tasks. (Ch. 1)

professionalism. Conduct that meets the standards of a profession. (Ch. 1)

prone position. The patient lies on the abdomen. (Ch. 16)

prosthesis. An artificial replacement of a body part. (Ch. 21)

proteins. Organic (carbon-containing) chemicals that are present in every body cell. Proteins are responsible for the development and rebuilding of cells and tissues. (Ch. 26)

protocols. Specific rules for how to do tasks at a health care facility. (Ch. 4)

psychosis. The general term for any severe disorder in which a person loses contact with reality. (Ch. 27)

puberty. The stage in which the sex organs mature and secondary sex characteristics develop. (Ch. 8)

pulse deficit. The difference between the apical and radial pulses. (Ch. 7)

pulse oximeter. An instrument that measures the percentage of oxygen in the blood. (Ch. 7)

pulse rate. The rate at which the heart beats. The pulse is felt over an artery as waves of blood pass through it. (Ch. 7)

Q

quadrants. A division into four parts, used to describe the areas of the abdomen. (Ch. 9)

quality of life. The ability to enjoy the activities of life or to be satisfied with everyday living. (Ch. 29)

R

R.A.C.E. The sequence of critical steps in a fire emergency. (Ch. 6)

radial pulse. The pulse measured at the wrist. (Ch. 7)

radiation therapy. A therapy that uses x-rays to destroy cancer cells. (Ch. 23)

range of motion (ROM). A joint's complete, normal range of movement. (Ch. 21)

range-of-motion exercises. Special exercises designed to move all muscles and joints through their complete range of motion and to build muscle. (Ch. 21)

reality orientation. A technique for guiding disoriented patients back to reality. It is based on constant repetition of information. (Ch. 27)

receiver. The person who receives a communication message. (Ch. 13)

receptor. A specialized cell or nerve ending that responds to specific stimuli, such as light, sound, or touch. (Ch. 9)

reciprocity. The recognition by one state of another state's certification, licensing, or registration. (Ch. 1)

recording. The process of writing down the observations you make and the treatments and procedures you perform. (Ch. 13)

rectal tube. A tube inserted into the rectum to relieve flatulence and abdominal distension. (Ch. 19)

reference. A person who knows you well and is willing to recommend you for a job. (Ch. 3)

reflex. An involuntary or automatic physical response. (Ch. 8)

registered nurse (RN). A trained health care provider with a nursing degree or diploma who carries out the orders of doctors, gives medications, performs some treatments and therapies, and sets up care plans. A registered nurse has passed a licensing exam given by a state board of nursing. (Ch. 1)

registry. An official record or listing of people who have successfully completed a state-approved nursing assistant training and evaluation program. (Ch. 1)

rehabilitation. The process of restoring patients to their highest possible physical, psychological, and social functioning after an injury or illness. (Ch. 1, Ch. 21)

rehabilitation center. A hospital or other facility devoted to retraining patients to enable them to function as fully as possible. (Ch. 2)

rehabilitation program. A structured series of activities designed to promote a patient's recovery. (Ch. 21)

reporting. The process of describing observations and care given. (Ch. 13)

rescue breathing. A step in basic life support, in which the rescuer forces oxygen into the patient's lungs to support or restore breathing. (Ch. 17)

reservoir. Any environment that allows a pathogen to live and grow. (Ch. 11)

resident. A person who lives in a long-term care facility. (Ch. 2)

Residents' Rights. Rights for home health care clients and residents of long-term care facilities provided by OBRA regulations. (Ch. 4)

resource management. Having resources on hand when they are needed and using them efficiently. (Ch. 25)

respiration. The process of inhaling (breathing in) and exhaling (breathing out). (Ch. 7)

respiratory arrest. The condition that occurs when breathing stops but the heart continues to work for several minutes. (Ch. 17)

respite care. Relief time for family caregivers to take care of personal needs or have time off. (Ch. 25)

restorative care. The everyday process of restoring patients to their highest possible physical, psychological, and social functioning on a long-term basis. (Ch. 1, Ch. 21)

résumé. A written summary of job qualifications, including education, skills, and work experience. (Ch. 3)

resuscitation. Lifesaving measures on a person whose breathing and/or heart has stopped. (Ch. 30)

reverse-Trendelenburg's position. A position in which the entire bed is tilted so that the patient's head is slightly higher than the feet. (Ch. 16)

rigor mortis. The stiffening of a body 2 to 4 hours after death. (Ch. 30)

ROM (range of motion). A joint's complete, normal range of movement. (Ch. 21)

rooting reflex. The natural response that causes a baby to look for something to suck when the cheek is touched. (Ch. 28)

root word. The basic part of a word that gives the word meaning. (Ch. 12)

S

sacraments. Rites or rituals, held to be sacred, to confer grace on an individual. (Ch. 29)

scales. Small, dry flakes of skin. (Ch. 22)

schizophrenia. A thought disorder that may include disorganized speech and behavior, irrational and illogical thoughts, social withdrawal, and an inability to make choices or decisions. (Ch. 27)

scope of practice. The things a health care worker can and cannot do by law. (Ch. 1)

secondary sex characteristics. Gender characteristics such as breasts in females and facial hair in males. (Ch. 8)

security needs. The group of needs that, when met, make one feel safe. (Ch. 5)

seizure. An electrical disturbance in the brain that results in uncontrollable spasms or jerking of the muscles of the body. (Ch. 17)

self-actualization needs. The psychological needs that, when met, enable a person to reach his or her highest potential. (Ch. 5)

semen. The fluid that transports sperm. (Ch. 10)

semi-Fowler's position. A semisitting position with the head raised to a 45° angle and the portion of the bed under the knee raised 15°, if possible. (Ch. 16)

sender. The person who sends a communication message. (Ch. 13)

shallow breathing. Partial breaths that do not fill the lungs with air. (Ch. 7)

shearing force. A combination of friction and pressure. (Ch. 16)

shift report. A summary of what went on during the previous shift that might affect patient care techniques and decisions. (Ch. 1)

shock. A condition that occurs when an inadequate blood supply is delivered to the body's tissues. (Ch. 17)

shroud. A cloth used to wrap a person's body for burial. (Ch. 30)

side rail. A rail attached to the side of a bed that can be raised to prevent falling out of bed. (Ch. 6)

sign. Something about a patient that you can see, hear, feel, or smell. (Ch. 13)

Sims' position. The patient lies in a semi-prone position on the left side with the right knee flexed up toward the abdomen. The left knee is also flexed, but not as much as the right knee. (Ch. 16)

sitz bath. A type of moist warm therapy in which the patient's perineal and anal regions are immersed in warm water in a special tub or seat. (Ch. 18)

slide board. A device used to assist in patient transfers at even levels. (Ch. 16)

social needs. The group of needs that, when met, make a person feel accepted and loved. (Ch. 5)

social well-being. A feeling of being able to form and maintain relationships with family and friends. (Ch. 5)

sphygmomanometer. A device used to measure blood pressure; often referred to as a blood pressure cuff. (Ch. 7)

sputum. The mucous secretion from the lungs, bronchi, and trachea. (Ch. 19)

standard precautions. A set of infection control guidelines designed to minimize the risk of transmitting microorganisms and disease. (Ch. 11)

sterile. Free from microorganisms. (Ch. 18)

sterilization. The use of extremely high temperatures to kill pathogens, nonpathogens, and spores. (Ch. 11)

stertorous breathing. Breaths accompanied by noises. (Ch. 7)

stethoscope. An instrument used to listen to the sounds produced by the heart, lungs, and other body organs. (Ch. 7)

stimulation. Activities that excite the senses. (Ch. 8)

stoma. An artificial opening in the body created by surgery. (Ch. 19)

stool. Feces that have been excreted from the body. (Ch. 19)

stress. The body's response to any emotional, social, or economic factor that produces tension or anxiety. (Ch. 1)

stretcher. A cart with wheels for transporting patients from one place to another while they are lying down. (Ch. 16)

strict bed rest. Confined to bed by a doctor's order and not allowed to do anything for oneself, including any form of exercise, unless ordered by a doctor. (Ch. 24)

stroke. A condition that occurs when there is damage to a blood vessel in the brain. (Ch. 17) A sudden interruption in the blood supply to the brain. (Ch. 23)

subacute care unit. An area in a long-term care facility that provides care for patients who are too ill to be in the general population but who have been released from the acute care of a hospital. (Ch. 2)

subjective information. Information the patient tells you. (Ch. 13)

substance abuse. Maladaptive behavior in which use of a chemical substance, such as alcohol, tobacco, or prescription or illegal drugs, has a negative impact on a person's life. (Ch. 27)

suctioning. The process of removing or sucking up fluid or body secretions. (Ch. 19)

suffix. A word part that comes after a root word or a combining form and modifies its meaning. (Ch. 12)

suicide. The taking of one's own life. (Ch. 27)

sundowning. Becoming upset, agitated, or disoriented in the late afternoon or evening. (Ch. 27)

supine position. The patient is positioned lying flat on the back. (Ch. 16)

suppository. Semisolid medication or lubricating agent that is inserted into the rectum for absorption by the body for prevention or treatment of constipation. (Ch. 19)

surgery. The use of manual procedures to diagnose and treat diseases, injuries, or deformities. (Ch. 20)

surgical asepsis. The practice of completely eliminating microorganisms. (Ch. 11)

surgical bed. A closed bed that has been opened to the side to allow safe, easy transfer of a patient who is being moved from a stretcher to a bed. (Ch. 14)

symbol. A written or printed sign that has meaning. (Ch. 12)

symptom. Something the patient tells you that he or she feels. (Ch. 13)

syndrome. A group of signs and symptoms that occur together. (Ch. 23)

system. Several organs working together to perform a particular function. (Ch. 9)

systole. The period during which the heart muscle contracts, pumping blood through the blood vessels. (Ch. 7)

systolic pressure. A measure of the pressure in the arteries when the heart contracts. (Ch. 7)

T

tachycardia. A rapid heart rate; more than 100 pulse beats per minute. (Ch. 7)

tachypnea. Fast breathing; more than 20 breaths per minute. (Ch. 7)

temperament. Each person's unique manner of thinking, reacting, and behaving. (Ch. 8)

terminal illness. An illness that is not curable and from which the person will eventually die. (Ch. 29)

thermometer. A device used to measure body temperature. (Ch. 7)

thrombophlebitis. A condition that occurs when a blood clot causes inflammation in a vein. (Ch. 18)

thrombus. A blood clot that stays at the site where it formed. (Ch. 20)

TIA (transient ischemic attack). A small stroke that temporarily reduces blood flow to the brain but results in less damage than a stroke; a ministroke. (Ch. 23)

time management. Planning and scheduling your time to do tasks efficiently. (Ch. 25)

time/travel record. A log that describes how the home health aide has spent time with the client, traveling to and from the client's home, and doing errands for the client. (Ch. 25)

tissue. A group of cells with similar structure and function. (Ch. 9)

toe pleat. A pleat made at the bottom of the bed linens to allow room for the toes and feet to move freely. (Ch. 14)

tort. A wrongful act that causes injury to another person or the person's property. (Ch. 4)

traction. A process of drawing or pulling used to promote and maintain proper bone alignment. A system of ropes, weights, and pulleys is used. (Ch. 21)

transfer. Moving a patient from one unit or room in a facility to another unit or room in the same facility or to a different facility. (Ch. 15) To move a patient from one item of furniture or equipment to another. (Ch. 16)

transfer belt. A belt that buckles around a patient's waist and provides a handle for the nursing assistant to hold onto when transferring a patient. (Ch. 16)

transfer form. A document that authorizes a patient's transfer and ensures that the patient's care plan is understood by the new staff. (Ch. 15)

transient ischemic attack (TIA). A small stroke that temporarily reduces blood flow to the brain but results in less damage than a stroke; a ministroke. (Ch. 23)

transmission-based precautions. Infection control guidelines used for patients with highly contagious infections. (Ch. 11)

transport. To move a patient from place to place using a transport device, such as a wheelchair or stretcher. (Ch. 16)

trapeze bar. A triangular device that hangs above a bed to help patients transfer and position themselves. (Ch. 21)

Trendelenburg's position. A position in which the entire bed is tilted so that the patient's feet are slightly higher than the head. (Ch. 16)

turning sheet. A sheet used by two nursing assistants to move or turn a patient in bed; also called a *draw sheet*. (Ch. 16)

U

umbilical cord. The structure that connects the fetus to the placenta during pregnancy. (Ch. 28)

unintentional tort. The act of causing harm or injury to a person or property without meaning to. (Ch. 4)

unit. A specialized area within a health care facility. (Ch. 15)

universal distress signal. A sign used to indicate that one is choking by clutching the neck with one or both hands. (Ch. 17)

unlawful restraint. Restraining or restricting the movements of another person without consent. (Ch. 4)

unoccupied bed. A bed that is empty. (Ch. 14)

urinal. A special container that men use for urinating when they are bedridden. (Ch. 19)

urinary catheter. A tube used to drain urine from the bladder. (Ch. 19)

urinary incontinence. The inability to control the passing of urine. (Ch. 19)

urinary retention. The incomplete emptying of the bladder. (Ch. 19)

urination. The passing of urine from the body. (Ch. 19)

urine. The waste material, or output, of the urinary system. (Ch. 19)

V–W

validation therapy. A communication technique that shows respect and maintains patients' dignity by acknowledging their reality. (Ch. 27)

vector. A nonhuman living organism that transmits pathogens. (Ch. 11)

vein. A blood vessel that carries deoxygenated blood and waste products back to the heart. (Ch. 10)

ventilation. The movement of air in and out of the lungs. (Ch. 10)

ventral. The front of the body. (Ch. 9)

ventricles. The two lower chambers of the heart. (Ch. 9)

verbal communication. Communication through the use of words. (Ch. 13)

vital signs. Important indicators of how body systems are functioning. The basic vital signs include temperature, pulse, respirations, and blood pressure. Pain level is often considered the "fifth" vital sign. In some cases, height and weight are also included. (Ch. 7)

vitamins. Important organic nutrients used by the body for a variety of body processes and functions. (Ch. 26)

walking aid. An assistive device that helps support the body while walking. (Ch. 6, Ch. 21)

warm compress. A folded and moistened piece of cloth or towel that is warmed and placed over a small area of the body for moist warm therapy. (Ch. 18)

warm pack. A heated moist treatment that is applied or wrapped around an area of the body. (Ch. 18)

well-baby checks. Regular visits to a doctor to monitor a baby's progress. (Ch. 8)

work ethic. A positive attitude about your work, including honesty, trustworthiness, reliability, and responsibility. (Ch. 3)

Credits

Design: Squarecrow Creative Graphics
Cover: Pete Saloutos/Corbis

Acknowledgements:
CNA/Health Occupations Program, Illinois Central College, East Peoria, Illinois; Handmaker Services, Villa Maria Care Center, Birth and Women's Health Center, Tucson, Arizona

Corbis/Pete Saloutos 1, Dynamic Graphics 3, Tony Stone/Getty Images 3, Punchstock 3, Index Stock/Thinkstock 3, Jim Cummins/Getty Images 3, Brad Wilson/Getty Images 5, John Coletti/Index Stock 5, Noel Hendrickson/Getty Images 5, Tom Stewart/Corbis 5, Bruce Ayres/Getty Images 6, Steve Puetzer/Getty Images 6, Stockbyte/Getty Images 6, Ole Grat/Corbis 6, Don Farrell/Getty Images 7, Ron Chapple/Getty Images 7, Marie/Corbis 7, Michael Barley/Corbis 8, Julie Fisher/Corbis 8, Scott Wilson/Getty Images 8, Corbis 9, Romilly Lockyear/Getty Images 9, Corbis 9, Richard Price/Getty Images 9, TEK Images/Photo Researchers, Inc. 10, Andersen Ross/Getty Images 10, Rolf Bruderer/Corbis 10, LWA-Dann Tardif 10, Flip Chalfant/Getty Images 11, Anderson Ross/Getty Images 11, Nancy Ney/Corbis 11, Tim Hill/Stock Food 11, Richard T. Nowitz/Photo Researchers, Inc. 12, Pete Saloutos/Corbis 12, Corbis 12, Ed Bock/Corbis 15, Tony Stone/Getty Images 16, Brad Wilson/Getty Images 18, Stockdisc/Getty Images 20, Scott Thompson 21, Scott Thompson 22, Chestnut Hill Enterprises, Inc. 22, Claire Artman/Corbis 23, Chestnut Hill Enterprises, Inc. 26, Ann Garvin 27, Taxi/Getty Images 29, Ronnie Kaufman/Corbis 29, Jeff Stoecker 34, Glencoe 35, Jeff Stoecker 37, John Coletti/Index Stock 42, Jeff Stoecker 44, Jeff Stoecker 45, George Disario/Corbis 47, The Image Works, Inc. 47, Bernard van Berg/Getty Images 48, Scott Thompson 48, Jeff Stoecker 48, Chestnut Hill Enterprises, Inc. 49, Ann Garvin 49, Kevin May 50, Thinkstock/Jupiter Images 51, M. Mollenberg/zefa/Corbis 51, Claire Artman/zefa/Corbis 52, Chestnut Hill Enterprises, Inc. 53, Jeff Stoecker 53, Spencer Grant/Photo Researchers, Inc. 55, Scott Thompson 57, Noel Hendrickson/Getty Images 62, Barbara Peacock/Getty Images 64, Graphic World 65, Jeff Stoecker 66, Graphic World 67, Frank Siteman/Index Stock 67, Jeff Stoecker 68, Graphic World 70, Zigy Kahizny/Getty Images 71, Scott Thompson 72, Digital Vision/Getty Images 73, Jeff Stoecker 74, Stockbyte/Getty Images 75, Internal Revenue Service 76, Barros & Barros/Getty Images 78, Graphic World 79, Tom Stewart/Corbis 84, Glencoe 86, American Hospital Association 87, Corbis 87, Glencoe 88, Jim Naughten/Getty Images 89, Glencoe 90, Jeff Stoecker 91, Graphic World 92, Scott Thompson 93, Stewart Cohen/Getty Images 94, Chestnut Hill Enterprises, Inc. 95, Glencoe 96, Jeff Stoecker 98, Bruce Ayres/Getty Images 104, Jeff Stoecker 106, Chestnut Hill Enterprises, Inc. 107, Tim Fuller 109, Brad Wilson/Getty Images 110, Jeff Stoecker 111, Tim Fuller 112, G. Baden/Zefa/Corbis 113, David Joel/Getty Images 114, Kevin May 115, Chestnut Hill Enterprises, Inc. 116, Corbis 116, Steven Puetzer/Getty Images 122, Floyd Dean/Getty Images 124, Tim Fuller 125, Ann Garvin 125, Scott Thompson 126, Glencoe 127, Tim Fuller 127, Jeff Stoecker 129, Alex Wilson/Getty Images 129, Jeff Stoecker 130, Ann Garvin 130, Graphic World 131, Wesley Bocxe/Photo Researchers, Inc. 133, Jim Reed/Corbis 133, Scott Thompson 135, Chestnut Hill Enterprises, Inc. 135, Keith Brofsky/Getty Images 136, Chestnut Hill Enterprises, Inc. 136, Chestnut Hill Enterprises, Inc. 137, Tim Fuller 137, Graphic World 138, Scott Thompson 139, Kevin May / Senior World 141, Scott Thompson 141, Graphic World 142, Graphic World 143, Graphic World 144, Scott Thompson 144, Scott Thompson 145, Scott Thompson 146, Graphic World 148, Stockbyte/Getty Images 154, Squarecrow Graphics 156, Jeff Stoecker 157, Scott Thompson 158, Graphic World 159, Scott Thompson 160, Graphic World 161, Scott Thompson 163, Graphic World 163, Chestnut Hill Enterprises, Inc. 164, Squarecrow Graphics 165, Graphic World 167, Chestnut Hill Enterprises, Inc. 168, Bernard van Berg/Getty Images 170, Scott Thompson 171, Scott Thompson 172, Scott Thompson 173, Graphic World 173, Wong-Baker 175, Graphic World 175, Graphic World 176, Thinkstock/Jupiter images 177, Graphic World 178, Thinkstock/Jupiter Images 178, Scott Thompson 179, Scott Thompson 180, Hans Neleman/Getty Images 181, Lee Powers/Photo Researchers, Inc. 181, Punchstock 186, Ole Graf/Corbis 188, Ben Edwards/Getty Images 191, Barbara Maurer/Getty Images 191, Mike Brinson/Getty Images 192, Graphic World 193, Arthur Tilley/Getty Images 194, Medioimages/Getty Images 195, Corbis 195, David W. Hamilton/Getty Images 197, Tim Fuller 197, Jeff Greenberg/Index Stock 198, Janet Bailey/Masterfile 199, Digital Vision/Getty Images 199, LaCoppola & Meier/Corbis 200, Don Farrell/Getty Images 206, Ian Worpole 208, Jeff Stoecker 209, Jeff Stoecker 210, Jeff Stoecker 211, Ian Worpole 211, Ian Worpole 212, Ian Worpole 213, Ian Worpole 214, Ian Worpole 215, Ian Worpole 216, Jeff Stoecker 217, Ian Worpole 218, Jeff Stoecker 219, Ian Worpole 220, Ken Clubb 220, Ron Chapple/Getty Images 226, Alfred Pasieka/Photo Researchers, Inc. 228, Ian Worpole 229, Ian Worpole 230, Ian Worpole 231, Ian Worpole 233, Ian Worpole 234, Ian Worpole 236, Ian Worpole 237, Ian Worpole 238, Jeff Stoecker 239, Ian Worpole 239, Jeff Stoecker 242, Ian Worpole 243, Ian Worpole 244, Ian Worpole 245, Marie/Corbis 250, Graphic World 252, Jeff Stoecker 253, Joseph Nettis/Photo Researchers, Inc. 255, Dr. P. Marazzi/Photo Researchers, Inc. 256, AJPhoto/Photo Researchers, Inc. 257, Ulrich Sapountsis/Photo Researchers, Inc. 257, Brevis Corporation 258, Chestnut Hill Enterprises, Inc. 259, Chestnut Hill Enterprises, Inc. 260, Chestnut Hill Enterprises, Inc. 261, Chestnut Hill Enterprises, Inc. 262, Scott Thompson 262, Scott Thompson 263, Scott Thompson 264, Brevis Corporation 265, Tim Fuller 267, Tim Fuller 268, Tim Fuller 269, Glencoe 272, Thinkstock 278, Michael Barley/Corbis 280, image100/Alamy 281, Ian Worpole 283, Ian Worpole 286, Chestnut Hill Enterprises, Inc. 291, Gorman & Assoc. 294, Corbis 298, Glencoe /Clip Art 299, Corbis 299, Julie Fisher/Corbis 304, Taxi/Getty Images 306, Digital Vision/Getty Images 307, Chestnut Hill Enterprises, Inc. 307, Jon Feingersh/

Index

A

abandonment, 625, 628, 740

abbreviation, 281, 293-298, 740

ABC assessment, 404

ABC Class (All Class) fire extinguisher, 123, 131, 740

abdominal cavity, 210

abdominal distension, 455, 470, 740

abduction, 520, 521, 522

absorbent pads and briefs, 465

abuse, 85, 96, 740
    abandonment as, 642
    and dementia, 688
    domestic violence, 625, 642
    emotional, 96
    from patients, 96
    and patients with dementia, 688
    physical, 96, 642
    reporting, 642-643
    signs of, 96, 642
    sexual, 96
    sexual harassment, 642
    substance, 675, 689-690
    suspecting, 642-643
    verbal, 96

accessory organs, 232

Acetest®, 483

acquired immunodeficiency syndrome (AIDS), 245, 577, 596–597, 740

acronym, 281, 293, 740

active listening, 89, 305, 307–308, 740
    clarification, 307
    reflection, 307
    restatement, 307

activities of daily living (ADLs), 105, 108–109, 740

acute illness, 46

adaptive behavior, 676

adduction, 520, 521, 522, 523

ADLs (activities of daily living), 105, 108–109, 740
    and rehabilitation, 518

admission, 351, 352–357, 740

admissions checklist, 351, 354–355, 740
    components of, 354

admissions process, 352–353, 357–358
    nursing assistant's role in, 352–353
    and personal belongings, 356
    and settling patient in room, 355

A.D.N. (associate degree of nursing), 34

adolescent period, of growth and development, 197–198

adrenal cortex, 236

adrenal gland, 236

adrenal medulla, 236

adult day-care center, 43, 50, 740

adulthood
    late, 200
    middle, 199
    young, 198–199

adult-onset diabetes, 216, 580

adult protective services, 642

advance directive, 85, 91–92, 402, 740
    analyzing, 403
    and dying patient, 717

advanced practice nurses (APNs), 52

AED (automated external defibrillator), 399, 408–409, 740
    signs indicating need for, 409

aerosol therapy, 123, 139, 740

age spots, 612

aging process, 606
    and nursing assistant, 612
    and OBRA competencies, 33
    in women, 27
    physical changes during, 611, 612–613
    psychological changes during, 616–617
    safety issues, 611
    social changes during, 616–617

agitation, 675, 679, 740
    causes of, 679

AHA (American Hospital Association), 87

AIDS (acquired immunodeficiency syndrome), 245, 577, 596–597, 740
    causes of, 596
    care requirements, 597
    symptoms, 596

airborne precautions, for infection control, 264–265

airborne transmission, 254

alcohol-based hand rubs, 258

All Class (ABC Class) fire extinguisher, 123, 131, 740

alternative medicine, 228

alveoli, 207, 214, 232, 740

Alzheimer's disease, 140, 207, 217, 675, 685–686, 740
    and movement restriction of, 140
    stages of, 686
    and validation therapy, 687, 688

ambulate, 605, 609, 740

ambulation, 524
    assisting with, 524

ambulatory, 123, 135, 740

ambulatory patient, 135
    using elimination equipment, 459
    weighing, 177–178

ambulatory surgery, 495, 511, 740

American Diabetes Association, 581, 669

Americans with Disabilities Act, 649, 654, 740

American Heart Association, 400
    2005 first aid guidelines, 400

American Hospital Association (AHA), 87

American Red Cross, 400

anal incontinence, 455, 459, 740

anatomical plane, 207, 211, 740
    types of, 211

anatomical position, 207, 212, 740
anatomy, 227, 228, 740
anesthesia, 495, 503, 740
   effects of, 503
   general, 503
   local, 503
   safety issues, 503
   spinal, 503
anesthesiologists, 503
anesthetic, 495, 503, 740
angina pectoris, 577, 585, 740
   care, 585
angles, estimating, 374
animal transmission, 255
anorexia, 649, 668, 740
anterior, 212
anterior tibial muscle, 243
antibodies, 227, 245
anticoagulants, 543
antiembolic stockings, 429, 448–449, 740
   applying, 449
   and postoperative patient, 508
antisepsis, 251, 256, 740
anus, 233, 457
anxiety, 675, 679, 741
   causes of, 679
aortic valve, 214
aphasia, 577, 590, 741
   expressive, 590
   receptive, 590
apical pulse, 155, 167, 741
   measuring, 168–169
apical-radial pulse, 155, 167, 741
APN (advanced practice nurse), 52
apnea, 155, 169, 741
appetite, 649, 667, 741
application form, 63, 69, 70, 741
   guidelines, 69
aquamatic pad, 429, 436, 438, 741
arachnoid, 239
arterial system, 229
artery, 227, 229, 741
   brachial, 167
   carotid, 167
   disease, 230
   dorsalis pedis, 166, 167

femoral, 167
popliteal, 167
posterior tibial, 167
radial, 167
renal, 234
temporal, 167
asepsis, 251, 256, 741
   medical, 251–256
   surgical, 256
as-needed medications, 700
aspiration, 649, 664, 741
assault, 85, 93–94, 741
assessment tools, 683
assisted-living facility, 43, 49–50, 741
associate degree of nursing (A.D.N.), 34
asthma, 232, 577, 587–588, 741
   causes of, 587
   treatments, 587–588
atelectasis, 495, 506, 741
atherosclerosis, 577, 585, 741
   risk factors, 585
atria, 207, 214, 741
atrophic skin, 541, 567, 741
auditory canal, 219
auricle, 219
autoclave, 251, 257, 741
automated external defibrillator (AED), 399, 408–409, 740, 741
   signs indicating need for, 409
autonomy, 605, 606, 741
averaging hourly urine output, 466
axillary crutches, 526
   safety issues, 527
axillary temperature, 162–163
   normal ranges for, 158
axon, 239

B

bachelor of science in nursing (B.S.N.), 34
bacteria, 252, 254–255, 271
   drug-resistant, 271
back rub, 562–563
back safety, 372–373
ball-and-socket joint, 242

bandages, elastic, 448
baseline information, of patient, 354
basic life support, 399, 402–411, 741
   for adults, 405–406
   for children, 406–408
   for infants, 406–408
   procedures, 404–421
bath blanket, 331, 335, 741
bath, 551–558
   bed, 553–554, 555–556
   benefits of, 551
   methods, 553–554
   observations, 553
   safety rules, 552
   temperatures
   tub, 553
   whirlpool, 554, 557–558
battery, 85, 93–94, 741
bed
   closed, 331, 336, 338–340, 743
   manual, 334
   occupied, 331, 336, 337, 342–345, 750
   open, 331, 336, 338–340, 750
   surgical, 331, 337
   unoccupied, 331, 336
bed bath, 553–554, 555–557
bed cradle, 605, 614, 741
bed linens, 335–336
   benefits of, 335
   changing schedule for, 336
   handling guidelines, 336
bedmaking, 335–345
   benefits of, 335
   OBRA competencies for, 31
bed pad, 331, 335–336, 741
   disposable, 336
bedpan, 455, 461, 462–463, 741
   fracture, 461, 462–463
bed rest, 605, 608, 741
   and exercise, 608
   strict, 605, 608, 754
bedridden patient, 371, 376, 741
   care of, 615
   moving or lifting guidelines, 376
   weighing, 179–180

bedside commode, 460
   usage guidelines, 460–461
benign prostatic hyperplasia, 239
bicep muscle, 243
bioethics, 43, 45, 741
bionics, 243
bladder, 234, 237, 456
   training, 465
bladder infection, 235. *See also*
   cystitis.
bland diet, 668
bleeding
   external, 399, 414
   internal, 399, 414
blood
   clot, 230
   diseases, 230–231
   handling safety, 230
   oxygen levels in, 173
   oxygen-poor, 230
   oxygen-rich, 230
bloodborne pathogen, 251, 257,
   741
Bloodborne Pathogen Standard
   (OSHA), 271–272
blood cells, 229
   red, 229
   white, 229
blood flow, 230. *See* circulation.
blood pressure, 155, 171, 741
   abnormal readings, 171
   high, 231, 585
   measuring, 171–173
   ranges in, 171
blood vessels, 229
body
   cavities, 210
   structure, 208–212
body alignment, 371, 372, 741
body composition fitness, 607
body fluids, 251, 253, 741
body language, 305, 306, 741
body mechanics, 371, 372–373,
   741
   for moving patients, 376
   principles of, 372–373
   safety issues, 376
body support, 371, 372, 741

body temperature, 155, 156–157,
   742. *See also* temperature.
bone marrow, 245
bones
categories of, 241–242
bottle-feeding, an infant, 706–707
bowel elimination, 457–459
   and aging process, 457
   changes in, 457
   and multiple sclerosis, 592
   problems, 458–459
   training, 465
bowel obstruction, 458
brace, 531
brachial artery, 167
bradycardia, 155, 168, 742
bradypnea, 155, 169, 742
brain, 216–217
   diseases, 217
brainstem, 207, 217, 742
breastfeeding, 697, 705–706, 742
   assisting with, 705–706
   standard precautions, 706
breathing
   rescue, 399, 402
   shallow, 169
   stertorous, 169
bronchi, 231–232
bronchioles, 232
bronchodilators, 587
B.S.N (bachelor of science in
   nursing), 34
buccal medications, 699
burns, 418–419
   chemical, 419
   major, 418
   minor, 418
   moderate, 418
   safety issues, 418
burn treatment
   chemical burn safety, 419
   safety, 418
burping, an infant, 706

C

calculating
   fluid intake, 684
   frequency of respirations, 732

   insurance payments, 56
   percentage of meals eaten, 581
   shift schedules, 323
   therapy times, 440
   time, 72
   urinary output, 235, 466, 468
   vaccination schedules, 273
   walking distances, 525
   weekly earnings, 629
calculi, 484
call signal, 305, 311, 356, 742
calorie requirements, 28
calorie-restricted diet, 669
cancer, 577, 594–595, 742
   causes, 594
   care requirements, 595
   common types of, 594
   reproductive system, 239
   safety issues, 595
   skin, 244
   symptoms, 595
   treatment, 595
cane, 527
   helping patient with, 528
capillary, 227, 229, 742
carbohydrates, 649, 650, 742
and MyPyramid, 652
cardiac arrest, 399, 403, 742
   signs of, 403
cardiac system, 156
cardiopulmonary resuscitation
   (CPR), 92, 399, 403, 404,
   742, 743
cardiovascular disease, 584–586
   care, 588–589
   causes, 584
cardiovascular fitness, 607
cardiovascular system, 228–231
   aging of, 612
   diseases, 230–231
care
   log, 633
   of opposite gender, 558
   neonate, 192, 193, 706
   perineal, 467, 541, 558–560, 751
   plan, 626
   postmortem, 32, 729, 733–735
   postoperative, 502–511
   postpartum, 697, 703–706, 751

prenatal, 697, 701–702, 751
preoperative patient, 498
principles of, 23
quality, 23
resident, 614–615
restorative, 19, 22, 517, 518, 752
subacute, 46
terminally ill, 717–718
caregiver, 19, 20, 742
career, 64. *See also* job.
career advancement, 78–79
career portfolio, 63, 78, 742
carotid artery, 167
carpals, 241–242
cartilage, 242
case manager, 625, 626, 742
cast, 531
    care guidelines, 531–532
catheter, 455, 465, 742
    assisting with, 465–467
    and bladder infection safety, 235
    care guidelines, 466
    condom, 455, 469, 743
    indwelling, 455, 468–469
    Texas®, 469
cavity, body, 207, 210, 742
    abdominal, 210
    cranial, 210
    spinal, 210
    thoracic, 210
CDC (Centers for Disease Control and Prevention), 251, 257, 742
cell, 207, 208–209, 742
    blood, 229
    body, 239
    division, 209
    membrane, 208, 209
Celsius scale, 157, 158
Centers for Disease Control and Prevention (CDC), 251, 257, 742
    and contaminated waste, 267
    standard precautions, 257–258
central nervous system, 239
cerebellum, 207, 217, 742
cerebrospinal fluid, 239

cerebrovascular accident (CVA), 240, 577, 590, 742, 743
cerebrum, 207, 217, 742
certification, 30
certified medication assistant, 698
certified nursing assistant (CNA), 34
cesarean section (c-section), 697, 703, 742
cervix, 238
chain of command, 19, 36–37, 742
chain of infection, 251, 253, 742
    and elimination devices, 460
    safety issues, 336
charge nurse, 19, 33, 53, 742
chart, 319. *See also* medical record.
    graphic, 305, 319–320
charting, 305, 318, 742. *See also* recording.
    by exception, 323
chemical burns, 419
    safety issues, 419
chemical restraints, 94, 123, 140, 742
chemoreceptor, 221
chemotherapy, 577, 595, 742
Cheyne-Stokes breathing, 155, 169, 742
    and dying patient, 731
CHF (congestive heart failure), 577, 585–586, 649, 660, 742
children
    basic life support for, 406–408
    communication with, 311
    meeting needs of, 112, 114
    parents identifying needs of, 112
    touch needs of, 114
chromosomes, 208, 209
chronic, 577, 578, 742
chronic bronchitis, 577, 587, 742
    symptoms, 587
chronic confusion, 683. *See* dementia.
chronic illness, 113, 568
    affects of, 578
    and attitude, 591

chronic obstructive pulmonary disease (COPD), 232, 577, 587, 588, 743
chronic productive cough, 587
chyme, 233
circulation, 230
    changes, in dying patient, 731
    in diabetes patient, 584
    in postoperative patient, 508–510
circumcision, 697, 709, 742
clarification, in active listening, 307
Class A fire extinguisher, 123, 130, 742
Class B fire extinguisher, 123, 130–131, 743
Class C fire extinguisher, 123, 131, 743
classified ads, as job lead, 68
clavical, 242
clean-catch (midstream) urine sample, 479–480
cleansing enema, 471
    giving a, 472–473
clean technique, 256. *See* medical asepsis.
clear liquid diet, 668
client, 43, 46, 743. *See also* patient or resident.
    care plan, 626
    goals, 630
    progress, 630–632
client care record, 91, 625, 633, 634, 743
clinic, 43, 48, 743
clinical thermometers, 158. *See also* glass thermometers.
Clinitest®, 483
clitoris, 238
closed bed, 331, 336, 338–340, 743
clot, 230
CNA (certified nursing assistant), 34
coccyx, 242
cochlea, 219
coercion, 85, 90, 743
cognitive, 518

cognitively impaired residents. *See also* mental retardation.
OBRA competencies for, 33
cold compress, 429, 441–442, 743
cold pack, 429, 444, 445, 743
applying, 445
cold soaks, 441, 443
cold therapy, 440–444
benefits, 440
dry, 444
guidelines, 440–441
moist, 441–443
safety issues, 440–441
sensitivity, 441
collaborating, 77
colon, 233
colostomy, 455, 474–475, 743
changing, appliance, 475–476
colostrum, 697, 705, 743
combining form, of word parts, 281, 282, 283, 284–286, 743
comfort devices, 614
commercial enema, 471
giving, 473–474
common vehicle transmission, 254
communication, 305, 306–313, 423, 743
active listening, 305, 307–308
adapting, to patient, 309–311
asking questions in, 436
barriers to, 309
call signal, 356
characteristics of good, 24
discussing long-term care in, 616
effective, 24, 307–308
in emergencies, 134
giving and following directions in, 337
with health care team, 311
language barriers in, 117
with neurological disorder patients, 594
nonverbal, 306, 308, 416
observation and, 519
in oral presentations, 599
patient, 308–309
pediatric patient, 196
plain language, 174

process, 306
sender-receiver model of, 74
and sensitivity, 464
with speech-impaired patients, 240
and standard precautions, 266
and teaching, 734
and teams, 704
telephone, 502
using technology, 311–313
and validation therapy, 687
verbal, 305, 306–308, 355
with visitors, 552
written, 306
comparing and contrasting, in writing, 254
compensation, as defense mechanism, 676
complementary medicine, 228
compound words, 282
comprehension, reading, 636
computed tomography (CT) scanning, 217
concept map, 365
conception, 238. *See* fertilization.
concise writing, 98, 401
condom catheter, 455, 469, 743
confidentiality, 85, 95, 743
confusion, 675, 678, 743
congestive heart failure (CHF), 577, 585–586, 649, 660, 743
care requirements, 586
causes, 585
connective tissue, 209
conscientiousness, 19, 24, 743
constipation, 455, 458, 743
constrict, 227, 229, 743
contact lens care, 569
contact precautions, for infection control, 264–265
contact transmission, 254, 264–265
contagious diseases, 254. *See also* infectious diseases.
contaminated waste, 267
in home care, 269
context clues, in reading, 283
continuing education, 63, 78–79
continuous traction, 532

continuum of care, 43, 45, 743
converting
fractions to percentages, 345
inches to feet and inches, 198
liquid measures, 662
temperatures, 422
COPD (chronic obstructive pulmonary disease), 232, 577, 587, 588, 743
care requirements, 588–589
and oxygen therapy, 588
coping mechanisms, 676
defense, 105, 133, 676, 743
negative, 676
positive, 676
cornea, 218
coronal plane, 211
coronary artery disease, 230
cortisol, 236
counting money, 359
courtesy, 54
cover letter, 63, 65, 743
CPR (cardiopulmonary resuscitation), 92, 399, 403, 404, 743
CPR certification, 400
cranial cavity, 210
cranium, 242
creative writing, 109
journal keeping, 353
croupette, 123, 139, 743
crutch, 526–527
axillary, 526
forearm, 527
safety issues, 527
c-section (cesarean section), 697, 703, 742
CT (computed tomography) scanning, 217
cultural strategies, 45
culture, 45, 105, 114, 743
valuing differences in, 114–115
Cushing's disease, 236
CVA (cerebrovascular accident), 240, 577, 590, 742, 743
cyanosis, 429, 441, 743
cystitis, 235
cytoplasm, 208, 209

D

daily report, 633. *See also* client care record.
dandruff, 541, 549, 743
dangle, 371, 377, 743
data, 305, 312, 743
death
    indications, of, 732
    signs of, 732
    signs of approaching, 730–732
death rattle, 729, 731, 743
decubitus ulcer, 541, 567, 743
defamation, 743
defecation, 455, 456, 743
defense mechanisms, 105, 113, 743
    types of, 676
defibrillation, 399, 408, 744
deficit, 518
degenerative, 217
dehydration, 110, 649, 660, 744
    signs of, 660
delegation, 19, 36, 744
    rights of, 37
delirium, 675, 679, 744
    causes of, 679
deltoid, 243
delusion, 675, 681–682, 744
dementia, 675, 683, 744
    symptoms, 683
    and validation therapy, 687, 688
dementia patient
    care guidelines, 688–689
    safety issues, 688
dendrites, 239
denial
    as defense mechanism, 676
    as grief stage, 716
dentifrice, 541, 543, 744
dentures, 541, 543, 744
    care of, 546–547
    problems of, 546
department head, 52
dependability, 24
depression, 675, 680–681, 744
    care guidelines, 680–681
    as grief stage, 716
    situational, 680
    symptoms, 680

dermatitis, 541, 567, 744
dermis, 207, 213, 243, 744
descriptive scale, of pain levels, 174
development, 189, 190, 744
    Erickson's stages of, 201
    stages of, 190–200
developmental tasks, 189, 190, 744
deviant, 679
devices
    assistive, 614
    comfort, 614
    elimination, 460
    eye appliances, 569–570
    feeding assistive, 657
    hearing aid, 571
    orthotic, 517, 531, 750
    oxygen delivery, 137–140
    support, 444–445, 448–449
diabetes mellitus (DM), 207, 216, 579–584, 744
    adult-onset, 580, 607
    care requirements, 583
    causes of, 579, 580
    circulation problems with, 584
    complications of, 579
    controlling, 580
    diet and, 581
    drugs, 580
    gestational, 702
    and glucose monitoring, 581, 582, 583
    juvenile-onset, 580
    symptoms, 579
    type 1 (insulin-dependent), 216, 580
    type 2 (noninsulin-dependent), 216, 580
diabetic coma, 583
diabetic diet, 581, 669
diagnosis
    illegal, 99
    of patient, 99
diarrhea, 455, 459
diaphragm, 210, 231
diastole, 155, 171, 744
diastolic pressure, 155, 171, 744
dictionary use, 290

diet
    balanced, 652–653
    bland, 668
    calorie-restricted, 669
    clear-liquid, 668
    controlling diabetes, 580
    diabetic, 669
    and discharge instructions, 363
    factors affecting, 667–668
    full liquid, 668
    high-fiber, 669
    light, 668
    low-fat/low-cholesterol, 669
    of nursing assistants, 27
    sodium-restricted, 669
    soft, 668
    special, 668–669
    vegetarian, 668
dietary preferences, 667–669
    age and, 667
    culture and, 667
    dental health and, 668
    financial situation and, 668
    geography and, 667
    illness and, 668
    personal choice and, 668
    religion and, 667
dietitian, 36, 363, 660, 669
    and discharge instructions, 363
digestion, 233, 744
digestive system, 210, 232–234.
    basic structure, 232
    changes, in aging, 612
    diseases, 233–234
digestive tract, 232
dilate, 227, 229, 744
dilation, 702
dilation stage, 703
dilemma, 90
directional terms, 207, 212, 744
    visualizing, 213
directions, giving and following, 337
disability, 517, 518, 744
    types of, 518
    rehabilitation program, 518

disaster, 123, 132, 744
   human-caused, 133
   natural, 132–133
   preparedness, 132–133
   response guidelines, 133
discharge, 351, 361–364, 744
discharge instructions, 351, 361, 363, 744
   components of, 362, 363
discharge interview, 351,361, 744
discharge plan, 351, 361, 744
discrimination, 85, 94, 744
   legal issues, 71
disease
   body's defense against, 255
   communicable, 254
   and discharge plan, 361
   emerging, 271
   exposure guidelines, 272–273
   infectious, 251, 254
   microorganisms and, 252
   noninfectious, 251, 254
disease transmission
   airborne, 254
   common vehicle, 254
   contact, 254
   droplet, 254
   employer's responsibility in, 271–272
methods of, 253, 254–255
nursing assistant's responsibility in, 272–273
   vector-borne (animal), 255
disinfection, 251, 256, 744
disorientation, 675, 678, 744
   causes of, 678
   safety issues, 688
disruptive patient, 113
distal, 212
diversity
   and language barriers, 117
   valuing, 114–115
DNR (do not resuscitate) order, 85, 92, 717, 732, 744
documents
   DNR, 92
   health care proxy, 91
   HIPAA, 88
   interviewing, 64–66, 67
   living will, 85, 92, 717, 748

   job, 76
   official, 66
   organ donation, 92
   tax, 76
   transfer form, 351, 358, 755
domestic violence, 625, 642, 744
do not resuscitate (DNR) order, 85, 92, 744
dopamine, 236
dorsal, 207, 210, 212, 744
dorsal cavity, 210
dorsalis pedis artery, 166, 167
dorsal recumbent position, 371, 374, 375, 744
dorsiflexion, 520, 521, 522
draping, 371, 373–374, 376, 744
draw sheet, 331, 335, 744
dress code policies, 29
dressings, 444–447
   applying, 447
   precautions, 446
droplet precautions, for infection control, 264–265
droplet transmission, 254
dry warm therapy, 436–439
   types of, 436
duodenum, 233
   ulcers, 234
dura mater, 239
dying patient, 716. *See also* terminally ill patient.
   and family reactions, 731
   grief stages for, 716
   grieving with, 730
   rights, 717
   stages of grief, 716
dyspnea, 155, 169, 744
dysuria, 457

E

ear, 219–220
   and aging, 219–220
   basic structure, 219
   diseases, 241
edema, 585, 649, 660, 744
   ankle, 660
   pulmonary, 586
ejaculation, 189, 197, 745
ejaculatory duct, 237, 238

elbow restraints, 146–147
elastic bandage, 429, 448–449, 745
   care guidelines, 448
elastic stockings. *See* antiembolic stockings.
elderly, 605, 606, 611, 745. *See also* geriatrics.
   and aging process, 606
   and dignity, 617
   care of, 606
   emotional well-being of, 616–617
elimination, 455, 456, 745
   assisting with, 459
   bowel, 457–459
   equipment, 459–463
   factors contributing to, 456
   of incontinent patient, 464–465
   need for, 110
   patient, 21, 110
   of terminally ill patient, 719
   urinary, 456–457
e-mail etiquette, 313
embolism, 495, 508, 745
embolus, 495, 508, 745
emergency, 123, 124, 399, 400, 745
   ABC assessment, 404
   assessing, 400
   cold, 423
   communicating in, 134
   fire, 128–132
   heat, 421–422
   home health care, 641–642
   initial care during, 402
   OBRA competencies for, 32
   patient conditions affecting, 641–642
   procedures, 400–402
   rapid response in, 404
   responding to, 22
   supportive care for, 402
   types of, 400
   weather, 421–423
emergency medical services (EMS) system, 399, 401, 745
emerging infectious diseases, 271
emesis, 649, 662, 745
emotional abuse, 96

emotional well-being, 105, 107, 745
   of elderly, 616–617
empathy, 19, 25, 745
emphysema, 232, 577, 587, 745
   causes of, 587
   symptoms, 587
Employee's Withholding
     Allowance Certificate (W-
     4), 76
employment. *See* job.
employment agencies, 68
employment application, 69, 70.
     See also application form.
EMS (emergency medical
     services) system, 399, 401,
     745
encourage fluids order, 661
end-of-shift report, 317, 318
endocardium, 214
endocrine gland, 235
endocrine system, 235–236
   basic structure, 235–236
   diseases, 236
   female, 236
   male, 236
endometrium, 238
endorphins, 27
enema, 455, 471, 745
   cleansing, 471, 472–473
   commercial, 471, 473–474
   giving, 471–474
   oil-retention, 471
   saline, 471
   soapsuds (SSE), 471
   tap water (TPE), 471
entrepreneur, 63, 79, 745
environmental
   general safety issues, 124–132
hazards, 124–125
home health safety, 640–641
   patient conditions, 332–334
epidermis, 207, 213, 745
epididymis, 237
epiglottis, 231
epilepsy, 399, 417, 745
epinephrine, 236
episiotomy, 697, 704, 745
epithelial tissue, 209, 210
Erickson, Erik, 200

Erickson's Development Stages,
   201
equipment
   cleaning isolation patient, 268
   elimination, 459–463
   examination room, 430–431
   hazards, 124–125
   personal protective, 123, 126,
     259–264, 751
   safety guidelines, 125
E-records, 323
escape route, 641
Escherichia coli bacteria, 271
esophagus, 233
esteem needs, 105, 106, 107, 745
   chronic illness affecting, 113
   meeting, 112–114
estrogen, 238
   aging changes in, 613
ethical behavior, 90, 108
ethical standards, 85, 86, 745
eustachian tube, 219
evacuation
   fire, 129–130
   of patients, 22, 129
   plan, 129, 641
   routes, 129
eversion, 520, 521
examinations
   assisting in, 430–431
   preparing examination room
     for, 430
   preparing patient for, 431
   supplies for, 430–431
excoriations, 541, 567, 745
exercise
   ambulatory resident, 609
   bedridden resident, 608
   benefits of, 607
   calculating length of, 611
   components of, 607
   effective, 608
   nursing assistant, 27
   repetitions, 510
   resident, 606–610
   stopping, 607–608
   wheelchair-confined resident,
     609
expenses, 635
   out-of-pocket, 55

expires, 729, 732, 745
exploitation, 85, 90, 745
exponential functions, and cell
     division, 209
expressive aphasia, 590
expulsion stage, 703
extension, 520, 521–524
external bleeding, 399, 414, 745
external oblique, 243
external rotation, 520, 521, 522,
   523
external traction, 532
eye appliances, 569–570
eyeglass care, 569, 570
eyes, 218–219
   and aging, 218–219
   artificial, 570
   basic structure of, 218

F

face mask, 123, 139, 745
faces (visual) scale, of pain levels,
     174, 175
facilities, 21
fact, vs. opinion, 97
falling, 530
   helping patient who is, 530
   legal issues, 530
fallopian tubes, 238
fall prevention, 135–136, 615, 640
   for elderly, 615
   guidelines, 136
   safety issues, 615
family
   of dying patient, 731
   and home health, 117, 632–633
   hospice guidelines for, 723
   of long-term care patient, 606
   of patients, 115–116
   of terminally ill patient, 722–
     723
fanfold, 331, 336, 745
Fahrenheit scale, 157, 158
fat, 649, 650, 745
fat-soluble vitamins, 651
FBAO (foreign body airway
     obstruction), 399, 410, 745
   symptoms of, 410
fecal impaction, 455, 458, 745

fecal occult blood slide, 486, 745
fecal occult blood test (FOBT), 455, 485, 745
feces, 233, 455, 457, 745
feedback, 305, 306, 745
   in systems, 44
fee-for-service insurance, 55
feeding, 656–659
   alternative methods to, 664–667
   bottle-feeding an infant, 706–707
   patient with sensory deficits, 221
   patient with swallowing problems, 658
femoral artery, 167
femur, 241–242
fibula, 241–242
fire
   elements necessary for, 130
   evacuation, 129–130
   emergencies, 128–132
   hazards, 640
   and late adulthood safety, 220
   moving patient in, 132
   plan, 641
   prevention, 128, 638
   response steps, 130
   safety issues, 130
fire blanket, 123, 132, 745
   moving patients, 132
fire extinguisher, 130–131
   ABC Class (All Class), 123, 131, 740
   Class A, 123, 130–131, 742
   Class B, 123, 131, 743
   Class C, 123, 131, 743
   using a, 131
first aid, 399, 400, 745
   goals of, 400
first trimester, 701–702
fitness, 607
   body composition, 607
   cardiovascular, 607
   flexibility, 607
   muscular, 607
flatulence, 455, 458, 745
flatus, 470
flexibility fitness, 607
flexion, 520, 521–524

flowmeter, 138
flow sheet, 305, 319, 321, 745
fluid intake. See intake.
fluid output. See output.
FOBT (fecal occult blood test), 455, 485, 745
Foley catheter, 468–469. See also indwelling catheter.
food. See also meals.
   assistive devices, 657
   and bacteria, 639
   documenting intake of, 660
   preparation guidelines, 638–640
   safety issues, 655, 657, 659
foot board, 605, 614, 745
food groups, 652–653
foot drop, 605, 614, 745
foreign body airway obstruction (FBAO), 399, 410, 745
forearm crutch, 527
formula, infant, 697, 706, 746
   mixing, 708
   safety issues, 708
Fowler's position, 371, 375, 746
fracture, 517, 531, 745
fracture pan, 455, 461, 462–463, 746
friction, 371, 376, 746
frontalis, 243
frontal plane, 211
fuel, 130
full liquid diet, 668
functional incontinence, 464
fungus, 252

G

gallbladder, 233
   diseases, 234
gangrene, 577, 584, 746
gas exchange, 227, 231, 746
gastrocnemius, 243
gastrointestinal system, 232. See also digestive system.
gastrostomy medications, 699
gastrostomy tube, 649, 664, 745
general anesthesia, 503
generalized seizure, 399, 416, 746

general practitioner (GP), 35
germs, preventing spread of, 26–27
geriatric assistant, 34
geriatric resident. See resident.
geriatrics, 605, 611, 746. See also elderly.
glands, 227, 235, 746
   adrenal, 236
   endocrine, 235
   mammary, 238
   pancreas, 215–216, 233, 236
   parathyroid, 236
   pineal, 236
   pituitary, 235
   prostate, 237, 239
   reproductive, 236
   salivary, 233
   thymus, 236, 245
glass thermometers, 158–163
   oral, 158
   mercury, 158
   reading, 159–160
   security issues, 158
gloving, 264–265, 260, 261–262
glucose, 483
   monitoring, 581
   normal levels, 581
   testing capillary blood, 582
gluteus maximus, 243
Google®, as job lead, 68
government-sponsored health care programs, 55
gowning, 264–265, 260, 262–263
GP (general practitioner), 35
graduate, 649, 662, 746
grains food group, 652
grand mal seizure, 416
graphic chart, 305, 319–320, 746
grasping reflex, 191
Grave's disease, 236
grief stages, 716
   acceptance, 716
   anger, 716
   bargaining, 716
   denial, 716
   depression, 716
grievance, 85, 89, 746

grooming, 541, 542, 746
group home, 43, 51, 746
group insurance, 55
growth, 189, 190, 746
    stages of, 190–200

H

hair
    care, 549
    of resident, 549–550
    shampooing, 550–551
halitosis, 541, 543, 746
hallucination, 675, 681–682, 746
hamstring muscle, 243
hand rail, 123, 136, 746
handwashing, 259–260, 258,
    264–265
    and patient transfer safety, 360
harassment, 85, 95, 746
hazardous material, 123, 125–
    127, 746
    MSDS for, 57, 126–127
    OSHA defined, 125
    and PPE, 126
    safety guidelines, 126–127
hazards
    environmental, 124–125
    and equipment, 125
    in home health care, 640
HBV (hepatitis B virus), 215, 269
    and safety issues, 77
HCV (hepatitis C virus), 215, 269
head nurse, 19, 33, 746
health, 105, 107, 746
    emotional, 107
    maintaining personal, 26–27
    social, 107
health care
    costs, 54–57
    government programs, 55
    preventive, 54
    regulating, 55–57
    terminology, 282
    trends, 44–45
health care delivery system, 44, 45
    components of, 44
    trends affecting, 44–45

health care facilities, 45–52
    as job leads, 68
health care proxy, 85, 91, 746
health care programs, 55
health care regulatory agencies,
    55–57
health care team, 19, 24, 33–36,
    746
    additional staff of, 35–36
    communication with, 311
    home, 54, 626
    nursing staff, 33–35
    rehabilitation program, 518
    support staff, 36
health insurance, 55
    calculating payments of, 56
    fee-for-service, 55
    long-term care, 55
    managed care, 55
    private, 55
    public, 55
Health Insurance Portability
    and Accountability Act
    (HIPAA), 43, 56, 746
hearing aid care, 571
hearing deficient patients,
    communicating with, 310
heart, 214
    attack, 207, 214, 403–404, 586
    basic structure, 214
    diseases, 214
heart attack, 214, 403–404
heat exhaustion, 399, 421, 746
heating pad, 429. See also
    aquamatic pad.
    safety issues, 438
heat lamp, 436, 439
    safety issues, 439
heat stroke, 399, 421–422, 746
    symptoms, 422
height, measuring, 175–180
    of ambulatory patient, 177–
    178
    of bedridden patient, 179–180
Heimlich maneuver, 399, 410,
    746
    with conscious patient, 410–
    411

    with unconscious patient,
    411–412
    OBRA competency for, 32
helpfulness, 25
hematuria, 457
hemiparesis, 541, 566, 746
hemiplegia, 592
Hemoccult®, 483
hemoglobin, 227, 229, 746
hemorrhage, 399, 414–415, 746
    standard precautions, 415
hemorrhoids, 455, 458, 746
hemostasis, 227, 229, 746
hepatitis, 207, 215, 746
    A, 215
    B, 77, 215, 269
    C, 215, 269
herbal remedies, 228
hierarchy, 106
high-fiber diet, 669
hinge joint, 242
HIPAA (Health Insurance
    Portability and
    Accountability Act), 43, 56,
    746
    privacy rule, 88
hip fractures, 533
hip replacement, 533
    care guidelines, 533
HIV (human immunodeficiency
    virus), 245, 577, 596, 746,
    747
home health aide, 43, 50, 624–
    643, 747
    effective, 628
    and family interaction, 117,
    632–633
    job benefits, 630
    possible tasks of, 626
    responsibilities of, 627
home health care, 50–51, 624–
    643
    additional safety issues, 638,
    640–641
    and client abuse, 642–643
    emergencies, 641–642
    and family interaction, 117,
    632–633

fire safety, 640
and infection control, 268–269
promoting independence in, 631
recording and reporting, 632–635
resource management in, 629–630
team, 54, 626
home safety plan, 641
homeostasis, 207, 208, 229, 747
honesty, 24, 628
horizontal plane, 211
horizontal recumbent position, 371, 374, 375, 747
hormone, 227, 235, 747
cortisol, 236
dopamine, 236
epinephrine, 236
insulin, 236, 577, 579, 747
melatonin, 236
norepinephrine, 236
parathyroid (PTH), 236
progesterone, 238, 611
testosterone, 237, 613
thyroxine, 236
hospice, 43, 51–52, 715, 747
as care option, 717–718
goals, 717–718
family guidelines, 723
hospital, 43, 47, 747
administrator, 52
care provided in, 47
private, 47
public, 47
specialized, 47
staff, 52–53
teaching, 47
hospital beds, 333. See bed.
host, 251, 747
human immunodeficiency virus (HIV), 245, 270, 577, 746, 747
human resources, 44
humerus, 241–242
hygiene, 19, 29, 541, 542, 747
nursing assistant, 29–30
oral, 29, 541, 542–548, 750
hyperextension, 520, 523
hyperglycemia, 577, 583, 747

symptoms, 583
hypertension, 155, 171, 231, 240, 585, 747
and exercise, 607
as risk factor, 585
hyperthermia, 399, 421, 747
safety issues, 422
hypoglycemia, 577, 583, 747
care requirements, 583
reactions, 416, 583
symptoms, 583
hypotension, 155, 171, 747
hypothalamus, 235
hypothermia, 399, 423
emergency care for, 423

I

identity, 189, 197, 747
in adolescents, 197–198
of patient, 134–135
ileostomy, 455, 476–477, 747
ileum, 233
ilium, 242
illegal diagnosis, 99
illness, 105, 108, 747
acute, 46
chronic, 113, 578
and dietary preferences, 668
and discharge plan, 361
food-related, 640
psychological reactions to, 112–113
terminal, 715, 716, 754
immobilize, 517, 531, 747
immune system, 244. See also lymphatic system.
safety issues, 244
immunity, 251, 255, 747
immunization, 189, 193, 255, 747
incentive spirometer, 495, 507, 747
incident, 123, 148, 747. See also variance.
incident report, 123, 148–149, 747
writing, 149
incontinence, 335, 464
aids, 465
anal, 455, 459, 740
causes of, 464

functional, 464
mixed, 464
overflow, 464
reflex, 464
stress, 464
training, 465
types of, 464
urge, 464
urinary, 464
independence, 190, 518
promoting, in home health care, 629
indwelling catheter, 455, 468–469, 747
urine samples from, 482
infant, 190–194. See also neonate.
basic life support, 406–408
bottle-feeding an, 706–707
burping an, 706
changing diaper of, 707–708
infection, 251, 253, 747
bladder, 235
chain of, 251, 253
nosocomial, 251, 255
opportunistic, 270
precautions, 257–265
risk factors, 255
symptoms, 255–256
transmission modes, 271
infection control, 256–265
and food preparation, 638–640
in home health care, 268–269, 636–640
and laundry, 638
techniques, 257–258
infectious agent, 253
infectious diseases, 251, 254, 269–271, 747
emerging, 271
inferior, 212
inflammatory response, 251, 255, 747
information
baseline, 354
objective, 305, 313, 314
subjective, 314, 316
informed consent, 85, 93, 747
inhaled medications, 700
inhaler, 588
inpatients, 46

inputs, of systems, 44
insulin, 236, 577, 579, 747
insulin-dependent diabetes (type 1), 216, 580
insulin resistance, 580
insulin shock, 583
insurance. *See* health insurance.
intake, 649, 661–663, 747
   calculating, 684
   documenting food, 660
   and disease, 110
   and drinking water, 663
   fluid, 660–663
   measuring, 661–662, 663
   minimum, 661
   required, 110
   special orders for, 661
intake and output (I & O), 661
intake records, 32
   fluid, 660
   food, 660
   OBRA competencies for, 32
integumentary system, 243–244
   changes, in aging, 612
intelligence quotient (IQ), 691
intentional tort, 85, 93–96, 747
   types of, 93–96
intercom, 305, 311, 747
intermittent pneumatic compression device, 495, 508, 747
intermittent positive pressure respiration (IPPR), 139
intermittent traction, 532
internal bleeding, 399, 414, 747
   symptoms, 414
internal rotation, 520, 522, 523
internal traction, 532
international time, 91
interview, 63, 71, 748. *See also* job interview.
   discharge, 361
intoxication, 689
intravenous (IV) nutrition therapy, 649, 665, 666–667, 747
   care requirements, 666
   dressing patients with, 666–667
invasive procedures, 256

invasion of privacy, 85, 95, 747
inversion, 520, 521
invoice, 635
involuntary muscles, 243
I & O (intake and output), 661
IPPR (intermittent positive pressure respiration) machine, 139
IQ (intelligence quotient), 691
iris, 218
islet cells, 207, 216, 747
isolation, 114
isolation patient, 265–268
   and cancer, 595
   cleaning supplies and equipment of, 268
   contaminated items of, 267
   food service of, 267
   personal care, 266
   psychological needs, 268
   specimen collection, 267
   transporting, 267
isolation precautions, 251, 257–265, 747
   standard, 257–264
   transmission-based, 257, 264–265
IV setup, 665

J

jacket restraint, 144
JCAHO (Joint Commission for Accreditation of Healthcare Organizations), 43, 56, 748
   abbreviation list, 293, 294
jejunum, 233
job
   advancement, 78–79
   applying for, 69
   health and safety, 77
   offers, 74–75
   orientation, 75–76
   starting new, 75–76
   transitions to new, 79
job interview, 63, 71, 748
   appearance for, 72
   following up, 74
   preparing for, 71–73
   researching for, 71

   successful, 73
job leads, 67–68
   sources for, 67
job safety, 127–128. *See also* environmental safety.
job search
   documents for, 64–66, 67
   organizing, 64–69
job shadowing, 63, 75, 748
joint, 242
   ball-and-socket, 242
   hinge, 242
   pivot, 242
Joint Commission for Accreditation of Healthcare Organizations (JCAHO), 43, 56, 748. *See also* JACHO.
journal keeping, 353
juvenile-onset diabetes, 580

K

Keto-Diastix®, 483
ketones, 483
kidney, 234
kidney dialysis, 577, 598, 748
   types of, 598
kidney (renal) failure, 577, 598–599, 748
   care for, 599
   causes of, 598
   symptoms, 598
   treatment, 598
kidney stones, 235
knee-chest position, 371, 375, 748

L

labia majora, 238
labia minora, 238
labor, 697, 702–703, 748
   pain relief during, 703
   signs of, 702
   stages, 702
language. *See also* communication.
   barriers, 117
   plain, 174
large intestine, 233, 457. *See also* colon.

larynx, 231
late adulthood period, of growth and development, 200
lateral, 212
lateral position, 371, 375, 748
latex allergies, 260
    and operating rooms, 498
latissimus dorsi muscle, 243
law violations, 93–98. *See also* tort.
learning log, 157
legal issues
    in employment, 71
    and falling, 530
    and medical records, 319
legal rights, 85, 86–92, 748. *See also* patients' legal rights.
lens, 218
lesion, 541, 543, 748
letdown reflex, 697, 705, 748
liability, 85, 93, 748
licensed nursing assistants, 30, 34–35
licensed practical nurse (LPN), 19, 34, 748
    duties of, 34
licensed vocational nurse (LVN), 19, 34, 748
    duties of, 34
lifting
    bedridden patient, 376
    proper, 372–373
light diet, 668
lightening, 702
listening, active, 89, 305, 307–308, 740
lithotomy position, 375, 376
liver, 215, 233
    diseases, 215
    functions, 215
living will, 85, 92, 717, 748
local anesthesia, 503
lochia, 697, 704, 748
log-in, 305, 323, 748
logrolling, 371, 376, 748
long-term care facility, 43, 48, 748
    autonomy in, 606
    discussing, 616
    and family, 606

levels, 616
    postmortem care procedures, 733
long-term care insurance, 55
long-term illness, 113. *See also* chronic illness.
lower respiratory tract, 231
low-fat/low-cholesterol diet, 669
LPN (licensed practical nurse), 19, 34
lungs, 214–215
    basic structure, 214, 215
    diseases, 214
LVN (licensed vocational nurse), 19, 34
lymph, 244
lymphatic system, 244–245
    central organs, 244
    basic structure, 244–245
    diseases, 245
    peripheral organs of, 245
lymphatic vessel, 245
lymph nodes, 245
lymphocytes, 245

M

malpractice, 85, 97, 748
mammary glands, 238
managed care insurance, 55
management
    of health care facilities, 52–54
    resource, 625, 629–630
    time, 628–629
mandible, 242
masking, for infection control, 264–265, 260, 264
Maslow, Abraham, 106
Maslow's hierarchy, 106
    as OBRA competency, 32
massage, 562–563
masseter muscle, 243
master gland. *See* pituitary gland.
material safety data sheet (MSDS), 57, 123, 126–127, 748
material safety guidelines, 126–127
MD (muscular dystrophy), 243

meals
    for blind patients, 656
    for isolation patients, 267
    in patient's room, 655
    percentage eaten, 581
    for residents, 653
    swallowing precautions during, 658
meat and beans food group, 652, 653
meatus, 234
mechanical lift, 371, 387–389, 748
medial, 212
Medicaid, 43, 55, 748
medical asepsis, 251, 256, 748
medical centers, 47. *See also* hospitals.
MedicAlert® bracelet, 423
medical record, 305, 319, 748
    and legal issues, 319
    recording guidelines, 320–323
medical terminology, 281, 282, 748
    abbreviations, 293–298
    combining forms, 282, 283, 284–286, 743
    interpreting, 291–292
    prefixes, 282, 286–288
    pronouncing, 288
    root words, 282, 284–286
    suffixes, 282, 289–290
    symbols, 299
Medicare, 43, 55, 748
medication, 99
    administration records, 700
    assisting with, 698–699
    buccal, 699
    determining times of, 293
    gastrostomy, 699
    inhaled, 700
    labels, 700
    nasal, 700
    PRN, 700
    routes, 699–700
    safety issues, 699
    storage, 701
    sublingual, 699
    times, 293
    topical, 699

medicine
   alternative, 228
   complementary, 228
   and discharge instructions, 363
medium, communication 305, 306, 748
meetings, formal, 643
melanoma, 244
melatonin, 236
membranes
   pleural, 214
   typanic, 219
menarche, 189, 197, 748
Meniere's disease, 241
menopause, 189, 199, 613, 749
menstruation, 227, 238, 748
mental disorder, 675, 676–679, 748
   care, 679
   categories, 677–679
   causes of, 678–679
   factors, 677
mental health, 675, 676, 749
mental health patient
   altered states of, 678–679
   behavior, 679
   care, 679
   treatment, 690
mental retardation, 675, 690–691, 749
   developmental levels of, 691
mental states, 677–679
   agitation, 675, 679, 740
   anxiety, 679
   causes of, 678–679
   confusion, 675, 678, 743
   delirium, 675, 679, 744
   disorientation, 675, 678, 744
   and dying patient, 731–732
mental status
   assessment, 683–684
   observations, 679
mercury thermometer safety, 158
message, 305, 306, 749
metatarsals, 241–242
methicillin-resistant
      Staphylococcus aureus
      (MRSA), 271

microorganisms, 251, 252, 749
   drug-resistant, 271
   growth of, 253
   types of, 252
middle adulthood period, of
      growth and development,
      199
midstream (clean-catch) urine
      sample, 479
military time, 91
milk food group, 652
minerals, 649, 651, 749
mitered corner, 331, 338, 749
mitral valve, 214
mitt restraint, 144
mixed incontinence, 464
morgue, 729, 733, 749
Moro reflex, 191
mottled, 729, 731
MRSA (methicillin-resistant
      Staphylococcus aureus), 271
MSDS (material safety data
      sheet), 57, 123, 126–127,
      749
multiple sclerosis (MS), 577, 592,
      749
   causes of, 592
   and elimination, 592
   symptoms, 592
muscle atrophy, 605, 606, 749
muscle contracture, 605, 606, 749
muscle tissue, 209, 210
muscles, 242–243
   anterior tibial, 243
   bicep, 243
   changes in, at death, 731
   hamstring, 243
   involuntary, 243
   latissimus dorsi, 243
   masseter, 243
   orbicularis oculi, 243
   orbicularis oris, 243
   pectoralis major, 243
   quadriceps, 243
   rhomboid, 243
   sternocleidomastoid, 243
   temporalis, 243
   trapezius, 243

   triceps, 243
   voluntary, 242
muscular dystrophy (MD), 243
muscular fitness, 607
muscular system, 242–243
   diseases, 243
musculoskeletal system, 241–243
   changes, in aging, 612
   of neonates, 192
myelin, 239
myocardium, 214
myocardial infarction, 207, 214,
      403–404, 586, 749
   care, 586
   symptoms of, 403–404, 586

N

NAGNA (National Association
      of Geriatric Nursing
      Assistants), 37
nail care, 560–562
nasal cannula, 123, 138, 139, 749
nasal catheter, 123, 138, 139, 749
nasal medications, 700
nasogastric tube, 649, 664, 749
   and oral care, 543
   observation of, 664
National Association of Geriatric
      Nursing Assistants
      (NAGNA), 37
National Network of Career
      Nursing Assistants
      (NNCNA), 37
natural disasters, 132–133
nebulizer, 139, 588
needle-stick injuries, 271
needs, 105, 106, 749
   basic, 106–107
   of children, 112,
   esteem, 105, 106, 107, 112–114
   meeting, 107–114
   physical, 105, 106, 108–112
   security, 105, 106, 107, 112
   self-actualization, 105, 106,
      107
   social, 105, 106, 107, 112–114
   touch, 114
negative coping mechanisms, 676

negligence, 85, 96, 749
neonate, 189, 190–194, 749
   development stages, 192–193
   musculoskeletal system, 192
   nervous system, 191
   safety issues, 192, 193
   sensory system, 192
nephrons, 234
nerves, 239
   cranial, 240
   optic, 218
   spinal, 240
nerve tissue, 209, 210
nervous system, 239–240
   central, 239
   changes, in aging, 612
   diseases, 240
   neonate, 191
   peripheral, 240
networking, 37, 63, 67–68, 749
neurological disorders, 590–594
   care of, 593
   communication approaches
      with, 594
   safety issues, 592
neuron, 239
newborn
   care, 706–709
   weighing a, 70
nil per os (NPO), 649, 661, 749
9-1-1, 129
   information, 401–402
nitroglycerin, 585
nits, 549
NNCNA (National Network of
   Career Nursing Assistants),
   37
no-code orders, 729, 732, 749.
   See also DNR order.
non-English speaking patients
   communication with, 311
noninfectious disease, 251, 254,
   749
noninsulin-dependent diabetes
   (Type 2), 216, 580
nonpathogen, 251, 252, 749
nonverbal communication, 305,
   306, 749
   and emergencies, 416

norepinephrine, 236
nose, 220–221
   and aging, 221
   basic structure, 220
nosocomial infection, 251, 255,
   749
notetaking, 709
nothing by mouth (NPO), 649,
   661, 749
   and oral care, 543
nucleus, 208, 209
numerical score, of pain levels,
   174
nurse anesthetists, 503
nurse
   charge, 33, 742
   head, 33
   licensed practical, 19, 34, 748
   licensed vocational, 19, 34, 748
   practitioner, 34
   recovery room, 502
   registered, 19, 30, 34
nurse's aide, 34
nurses' notes, 305, 319–320, 749
nursing assistant, 19, 20, 34–35,
   749
   ambulatory surgery, 511
   basic duties, 20–22
   ethical behavior of, 90, 108
   expanding roles of, 698–699
   and grief, 730
   health and wellness, 26–28,
      271–273
   health care facility, 45–52
   hygiene, 29–30
   illegal tasks of, 99
   job options, 67
   licensed, 30, 34–35
   OBRA requirements, 30–33
   protocols, 99
   qualities of effective, 24–26
   and rehabilitation, 519
   responses to residential
      behavior, 32
   rules of conduct, 90
   safe behaviors, 28
   specialty training, 698
   training requirements, 30
nursing career, choosing, 37

nursing care plan, 305, 316, 749
nursing home, 48. See long-term
   care facility.
nursing staff, 33–35. See also
   nurse.
nursing supervisors, 53
nursing technician, 34
nutrient, 649, 650–651, 749
   categories, 650
   functions of, 650–651
nutrition, 639, 649, 650, 749
   as basic need, 110
   for geriatric patients, 615
   for home health patient, 638–
      639
   and MyPyramid, 652
   patient, 21
   for terminally ill patient, 719
nutrition facts label, 639

O

objective information, 305, 313,
   314, 749
   vs. subjective, 314
objectivity, 19, 26, 749
OBRA (Omnibus Budget
   Reconciliation Act of 1987),
   19, 30, 57, 750
   rights for patients, 87–88
OBRA competencies
   for bedmaking, 31
   cognitively impaired residents,
      33
   for emergencies, 32
   Heimlich maneuver, 32
   intake records, 32
   Maslow's hierarchy, 106
   for nursing assistants, 30–33
   ouput records, 32
   personal care, 32
   postmortem care, 32
   resident behavior, 32–33
   resident environment, 31
   safety precautions, 31
   for vital signs, 31
OBRA Procedures. See
   Procedures.
observation, 305, 313–316, 750
   guidelines, 315

patient, 313–316
of resident, 614
reporting, 22, 317–323
Occupational Safety and Health Administration (OSHA), 43, 56, 271, 750
Bloodborne Pathogen Standard, 271–272
occupational therapy, 687
occupied bed, 331, 336, 337, 342–345, 750
oil-retention enema, 471
oils food group, 653
Older Americans Act, 88–89
ombudsman, 85, 88–89, 642, 750
Omnibus Budget Reconciliation Act of 1987 (OBRA), 19, 30, 57, 750. *See also* OBRA.
online searches, 68
open bed, 331, 336, 338–340, 750
operation, 496. *See also* surgery.
ophthalmoscope, 430
opinion, vs. fact, 97
opportunistic, 270
opposition, 522
optic nerve, 218
oral hygiene, 29, 541–548, 750
benefits of, 542–543
care, 543
for dependent residents, 547–548
disorders, 543
observations, 543
safety issues, 543
signs, 543
for unconscious residents, 547–548
oral medications, 699
oral presentations, 599
oral suctioning, 489
oral swab, 541, 543, 715, 720, 750
oral temperature, 158, 160
measurement guidelines, 160–161
normal range, 158
orbicularis oculi muscle, 243
orbicularis oris muscle, 243
organ donation form, 85, 92, 750

organ donor, 729, 732, 750
organic, 650
organs, 207, 210, 750
accessory, 232
donation of, 92
of dying patient, 731
major, 213–218
sensory, 218–221
orientation, 63, 75–76, 750
orthopedics, 531–533
orthostatic hypotension, 371, 377, 750
prevention, 377
orthotic device, 517, 531, 750
types of, 531
problems signs of, 532
OSHA (Occupational Safety and Health Administration), 43, 56, 271, 750
ossicles, 219
osteoarthritis, 243
osteoporosis, 605, 612, 750
and exercise, 607
ostomy, 455, 474, 750
assisting with, 474–477
otoscope, 430
outcomes, of systems, 44
outer ear, 219
out-of-pocket expenses, 55
outlines, 615
outpatients, 46
outpatient surgery, 511
output, 649, 662, 750
measuring, 661–662
output records
OBRA competencies for, 32
ova, 238
ovaries, 236, 238
overflow incontinence, 464
ovulation, 238
oxygen, 123, 137, 750
delivery devices, 137–140
and fire safety, 130
levels in blood, 173
mask, 138, 139
as medication, 137
need for, 109
oxygen pressure gauge, 138

oxygen tent, 123, 139, 750
oxygen therapy, 137
and COPD, 588
safety guidelines, 139–140

P

pain level
affect on patient, 174
determining, 174
descriptive, 174
numerical score of, 174
visual scale, 174, 175
pain management, 718
pancreas, 215–216, 233, 236
diseases, 216
paralysis, 592
symptoms, 592
paranoia, 675, 681–682, 750
paraplegia, 592
parasites, 485
parathyroid gland, 236
parathyroid hormone (PTH), 236
paresis, 541, 566, 750
Parkinson's disease, 577, 591, 750
causes of, 591
symptoms, 591
parliamentary procedure, 643
partial seizure, 399, 417, 750
P.A.S.S., 123, 131, 750
password, 305, 323, 750
patella, 242
pathogen, 251, 252, 750
bloodborne, 251, 257
patience, 25
patient, 43, 46, 750. *See also* client or resident.
additional safety issues, 21, 134–142
clothing, 336
communication, 308–311
diagnosis of, 99
discharge, 351, 361–364, 744
disruptive, 113
diversity, 114–115
education, 312
emergency care for, 32, 402
environment, 21, 31, 332–334, 640–641

evacuation of, 22
general needs of, 107–114
home safety of, 21, 269
identity, 134–135
isolation, 265–268
legal rights, 86–92
measuring weight, 175–182
movement, 31, 132, 379–393
needs, 106–107
nutrition, 21
observation, 313–316, 519
personal care, 21, 32
postmortem care, 32, 729, 733–735
psychological needs, 33, 352
rehabilitation, 19, 22, 517, 518, 752
sensory-deficit, 221
standard precautions, 31
stress, 113
transfer, 31, 359–360, 385–387
types, 46
violent, 113
vital signs, 22, 31
waste elimination, 21, 110
patient care
isolation, 265–268
principles of, 23
patient care assistant, 34
Patient Care Partnership, The, 87
patient consent form, 497
patient-controlled anesthesia (PCA), 715, 718, 750, 751
patient record, 91, 319. *See also* medical record.
Patient's Bill of Rights, 85, 86, 750
patients' legal rights, 86
federal protection of, 86, 89–97
PCA (patient controlled anesthesia), 715, 718, 750, 751
pectoralis major muscle, 243
pedal pulse, 155, 166, 751
pediatric patient
basic life support, 406–408
communicating with, 196
physical needs of, 114
security needs, 112
social needs, 114

pediculosis, 541, 549, 751
peer editing, 245
peer groups, 197
pelvic bone, 242
penis, 237
pericardium, 214
perineal, 435
perineal care, 467, 541, 558–560, 751
perineum, 541, 558, 751
periodontal disease, 541, 542, 751
and oral care, 543
peripheral nervous system, 240
peripheral vascular disease (PVD), 166
peristalsis, 227, 233, 751
in dying patient, 731
perseverance, 19, 25
personal belongings, of patients, 334
inventory, 356
personal care
OBRA competencies for, 32
of isolation patient, 266
of patients, 21
personal data sheet, 63, 66, 67, 751
personal growth, 77–79
personality, 189, 200, 751
development, 200–201
personal protective equipment (PPE), 123, 126, 751
and standard precautions, 259–264
pertussis, 271
phalanges, 242
pharynx, 231, 233
phlebitis, 429, 448, 751
phlebotomy, 698
physical abuse, 96
physical movement, 111–112
and discharge instructions, 363
physical needs, 105, 106, 751
of children, 114
meeting, 108–112
physical restraints, 94, 123, 140, 751
physiological, 518
physiology, 227, 228, 751

pia mater, 239
pineal gland, 236
pituitary gland, 235
pivot joint, 242
placenta, 697, 703, 751
placental stage, 703
plagiarism, 632
plantar flexion, 520, 521, 605, 614, 751
plasma, 227, 229, 751
platelets, 227, 229, 751
pneumonia, 588
poison, 399, 420–421, 751
and conscious patient, 420
and home health care prevention, 420
and inducing vomiting, 420
information, 421
symptoms, 420
and unconscious patient, 421
poison control, 127
poison control hotline, 421
policies
dress code, 29
no-lift, 372
popliteal artery, 167
portal of entry, 253
portal of exit, 253
positions, of patient, 373–376
common, 374–376
dorsal recumbent, 371, 374, 375
Fowler's, 371, 375
horizontal recumbent, 371, 374, 375
knee-chest, 371, 375
lateral, 371, 375
lithotomy, 375, 376
prone, 371, 375
reverse-Trendelenburg's, 371, 376
semi-Fowler's, 371, 375
Sims', 371, 375
supine, 371, 374
Trendelenburg's, 371, 376
positive attitude, 25
positive coping mechanisms, 676
posterior, 212
posterior tibial artery, 167

postictal state, 417

postmortem care, 729, 733–735, 751

OBRA competencies for, 32

postoperatively, 429, 448, 751

postoperative patient, 502–511

assisting circulation of, 508–510

assisting respiratory functions of, 506

general care, 504

observation, 504

psychological needs, 504

turning, 505

postoperative period, 495, 502–511, 751

preparing patient's room for, 501

postpartum care, 697, 703–706, 751

in home, 706

potential, 518

PPE (personal protective equipment), 123, 126, 751

and standard precautions, 259–264

preadolescent period, of growth and development, 196–197

prefix, in medical terminology, 281, 286–288, 751

pregnancy, 701–703

signs of complications in, 702

trimesters, 701–702

prehypertension, 155, 171, 751

prenatal care, 697, 701–702, 751

tests during, 701–702

preoperative checklist, 499

preoperative patient

care, 498

easing fears of, 498

educating, 496–497

physical preparation, 498–500

skin preparation, 499–500

preoperative period, 495, 496–500, 751

preschool stage, of growth and development, 195

pressure sores, 371, 377, 541, 567–569, 751

avoiding, 376–377

and planned movement, 384

prevention, 568–569

risk factors, 567

stages of, 568

and wheelchair patient, 569

preventive health programs, 54

primary caregiver, 189, 191, 751

primary period, of growth and development, 196

principles, of patient care, 23

privacy, 85, 88, 751

invasion of, 95

private health insurance, 55

private hospitals, 47

PRN medications, 700

Procedures, 19, 20, 751

Admitting a New Patient, (Procedure 15-2, OBRA), 357–358

Applying Antiembolic Stockings (Procedure 18-12), 449

Applying an Aquamatic Pad (Procedure 18-6, OBRA), 438

Applying a Cold Compress (Procedure 18-8, OBRA), 442

Applying a Cold Pack (Procedure 18-10, OBRA), 445

Applying a Dressing (Procedure 18-11, OBRA), 447

Applying Elbow restraints (Procedure 6-7), 147

Applying a Jacket or Vest Restraint (Procedure 6-5, OBRA), 145

Applying a Mitt Restraint (Procedure 6-4), 144

Applying a Safety Belt Restraint (Procedure 6-6), 146

Applying a Transfer Belt (Procedure 16-7), 385

Applying a Warm Compress (Procedure 18-2, OBRA), 433–434

Applying a Warm Water Bottle (Procedure 18-5, OBRA), 437

Applying a Wrist or Ankle Restraint (Procedure 6-3), 143

Assisting in an Examination (Procedure 18-1), 431

Assisting a Patient with a Bedside Commode (Procedure 19-1, OBRA), 460

Assisting the Patient with Deep-Breathing and Coughing Exercises (Procedure 20-3, OBRA), 506–507

Assisting the Patient with an Incentive Spirometer (Procedure 20-4), 507

Assisting with Range-of-Motion Exercises (Procedure 21-1, OBRA), 521–524

Basic Life Support for Adults (Procedure 17-1, OBRA), 405–406

Basic Life Support for Infants and Children (Procedure 17-2, OBRA), 406–408

Brushing or Combing a Resident's Hair (Procedure 22-5, OBRA), 549–550

Caring for Dentures (Procedure 22-3, OBRA), 546–547

Caring for a Resident's Eyeglasses (Procedure 22-16, OBRA), 570

Changing a Colostomy Appliance (Procedure 19-9, OBRA), 475–476

Cleaning an Ileostomy Appliance (Procedure 19-10, OBRA), 476–477

Cleaning the Perineal Area (Procedure 22-10, OBRA), 559–560

Cleaning and Trimming Nails (Procedure 22-11, OBRA), 561–562

Collecting a Clean-Catch (Midstream) Sample (Procedure 19-12, OBRA), 479–480

Collecting a Fecal Occult Blood Slide (Procedure 19-18), 487

Collecting and Preserving a Sputum Sample (Procedure 19-19, OBRA), 488–489

Collecting a Routine Urine Sample (Procedure 19-11, OBRA), 478–479

Collecting a Stool Sample (Procedure 19-17, OBRA), 486

Collecting a 24-Hour Urine Specimen (Procedure 19-13, OBRA), 480–481

Collecting Urine from an Infant or Toddler (Procedure 19-14, OBRA), 482

Discharging a Patient (Procedure 15-4, OBRA), 363–364

Dressing a Patient Who Has an IV (Procedure 26-6), 666–667

Dressing a Resident Who Has Limited Use of Limbs (Procedure 22-14, OBRA), 566–567

Emptying a Urine Drainage Bag and Measuring Urinary Output (Procedure 19-5, OBRA), 468

Feeding Patients Who Cannot Feed Themselves (Procedure 26-4, OBRA), 659

Flossing a Dependent Resident's Teeth (Procedure 22-2, OBRA), 545

Giving a Back Rub (Procedure 22-12, OBRA), 562–563

Giving a Bedpan or Fracture Pan to a Patient (Procedure 19-2, OBRA), 462–463

Giving a Cleansing Enema (Procedure 19-7, OBRA), 472–473

Giving a Cold Soak (Procedure 18-9, OBRA), 443

Giving a Commercial Enema (Procedure 19-8, OBRA), 473–474

Giving a Complete Bed Bath (Procedure 22-8, OBRA), 555–557

Giving a Sitz Bath (Procedure 18-4, OBRA), 435–436

Giving a Warm Soak (Procedure 18-3, OBRA), 434

Giving a Whirlpool Bath (Procedure 22-9, OBRA), 557–558

Helping an Ambulatory Resident Bath or Shower (Procedure 22-7, OBRA), 554–555

Helping a Conscious Patient Who Has Been Poisoned (Procedure 17-11), 420

Helping a Nonambulatory Resident Shave (Procedure 22-13, OBRA), 564

Helping a Patient with an Obstructed Airway (Procedure 17-4), 410–411

Helping a Patient with Burns (Procedure 17-10), 419

Helping the Patient Perform Leg Exercises (Procedure 20-5, OBRA), 509–510

Helping a Patient in Shock (Procedure 17-6), 413

Helping a Patient Sit and Dangle (Procedure 16-1, OBRA), 378

Helping a Patient Walk with a Cane (Procedure 21-3, OBRA), 528

Helping a Patient with a Walker (Procedure 21-4, OBRA), 529

Helping a Patient Who Is Falling (Procedure 21-5, OBRA), 530

Helping a Patient Who Is Having a Seizure (Procedure 17-9), 417

Helping a Patient Who Seems to Be Having a Stroke (Procedure 17-7), 414

Helping a Resident on Bed Rest Brush the Teeth (Procedure 22-1, OBRA), 544

Helping Stop a Hemorrhage (Procedure 17-8), 415

Helping an Unconscious Patient Who Has Been Poisoned (Procedure 17-12, OBRA), 421

Helping an Unconscious Person with an Obstructed Airway (Procedure 17-5, OBRA), 411–412

Inserting a Rectal Tube (Procedure 19-6, OBRA), 470–471

Inserting and Removing a Hearing Aid (Procedure 22-17, OBRA), 571

Logrolling a Patient and Positioning onto Side (Procedure 16-6, OBRA), 383–384

Making a Closed Bed and Making an Open Bed (Procedure 14-1, OBRA), 338–340

Making an Occupied Bed (Procedure 14-3, OBRA), 342–345

Making a Surgical Bed (Procedure 14-2, OBRA), 341–342

Measuring an Apical Pulse (Procedure 7-8), 168–169

Measuring Axillary Temperature with a Glass Thermometer (Procedure 7-4, OBRA), 162–163

Measuring Blood Pressure (Procedure 7-10, OBRA), 172–173

Measuring Height and Weight of a Bedridden Patient (Procedure 7-12, OBRA), 179–180

Measuring Oral Temperature with a Glass Thermometer (Procedure 7-2, OBRA), 160

Measuring a Radial Pulse (Procedure 7-7, OBRA), 168

Measuring Rectal Temperature with a Glass Thermometer (Procedure 7-3, OBRA), 161–162

Measuring Temperature with a Digital Thermometer (Procedure 7-6, OBRA), 164–165

Measuring Temperature with a Tympanic Thermometer (Procedure 7-5, OBRA), 164

Moving a Helpless Patient in Bed (Procedure 16-3, OBRA), 380

Moving a Helpless Patient Using a Turning Sheet (Procedure 16-4, OBRA), 381

Moving a Patient Who Can Assist You Up in Bed (Procedure 16-2, OBRA), 379

Observing and Measuring Respirations (Procedure 7-9, OBRA), 170

Offering a Urinal to a Male Patient (Procedure 19-3, OBRA), 463

Performing Oral Care for an Unconscious Resident (Procedure 22-4, OBRA), 548

Perineal Care for the Catheterized Patient (Procedure 19-4, OBRA), 467

Positioning the Postoperative Patient (Procedure 20-2, OBRA), 505

Preparing a Patient for a Meal (Procedure 26-1, OBRA), 654

Preparing a Room for a New Admission (Procedure 15-1, OBRA), 354

Providing Postmortem Care (Procedure 30-1, OBRA), 734–735

Pulse Oximetry (Procedure 7-11, OBRA), 173–174

Reading a Glass Thermometer (Procedure 7-1, OBRA), 159–160

Serving a Meal to a Blind Patient (Procedure 26-3, OBRA), 656–657

Serving a Meal in a Patient's Room (Procedure 26-2, OBRA), 655

Shampooing a Bedridden Resident's Hair (Procedure 22-6, OBRA), 550–551

Shaving a Dependent Resident (Procedure 22-14, OBRA), 564–565

Shaving the Preoperative Patient (Procedure 20-1, OBRA), 500

Standard Precautions: Gloving (Procedure 11-2, OBRA), 261–262

Standard Precautions: Gowning (Procedure 11-3, OBRA), 262–263

Standard Precautions: Handwashing (Procedure 11-1, OBRA), 259–260

Standard Precautions: Masking (Procedure 11-4, OBRA), 264

Straining Urine for Stones (Procedure 19-16), 484

Testing Capillary Blood Glucose (Procedure 23-1), 582

Testing a Urine Sample (Procedure 19-15), 483

Transferring a Conscious Patient to a Stretcher (Procedure 16-11, OBRA), 391–392

Transferring a Patient (Procedure 15-3, OBRA), 359–360

Transferring a Patient Using a Slide Board (Procedure 16-8, OBRA), 386

Transferring a Patient to a Wheelchair (Procedure 16-10, OBRA), 389–391

Transferring an Unconscious Patient to a Stretcher (Procedure 16-12, OBRA), 392–393

Turning or Rolling a Patient to Position onto Side (Procedure 16-5, OBRA), 382–383

Using the Automated External Defibrillator (Procedure 17-3), 409

Using a Fire Blanket to Move a Patient (Procedure 6-2), 132

Using a Fire Extinguisher (Procedure 6-1), 131

Using a Heat Lamp (Procedure 18-7, OBRA), 439

Using a Mechanical Lift (Procedure 16-9, OBRA), 387–389

Using a Transfer Belt to Help a Patient Walk (Procedure 21-2, OBRA), 525–526

Weighing a Patient in a Wheelchair (Procedure 7-13), 181

procedures, 19, 20

process analysis list, 340

processes, of systems, 44

professional growth, 77–79

professionalism, 19, 26, 751
    in appearance, 29–30

progesterone, 238
    changes, in aging, 611

projection, as defense mechanism, 676

pronation, 520, 523

prone position, 371, 375, 751

proofreading, 66

prostate gland, 237

prosthesis, 517, 533, 751
    care guidelines, 533

protective eyewear, 264

proteins, 649, 650, 751

protocols, 85, 99, 751

protozoa, 252
proximal, 212
psi, 138
psychiatry, 677
psychological, 518, 677
psychological dependence, 689
psychology, 677
psychosis, 675, 681–682, 751
PTH (parathyroid hormone), 236
puberty, 189, 197, 751
pubis, 242
public health insurance, 55
public hospitals, 47
pulmonary valve, 214
pulmonary vein, 230
pulse deficit, 155, 167, 751
pulse force, 166
pulse oximeter, 155, 173, 752
pulse rate, 155, 166, 752
  abnormal, 166
  apical, 155, 167, 168–169, 741
  apical-radial, 155, 167, 741
  measuring, 166–169
  normal, 166
  pedal, 155, 166
  radial, 155, 166, 168
  rhythm, 166
  variance, 166
  volume, 166
puncture safety issues, 415
pupil, 218
PVD (peripheral vascular disease), 166

Q

quadrants, 207, 211, 752
quadriceps muscle, 243
quadriplegia, 592
quality care, providing, 23
quality of life, 715, 718, 752
questions
  asking, 436
  closed-ended, 307
  open-ended, 307

R

R.A.C.E., 123, 129, 752
radial artery, 167

radial flexion, 522
radial pulse, 155, 166, 752
  measuring, 168
radiation therapy, 577, 595, 752
radius, 241–242
range of motion (ROM), 517, 520, 752
range-of-motion exercises, 517, 520, 752
  active assist level, 520
  active level, 520
  assisting with, 521–524
  guidelines, 520
  passive, 520
  safety issues, 524
rationalization, as defense mechanism, 676
reality orientation, 675, 678–679, 752
receiver, 305, 306, 752
receptive aphasia, 590
receptor, 207, 218, 752
  muscle, 241
  visceral, 241
reciprocity, 19, 30, 752
recording, 305, 318–323, 752
  on computers, 323
  fluid intake, 663
  home health care, 632–635
records
  client, 91
  client care, 625, 633, 634, 743
  computers, 323
  E-, 323
  intake, 32
  medical, 305, 319, 320–323, 748
  medication administration, 700
  output, 32
  patient, 91, 319
  time/travel, 634–635
rectal temperature, 158
  measurement guidelines, 161–162
  normal ranges for, 158
  safety issues, 161
rectal tube, 455, 470, 752
  inserting, 470–471
rectum, 233, 457
red blood cells, 229
reference, 63, 65, 752

referral agencies, 363
reflection, in active listening, 307
reflex, 189, 191, 752
  grasping, 191
  letdown, 697, 705, 748
  Moro, 191
  rooting, 191, 697, 705
  sucking, 191
reflex hammer, 430
reflex incontinence, 464
reflux, 655, 657, 659
registered nurse (RN), 19, 30, 34, 752
  duties of, 34
registry, 19, 30, 752
regression, as defense mechanism, 676
rehabilitation, 19, 22, 517, 518, 752
rehabilitation center, 43, 47, 752
rehabilitation program, 517, 518, 752
  guidelines, 518–519
  health care team, 518
  and nursing assistant, 519
religion, 114, 667
reminiscing therapy, 721
renal artery, 234
renal failure, 577, 598–599, 748
  care for, 599
  symptoms, 598
  treatment, 598
repetitions, 510
reportable event, 317
reporting, 305, 317, 752, 632–635
  abuse, 642–643
  daily,
  end-of-shift, 317, 318
  guidelines, 318
  home health, 633
  incident, 123, 148–149, 747
  observations, 22, 317–323
  restraint, 147
  shift, 19, 20
  stool, 459
  urine, 459
reproductive system, 210, 236–239
  changes, in aging, 613

diseases, 239
female, 238–239
male, 237–238
rescue breathing, 399, 402, 752
reservoir, 251, 253, 752
resident, 43, 46, 752. *See also*
client or patient.
ambulatory, 609
bathing a, 551–558
dressing, 566–567
exercise, 606–610
eye appliances, 569–570
grooming, 541, 542, 746
hair care, 549–550
hearing aid of, 571
hygiene, 541, 542, 747
massage, 562–563
nail care, 560–562
and oral hygiene, 541–548
physical care, 614–615
recreation, 610
serving food to, 653
shaving, 563–565
skin care, 567–569
transfer, to hospital, 358
wheelchair-confined, 609
resident behavior
OBRA competencies for,
32–33
resident environment
OBRA competencies for, 31
Residents' Rights, 85, 87–88, 752
resource management, 625,
629–630, 752
respiration, 155, 169, 214, 231–
232, 752
abnormal, 169
calculating frequency of, 732
changes, in dying patient, 731
counting, 170
measuring, 169–170
normal, 169
observing, 170
patterns, 169
respiratory arrest, 399, 402, 752
respiratory care
infection control in, 269
of postoperative patient, 506–
507

respiratory disorders, 587–589
care, 588
treatments, 587–588
types of, 587
respiratory distress, 587
respiratory system, 156, 231–232
changes, in aging, 612
diseases, 232, 587–589
respiratory tract
lower, 231
upper, 231
respite care, 625, 626, 752
restatement, in active listening,
307
restorative care, 19, 22, 517, 518,
752
restraint
additional safety issues, 140–
147
alternatives to, 140
belt, 145–146
chemical, 94, 123, 140, 742
closure safety, 147
elbow, 146–147
guidelines, 141
jacket, 144–145
mitt, 144
orders, 140
physical, 94, 140
reports, 147
unlawful, 85, 94
wrist and ankle, 142–143
restrict fluids order, 661
résumé, 63, 64–65, 752
formatting a, 65
sample, 65
resuscitation, 729, 732, 752
retention catheter, 468–469. *See
also* indwelling catheter.
retina, 218
reverse-Trendelenburg's
position, 371, 376, 752
rhomboid muscle, 243
ribs, 242
rigor mortis, 729, 733, 753
Robert's Rules of Order Newly
Revised, 641
ROM (range of motion), 517,
520, 753

room,
comfort of, 355
preparation of, 353–354
preparing, after surgery, 501
settling patient in, 355
rooting reflex, 191, 697, 705, 753
root word, in medical
terminology, 281, 282,
284–286, 753
rotation, 520, 524
external, 520
internal, 520
right/left, 524
rules of conduct for nursing
assistants, 90

S

sacraments, 715, 722, 753
sacrum, 384
safety
belts, 145–146
environmental, 124–125
fire, 128–132
job, 127–128
patient, 21, 134–142
restraint, 140–147
safety guidelines
disaster, 133
environmental, 640–641
equipment, 125
fall prevention, 136
and food-related illness, 639–
640
hazardous material, 126–127
material safety, 126–127
oxygen therapy, 137, 139–140
restraint, 141
safety measures
environmental, 124–125
safety plan, home, 641
safety precautions
OBRA competencies for, 31
safety surveys, 640
sagittal plane, 211
saline enema, 471
salivary gland, 233
Salmonella bacteria, 254, 639
same-day surgery, 511

SARS (severe acute respiratory syndrome), 271
scales, 541, 567, 753
scales, height and weight
    lift, 175
    overbed, 179–180
    upright, 175, 176, 177–178
    wheelchair, 175, 181
scheduling, 323
schizophrenia, 675, 681–682, 753
scope of practice, 19, 23, 753
scrotum, 237
search engines, 68
sebum, 244
secondary sex characteristics, 189, 197, 238, 753
second trimester, 702
security needs, 105, 106, 107, 753
    of children, 112
    meeting, 112
seizure, 399, 416, 753
    causes of, 416
    in epilepsy, 399, 417
    generalized, 399, 416, 746
    grand mal, 416
    helping patient during, 417
    partial, 399, 417, 750
    symptoms, 416–417
    tonic-clonic, 416
self-actualization needs, 105, 106, 107, 753
self-esteem. See esteem.
semen, 227, 237–238, 753
semi-Fowler's position, 371, 375, 753
seminal vesicles, 237
sender, 305, 306, 753
sender-receiver communication model, 74
senses
    muscle, 241
    visceral, 241
sensitivity, heat and cold, 441
sensory organs, 218–221
sensory system, 218–221, 240–241
    changes, in aging, 612
    diseases, 241
    of neonates, 192

serum test, 701
severe acute respiratory syndrome (SARS), 271
sexual abuse, 96
sexuality, 199
shallow breathing, 155, 169, 753
sharps, 269
    and bedmaking, 337
    disposal box, 638
shave prep, 499
shaving, 563–565
    electric razor and safety, 563
shearing force, 371, 376, 753
shift report, 19, 20, 753
shock, 399, 412–413, 753
    symptoms of, 412
short-term memory, 200, 686
shroud, 729, 734, 753
side rail, 123, 135, 753
sign, 305, 313, 753
Sims' position, 371, 375, 753
sitz bath, 429, 435–436, 753
skeletal system, 241–242
    major bones of, 241–242
skilled nursing facilities, 48. See long-term care facility.
skin, 221, 243–244
    atrophic, 541, 567, 741
    care, for resident, 567–569
    diseases, 221, 244
    mottled, 731
    prepping, for surgery, 499–500
    structures, 244
skin prep, 499
sleep
    need for, 110–111
slide board, 371, 386, 753
small intestine, 233, 457
smoke detector safety, 128, 129
smoking
    and fire prevention, 128
    and oxygen therapy, 139–140
    as personal habit, 28
    safety issues, 28
soapsuds enema (SSE), 471
social needs, 105, 106, 107, 753
    of children, 114
    chronic illness affecting, 113

meeting, 112–114
social well-being, 105, 107, 753
sodium-restricted diet, 669
soft diet, 668
specialist, 35
specimen collection, 477
    of isolated patient, 267
    products, 483
    sputum, 488–489
    stool, 485–487
    urine, 477–483
Specipan®, 483
speech-deficient patients, 240
    communication with, 240, 310–311
spell-checkers, and writing, 485
sphygmomanometer, 155, 171, 430, 753
    aneroid, 171
    mercury, 171
spinal cavity, 210
spinal cord
    injuries, 240
    and nerves, 239
spleen, 245
splint, 531
spiral anesthesia, 503
spiritual healing, 228
spiritual needs, of the dying, 721
sponge bath, 442
sputum, 455, 488, 753
SSE (soapsuds enema), 471
standard precautions, for infection control, 251, 257–264, 265, 753
    and communication, 266
Staphylococcus aureus, methicillin-resistant (MRSA), 271
sterile, 429, 446, 753
sterile technique, 256. See surgical technique.
sterilization, 251, 257, 753
sternocleidomastoid muscle, 243
sternum, 242
stertorous breathing, 155, 169, 753
stethoscope, 155, 167, 430, 753
    and blood pressure, 171
    parts of, 167

stimulation, 189, 192, 753

stoma, 455, 474, 753

stomach, 233, 457

    ulcers, 234

stool, 455, 457, 753

    collection, 485–487

    reports on, 459

    samples, 486–487

stress, 19, 28, 753

    long–term, 28

    managing, 28

    patient, 113

stress incontinence, 464

stretcher, 371, 391, 753

    transferring conscious patient to, 391–392

    transferring unconscious patient to, 392–393

    transporting on stretchers, 393

strict bed rest, 605, 608, 754

stroke, 240, 399, 413–414, 577, 590–591, 754

    causes of, 590

    heat, 399, 421–422, 746

    symptoms of, 413, 590–591

subacute care, 46

subacute care unit, 43, 49, 754

subjective information, 305, 314, 316, 754

    vs. objective information, 314

sublingual medications, 699

substance abuse, 675, 689–690, 754

    effects of, 689

    symptoms of, 689

    treatment of, 690

subtraction, with months, 719

sucking reflex, 191

suctioning, 455, 489, 754

    oral, 489

    tonsillar, 489

    tracheal, 489

suffix, 281, 289–290, 754

suicide, 675, 679, 754

    preventing, 680

summary, 35, 270

sundowning, 675, 685, 754

superior, 212

supervisors, nursing, 53

supination, 520, 523

supine position, 371, 374, 754

support devices, 444–445, 448–449

supporting details, 25

suppository, 455, 470, 754

support services, 36

surgery, 495, 496, 754

    ambulatory, 495, 511, 740

    educating patient about, 496–497

    elective, 496

    general, 496

    guidelines for transporting patient to, 501

    outpatient, 511

    patient fears of, 498

    patient preparation for, 498–500

    preparing patient's room after, 501

    preparing patient's skin for, 499–500

    same-day, 511

surgical asepsis, 251, 256, 754

surgical bed, 331, 337, 341–342, 754

surgical techniques, 511

susceptible host, 253

suture, 704

swallowing problems, 658

symbol, in medical terminology, 281, 299, 754

symptom, 305, 314, 754

    of infection, 255–256

    for stopping exercise, 609–610

synapse, 239

syndrome, 577, 596, 754

system, 44, 207, 210, 228, 754

    arterial, 229

    cardiovascular, 228–231

    digestive, 210, 232–234

    endocrine, 235–236

    integumentary, 243–244

    lymphatic, 244–245

    muscular, 242–243

    musculoskeletal, 241–243

    nervous, 239–240

    reproductive, 210, 236–239

    respiratory, 231–232

    sensory, 218–221, 240–241

    skeletal, 241–242

    urinary, 210, 234–235

    venous, 229

systems theory, 44

    trends affecting, 44–45

systole, 155, 171, 754

systolic pressure, 155, 171, 754

T

tachycardia, 155, 168, 583, 754

tachypnea, 155, 169, 754

tactile, 221

tap water enema (TPE), 471

tarsals, 242

taste buds, 220

    chemoreceptors of, 221

    diminished sense in, 221

teaching hospitals, 47

team, 704

teamwork, 704

technology, 311–313

teeth

    brushing, 544

    flossing, 545

telecommunication, 311–313

telemedicine, 98

telephone messages, 502

temperament, 189, 200

temperature, 156–157, 158, 754

    axillary, 158, 162–163

    converting, 422

    oral, 158, 160

    rectal, 158, 161–162

    tympanic, 158, 164

temporal artery, 167

temporalis muscle, 243

terminal illness, 715, 716, 754

terminally ill patient, 717

    care options for, 717–718

    elimination needs, 719

    emotional and social needs, 721

    helping family of, 722–723

    hospice care for, 717

    mouth and nose care, 720

    nutritional needs, 719

    physical needs, 718–720

    psychological care, 720

spiritual and cultural needs, 721–722

vision and hearing, 720

Tes-Tape®, 483

testes, 236, 237

testosterone, 237

change, in aging, 613

Texas® catheter, 469

theft, 94

therapy

aerosol, 123, 139, 740

cold, 440–444

cold dry, 444

dry warm, 436–439

IV nutrition, 649, 665, 666–667, 747

occupational, 687

oxygen, 137, 139–140

radiation, 577, 595, 752

reality, 675

reminiscing, 721

times, 440

validation, 675, 687, 688, 755

warm, 432–439

warm dry, 436–439

warm moist, 432–436

thermometer, 157, 430

and bathing, 560

clinical, 158

digital, 164–165

disposable, 163

electronic, 163

glass, 158–163

mercury, 158

oral, 158, 160–161

reading glass, 159–160

safety issues, 158, 161

security, 158

tympanic, 164

thiamine, 653

third trimester, 702

thoracic cavity, 210

thrombophlebitis, 429, 448, 754

thrombus, 495, 508, 754

thrush, 543

thymus, 236, 245

thyroxine, 236

TIA (transient ischemic attacks), 414, 577, 590, 755

tibia, 242

time management, 625, 628–629, 754

time/travel record, 625, 634–635, 754

tissue, 207, 209–210, 754

connective, 209

epithelial, 209, 210

muscle, 209, 210

nerve, 209, 210

toddler period, of growth and development, 194–195

development stages of, 194

growth, 194

safety issues, 195

toe pleat, 331, 345, 754

tonic-clonic seizure, 416

tonsillar suctioning, 489

tonsils, 245

topical medications, 699

tort, 85, 93, 754

intentional, 85, 93–96, 747

types of, 93–98

unintentional, 85, 96–98, 755

toxins, 252

TPE (tap water enema), 471

trachea, 231

tracheal suctioning, 489

traction, 517, 532–533, 754

care guidelines, 533

continuous, 532

external, 532

intermittent, 532

internal, 532

reasons for, 532

transfer, 351, 358, 371, 385, 754

conscious patient to stretcher, 391–392

with mechanical lift, 387–389

patient, 31, 359–360, 385–387

reasons for, 358

of resident, to hospital, 358

safety issues, 386

with slide board, 386

unconscious patient, to stretcher, 392

of wheelchair patients, 393

transfer belt, 371, 385, 754

and walking, 525–526

and wheelchair patient, 390

transfer form, 351, 358, 755

transient ischemic attacks (TIA), 414, 577, 590, 755

transmission-based precautions, 251, 257, 264–265, 755

types of, 264–265

transmission, of diseases

airborne, 254

common vehicle, 254

contact, 254

droplet, 254

employer's responsibility in, 271–272

methods of, 253, 254–255

nursing assistant's responsibility in, 272–273

vector-borne (animal), 255

transport, 371, 393, 755

to stretcher, 393

to surgery, 501

in wheelchairs, 393

transverse, 211

trapeze bar, 517, 532, 755

trapezius muscle, 243

Trendelenburg's position, 371, 376, 755

triceps muscle, 243

tricuspid valve, 214

tube feedings. See nasogastric tube.

tuning fork, 430

turning sheet, 371, 376, 755

24-hour time, 91, 317

24-hour urine specimen, 480–481

tympanic membrane, 219

tympanic temperature, 163–164

normal temperature ranges, 158, 164

tympanic thermometer, 164

type 1 (insulin-dependent) diabetes, 216, 580

type 2 (noninsulin-dependent) diabetes, 216, 580

U

ulcers, 233–234
    decubitus, 541, 567, 743
    duodenum, 234
    gastric, 234
    stomach, 234
ulna, 241–242
ulnar flexion, 522
umbilical cord, 697, 708, 755
    care, 708
unconscious patient
    and Heimlich maneuver, 411–412
    with obstructed airway, 411–412
    oral care, 547–548
    poisoned, 421
    transferring, 392–393
unintentional tort, 85, 96–98, 755
unit, in health care facility, 351, 358, 755
universal distress signal, 399, 410, 755
unlawful restraint, 85, 94, 755
unoccupied bed, 331, 336, 755
upper respiratory tract, 231
upright scale
    reading, 176
    using, 177–178
ureter, 234, 456
urethra, 234, 456
    male, 237–238
urge incontinence, 464
urinal, 455, 463, 755
urinary catheter, 455, 465, 755. See also catheter.
urinary incontinence, 455, 457, 755
urinary meatus, 238
urinary retention, 455, 457, 755
urinary system, 210, 234–235
    basic structure, 234
    calculating output of, 235, 466, 468
    changes, in aging, 613
    common problems, 456
    diseases, 235
    elimination process, 456–457
    functions of, 234

urinary tract infection, 457
urination, 455, 456, 755
urine, 234, 455, 456, 755
    collecting and testing products, 483
    drainage bag, 468, 469
    elimination, 234
    formation, 234
    output, 235, 466
    reporting on, 459
    straining, 484
    testing, 483
urine samples, 477–483
    clean-catch (midstream), 479–480
    closed urinary drainage system, 482
    collecting and testing, 477–479
    collection guidelines, 478
    infant and toddler, 481–482
    reasons for collecting, 477
    routine, 478
    24-hour, 480–481
USDA's MyPyramid, 652–653
U.S. Department of Agriculture (USDA), 652
U.S. Department of Labor, 64
uterus, 238

V

vagina, 238
vaginal speculum, 430
validate, 688
validation therapy, 675, 687, 688, 755
valves
    aortic, 214
    mitral, 214
    pulmonary, 214
    tricuspid, 214
variance, 148. See also incident.
variance report. See incident report.
vas deferens, 237
vector, 251, 255, 755
vector-borne transmission, 255
vegetables food group, 652
vegetarianism, 668

vein, 227, 229, 755
    pulmonary, 230
venous system, 229
ventilation, 227, 231, 755
ventral, 207, 210, 212, 755
ventral cavity, 210
ventricles, 207, 214, 755
ventricular fibrillation, 408
verbal abuse, 96
verbal communication, 305, 306–308, 755
vertebrae, 242
vertigo, 241
vest restraint, 144
vibropercussion, 508
villi, 233
violent patient, 113
virus, 252
    West Nile, 271
    HBV (hepatitis B), 77, 215, 269
    HCV (hepatitis C), 215, 269
    HIV (human immunodeficiency), 245, 577, 596, 746, 747
visitors
    informing, 116
    interacting with, 115–117
    and privacy, 115
    responding to challenging, 116–117
visual ("faces") scale, of pain levels, 174, 175
visually impaired patients
    communication with, 310, 658
vital signs, 22, 155, 156, 755
    abnormal, 156
    communication and, 174
    components of, 156
    flow sheet, 156, 319, 321
    life-threatening, 402
    OBRA competencies for, 31
    working with, 156
vitamins, 649, 650–651, 755
    fat-soluble, 651
    water-soluble, 651
vocabulary log, 237
voluntary muscles, 242
vulva, 238

W

walking. *See also* ambulation.
  with cane, 528
  distances, 525
  with transfer belt, 525–526
  with walker, 529
walker, 527
  assisting patient with, 529
  front-wheeled, 527
walking aids, 123, 135, 517, 526–527, 755
  safety guidelines, 526
  types of, 526–527
warm compress, 429, 433–434, 755
warm pack, 429, 433, 755
warm soaks, 433, 434–435
warm therapy, 432–439
  benefits, 432
  dry, 436–439
  guidelines, 432
  moist, 432–436
  safety issues, 432
  sensitivity, 441

warm water bottle, 437
water
  daily requirements, 110
  enema, 471
  intake, 663
  need, 110
water-soluble vitamins, 651
weigh schedules, 175
weight, measuring, 175–182
  of ambulatory patient, 177–178
  of bedridden patient, 179–180
  of patient in wheelchair, 181
well-baby checks, 189, 193, 755
West Nile virus, 271
W-4 (Employee's Withholding Allowance Certificate), 76
wheelchair patient
  transferring a, 389–391
  weighing, 181
white blood cells, 229
whooping cough, 271
will. *See* living will.

Wong-Baker FACES Pain Rating Scale, 175
word parts, 282
  combining forms, 282, 283, 284–286
  correct usage, 441
  prefixes, 282, 286–288
  root words, 282, 284–286
  suffixes, 282, 289–290
work ethic, 63, 78, 755
wrist and ankle restraints, 142–143

Y

Yahoo®, as job lead, 68
young adulthood period, of growth and development, 198